Nursing Diagnosis Index

i

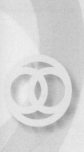

Handbook of
Nursing
Diagnosis

15TH EDITION

Lynda Juall Carpenito, RN, MSN, CRNP
Family Nurse Practitioner
ChesPenn Health Services
Chester, Pennsylvania
Nursing Consultant
Mullica Hill, New Jersey

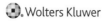 Wolters Kluwer

Philadelphia • Baltimore • New York • London
Buenos Aires • Hong Kong • Sydney • Tokyo

Acquisitions Editor: Natasha McIntyre
Product Development Editor: Annette Ferran
Director of Product Development: Jennifer Forestieri
Editorial Assistant: Dan Reilly
Design Coordinator: Holly McLaughlin
Senior Production Project Manager: Cynthia Rudy
Manufacturing Coordinator: Karin Duffield
Prepress Vendor: S4Carlisle Publishing Services

15th Edition

Library of Congress Cataloging-in-Publication Data
Names: Carpenito, Lynda Juall, author.
Title: Handbook of nursing diagnosis / Lynda Juall Carpenito, RN, MSN, CRNP Family Nurse Practitioner, ChesPenn Health Services, Chester, Pennsylvania, Nursing Consultant, Mullica Hill, New Jersey.
Description: 15th edition. | Philadelphia : Wolters Kluwer, [2017] | Includes bibliographical references and index.
Identifiers: LCCN 2016021464 | ISBN 9781496338396
Subjects: LCSH: Nursing diagnosis--Handbooks, manuals, etc.
Classification: LCC RT48.6 .C385 2017 | DDC 616.07/5—dc23 LC record available at https://lccn.loc.gov/2016021464

CCS0717

To Olen, my son

for your wisdom and commitment to justice

for our quiet moments and embraces

for Olen Jr. and Aiden

for your presence in my life

. . . I am grateful

for you are my daily reminder of what is

really important . . .

love, health, and human trust

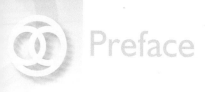

Preface

Many nurses, and even some faculty, question the usefulness of nursing diagnosis. Unfortunately, nursing diagnosis is still joined at the hip with traditional care planning. It is time to separate these conjoined twins so that both can function separately. Nursing diagnosis defines the science and art of nursing. It is as imperative to nurses and the nursing profession as medical diagnoses are to physicians. It serves to organize nursing's knowledge in the literature, in research, and in the clinician's mind. Do not underestimate the importance of this classification. A clinician with expertise in nursing diagnoses can hypothesize several explanations for a client's anger, such as fear, anxiety, grieving, powerlessness, or spiritual distress. Without this knowledge, the client is simply angry.

Care planning as it is taught in schools of nursing is an academic exercise. This is not wrong, but as the student progresses into the senior year, this academic care plan must be transformed into a clinically useful product. Students will progress to utilizing a standardized care plan *rather* than creating them. Copying from books, such as this one, does not enhance one's knowledge of nursing diagnosis and critical analysis. Students should start with a standardized document (electronic or preprinted) and then revise it according to the specific data they have acquired while caring for their client. For example, each student would have a standardized care plan for an individual experiencing abdominal surgery. If the person also has diabetes mellitus, then the collaborative problem *Risk for Complications of Hypoglycemia/Hyperglycemia* would be added with monitoring interventions. If another client, after emergency abdominal surgery from motor vehicle trauma, lost his wife in the accident, then *Grieving* would be added.

Faculty, nurse managers, administrators, and clinicians need to do their part. Change is imperative. Nursing must defend its right to determine its documentation requirements, just as medicine has done. If nursing continues to do business as usual, nursing as we want it—nursing as clients need it—will cease to exist. Nursing will continue to be defined by what we do and write and not by what we know.

From goals to specific interventions, *Handbook of Nursing Diagnosis* focuses on nursing. It provides a condensed, organized outline of clinical nursing practice designed to communicate creative clinical nursing. It is not meant to replace nursing textbooks, but rather to provide nurses who work in a variety of settings with the information they need without requiring a time-consuming review of the literature. It will assist students in transferring their theoretical knowledge to clinical practice; it can also be used by experienced nurses to recall past learning and to intervene in those clinical situations that previously went ignored or unrecognized.

The 15th edition is organized in four sections, with additional content available online. Section 1, Nursing Diagnoses, provides an alphabetical reference to nursing diagnoses, including Author's Notes and interventions for nursing care. Section 2 focuses on Health Promotion/Nursing Diagnoses. Section 3, Manual of Collaborative Problems, is new to this edition and presents certain physiologic complications that nurses monitor to detect onset or changes in status. Section 4 introduces the idea of Diagnostic Clusters, presenting sample medical conditions with associated collaborative problems and nursing diagnoses, and directing readers to additional content online at thePoint®. thePoint® also contains other useful information for users of this text and can be accessed with the code printed inside the front cover of the book.

Lynda Juall Carpenito

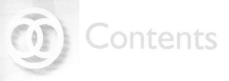
Contents

Section 2

Health-Promotion Nursing Diagnoses 653

Section 3

Manual of Collaborative Problems 693

Section 4

Diagnostic Clusters 755

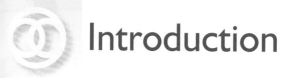

Introduction

Creating a Care Plan for Your Assigned Client

Step 1: Complete the Assessment From Your Course or the Agency

Ask your instructor which format to use.

Step 2: Refer to Diagnostic Clusters in Section 4 of This Book and on thePoint for the Primary Medical Diagnosis of Your Assigned Client

Diagnoses such as:

- Diabetes mellitus
- Pneumonia
- Heart failure

OR

The surgical procedure the individual has had such as:

- Abdominal surgery
- Hysterectomy
- Total joint replacement

Note: If a diagnostic cluster is not relevant to your assigned client, proceed to Step 3.

Step 3: Refer to thePoint for Sample Generic Care Plans

For a generic care plan with goals, interventions, and rationales for all hospitalized persons or a generic care plan for all persons having surgery, go to thePoint. These plans focus on the usual nursing diagnoses and collaborative problems present for persons admitted for medical problems or surgical procedures. Save the care plan to your computer so you can do the following:

- Add risk factors to the general care plan from your assessment data of your client.
- Delete or revise goals/interventions not useful for your client.

- Add additional priority diagnoses not on the general care plan, such as *Risk for Complications of Unstable Blood Glucose Level* if the person has diabetes mellitus and has had abdominal surgery.
- You can start your care plan with one of these plans. Now you will review the assessment data on your assigned client in Step 4.

 Carp's Cues

You can find generic medical and surgical care plans on thePoint. Consult your instructor on how you can use these generic care plans.

Step 4: Identify the Client's Risk

Factors

Risk factors are situations, personal characteristics, disabilities, or medical conditions that can hinder the person's ability to heal, cope with stressors, and progress to his or her original health prior to hospitalization, illness, or surgery.

Before hospitalization:

- Did the individual have an effective support system?
- Could the individual perform self-care? Bathing? Feeding self?
- Did the individual need assistance (e.g., ADLs, housekeeping, transportation)?
- Could the individual walk unassisted?
- Did the individual have memory problems?
- Did the individual have hearing problems?
- Did the individual smoke cigarettes?
- Did the individual abuse alcohol or drugs?

What conditions or diseases does the individual have that make him or her more vulnerable to:

- Falling
- Infection
- Nutrition/fluid imbalance
- Pressure ulcers
- High anxiety
- Physiologic instability (e.g., electrolytes, blood glucose, blood pressure, respiratory function, healing problems)

When you meet your assigned client, determine if any of the risk factors are present:

- Obesity
- Communication problems
- Movement difficulties
- Inadequate nutritional status
- Recent or ongoing stress (e.g., financial, death in family)

Write significant data on index card:

- Hearing problems
- No or ineffective support system
- Unhealthy lifestyle (e.g., little regular exercise, smokes, poor nutritional habits)
- Learning difficulties
- Ineffective coping skills (e.g., angry, depressed, unmotivated, denial)
- Obesity
- Fatigue
- Financial problems
- Negative self-efficacy (belief that they will not improve)
- Self-care difficulties

 Carp's Cues

Risk factors can be used as additional related factors for a nursing diagnosis on the general plan such as:

- *Anxiety* related to loss of job and hospital costs
- *Risk for Infection* related to compromised healing secondary to excess adipose tissue (obesity)

OR

An additional nursing diagnosis not on the general plan as:

- *Ineffective Health Management* related to insufficient knowledge of risks and strategies to quit smoking
- *Impaired Verbal Communication* related to unavailable interpreter and compromised hearing
- *Ineffective Denial* related to continued smoking despite recent deep vein thrombosis
- *Fatigue* (refer to Related Factors under *Fatigue*)
- *Impaired Memory* (refer to Related Factors under *Impaired Memory*)

Step 5: Identify Strengths

Strengths are qualities or factors that will help the person to recover, cope with stressors, and progress to his or her original health (or as close as possible) prior to hospitalization, illness, or surgery. Examples of strengths are as follows:

- Positive spiritual framework
- Positive support system
- Ability to perform self-care
- No eating difficulties
- Effective sleep habits
- Alertness and good memory

- Financial stability
- Ability to relax most of the time
- Motivation, resiliency
- Positive self-esteem
- Internal locus of control
- Self-responsibility
- Positive belief that they will improve (self-efficacy)

Write a list on a card of the strengths of your assigned client and of their support systems.

The strengths of the individual and of their support systems can be used to motivate them to cope with some difficult activities. Strengths are not nursing diagnoses, risks, or related factors. They are to be considered in planning care. For example, a person with a strong religious affiliation and a new cancer diagnosis may benefit from a dialogue session with their religious leader.

Step 6: Create Your Initial Care Plan

Print the generic care plan (medical, surgical) for your assigned client. These generic care plans reflect the usual, predicted care an individual needs. Ask your instructor how you can use them to avoid excessive writing.

❯❯ Carp's Cues

In the remaining steps, collaborative problems are discussed. If you do not know about them, please refer to the section that follows care planning on the Bifocal Clinical Practice Model.

Step 7: Review the Collaborative Problems on the Generic Plan

Review the collaborative problems listed. These are the physiologic complications that you need to monitor. Do not delete any because they all relate to the condition or procedure that your assigned client has had. You will need to add how often you should take vital signs, record intake and output, change dressings, etc. Ask the nurse to whom you are assigned for the frequency of monitoring.

Review each intervention for collaborative problems. Are any interventions unsafe or contraindicated for your client? For example, if your client has edema and renal problems, the fluid requirements may be too high for him or her. Ask a nurse or instructor for help here.

Review the collaborative problems on the general plan. Also review all additional collaborative problems that you found that are related to any medical or treatment problems. For example, if your assigned client has diabetes mellitus, you need to add *Risk for Complications of Unstable Blood Glucose Level*.

Step 8: Review the Nursing Diagnoses
on the Generic Plan

Review each nursing diagnosis on the plan.

- Does it apply to your assigned client?
- Does your assigned client have any risk factors (see your index card) that could make this diagnosis worse?

An example on the Generic Medical Care Plan is Risk for Injury related to unfamiliar environment and physical or mental limitations secondary to condition, medication, therapies, or diagnostic tests.

Now look at your list of risk factors for your assigned client. Can any factors listed contribute to the individual sustaining an injury? For example, is he or she having problems walking or seeing? Is he or she experiencing dizziness?

If the individual has an unstable gait related to peripheral vascular disease (PVD), you would add the following diagnosis: *Risk for Injury related to unfamiliar environment and unstable gait secondary to peripheral vascular disease.*

Review each intervention for each nursing diagnosis:

- Are they relevant for your client?
- Will you have time to provide them?
- Are any interventions not appropriate or contraindicated for your assigned client?
- Can you add any specific interventions?
- Do you need to modify any interventions because of risk factors (see index card)?

Review the goals listed for the nursing diagnosis:

- Are they pertinent to your client?
- Can the individual demonstrate achievement of the goal on the day you provide care?
- Do you need more time?
- Do you need to make the goal more specific for your client?

Delete goals that are inappropriate for this individual. If your assigned client will need more time to meet the goal, add "by discharge." If the individual can accomplish the goal this day, write "by (insert date)" after the goal.

Using the same diagnosis, Risk for Injury related to unfamiliar environment and physical and mental limitations secondary to the condition, therapies, and diagnostic tests, consider this goal:

- The individual will request assistance with ADLs.

Indicators

- Identify factors that increase risk of injury
- Describe appropriate safety measures

If it is realistic for the individual to achieve all the goals on the day of your care, you should add the date to all of them. If the individual is confused, you can add the date to the main goal, but you would delete all the indicators because the person is confused. Or you could modify the goal by writing:

- Family member will identify factors that increase the individual's risk of injury.

Remember that you cannot individualize a care plan for an individual until you spend time with him or her, but you can add or delete interventions based on your preclinical knowledge of the individual (e.g., medical diagnosis, coexisting medical conditions).

Step 9: Prepare the Care Plan (Written or Printed)

You can prepare the care plan by:

- Saving the online general care plan onto your computer, then deleting or adding specifics for your assigned client (use another color or a different type font for additions/deletions), and printing it.
- Writing the care plan
- Adding to the electronic care plan in the facility

Ask your faculty person what options are acceptable. Using different colors or fonts allows your instructor to clearly see your analysis. Be prepared to provide rationales for why you added or deleted items.

Step 10: Initial Care Plan Completed

Now that you have a care plan of the collaborative problems and nursing diagnoses, which ones are associated with the primary condition for which your client was admitted? If your assigned client is a healthy adult undergoing surgery or was admitted for an acute medical problem and you have not assessed any significant factors in Step 1, you have completed the initial care plan. Go to Step 12.

Step 11: Additional Risk Factors

If your assigned client has risk factors (on the index card) that you identified in Steps 1 and 2, evaluate if these risk factors make your assigned client more vulnerable to develop a problem. The following questions can help to determine if the individual or family has additional diagnoses that need nursing interventions:

- Are additional collaborative problems associated with coexisting medical conditions that require monitoring? For example, if the individual has diabetes mellitus, add *Risk for Complications of Hyper/hypoglycemia*.
- Are there additional nursing diagnoses that, if not managed or prevented now, will deter recovery or affect the individual's functional status? For example, an individual who has recently experienced a death of a significant person needs *Grieving* added to the plan.

You can address nursing diagnoses not on the priority list by referring the individual/family for assistance after discharge (e.g., counseling, weight loss program).

Step 12: Evaluate the Status of Your Assigned Client (After You Provide Care)

Collaborative Problems
Review the collaborative goals for the collaborative problems:

- Assess the individual's status
- Compare the data to established norms (indicators)
- Judge if the data fall within acceptable ranges
- Conclude if the individual is stable, improved, unimproved, or worse

Is your assigned client stable or improved?

- If yes, continue to monitor the individual and provide interventions indicated.
- If not, has there been a dramatic change (e.g., elevated blood pressure and decreased urinary output)? Have you notified the physician or advanced practice nurse? Have you increased your monitoring of the individual? Communicate your evaluations of the status of collaborative problems to your clinical faculty and to the nurse assigned to your client.

Nursing Diagnosis
Review the goals or outcome criteria for each nursing diagnosis. Did the individual demonstrate or state the activity defined in the goal? If yes, then document the achievement on your plan. If not and the individual needs more time, change the target date. If time is not the issue, evaluate why the individual did not achieve the goal. Was the goal:

- Not realistic because of other priorities?
- Not acceptable to the individuals?

Step 13: Document the Care You Provided and the Individual's Responses on the Agency's Forms, Flow Records, and Progress Notes

Nursing Diagnoses versus Collaborative Problems[1]

In 1983, Carpenito published the Bifocal Clinical Practice Model. In this model, nurses are accountable to treat two types of clinical judgments or diagnoses: nursing diagnoses and collaborative problems.

Nursing diagnoses are clinical judgments about individual, family, or community responses to actual or potential health problems/life processes. Nursing diagnoses provide the basis for selection of nursing interventions to achieve outcomes for which the nurse has accountability (NANDA, 1998; NANDA-I, 2012).

Collaborative problems are certain physiologic complications that nurses monitor to detect onset or changes in status. Nurses manage collaborative problems using physician-prescribed and nurse-prescribed interventions to minimize the complications of the events (Carpenito, 2016).

Nursing interventions are classified as nurse-prescribed or physician-prescribed. Nurse-prescribed interventions are those that the nurse can legally order for nursing staff to implement. Nurse-prescribed interventions treat, prevent, and monitor nursing diagnoses. Nurse-prescribed interventions manage and monitor collaborative problems. Physician-prescribed interventions represent treatments for collaborative problems that the nurse initiates and manages. Collaborative problems require both nursing-prescribed and physician-prescribed interventions. Box 1 represents these relationships.

The following illustrates the types of interventions associated with the collaborative problem *Risk for Complications of Hypoxemia:*

NP	1. Monitor for signs of acid–base imbalance
NP/PP	2. Administer low flow oxygen as needed
NP	3. Ensure adequate hydration
NP	4. Evaluate the effects of positioning on oxygenation
NP/PP	5. Administer medications as needed

NP, Nurse-prescribed; PP, Physician/Nurse-Practitioner-prescribed.

---

[1]The terminology for collaborative problems has been changed to Risk for Complications of (specify) from Potential Complications: (specify).

Box 1 RELATIONSHIP BETWEEN NURSING-PRESCRIBED INTERVENTIONS AND PHYSICIAN-PRESCRIBED INTERVENTIONS

*Nursing-Prescribed
Interventions*

- Reposition q2h
- Lightly massage vulnerable areas
- Teach how to reduce pressure when sitting

Nursing Diagnoses

*Risk for Pressure Ulcers related to
immobility secondary to fatigue*

*Physician-Prescribed
Interventions*

- Usually not needed

*Nursing-Prescribed
Interventions*

- Maintain NPO state
- Monitor:
  Hydration
  Vital signs
  Intake/output
  Specific gravity
- Monitor electrolytes
- Maintain IV at prescribed rate
- Provide/encourage mouth care

Collaborative Problems

Risk for Complications of Fluid and
Electrolyte Imbalances

*Physician-Prescribed
Interventions*

- IV (type, amount)
- Laboratory studies

Selection of Collaborative Problems

As mentioned earlier, collaborative problems are different from nursing diagnoses. The nurse makes independent decisions regarding both collaborative problems and nursing diagnoses. The decisions differ in that, for nursing diagnoses, the nurse prescribes the definitive treatment for the situation and is responsible for outcome achievement; for collaborative problems, the nurse monitors the individual's condition to detect onset or status of physiologic complications and manages the events with nursing- and physician-prescribed interventions. Collaborative problems are as follows:

Risk for Complications of Bleeding
Risk for Complications of Kidney Failure

The physiologic complications that nurses monitor usually are related to disease, trauma, treatments, and diagnostic studies. The following examples illustrate some collaborative problems:

Situation	Collaborative Problem
Anticoagulant therapy	*Risk for Complications of Bleeding*
Pneumonia	*Risk for Complications of Hypoxemia*

Outcome criteria or client goals are used to measure the effectiveness of nursing care. When a client is not progressing to goal achievement or has worsened, the nurse must reevaluate the situation. Box 2 represents the questions to be considered. If none of these options is appropriate, the situation may not be a nursing diagnosis.

Collaborative problems have collaborative goals that represent the accountability of the nurse—to detect early changes and to co-manage with physicians/nurse practitioners/physician assistants. Nursing diagnoses have goals that represent the accountability of the nurse—to achieve or maintain a favorable status after nursing care. Box 3 includes frequently used collaborative problems.

Some physiologic complications, such as pressure ulcers and infection from invasive lines, are problems that nurses can prevent. Prevention is different from detection. Nurses do not prevent

---

Box 2 EVALUATION QUESTIONS

Is the diagnosis correct?
Has the goal been mutually set?
Is more time needed for the plan to work?
Does the goal need to be revised?
Do the interventions need to be revised?

Box 3 CONDITIONS THAT NECESSITATE NURSING CARE

Nursing Diagnoses*

1. Health Perception—Health Management

Contamination
 Contamination, Risk for
†Energy Field, Disturbed
Development, Risk for Delayed
 †Failure to Thrive, Adult
 Growth, Risk for Disproportionate
Frail Elderly Syndrome
 Frail Elderly Syndrome, Risk for
Health, Deficient Community
Health Behavior, Risk-Prone
Health Maintenance, Ineffective
Injury, Risk for
 Aspiration, Risk for
 Falls, Risk for
 Perioperative Positioning Injury, Risk for
 Poisoning, Risk for
 Suffocation, Risk for
 Thermal Injury, Risk for
 Trauma, Risk for
 Urinary Tract Injury, Risk for
Noncompliance
Obesity
 Overweight
 Overweight, Risk for
Health Management, Ineffective
†Health Management, Ineffective Community
†Health Management, Ineffective Family
Health Management, Readiness for Enhanced
Surgical Recovery, Delayed
 Surgical Recovery, Risk for Delayed

2. Nutritional—Metabolic

Adverse Reaction to Iodinated Contrast Media, Risk for
Allergy Response, Risk for
Blood Glucose Level, Risk for Unstable

(continued)

Box 3   CONDITIONS THAT NECESSITATE NURSING CARE (*continued*)

Body Temperature, Risk for Imbalanced
 Hyperthermia
 Hypothermia
 Hypothermia, Risk for Perioperative
 Thermoregulation, Ineffective
Breastfeeding, Ineffective
Breastfeeding, Interrupted
Breastfeeding, Readiness for Enhanced
Breast Milk, Insufficient
Electrolyte Imbalances, Risk for
Fluid Balance, Readiness for Enhanced
Fluid Volume, Deficient
 Fluid Volume, Risk for Deficient
Fluid Volume, Excess
Fluid Volume, Risk for Imbalanced
Infection, Risk for
†Infection Transmission, Risk for
Jaundice, Neonatal
 Jaundice, Risk for Neonatal
Latex Allergy Response
 Latex Allergy Response, Risk for
Nutrition, Imbalanced
 Dentition, Impaired
 Infant Feeding Pattern, Ineffective
 Swallowing, Impaired
Nutrition, Readiness for Enhanced
Protection, Ineffective
 Corneal Injury ,Risk for
 Dry Eye, Risk for
 Oral Mucous Membrane, Impaired
 Skin Integrity, Impaired
 Skin Integrity, Risk for Impaired
 Pressure Ulcer
 Pressure Ulcer, Risk for
 Tissue Integrity, Impaired
 Tissue Integrity, Risk for Impaired

3. Elimination

Bowel Incontinence

Box 3   CONDITIONS THAT NECESSITATE NURSING CARE (continued)

Constipation
  Constipation, Chronic Functional
  Constipation, Risk for Chronic Function
  Constipation, Perceived
Diarrhea
Gastrointestinal Motility, Dysfunctional
  Gastrointestinal Motility, Risk for Dysfunctional
Urinary Elimination, Impaired
  †Continuous Urinary Incontinence
  Functional Urinary Incontinence
  Maturational Enuresis
  Overflow Urinary Incontinence
  Reflex Urinary Incontinence
  Stress Urinary Incontinence
  Urge Urinary Incontinence
  Urge Urinary Incontinence, Risk for
Urinary Elimination, Readiness for Enhanced

4. Activity—Exercise

Activity Intolerance
Activity Planning, Ineffective
  Activity Planning, Risk for Ineffective
Bleeding, Risk for
Cardiac Output, Decreased
Disuse Syndrome, Risk for
Diversional Activity, Deficient
Home Maintenance, Impaired
Infant Behavior, Disorganized
  Infant Behavior, Risk for Disorganized
Infant Behavior, Readiness for Enhanced Organized
Intracranial Adaptive Capacity, Decreased
Lifestyle, Sedentary
Liver Function, Risk for Impaired
Mobility, Impaired Physical
  Bed Mobility, Impaired
  Sitting, Impaired
  Standing, Impaired
  Transfer Ability, Impaired
  Walking, Impaired
  Wheelchair Mobility, Impaired

(continued)

Box 3   CONDITIONS THAT NECESSITATE NURSING CARE (*continued*)

†Respiratory Function, Risk for Ineffective
    Airway Clearance, Ineffective
    Breathing Pattern, Ineffective
    Gas Exchange, Impaired
    Spontaneous Ventilation, Impaired
    Ventilatory Weaning Response, Dysfunctional
    †Ventilatory Weaning Response, Risk for Dysfunctional
Self-Care, Readiness for Enhanced
†Self-Care Deficit Syndrome
    Feeding Self-Care Deficit
    Bathing Self-Care Deficit
    Dressing Self-Care Deficit
    †Instrumental Self-Care Deficit
    Toileting Self-Care Deficit
Shock, Risk for
Sudden Infant Death Syndrome, Risk for
Tissue Perfusion, Ineffective
    Cardiac Tissue Perfusion, Risk for Decreased
    Cardiovascular Function, Risk for Impaired
    Cerebral Tissue Perfusion, Risk for Ineffective
    Gastrointestinal Tissue Perfusion, Risk for Ineffective
    Peripheral Neurovascular Dysfunction, Risk for
    Peripheral Tissue Perfusion, Ineffective
    Peripheral Tissue Perfusion, Risk for Ineffective
    Renal Perfusion, Risk for Ineffective
Vascular Trauma, Risk for
Wandering

5. Sleep—Rest

Sleep, Readiness for Enhanced
Sleep Pattern, Disturbed
    Insomnia
    Sleep Deprivation

6. Cognitive—Perceptual

Aspiration, Risk for
Comfort, Impaired
    Nausea
    Pain, Acute
    Pain, Chronic

Box 3   CONDITIONS THAT NECESSITATE NURSING CARE (continued)

Pain, Labor
Pain Syndrome, Chronic
Comfort, Readiness for Enhanced
Confusion, Acute
Confusion, Risk for Acute
Confusion, Chronic
Decisional Conflict
Decision Making, Impaired Emancipated
Decision Making, Risk for Impaired Emancipated
Decision Making, Readiness for Impaired Emancipated
Decision Making, Readiness for Enhanced
Dysreflexia, Autonomic
Dysreflexia, Risk for Autonomic
Knowledge, Deficient
Knowledge (Specify), Readiness for Enhanced
Memory, Impaired
Neglect, Unilateral

7. Self-Perception

Anxiety
Anxiety, Death
Fatigue
Fear
Hope, Readiness for Enhanced
Hopelessness
Human Dignity, Risk for Compromised
Neglect, Self
Power, Readiness for Enhanced
Powerlessness
Powerlessness, Risk for
†Self-Concept, Disturbed
Body Image, Disturbed
Personal Identity, Disturbed
Personal Identity, Risk for Disturbed
Self-Esteem, Chronic Low
Self-Esteem, Risk for Chronic Low
†Self-Esteem, Disturbed
Self-Esteem, Situational Low
Self-Esteem, Risk for Situational Low
Self-Concept, Readiness for Enhanced

(continued)

Box 3   CONDITIONS THAT NECESSITATE NURSING CARE (continued)

8. Role—Relationship

Childbearing Process, Ineffective
  Childbearing Process, Risk for Ineffective
†Communication, Impaired
  Communication, Impaired Verbal
Communication, Readiness for Enhanced
Family Processes, Dysfunctional
Family Processes, Interrupted
Family Processes, Readiness for Enhanced
Grieving
  †Grieving, Anticipatory
  Grieving, Complicated
  Grieving, Risk for Complicated
Loneliness, Risk for
Parental Role Conflict
Parenting, Impaired
  Attachment, Risk for Impaired
Parenting, Readiness for Enhanced
Relationship, Ineffective
  Relationship, Risk for Ineffective
Relationship, Readiness for Enhanced
Role Performance, Ineffective
Social Interaction, Impaired
Social Isolation
Sorrow, Chronic

9. Sexuality—Reproductive

Childbearing Process, Readiness for Enhanced
Maternal/Fetal Dyad, Risk for Disturbed
Sexuality Patterns, Ineffective
  Sexual Dysfunction

10. Coping—Stress Tolerance

Caregiver Role Strain
  Caregiver Role Strain, Risk for
Coping, Compromised Family
Coping, Disabled Family
Coping, Ineffective
  Coping, Defensive
  Denial, Ineffective

Box 3 CONDITIONS THAT NECESSITATE NURSING CARE (*continued*)

    Impulse Control, Ineffective
    Labile Emotional Control
    Mood Regulation, Impaired
Coping, Ineffective Community
Coping, Readiness for Enhanced
Coping, Readiness for Enhanced Community
Coping, Readiness for Enhanced Family
Post-Trauma Syndrome
Post-Trauma Syndrome, Risk for
Rape-Trauma Syndrome
Relocation Stress [Syndrome]
Relocation Stress [Syndrome], Risk for
Resilience, Impaired Individual
Resilience, Readiness for Enhanced
Resilience, Risk for Compromised
†Self-Harm, Risk for
    Self-Mutilation
    Self-Mutilation, Risk for
    Suicide, Risk for
Stress Overload
Violence, Risk for Other-Directed
Violence, Risk for Self-Directed

I I. Value—Belief

Moral Distress
    †Moral Distress, Risk for
Religiosity, Readiness for Enhanced
Spiritual Distress
    Religiosity, Impaired
    Religiosity, Risk for Impaired
    Spiritual Distress, Risk for
Spiritual Well-Being, Readiness for Enhanced

‡Collaborative Problems

Risk for Complications of Cardiac/Vascular Dysfunction

RC of Decreased Cardiac Output
RC of Arrhythmias
RC of Pulmonary Edema
RC of Cardiogenic Shock

(*continued*)

Box 3   CONDITIONS THAT NECESSITATE NURSING CARE *(continued)*

RC of Deep Vein Thrombosis
RC of Hypovolemia
RC of Peripheral Vascular Insufficiency
RC of Hypertension
RC of Congenital Heart Disease
RC of Abdominal Hypertension
RC of Endocarditis
RC of Pulmonary Embolism
RC of Spinal Shock
RC of Ischemic Ulcers

Risk for Complications of Respiratory Dysfunction

RC of Hypoxemia
RC of Atelectasis/Pneumonia
RC of Tracheobronchial Constriction
RC of Pleural Effusion
RC of Tracheal Necrosis
RC of Pneumothorax
RC of Laryngeal Edema

Risk for Complications of Renal/Urinary Dysfunction

RC of Acute Urinary Retention
RC of Renal Failure
RC of Bladder Perforation
RC of Renal Calculi

Risk for Complications of Gastrointestinal/Hepatic/Biliary Dysfunction

RC of Paralytic Ileus/Small Bowel Obstruction
RC of Hepatic Failure
RC of Hyperbilirubinemia
RC of Evisceration
RC of Hepatosplenomegaly
RC of Curling's Ulcer
RC of Ascites
RC of Gastrointestinal Bleeding

Risk for Complications of Metabolic/Immune/Hematopoietic Dysfunction

RC of Hypoglycemia/Hyperglycemia
RC of Negative Nitrogen Balance

Box 3 CONDITIONS THAT NECESSITATE NURSING CARE (continued)

RC of Electrolyte Imbalances
RC of Thyroid Dysfunction
RC of Hypothermia (Severe)
RC of Hyperthermia (Severe)
RC of Sepsis
RC of Acidosis (Metabolic, Respiratory)
RC of Alkalosis (Metabolic, Respiratory)
RC of Hypo/Hyperthyroidism
RC of Allergic Reaction
RC of Donor Tissue Rejection
RC of Adrenal Insufficiency
RC of Anemia
RC of Thrombocytopenia
RC of Opportunistic Infection
RC of Polycythemia
RC of Sickling Crisis
RC of Disseminated Intravascular Coagulation

Risk for Complications of Neurological/Sensory Dysfunction

RC of Increased Intracranial Pressure
RC of Stroke
RC of Seizures
RC of Spinal Cord Compression
RC of Meningitis
RC of Cranial Nerve Impairment (Specify)
RC of Paralysis
RC of Peripheral Nerve Impairment
RC of Increased Intraocular Pressure
RC of Corneal Ulceration
RC of Neuropathies

Risk for Complications of Muscular/Skeletal Dysfunction

RC of Osteoporosis
RC of Joint Dislocation
RC of Compartment Syndrome
RC of Pathologic Fractures

Risk for Complications of Reproductive Dysfunction

RC of Fetal Distress
RC of Postpartum Bleeding

(continued)

Box 3   CONDITIONS THAT NECESSITATE NURSING CARE *(continued)*

RC of Gestational Hypertension

RC of Hypermenorrhea

RC of Polymenorrhea

RC of Syphilis

RC of Pelvic Inflammatory Disease

RC of Prenatal Bleeding

RC of Preterm Labor

Risk for Complications of Medication Therapy Adverse Effects

RC of Adrenocorticosteroid Therapy Adverse Effects

RC of Antianxiety Therapy Adverse Effects

RC of Antiarrhythmic Therapy Adverse Effects

RC of Anticoagulant Therapy Adverse Effects

RC of Anticonvulsant Therapy Adverse Effects

RC of Antidepressant Therapy Adverse Effects

RC of Antihypertensive Therapy Adverse Effects

RC of Beta-Adrenergic Blocker Therapy Adverse Effects

RC of Calcium-Channel Blocker Therapy Adverse Effects

RC of Angiotensin-Converting Enzyme Therapy Adverse Effects

RC of Antineoplastic Therapy Adverse Effects

RC of Antipsychotic Therapy Adverse Effects

RC of Diuretic Therapy Adverse Effects

---

* The Functional Health Patterns were identified in Gordon, M. (1994). *Nursing diagnosis: Process and application.* New York: McGraw-Hill, with minor changes by the author.
† These diagnoses are not currently on the NANDA-I list but have been included for clarity and usefulness or retained after NANDA-I deletion.
‡ Frequently used collaborative problems are represented on this list. Other situations not listed here could also qualify as collaborative problems.

paralytic ileus but, instead, detect its presence early to prevent greater severity or even death. Physicians cannot treat collaborative problems without nursing knowledge, vigilance, and judgment.

Formulate Nursing Diagnoses Correctly

Types of Nursing Diagnoses

A nursing diagnosis can be a problem, risk, health promotion, or syndrome type.

- *Problem:* A problem nursing diagnosis describes a clinical judgment that the nurse has validated because of the presence of major defining characteristics.
- *Risk:* A risk nursing diagnosis describes a clinical judgment that an individual/group is more vulnerable to develop the problem than others in the same or a similar situation because of risk factors.
- *Health Promotion:* A health promotion nursing diagnosis is a clinical judgment about an individual, family, or community in transition from a specific level of wellness to a higher level of wellness (NANDA-I, 2012).
- *Syndrome:* A syndrome diagnosis comprises a cluster of problem or risk nursing diagnoses that are predicted to present because of a certain situation or event.
- Possible nursing diagnosis is not a type of diagnosis as are problem, risk, and syndrome. Possible nursing diagnoses are a diagnostician's option to indicate that some data are present to confirm a diagnosis but are insufficient at this time.

Diagnostic Statements

The diagnostic statement describes the health status of an individual or group and the factors that have contributed to the status.

One-Part Statements

Health Promotion nursing diagnoses will be written as one-part statements: *Readiness for Enhanced* _____ (e.g., *Readiness for Enhanced Parenting*). Related factors are not present for wellness nursing diagnoses because they would all be the same: motivated to achieve a higher level of wellness. Syndrome diagnoses, such as *Rape-Trauma Syndrome*, have no "related to" designations.

Two-Part Statements

Risk and possible nursing diagnoses have two parts. The validation for a risk nursing diagnosis is the presence of risk factors. The risk factors are the second part, as in:

Risk Nursing Diagnosis Related to Risk Factors
Possible nursing diagnoses are suspected because of the presence of certain factors.

Two-Part Statement Examples
Risk for Impaired Skin Integrity related to immobility secondary to fractured hip
Possible Self-Care Deficit related to impaired ability to use left hand secondary to IV
Designating a diagnosis as possible provides the nurse with a method to communicate to other nurses that a diagnosis may be present. Additional data collection is indicated to rule out or confirm the tentative diagnosis.

Three-Part Statements
A problem nursing diagnosis consists of three parts.

Diagnostic label + contributing factors + signs and symptoms

The presence of major signs and symptoms (defining characteristics) validates that a problem diagnosis is present. This is the third part. It is not possible to have a third part for risk or possible diagnoses because signs and symptoms do not exist.

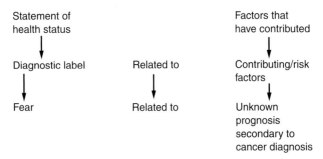

Statement of health status		Factors that have contributed
↓		↓
Diagnostic label	Related to	Contributing/risk factors
↓	↓	↓
Fear	Related to	Unknown prognosis secondary to cancer diagnosis

Three-Part Statement Examples
*Anxiety related to unpredictable nature of asthmatic episodes as evident
     by statements of "I'm afraid I won't be able to breathe"*
*Urge Incontinence related to diminished bladder capacity secondary to
     habitual frequent voiding as evident by inability to hold off urination
     after desire to void and report of voiding out of habit, not need*

The presence of a nursing diagnosis is determined by assessing the individual's health status and ability to function. Functional health patterns and the corresponding nursing diagnoses are listed in Box 3. If significant data are collected in a particular functional pattern, the next step is to check the related nursing diagnoses to see whether any of them are substantiated by the data that are collected.

Validation

The process of validating a nursing diagnosis should not be done in isolation from the individual or family. Individuals are the experts on themselves. During assessments and interactions, nurses are provided a small glimpse of their clients. Diagnostic hunches or inferences about data should be discussed with clients for their input. Individuals are given opportunities to select what they want assistance with, which problems are important to them, and which ones are not.

Clinical Example

After the screening assessment has been completed, the nurse applies each of the following questions to each functional or need area:

- Is there a possible problem in a specific area?
- Is the person at risk (or high risk) for a problem?
- Does the person desire to improve his/her health?

For example, after assessing an individual's elimination pattern, the nurse would then analyze the data. Does this person have a possible problem with constipation or diarrhea? If yes, the nurse would then ask the person more focused questions to confirm the presence of the defining characteristics of constipation or diarrhea. If these defining characteristics are not present, then there is no problem in diagnosis of *Constipation or Diarrhea*. Is there a risk

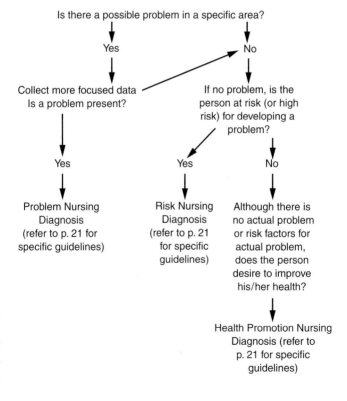

Is there a possible problem in a specific area?

Yes   No

Collect more focused data
Is a problem present?

If no problem, is the person at risk (or high risk) for developing a problem?

Yes   Yes   No

Problem Nursing Diagnosis (refer to p. 21 for specific guidelines)

Risk Nursing Diagnosis (refer to p. 21 for specific guidelines)

Although there is no actual problem or risk factors for actual problem, does the person desire to improve his/her health?

Health Promotion Nursing Diagnosis (refer to p. 21 for specific guidelines)

diagnosis? To determine this, the nurse will assess for risk factors of *Constipation or Diarrhea* (listed under related/risk factors). If none of these are present, there is no risk for *Constipation or Diarrhea*.

Problem Nursing Diagnoses

Problem nursing diagnoses are written in two- or three-part statements:

1st part	2nd part	3rd part
Diagnostic Label	related to *factors that have caused or contributed*	as evident by *signs and symptoms in the individual that indicate the diagnosis is present*

Now that the defining characteristics have been confirmed to be present in the individual, you have:

Label	Constipation
Causative/contributing factors:	related to inadequate fiber and fluid intake
Signs/symptoms: (defining characteristics)	as evident by reports of dry, hard stools, q3–4 days

Clinical Example

As part of the screening assessment under nutrition you elicit:

Usual food intake	Usual fluid intake
BMI	Current weight
Appearance of skin, nails, and hair	

You then analyze the data to determine which data are within a normal range, and which are not:

- Are there sufficient servings of five food groups?
- Is there sufficient intake of calcium, protein, and vitamins?
- Is the fat intake <30% of total caloric intake?
- Does the person drink at least six to eight cups of water besides coffee or soft drinks?
- Does the appearance of skin, hair, and nails reflect a healthy nutrition pattern?
- Is the person's weight within normal limits for height?

For example, in a specific person, Mr. Jewel, you find there is:

- Appropriate weight for height
- Insufficient fluid intake (four 8-oz glasses of water/juice)
- Insufficient vegetable intake (two servings)
- Excess intake of bread, cereal, rice, and pasta (eight servings)
- Dry skin and hair

From your assessment, you have confirmed that a nursing diagnosis is present because the person has signs or reports symptoms that represent those listed as defining characteristics under that specific diagnosis. These are usually the person's complaints.

At this point, you have two parts of the diagnostic statement—the first and third, but not the second:

Imbalanced Nutrition related to _____, as evident from dry skin and hair, dietary intake (low in fiber, vegetables, fluids, and high in CHO)

Now you want to determine what has caused or contributed to Mr. Jewel's imbalanced nutrition. Look at the list of related factors or risk factors under *Imbalanced Nutrition*. Do any relate to Mr. Jewel's situation? Does Mr. Jewel think his diet is inadequate? If he says no, "lack of knowledge" would be the third part of your diagnostic statement. If he says yes, but it is not important to him to change his habits at his age, you will need to talk with him. Perhaps he has a problem with constipation or energy. Maybe a change of diet could help. When you are assured that Mr. Jewel understands the reasons for a balanced diet, but see that he has decided to continue his present diet, record his decision and your attempts to influence that decision.

Select Priority Diagnoses

Priority Criteria

Nurses cannot treat all the nursing diagnoses and collaborative problems that an individual client, family, or community has. Attempts to do this will result in frustration for the nurse and the client. By identifying a priority set—a group of nursing diagnoses and collaborative problems that take precedence over other nursing diagnoses or collaborative problems—the nurse can best direct resources toward goal achievement. It is useful to differentiate priority diagnoses from those that are important, but not priority.

Priority diagnoses are those nursing diagnoses or collaborative problems that, if not managed now, will deter progress to achieve outcomes or will negatively affect the individual's functional status.

Nonpriority diagnoses are those nursing diagnoses or collaborative problems for which treatment can be delayed to a later time without compromising present functional status. How does the nurse identify a priority set? In an acute-care setting, the individual enters the hospital for specific purpose, such as surgery or other treatments for acute illness.

- What are the nursing diagnoses or collaborative problems associated with the primary condition or treatments (e.g., surgery)?
- Are there additional collaborative problems associated with coexisting medical conditions that require monitoring (e.g., hypoglycemia)?
- Are there additional nursing diagnoses that, if not managed now, will deter recovery or affect the individual's functional status (e.g., *High Risk for Constipation*)?
- What problems do the individual perceive as priority?

Use of Consultants/Referrals

How are other diagnoses not on the diagnostic cluster selected for an individual's problem list? Limited nursing resources and increasingly reduced care time mandate that nurses identify important nursing diagnoses that can be addressed later and do not need to be included on the individual's problem list. For example, for an individual hospitalized after myocardial infarction who is 50 pounds overweight, the nurse would want to explain the effects of obesity on cardiac function and refer the individual to community resources for a weight-reduction program after discharge. The discharge summary record would reflect the teaching and the referral; a nursing diagnosis related to weight reduction would not need to appear on the individual's problem list.

Summary

Making accurate nursing diagnoses takes knowledge and practice. If the nurse uses a systematic approach to nursing diagnosis validation, then accuracy will increase. The process of making nursing diagnoses is difficult because nurses are attempting to diagnose human responses. Humans are unique, complex, and ever-changing; thus, attempts to classify these responses have been difficult.

References

Carpenito, L. J. (2016). *Nursing diagnosis: Application to clinical practice* (15th ed.). Philadelphia: Wolters Kluwer.
North American Nursing Diagnosis Association (NANDA). (2008). National conference, Miami, FL.
NANDA International. (2012). *Nursing diagnoses: Definitions and classification 2012–2014*. Ames, IA: Wiley-Blackwell.

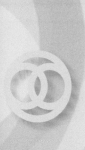

Section I

Nursing Diagnoses[1]

ACTIVITY INTOLERANCE

NANDA-I Definition

Insufficient physiologic or psychological energy to endure or complete required or desired daily activities

Defining Characteristics

Major (Must Be Present)

An altered physiologic response to activity

Respiratory
Exertional dyspnea*   Shortness of breath
Excessively increased rate   Decreased rate

Pulse
Weak   Failure to return to preactivity
Excessively increased   level after 3 minutes
Rhythm change   EKG changes reflecting
Decreased   arrhythmias or ischemia*

Blood Pressure
Abnormal blood pressure response to activity
Failure to increase with activity
Increased diastolic pressure (greater than 15 mm Hg)

Minor (May Be Present)

Verbal report of weakness*   Verbal report of fatigue*
Pallor or cyanosis   Confusion
Verbal report of vertigo

Related Factors

Any factors that compromise oxygen transport orphysical conditioning or create excessive energy demands that outstrip the individual's physical and psychological abilities can cause activity intolerance. Some common factors follow.

Pathophysiologic

Related to deconditioning secondary to prolonged immobilization and pain

*Related to imbalance between oxygen supply and demand**

Related to compromised oxygen transport system secondary to:

Cardiac
Cardiomyopathies   Congestive heart failure
Dysrhythmias   Angina
Myocardial infarction   Valvular disease
Congenital heart disease

Respiratory
Chronic obstructive pulmonary disease (COPD)
Bronchopulmonary dysplasia
Atelectasis

Circulatory
Anemia
Hypovolemia
Peripheral arterial disease

Related to increased metabolic demands secondary to:

Acute or Chronic Infections
Viral infection   Mononucleosis
Endocrine or metabolic disorders   Hepatitis

Chronic Diseases
Renal   Hepatic
Inflammatory   Musculoskeletal
Neurologic

Related to inadequate energy sources secondary to:
Obesity   Inadequate diet
Malnourishment

Treatment Related

Related to inactivity secondary to assistive equipment (walkers, crutches, braces)

Related to increased metabolic demands secondary to:
Malignancies   Surgery
Diagnostic studies   Treatment schedule/frequency

Related to compromised oxygen transport secondary to:
Hypovolemia   Immobility*
Bed rest*

Situational (Personal, Environmental)

Related to inactivity secondary to:
Depression   Sedentary lifestyle*
Inadequate social support

Related to increased metabolic demands secondary to:
Environmental barriers (e.g., stairs)
Climate extremes (especially hot, humid climates)
Air pollution (e.g., smog)
Atmospheric pressure (e.g., recent relocation to high-altitude
  living)

Related to inadequate motivation secondary to:

Fear of falling	Pain
Depression	Dyspnea
Obesity	Generalized weakness*

Maturational

Older adults may have decreased muscle strength and flexibility, as well as sensory deficits. These factors can undermine body confidence and may contribute directly or indirectly to activity intolerance.

 Author's Note

Activity Intolerance is a diagnostic judgment that describes an individual with compromised physical conditioning. This individual can engage in therapies to increase strength and endurance. *Activity Intolerance* is different from *Fatigue*; *Fatigue* is a pervasive, subjective draining feeling. Rest does treat *Fatigue*, but it can also cause tiredness. Moreover, in *Activity Intolerance*, the goal is to increase tolerance for and endurance of activity; in *Fatigue*, the goal is to assist the individual to adapt to the fatigue, not to increase endurance.

Activity Intolerance

Goals

The individual will progress to (specify level of activity desired), evidenced by these indicators:

- Identify factors that aggravate activity intolerance
- Identify methods to reduce activity intolerance
- Maintain blood pressure within normal limits 3 minutes after activity

Activity Tolerance, Energy Management, Exercise Promotion, Sleep Enhancement, Mutual Goal Setting

Interventions

Elicit From the Individual Their Personal Goals to Improve Their Health

Explain the Risks of Inactivity

Monitor the Individual's Response to Activity and Record Response

- Take resting pulse, blood pressure, and respirations.
- Consider rate, rhythm, and quality (if signs are abnormal—e.g., pulse above 100—consult with physician about advisability of increasing activity).
- If signs are normal or if physician approves, have the individual perform the activity.
- Take vital signs immediately after activity.
- Have the individual rest for 3 minutes; take vital signs again.
- Discontinue the activity if the individual responds with
  - Complaints of chest pain, vertigo, or confusion
  - Decreased pulse rate
  - Failure of systolic blood pressure to increase
  - Decreased systolic blood pressure
  - Increased diastolic blood pressure (by more than 15 mm Hg)
  - Decreased respiratory response
- Reduce the intensity or duration of the activity if
  - The pulse takes longer than 3 to 4 minutes to return to within 6 beats of the resting pulse.
  - The respiratory rate increase is excessive after the activity.

Increase the Activity Gradually

- Increase tolerance for activity by having the individual perform the activity more slowly, for a shorter time, with more rest pauses, or with more assistance.
- Minimize the deconditioning effects of prolonged bed rest and imposed immobility:
  - Begin active range of motion (ROM) at least twice a day. For the individual who is unable, the nurse should perform passive ROM.
  - Encourage isometric exercise.
  - Encourage the individual to turn and lift the body actively, unless contraindicated.
  - Gradually increase tolerance, starting with 15 minutes the first time out of bed.
  - If the individual cannot stand without buckling the knees, he or she is not ready for ambulation; help the individual to practice standing in place with assistance.
  - Choose a safe gait. (If the gait appears awkward but stable, continue; stay close by and give clear coaching messages, e.g., "Look straight ahead, not down.")

- Allow the individual to gauge the rate of ambulation.
- Provide sufficient support to ensure safety and prevent falling.
- Encourage the individual to wear comfortable walking shoes (slippers do not support the feet properly).

Plan Rest Periods According to the Person's Daily Schedule

Promote a Sincere "Can-Do" Attitude

- Identify factors that undermine the individual's confidence, such as fear of falling, perceived weakness, and visual impairment.
- Explore possible incentives with the individual and the family; consider what the individual values (e.g., playing with grandchildren, returning to work, going fishing, performing a task or craft).
- Allow the individual to set the activity schedule and functional activity goals. If the goal is too low, negotiate (e.g., "Walking 25 feet seems low. Let's increase it to 50 feet. I'll walk with you.")
- Plan a purpose for the activity, such as sitting up in a chair to eat lunch, walking to a window to see the view, or walking to the kitchen to get some juice.
- Help the individual to identify progress. Do not underestimate the value of praise and encouragement as effective motivational techniques. In selected cases, assisting the individual to keep a written record of activities may help to demonstrate progress.

Interventions for Individuals With Chronic Pulmonary Insufficiency

- Encourage conscious controlled-breathing techniques during increased activity and times of emotional and physical stress (techniques include pursed-lip and diaphragmatic breathing).
- Teach pursed-lip breathing. The person should breathe in through the nose, then breathe out slowly through partially closed lips while counting to seven and making a "pu" sound. (Often, people with progressive lung disease learn this naturally.)
- Teach diaphragmatic breathing:
  - Place your hands on their abdomen below the base of the ribs, and keep them there while he or she inhales.
  - To inhale, the individual relaxes the shoulders, breathes in through the nose, and pushes the stomach outward against your hands. The individual holds the breath for 1 to 2 seconds to keep the alveoli open, then exhales.
  - To exhale, the individual breathes out slowly through the mouth while you apply slight pressure at the base of the ribs.
  - Have the individual practice this breathing technique several times with you; then, the individual should place his or her own hands at the base of the ribs to practice alone.

- Once the technique has been learned, have the individual practice it a few times each hour.
- Encourage the use of adaptive breathing techniques to decrease the work of breathing.
- "Explain that the tripod position, in which the patient sits or stands leaning forward with the arms supported, forces the diaphragm down and forward and stabilizes the chest while reducing the work of breathing. Point out that this reduces competing demands of the arm, chest, and neck muscles needed for breathing" (Bauldoff, 2015; *Bauldoff, Hoffman, Sciurba, & Zullo, 1996; *Breslin, 1992).
- Providing arm support (e.g., resting elbows on a tabletop while shaving or eating) may enhance independence and improve functional capacity.
- While in the hospital, discuss the effects of smoking on the cardiovascular, respiratory, circulatory, and musculoskeletal systems with a focus on the specific health problems of the individual (e.g., frequent infections, leg cramps, worsening of COPD, cardiac problems).

INEFFECTIVE ACTIVITY PLANNING

Risk for Ineffective Activity Planning

NANDA-I Definition

Inability to prepare for a set of actions fixed in time and under certain conditions

Defining Characteristics*

Verbalization of fear toward a task to be undertaken
Verbalization of worries toward a task to be undertaken
Excessive anxieties toward a task to be undertaken
Failure pattern of behavior
Lack of plan
Lack of resources
Lack of sequential organization
Procrastination
Unmet goals for chosen activity

Related Factors*

Compromised ability to process information

Defensive flight behavior when faced with proposed solution

Hedonism

Lack of family support

Lack of support from friends

Unrealistic perception of events

Unrealistic perception of personal competence

 Author's Note

This newly accepted NANDA-I nursing diagnosis can represent a problematic response that relates to many existing nursing diagnoses such as *Chronic Confusion, Self-Care Deficit, Anxiety, Ineffective Denial, Ineffective Coping,* and *Ineffective Self-Health Management. This author recommends that Ineffective Activity Planning should be seen as a sign or symptom. The questions are as follows:*

- What activities are not being planned effectively? Self-care? Self-health management?
- What is preventing effective activity planning? Confusion? Anxiety? Fear? Denial? Stress overload? Examples are as follows:
  - Stress Overload related to unrealistic perception of events as evidenced by impaired ability to plan ... (specify activity)
  - Ineffective Self-Health Management related to lack of plan, lack of resources, lack of social support as evidenced by impaired ability to plan ... (specify activity)
  - Anxiety related to compromised ability to process information and unrealistic perception of personal competence as evidenced by impaired ability to plan ... (specify activity)

Risk for Ineffective Activity Planning

NANDA-I Definition

Vulnerable to an inability to prepare for a set of actions fixed in time and under certain conditions which can compromise functioning.

Risk Factors*

Compromised ability to process information
Defensive flight behavior when faced with proposed solution
Hedonism
History of procrastination

Ineffective support system
Insufficient support system
Unrealistic perception of events
Unrealistic perception of personal competence

 Author's Note

Refer to *Ineffective Activity Planning.*

RISK FOR ADVERSE REACTION TO IODINATED CONTRAST MEDIA

NANDA-I Definition

Vulnerable to noxious or unintended reaction associated with the use of iodinated contrast media that can occur within seven (7) days after contrast agent injection, which may compromise health

Risk Factors

Pathophysiologic

For Acute Reaction
History of asthma
Prior reaction to contrast
Atrophy (typically associated with heightened immune responses to common allergens, especially inhaled allergens and food allergens)

For Delayed Reaction
Prior reaction to contrasts
Those being treated with interleukin-2
Sun exposure

For Contrast-Induced Nephropathy

Preexisting renal dysfunction
Concurrent use of nephrotoxic drugs
Use of a high-osmolality contrast
    agent
High volumes of contrast agent
Hypertension
Heart failure

Hemodynamic instability
ACE inhibitors
Dehydration
Diabetes mellitus
Poor renal perfusion
Myocardial infarction

Underlying disease (e.g., heart disease, pulmonary disease, blood
    dyscrasias, endocrine disease, pheochromocytoma, autoim-
    mune disease)*
Collagen vascular disease
Sickle cell disease
Myeloma
Polycythemia
Paraproteinemia syndrome/disease (e.g., multiple myeloma)
History of a kidney transplant, renal tumor, renal surgery, or
    single kidney
History of end-stage liver disease
Dehydration*
Elevated creatinine levels
Recent history (1 month) of (Robbins & Pozniak, 2010)
    Major infection (e.g., pneumonia, sepsis, osteomyelitis)
    Vascular ischemia of extremities (e.g., amputation, arterial
        thrombosis)
    Venous or arterial thrombosis
    Major surgery or vascular procedure (e.g., amputation, trans-
        plantation, coronary artery bypass grafting)
    Multiorgan system failure

Treatment Related

More than 20 mg iodine
Chemotherapy or amino glycoside within past month
Concurrent use of medications (e.g., ACE inhibitors,
    beta-blockers, interleukin-2, metformin, nephrotoxic medica-
    tions,* NSAIDs, aminoglycosides)
Fragile veins (e.g., prior or actual chemotherapy treatment or ra-
    diation in the limb to be injected, multiple attempts, to obtain
    intravenous access, indwelling intravenous lines in place for
    more than 24 hours, previous axillary lymph node dissection
    in the limb to be injected, distal intravenous access sites: hand,
    wrist, foot, ankle)*

Physical and chemical properties of the contrast media
   (e.g., iodine concentration, viscosity, high osmolality, ion
   toxicity, unconsciousness)*

Situational (Personal, Environmental)

Females more than males
Anxiety*
Generalized debilitation*
History of previous adverse effect from iodinated contrast
   media*

Maturational

Older than 60 years
Extremes of age*

 Author's Note

This NANDA-I nursing diagnosis represents a clinical situation in which
iodinated contrast media is infused for radiographic diagnostic tests.
Complications of intravascular injection of iodinated contrast include ana-
phylactoid contrast reaction, contrast-induced nephropathy, and contrast
media extravasation (Pasternak & Williamson, 2012).

   Reactions can be mild and self-limiting (e.g., scattered urticaria,
nausea) to severe and life-threatening (e.g., cardiac arrhythmias, seizures). Nurses caring for individuals scheduled for these tests must be
aware of individuals who are at higher risk for adverse events. Nurses
in radiology departments are responsible for assessing for high-risk individuals, reviewing renal function status of individual prior to the procedure, monitoring for early signs or reactions, and using protocols when
indicated.

   This clinical situation can be described with this nursing diagnosis.
In contrast, *Risk for Complications of Contrast Media* is more appropriate
as a collaborative problem, since interventions required are nurse- and
physician-prescribed with protocols for treatment of adverse events. The
interventions included with this diagnosis can be used with *Risk for Adverse
Reaction to Iodinated Contrast Media* or *Risk for Complications of Contrast
Media*.

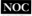 **NOC**

Vital Signs, Coping, Medication Response, Peripheral Vascular Access, Peripheral
Tissue Perfusion, Allergic Response, Symptom Severity, Risk Detection

Goals

The individual will report risk factors for adverse reaction and any symptoms experienced during infusion, as evidenced by the following indicators:

- State risk factors for adverse reactions
- Report any sensations that are felt during and after infusion
- Describe delayed reactions and the need to report

NIC
Teaching: Individual, Vital Sign Monitoring Venous Access Device, Maintenance, Anxiety Reduction, Circulatory Precautions, Peripheral Sensation Management, Preparatory Sensory Information: Procedure, Allergy Management, Risk Identification, Surveillance

Interventions

Assess for Factors That Increase Risk for Contrast Medium Adverse Reactions

- Refer to Risk Factors.
- Review with the individual/significant others previous experiences with contrast media infusions.
- Consult with radiologist if indicated.

Prepare the Individual for the Procedure

On Unit
- Explain the procedure (e.g., administration, sensations that may be felt such as mild, warm flushing at site of injection, which may spread over body and may be more intense in perineum, metallic taste).
- Evaluate level of anxiety. Consult with prescribing physician and/or NP if anxiety is high.
- Ensure that the individual is well hydrated prior to procedure. Consult with physician and/or NP for hydration ordered, if indicated. Follow protocol for
  - Hydration
  - Withholding certain medications (e.g., metformin or other oral hyperglycemic agents)
  - Determining when the last contrast media was infused

In Radiology Department
- Ensure that the individual is well hydrated prior to procedure.

- Explain the procedure (e.g., administration, sensations that may be felt such as mild, warm flushing at site of injection, which may spread over body, may be more intense in perineum, metallic taste).
- Evaluate the level of anxiety. Consult with prescribing physician, PA, or NP if anxiety is high.
- Encourage continuous conversation with and feedback from the individual during the procedure (Singh & Daftary, 2008).
- Follow protocol for administration of contrast media (e.g., site preparation, rate of infusion, warming of intravenous contrast medium (ICM)).
- Monitor the individual's emotional and physiologic response continuously during infusion.
- Refer to Table I.1 for signs and symptoms of adverse reactions.
- Monitor for extravasation of contrast by assessing for swelling, erythema, and pain that usually abates with no residual problems.
- If extravasation is suspected (Robbins & Pozniak, 2010):
  - Discontinue injection/infusion.
  - Notify prescribing professional.

Table I.1	CONTRAST MEDIUM REACTIONS

Idiosyncratic

Mild Reactions (Self-Limited)

Limited cutaneous edema	Transient flushing	"Scratchy" sore throat
Scattered urticaria	Limited itching	Nasal congestion
Limited nausea/vomiting	Anxiety	Chills
Sneezing	Mild hypertension	Dizziness

Moderate Reactions

Persistent nausea/vomiting	Diffuse urticarial/pruritus	Wheezing/bronchospasm
Facial edema, no dyspnea	Tachycardia	Hypertension urgency
Palpitations	Throat tightness/hoarseness	Abdominal cramps
Vasovagal reaction (bradycardia, fainting) that requires and is responsive to treatment		

(continued)

Table I.I *(continued)*		
Idiosyncratic		
Severe Reactions[a]		
Bronchospasm, significant hypoxia	Anaphylactic shock (hypotension + tachycardia)	Overt broncho-spasm
Life-threatening arrhythmias	Laryngeal edema	Syncope
Pulmonary edema	Seizures	Hypertensive emergency
Nonidiosyncratic		
Bradycardia	Hypotension	Vasovagal reactions
Neuropathy	Cardiovascular reactions	Extravasation
Delayed reactions	Sensations of warmth	Metallic taste in mouth
Nausea/vomiting		

[a]Signs and symptoms are often life-threatening and can result in permanent morbidity or death if not managed appropriately.

Sources: Siddiqi, N. (2015). Contrast medium reactions. In *Medscape.* Retrieved from http://emedicine.medscape.com/article/422855-overview; American College of Radiology Committee on Drugs and Contrast Media. (2013). *ACR manual on contrast media: Version 9.* Reston, VA: American College of Radiology. Retrieved from www. acr.org/quality-%20safety/resources/~/media/37D84428BF1D4E1B9A3A2918DA9 E27A3.pdf/.

- Elevate the affected extremity above the heart.
- Provide brief compression for no more than 1 minute.
- Follow agency protocol for documentation and reporting.
- Consult with plastic surgeon if swelling or pain progresses, decreased capillary refill is present, sensation alters, and/or skin ulcers or blisters are present.

Explain Delayed Contrast Reactions

- Advise the individual/family that a delayed contrast reaction can occur anytime between 3 hours and 7 days following the administration of contrast.
- Advise to avoid direct sun exposure for 1 week.
- Explain that delayed reaction can be cutaneous exanthem, pruritus without urticaria, nausea, vomiting, drowsiness, and headache.
- Advise them to report signs and symptoms to responsible physician/NP/PA.
- Advise to go to ER if symptoms increase or difficulty in swallowing or breathing occurs (Siddiqi, 2011).

RISK FOR ALLERGY RESPONSE

NANDA-I Definition

Vulnerable to an exaggerated immune response or reaction to substances, which may compromise health

Risk Factors

Treatment Related

Pharmaceutical agents (e.g., penicillin*, sulfa)
Adhesive tape
Latex

Situational (Personal, Environmental)

Chemical products (e.g., bleach*, solvents, paint, glue)
Animals (e.g., dander)
Environmental substances* (e.g., mold, dust mites, hay)
Food (e.g., peanuts, shellfish, mushrooms*, citrus fruits, sulfites)
Insect stings*
Repeated exposure to environmental substances*
Down pillows, quilts
Cosmetics*, lotions, creams, perfumes
Nickel
Plants (e.g., tomato, poison ivy)

Maturational

Genetic predisposition to atopic disease

 Author's Note

This new NANDA-I diagnosis can represent a diagnosis with the nursing assessments and educational interventions that can assist individuals and families with the prevention of allergic responses. The collaborative problem *Risk for Complications of Allergic Reaction* that can be found in Section 3 Collaborative Problems when nursing and medical interventions are needed for an allergic reaction.

 NOC
Immune Hypersensitivity Control, Allergic Response: Localized, Allergic Response: Systemic, Symptom Severity

Goals

The individual will report less or no allergy symptoms, as evidenced by the following indicators:

- Describe strategies to avoid exposure
- Describe methods to reduce environmental exposure
- Describe pharmaceutical management of a reaction

NIC
Allergy Management, Risk Identification, Surveillance, Teaching Environmental Risk Protection

Interventions

Refer the Individual to Allergy Specialist for Testing and Treatment If the Individual Has Food Allergies

Instruct the Individual on How to Reduce Allergens in Home
(Asthma and Allergy Foundation of America, 2011; Mayo Clinic Staff, 2011)

Develop Weekly/Monthly Cleaning Routine

- Damp-mop wood or linoleum flooring and vacuum carpeting. Use a vacuum cleaner with a small-particle or a high-efficiency particulate air (HEPA) filter.
- Use a damp cloth to clean other surfaces, including the tops of doors, windowsills, and window frames.
- Vacuum weekly with a vacuum cleaner that has a small-particle or HEPA filter. Wash area rugs and floor mats weekly. Shampoo wall-to-wall carpets periodically.
- If you have allergies, either wear a dust mask while cleaning or ask someone who does not have allergies to do the cleaning.
- Change or clean heating and cooling system filters once a month.
- Use HEPA filters in your whole-house central-air system, or in room air-cleaning devices. Replace filters regularly.

Bedroom
- Encase pillows, mattresses, and box springs in dust-mite-proof covers.
- Wash sheets once a week in 130° C hot water to kill mites and their eggs.
- Replace mattresses every 10 years.
- Replace pillows every 5 years.
- Remove, wash, or cover comforters. Choose bedding made of synthetic materials, not down.

Kitchen

- Install and use a vented exhaust fan. Most stovetop hoods simply filter cooking particulates without venting outside.
- Wash dishes daily. Scrub the sink and faucets as well.
- Wipe excessive moisture. Discard moldy or out-of-date food.
- Regularly empty and clean dripping pan, and clean or replace moldy rubber seals around doors.
- Place garbage in a can with an insect-proof lid, and empty trash daily. Keep the kitchen free of food crumbs.
- Clean cabinets and countertops with detergent and water. Check under-sink cabinets for plumbing leaks. Store food, including pet food, in sealed containers.
- Never leave food or garbage out to attract roaches.
- Store food in airtight containers in or out of the refrigerator.
- Wipe the stovetop right after cooking to remove food particles that attract insects, and remove crumbs and/or spilled items on countertops right away.
- Use poison baits, boric acid, and insect traps to kill cockroaches. People with asthma should avoid using liquid or spray pesticides.
- Wash dishes immediately after eating; avoid piling dishes in the sink.
- Use a covered/sealed trash can in the kitchen.
- Keep stovetop items covered. Use the kitchen fan when cooking to keep steam and moisture from condensing on kitchen surfaces.
- Use easy-to-clean kitchen flooring. Wash floor mats weekly to remove small food particles.

Bathroom

- Install and use an exhaust fan to reduce moisture while taking baths or showers.
- Towel-dry the tub and enclosure after use. Scrub mold from tub, shower, and faucets with bleach. Clean or replace moldy shower curtains and bathmats.
- Scrub mold from plumbing fixtures. Repair leaks.
- Remove wallpaper and install tile, or paint walls with mold-resistant enamel paint.
- Remove mold as soon as you see it anywhere in the bathroom.
- Fix leaky pipes under the sink, in the shower/tub, and behind the toilet.
- Use the fan/vent when showering to keep air circulating.
- Use washable floor mats, and wash them weekly.
- Use a mold/mildew spray to clean moldy areas, including shower curtains, tiles, and others.

- Wash the "show towels" and bath towels weekly.
- Wipe the sink and counter every day to remove puddles of water and moisture.

Windows/Doors
- Close windows and rely on air conditioning during pollen season. Clean mold and condensation from window frames and sills. Use double-paned windows, if you live in a cold climate.
- Use washable curtains made of plain cotton or synthetic fabric. Replace horizontal blinds with washable roller-type shades.

Humidity
- Vent clothes dryer outside.
- Choose an air filter that has a small-particle or HEPA filter. Try adjusting your air filter so that it directs clean air toward your head when you sleep.
- Maintain temperature at 70° F (21° C) and keep relative humidity no higher than 50%. Clean or replace small-particle filters in central heating and cooling systems and in room air conditioners at least once a month.

Pets
- Never allow pets on the bed.
- Keep pet sleeping areas and/or bird cages out of bedrooms.
- Bath pets at least twice a week which may reduce the amount of allergen in the dander they shed.

Fireplaces
- Avoid use of wood-burning fireplaces or stoves.

Child's Room
- Create a "healthy room" for your child.
- Use special mite-proof mattress and pillow covers.
- Wash sheets once a week in 130° F hot water to kill dust mites and their eggs, with bleach to kill mold.
- Wash stuffed toys every week in 130° F hot water to kill dust mites and their eggs, with bleach to kill mold.
- Place nonwashable stuffed toys in the freezer once a week for 24-hours to kill dust mites, then rinse them in cold water to remove dead mites.
- Keep kids' toys away from pets and store them in a covered, dry place where pets cannot get them.
- Do not allow your kids to sleep with stuffed toys (mites from the bed will get onto the toys, and vice versa).
- Make sure all clothes are fully dry before putting them in drawers and closets.

- Tell kids to wipe their feet and shake out their coats before coming inside, to keep any outside pollen from coming in on their clothes.
- Tell kids to put their clothes in the laundry immediately after coming in from outdoors, rather than on the floor or back in drawers, to minimize pollen exposure.

Living Room
- Vacuum furniture and curtains/drapes once a week.
- Use washable slip covers and cushions. Wash them in 130° F hot water once a week.
- Keep pets off of the furniture.
- Use easy-to-clean flooring, and avoid carpeting where moisture can get trapped.
- Use blinds and other easy-to-clean window treatments, or wash and dry curtains once a month.
- Never eat on the floor or on furniture.

Basement
- Find and fix all leaks, seams, and cracks in the foundation that let moisture seep in.
- Fix leaks and drips in pipes in and around the water heater and central HVAC (heating, ventilation, and air conditioning) system.
- Remove and clean mold wherever it appears. Apply mold prevention paint sealer.

Flooring
- Be vigilant about keeping flooring surfaces clean. Every type of flooring is a potential breeding ground for allergens, whether it is carpet, tile, or hardwood.
- Do not install wall-to-wall carpeting if you do not have to. It is harder to remove moisture, mold, and other allergens that are hidden in it.
- Vacuum all flooring weekly.

Instruct on Treatments at Home If Symptoms Occur

- Instruct to consult with allergist or primary care provider (physician, NP) regarding medical management of symptoms at home (e.g., Benadryl).
- Ensure that the individual has an Epi-pen, knows when and how to use it, and has transportation to the ER.
- Advise of the need to check expiration dates.

Do Not Allow Smoking Anywhere Inside Your House

Seek Immediate Emergency Care If

- Facial edema occurs
- Change in voice
- Difficulty breathing or swallowing

Call 911; Do Not Drive to the ER

Wear an Allergy ID Bracelet, Carry a List of Allergies, and/or Store a List of Allergies in Cell Phone in Designated Site

Refer to Allergy Specialist for Skin Testing and Treatment

ANXIETY

Anxiety

Death Anxiety

NANDA-I Definition

Vague uneasy feeling of discomfort or dread accompanied by an autonomic response (the source often unspecific or unknown to the individual); a feeling of apprehension caused by anticipation of danger. It is an alerting signal that warns of impending danger and enables the individual to take measures to deal with threat.

Defining Characteristics

Major (Must Be Present)

Manifested by symptoms from each category—physiologic, emotional, and cognitive; symptoms vary according to level of anxiety (*Whitley, 1994).

Physiologic
Increased pulse[2]   Increased blood pressure[2]
Increased respiration[2]   Pupil dilation[2]

---

[2] The items represent the results of concept analysis research of anxiety by Georgia Whitley in 1994.

Diaphoresis[2]
Voice quivering[2]
Palpitations
Urinary frequency, hesitancy, urgency[2]
Insomnia[2]
Facial flushing[2] or pallor
Body aches and pains (especially chest, back, neck)

Trembling, twitching[2]
Nausea[2]
Diarrhea[2]
Fatigue[2]
Dry mouth[2]
Restlessness[2]
Faintness[2]/dizziness

Emotional
Individual states feeling:
Apprehensive[2]
Jittery[2]
Loss of control
Persistent increased helplessness[2]

Vigilance[2]
Tension or being "keyed up"
Anticipation of misfortune

Individual exhibits:
Irritability[2]/impatience
Crying
Startle reaction
Withdrawal
Self-deprecation

Angry outbursts
Tendency to blame others[2]
Criticism of self and others
Lack of initiative
Poor eye contact[2]

Cognitive
Impaired attention[2]; difficulty concentrating[2]
Forgetfulness[2]
Orientation to past
Hyperattentiveness
Diminished ability to learn[2]
Confusion[2]

Lack of awareness of surroundings
Rumination[2]
Blocking of thoughts (inability to remember)
Preoccupation[2]

Related Factors

Pathophysiologic

Any factor that interferes with physiologic stability.

Related to respiratory distress secondary to:
Chest pain   Cancer diagnosis
Mind-altering drugs

Treatment Related

Related to (examples):
Impending surgery   Invasive procedure
Effects of chemotherapy

Situational (Personal, Environmental)

Related to threat to self-concept secondary to:

Change in or threat to role status/function* and prestige

Failure (or success)

Ethical dilemma (Halter, 2014; Varcarolis, 2011)

Exposure to phobic object or situation

Intrusive, unwanted thoughts

Flashbacks

Lack of recognition from others

Loss of valued possessions

Fear of panic attack

Unmet needs

Cessation of ritualistic behavior

Related to loss of significant others secondary to:

Threat of death*   Divorce
Cultural pressures   Moving
Temporary or permanent   Death
  separation

Related to threat to biologic integrity secondary to:

Dying   Assault
Invasive procedures   Disease (specify)

Related to change in environment secondary to:

Hospitalization   Incarceration
Retirement   Natural disasters
Environmental pollutants Refugee issues
Moving   Military or political deployment
Safety hazards   Airline travel

Related to change in socioeconomic status secondary to:

Unemployment   New job
Promotion   Displacement

Related to idealistic expectations of self and unrealistic goals (specify)

Maturational

Infant/Child
Related to separation

Related to unfamiliar environment or people

Related to changes in peer relationships

Related to death of (specify) with unfamiliar rituals and grieving adults

Adolescent
Related to death of (specify)

Related to threat to self-concept secondary to:
Sexual development   Peer relationship changes
Academic failure

Adult
Related to threat to self-concept secondary to:
Pregnancy   Parenting
Career changes   Effects of aging

Related to previous pregnancy complications, miscarriage, or fetal death

Related to lack of knowledge of changes associated with pregnancy

Related to lack of knowledge about labor experience

Older Adult
Related to threat to self-concept secondary to:
Sensory losers   Motor losses
Financial problems   Retirement changes

 Author's Note

Several researchers have examined the nursing diagnoses of *Anxiety* and *Fear* (*Jones & Jakob, 1984; *Taylor-Loughran, O'Brien, LaChapelle, & Rangel, 1989; Whitley, 1994; *Yokom, 1984). Differentiation of these diagnoses focuses on whether the threat can be identified. If so, the diagnosis is *Fear*; if not, it is *Anxiety* (NANDA, 2002). This differentiation, however, has not proved useful for clinicians (Taylor-Loughran et al., 1989).

Anxiety is a vague feeling of apprehension and uneasiness in response to a threat to one's value system or security pattern (*May, 1977). The individual may be able to identify the situation (e.g., surgery, cancer), but actually the threat to oneself relates to the enmeshed uneasiness and apprehension. In other words, the situation is the source of, but is not itself, the threat. In contrast, fear is feelings of apprehension related to a specific threat or danger to which one's security patterns respond (e.g., flying, heights, snakes). When the threat is removed, fear dissipates (May, 1977). Anxiety is distinguished from fear, which is feeling afraid or threatened by a clearly identifiable external stimulus that represents danger to the person. "Anxiety affects us at a deeper level . . . invades the central core of the personality and erodes feelings of self-esteem and personal worth" (Halter, 2014, p. 279; Varcarolis, 2011). Anxiety is unavoidable in life and can serve many positive functions by motivating the person to take action to solve a problem or to resolve a crisis (*Varcarolis, Carson, & Shoemaker, 2005).

Clinically, both anxiety and fear may coexist in a response to a situation. For example, an individual facing surgery may be fearful of pain and anxious about possible cancer. According to Yokom (*1984), "Fear can be allayed by withdrawal from the situation, removal of the offending object, or by reassurance. Anxiety is reduced by admitting its presence and by being convinced that the values to be gained by moving ahead are greater than those to be gained by escape."

Anxiety Level, Coping, Social Anxiety Level, Coping, Anxiety Self-Control

Goals

The individual will relate increased psychological and physiologic comfort, as evidenced by the following indicators:

- Describe own anxiety and coping patterns
- Identify two strategies to reduce anxiety

NIC

Anxiety Reduction, Impulse Control Training, Anticipatory Guidance, Calming Enhancement, Relaxation Therapy

Interventions

Nursing interventions for *Anxiety* can apply to any individual with anxiety, regardless of etiologic and contributing factors.

Assist the Individual to Reduce Present Level of Anxiety

- Assess level of anxiety: mild, moderate, severe, or panic.
  - Provide reassurance and comfort.
  - Stay with the individual.
  - Support present coping mechanisms (e.g., allow the individual to talk, cry); do not confront or argue with defenses or rationalizations.
  - Speak slowly and calmly.
  - Be aware of your own concern and avoid reciprocal anxiety.
  - Convey empathic understanding (e.g., quiet presence, touch, allowing crying, talking).
  - Provide reassurance that a solution can be found.

- Remind the individual that feelings are not harmful.
- Respect personal space.
- If anxiety is at severe or panic level:
  - Ensure someone stays with the person with severe or panic levels of anxiety.
  - Do not make demands or ask the person to make decision.
  - Provide a quiet, nonstimulating environment with soft lighting.
  - Use short, simple sentences; speak slowly and calmly.
  - Focus on the present.
  - Remove excess stimulation (e.g., take the individual to a quieter room); limit contact with others who are also anxious (e.g., other individuals, family).
  - Avoid suggesting that the individual "relax." Do not leave the individual alone.
  - Provide assistance with all tasks during acute episodes of dyspnea.
  - During an acute episode, do not discuss preventive measures.
  - During nonacute episodes, teach relaxation techniques (e.g., tapes, guided imagery).
  - Consult a physician/NP/PA for possible pharmacologic therapy, if indicated.
- If the individual is hyperventilating or experiencing dyspnea:
  - Demonstrate breathing techniques; ask the individual to practice the technique with you.
  - Acknowledge the individual's fear, and give positive reinforcement for efforts.
  - Acknowledge feelings of helplessness.
  - Avoid suggesting that the individual "relax." Do not leave the individual alone.
  - Provide assistance with all tasks during acute episodes of dyspnea.
  - During an acute episode, do not discuss preventive measures.
  - During nonacute episodes, teach relaxation techniques (e.g., tapes, guided imagery).
- If the individual is hyperventilating or experiencing dyspnea:
  - Ask the person to breathe with you (e.g., slow abdominal breathing rhythm)

When Anxiety Diminishes, Assist in Recognizing Anxiety and Causes

- Help to see that mild anxiety can be a positive catalyst for change and does not need to be avoided.
- Request validation of your assessment of anxiety (e.g., "Are you uncomfortable now?").

- If the individual says yes, continue with the learning process; if the person cannot acknowledge anxiety, continue supportive measures until he or she can.
- When the individual can learn, determine usual coping mechanisms: "What do you usually do when you get upset?" (e.g., read, discuss problems, distance, use substances, seek social support).
- Assess for unmet needs or expectations; encourage recall and description of what individual experienced immediately before feeling anxious.
- Assist in reevaluation of perceived threat by discussing the following:
  - Were expectations realistic? Too idealistic?
  - Was it possible to meet expectations?
  - Where in the sequence of events was change possible?
- "Keep focused on manageable problems; define them simply and concretely" (Varcarolis, 2011).
- Teach anxiety interrupters to use when the individual cannot avoid stressful situations:
  - Look up. Lower shoulders.
  - Control breathing.
  - Slow thoughts. Alter voice.
  - Give self-directions (out loud, if possible).
  - Exercise.
  - "Scruff your face"—changes facial expression.
  - Change perspective: Imagine watching a situation from a distance (*Grainger, 1990).

Reduce or Eliminate Problematic Coping Mechanisms

- Refer to *Ineffective Coping.*

Promote Resiliency

- Avoid minimizing positive experiences.
- Gently encourage humor.
- Encourage optimism.
- Encourage discussion with significant others.
- Encourage the individual to seek spiritual comfort through religion, nature, prayer, meditation, or other methods.

Initiate Health Teaching and Referrals as Indicated

- Refer people identified as having chronic anxiety and maladaptive coping mechanisms for ongoing mental health counseling and treatment.
- Instruct in nontechnical, understandable terms regarding illness and associated treatments.

- Instruct (or refer) the individual for assertiveness training.
- Instruct the individual to increase exercise and reduce TV watching (refer to *Risk-Prone Health Behavior* for specific interventions).
- Instruct in use of relaxation techniques (e.g., aromatherapy [orange, lavender], hydrotherapy, music therapy, massage).
- Explain the benefits of foot massage and reflexology (*Grealish, Lomasney, & Whiteman, 2000; *Stephenson, Weinrich, & Tavakoli, 2000).
- Provide telephone numbers for emergency intervention: hotlines, psychiatric emergency room, and on-call staff, if available.

Pediatric Interventions

- Explain events that are sources of anxiety using simple, age-appropriate terms and illustrations, such as puppets, dolls, and sample equipment.
- Allow child to wear underwear and have familiar toys or objects.
- Assist the child to cope with anxiety (Hockenberry & Wilson, 2015):
  - Establish a trusting relationship.
  - Minimize separation from parents.
  - Encourage expression of feelings.
  - Involve the child in play.
  - Prepare the child for new experiences (e.g., procedures, surgery).
  - Provide comfort measures.
  - Allow for regression.
  - Encourage parental involvement in care.
  - Allay parental apprehension and provide them information.
- Assist a child with anger.
  - Encourage the child to share anger (e.g., "How did you feel, when you had your injection?").
  - Tell the child that being angry is okay (e.g., "I sometimes get angry when I can't have what I want.").
  - Encourage and allow the child to express anger in acceptable ways (e.g., loud talking, running outside around the house).

Maternal Interventions

- Screen for pregnancy anxiety in prenatal care settings.
- Discuss expectations and concerns regarding pregnancy and parenthood with the woman alone, her partner alone, and then together, if indicated.
- Refer women with high levels of anxiety or clinically significant anxiety disorders and other psychiatric conditions to mental health professionals.

- Stress the importance of attending childbirth classes.
- Researchers have found certain factors that contribute to more anxiety in pregnant woman as follows (Guardino & Schetter, 2014; Gurung, Dunkel-Schetter, Collins, Rini, & Hobel, 2005; *Lobel, DeVincent, Kaminer, & Meyer, 2000):
  - Those who are of youngest and oldest maternal age
  - African-American and Latina women as compared to White
  - Those who are anxious in general tend to score higher on measures of pregnancy anxiety.
  - Those with lower personal resources (generalized beliefs about oneself [self-esteem], one's future [dispositional optimism], and one's perceived ability to control important outcomes)
  - Those with poorer marital satisfaction and those who reported greater social support from the baby's father
  - Those with higher medical risks as diabetes mellitus and cardiac disease
  - Those who are pregnant for the first time
  - Those whose previous delivery experiences were negative or who has a history of miscarriages.
- Acknowledge anxieties and their normality (Guardino & Schetter, 2014; *Lugina, Christensson, Massawe, Nystrom, & Lindmark, 2001):
  - *1 week postpartum*: worried about self (e.g., feeling tired and nervous about breasts, perineum, and infection)
  - *1 week postpartum*: worried about baby's health (e.g., baby's eyes, respirations, temperature, safety, and crying)
  - *6 weeks postpartum*: worried about partner's reaction to her and baby
- Provide support before and after diagnostic tests, and explain why they are being done.

Geriatric Interventions

- Explore the individual's worries (e.g., financial, security, health, living arrangements, crime, violence).

Death Anxiety

NANDA-I Definition

Vague uneasy feeling of discomfort or dread generated by perceptions of a real or imagined threat to one's existence

Defining Characteristics*

Individual reports:

Worry about the impact of
one's own death on
significant others
Feeling powerless over dying
Fear of loss of mental
abilities when dying
Fear of pain related to dying
Fear of suffering related to
dying
Deep sadness

Fear of the process of dying
Concerns of overworking the
caregiver
Negative thoughts related to
death and dying
Fear of prolonged dying
Fear of premature death
Fear of developing a terminal
illness

Related Factors

A diagnosis of a potentially terminal condition or impending
death can cause this diagnosis. Additional factors can contribute
to death anxiety.

Situational (Personal, Environmental)

Related to discussions on topic of death*

Related to near-death experience*

Related to perceived proximity of death*

Related to uncertainty of prognosis*

Related to anticipating suffering*

Related to confronting reality of terminal disease*

Related to observations related to death*

Related to anticipating pain*

Related to nonacceptance of own mortality*

Related to uncertainty about life after death*

Related to uncertainty about an encounter with a higher power*

Related to uncertainty about the existence of a higher power*

Related to experiencing the dying process*

Related to anticipating impact of death on others*

Related to anticipating adverse consequences of general anesthesia*

Related to personal conflict with palliative versus curative care

Related to conflict with family regarding palliative versus curative care

Related to fear of being a burden

Related to fear of unmanageable pain

Related to fear of abandonment

Related to unresolved conflict (family, friends)

Related to fear that one's life lacked meaning

Related to social disengagement

Related to powerlessness and vulnerability

 Author's Note

The inclusion of *Death Anxiety* in the NANDA-I classification creates a diagnostic category with the etiology in the label. This opens the NANDA-I list to many diagnostic labels with etiology (e.g., separation anxiety, failure anxiety, and travel anxiety). Many diagnostic labels can take this same path: fear as claustrophobic fear, diarrhea as traveler's diarrhea, decisional conflict as end-of-life decisional conflict.

Specifically, end-of-life situations create multiple responses in individuals and significant others. Some of these are shared and expected of those involved. These responses could be described with a syndrome diagnosis as End-of-Life Syndrome. This author recommends its development by nurses engaged in palliative and hospice care.

NOC

Dignified Life Closure, Fear Level, Self-Control, Individual Satisfaction, Decision-Making, Family Coping, Comfortable Death, Coping, Suffering Severity

Goals

The individual will report diminished anxiety or fear, as evidenced by the following indicators:

- Share feelings regarding dying
- Identify specific requests that will increase psychological comfort

NIC

Anxiety Reduction Patient Rights Protection, Family Support, Dying Care, Coping Enhancement, Active Listening, Emotional Support, Spiritual Support

Interventions

Explore Your Own Feelings Regarding Your Dying or Those You Love. Examine If You or Your Nurse/Physician Colleagues Engage in "Death Avoidance" (Braun, Gordon, & Uziely, 2010)

- Braun et al. (2010) found that nurses' attitudes to caring for dying patients was related to personal attitudes toward death. Those demonstrating positive attitudes reported more engagement with dying individuals. A mediating role was found for death avoidance, suggesting some may use avoidance to cope with fear of death. Culture and religion may be key to attitudes (most were Jewish).

For an Individual With New or Early Diagnosis of a Potentially Terminal Condition Explore Their Feelings and Levels of Anxiety

- Allow the individual and family separate opportunities to discuss their understanding of the condition. Correct misinformation.
- Access valid information regarding condition, treatment options, and stage of condition from primary provider (physician, nurse practitioner).
- Ensure a discussion of the prognosis if known.

For the Individual Experiencing a Progression of a Terminal Illness

- Explore with the individual his or her understanding of the situation and feelings.
- Ensure that the primary physician/ NP/PA has had discussions regarding the situation and options desired by the individual/ family.
- Encourage the sharing of fears about what their death will look like and what events will lead up to it.
- Elicit from the individual and family specific requests for end-of-life care.
- Provide family with explanation of changes in their loved one that may occur as death nears (e.g., death rattle, anorexia, nausea, weakness, withdrawal, decreased perfusion in extremities) (Yarbro, Wujcik, & Gobel, 2013).
- Encourage the individual to reconstruct his or her world view:
  - Allow the individual to verbalize feelings about the meaning of death.
  - Advise the individual that there are no right or wrong feelings.
  - Advise the individual that responses are his or her choice.
  - Acknowledge struggles.
  - Encourage dialogue with a spiritual mentor or close friend.

- Allow significant others opportunities to share their perceptions and concerns. Advise them that sadness is expected and normal.
- Discuss the value of truthful conversations (e.g., sorrow, mistakes, disagreements).
- If appropriate, offer to help the individual contact others to resolve conflicts (old or new) verbally or in writing. Validate that forgiveness is not a seeking reconciliation, "but a letting go of a hurt" (Yakimo, 2008).
- Review what their life has meant.
- Reflect on life review and sorrow of impeding losses.
- Encourage significant others to allow for life review and sorrow and not to try and cheer him or her up.
- Respect the dying individual's wishes (e.g., few or no visitors, modifications in care, no heroic measures, food or liquid preferences). Actively support the individual's requests over family desires.
- Initiate referrals and health teaching as indicated to explain hospice care:
  - Hospice has designated caregivers, nurses, social service, physicians, and nurse practitioners in the program.
  - Hospice provides palliative care in homes and health-care settings.
  - Refer to educational resources (e.g., National Hospice and Palliative Care Organization, www.nhpco.org).

RISK FOR BLEEDING

See also *Risk for Complications of Bleeding* in Section 3.

NANDA-I Definition

At risk for a decrease in blood volume that may compromise health

Risk Factors*

Aneurysm	Impaired liver function (e.g., cirrhosis, hepatitis)

Circumcision
Deficient knowledge
Disseminated intravascular coagulopathy
History of falls
Gastrointestinal disorders (e.g., gastric ulcer disease, polyps, varices)

Inherent coagulopathies (e.g., thrombocytopenia)
Postpartum complications (e.g., uterine atony, retained placenta)
Pregnancy-related complications (e.g., placenta previa, molar pregnancy, placenta abruptio [placental abruption])
Trauma
Treatment-related side effects (e.g., surgery, medications, administration of platelet-deficient blood products, chemotherapy)

 Author's Note

This NANDA-I diagnosis represents several collaborative problems.

Goals/Interventions

Refer to Section 3 for the specific collaborative problems such as *Risk for Complications of Hypovolemia, Risk for Complications of Bleeding, Risk for Complications of GI Bleeding, Risk for Complications of Prenatal Bleeding, Risk for Complications of Postpartum Hemorrhage,* or *Risk for Complications of Anticoagulant Therapy Adverse Effects.*

RISK FOR UNSTABLE BLOOD GLUCOSE LEVEL

See also *Risk for Complications of Hypo/Hyperglycemia* in Section 3, Collaborative Problems.

NANDA-I Definition

At risk for variation of blood glucose/sugar levels from the normal range that may compromise health

Risk Factors*

Deficient knowledge of diabetes man-
agement (e.g., action plan)
Developmental level
Dietary intake
Inadequate blood glucose monitoring
Lack of acceptance of diagnosis
Lack of adherence to diabetes manage-
ment (e.g., adhering to action plan)
Lack of diabetes management (e.g.,
action plan)
Medication management

Physical activity level
Physical health status
Pregnancy
Rapid growth periods
Stress
Weight gain
Weight loss

 Author's Note

This nursing diagnosis represents a situation that requires collaborative
intervention with medicine. This author recommends that the collaborative problem *Risk for Complications of Hypo/Hyperglycemia* be used instead. Students should consult with their faculty for advice about whether
to use *Risk for Unstable Blood Glucose Level* or *Risk for Complications of
Hypo/Hyperglycemia*. Refer to thePoint* for interventions for these specific
diagnoses. In addition, the nursing diagnosis of *Ineffective Self-Health Management* relates to insufficient knowledge of blood glucose monitoring,
dietary requirements of diabetes mellitus, need for exercise and prevention of complications, and risk of infection. Refer to *Ineffective Self-Health
Management* for more information.

BOWEL INCONTINENCE

NANDA-I Definition

Change in normal bowel habits characterized by involuntary passage of stool

Defining Characteristics*

Constant dribbling of soft
stool

Inability to recognize urge to
defecate

Constant dribbling of soft stool
Fecal odor
Fecal staining of bedding
Fecal staining of clothing
Inability to delay defecation
Urgency

Inability to recognize urge to defecate
Inattention to urge to defecate
Recognizes rectal fullness but reports inability to expel formed stool
Red perianal skin
Self-report of inability to recognize rectal fullness

Related Factors

Pathophysiologic

Related to rectal sphincter abnormality secondary to:
Anal or rectal surgery
Anal or rectal injury
Obstetric injuries
Peripheral neuropathy

Related to overdistention of rectum secondary to chronic constipation

Related to loss of rectal sphincter control* secondary to:
Progressive neuromuscular disorder
Spinal cord compression
Cerebrovascular accident
Spinal cord injury
Multiple sclerosis

Related to impaired reservoir capacity* secondary to:
Inflammatory bowel disease
Chronic rectal ischemia

Treatment Related

Related to impaired reservoir capacity* secondary to:
Colectomy
Radiation proctitis

Situational (Personal, Environmental)

Related to inability to recognize, interpret, or respond to rectal cues secondary to:
Depression
Impaired cognition*

 Author's Note

This diagnosis represents a situation in which nurses have multiple responsibilities. Individuals experiencing bowel incontinence have various responses that disrupt functioning, such as embarrassment and skin problems related to the irritative nature of feces on skin.

For some spinal cord–injured individuals, *Bowel Incontinence* related to lack of voluntary control over rectal sphincter would be descriptive.

NOC
Bowel Continence, Tissue Integrity

Goals

The individual will evacuate a soft, formed stool every other day or every third day:

- Relate bowel elimination techniques
- Describe fluid and dietary requirements

NIC
Bowel Incontinence Care, Bowel Training, Bowel Management, and Skin Surveillance

Interventions

Assess Contributing Factors

- Refer to Related Factors.

Assess the Individual's Ability to Participate in Bowel Continence

- Ability to reach toilet
- Control of rectal sphincter
- Intact anorectal sensation
- Orientation and motivation

Plan a Consistent, Appropriate Time for Elimination

- Institute a daily bowel program for 5 days or until a pattern develops, then move to an alternate-day program (morning or evening).
- Provide privacy and a nonstressful environment.
- Offer reassurance and protect from embarrassment while establishing the bowel program.
- Implement prompted voiding program.

Teach Effective Bowel Elimination Techniques

- Position a functionally able individual upright or sitting. If he or she is not functionally able (e.g., quadriplegic), place the individual in left-side-lying position.
- For a functionally able individual, use assistive devices (e.g., dil stick, digital stimulator, raised commode seat, lubricant, gloves) as appropriate.

- For an individual with impaired upper extremity mobility and decreased abdominal muscle function, teach bowel elimination facilitation techniques as appropriate:
  - Abdominal massage
  - Forward bends
  - Pelvic floor exercises
  - Sitting push-ups
  - Valsalva maneuver
- Maintain an elimination record or a flow sheet of the bowel schedule that includes time, stool characteristics, assistive methods used, and number of involuntary stools, if any

Explain Fluid and Dietary Requirements for Good Bowel Movements

- Ensure individual drinks 8 to 10 glasses of water daily.
- Design a diet high in bulk and fiber. Refer to *Constipation* for specific dietary instructions.
- Teach the individual about caffeine and explain why it should be avoided.

Explain Effects of Activity on Peristalsis

- Assist in determining the appropriate exercises for the individual's functional ability.

Initiate Health Teaching, as Indicated

- Explain the hazards of using stool softeners, laxatives, suppositories, and enemas.
- Explain the signs and symptoms of fecal impaction and constipation. Refer to *Autonomic Dysreflexia* for additional information.
- Initiate teaching of a bowel program before discharge. If the individual is functionally able, encourage independence with the bowel program; if not, incorporate assistive devices or attendant care, as needed.
- Explain the effects of stool on the skin and ways to protect the skin. Refer to *Diarrhea* for interventions.

INEFFECTIVE BREASTFEEDING

NANDA-I Definition

Dissatisfaction or difficulty a mother, infant, or child experiences with the breastfeeding process

Defining Characteristics

Unsatisfactory breastfeeding process*
Perceived inadequate milk supply*
Infant inability to latch on to maternal breast correctly*
Observable signs of inadequate infant intake*; poor weight gain, voids, or stools
No observable signs of oxytocin release*
Nonsustained or insufficient opportunity for suckling at the breast*
Persistence of sore nipples beyond the first week of breastfeeding
Infant exhibiting fussiness and/or crying within the first hour after breastfeeding*, unresponsive to other comfort measures*
Infant arching or crying at the breast, resisting latching on*

Related Factors
(Evans, Marinelli, Taylor, & ABM, 2014)

Physiologic
Related to difficulty of neonate to attach or suck secondary to:*
Poor infant sucking reflex*
Prematurity*, late preterm
Low birth weight
Sleepy infant
Oral anatomic abnormality (cleft lip/palate, tight frenulum, microglossia)
Infant medical problem (hypoglycemia, jaundice, infection, respiratory distress)
Previous breast surgery*
Flat, inverted, or very large nipples
Extremely or previously sore nipples
Previous breast abscess
Inadequate let-down reflex
Lack of noticeable breast enlargement during puberty or pregnancy

Situational (Personal, Environmental)

Related to maternal fatigue

Related to peripartum complication

*Related to maternal anxiety**

*Related to maternal ambivalence**

Related to multiple birth

Related to inadequate nutrition intake

Related to inadequate fluid intake

Related to previous history of unsuccessful breastfeeding*

Related to nonsupportive partner/family*

Related to knowledge deficit*

Related to interruption in breastfeeding* secondary to ill mother and ill infant

Related to work schedule and/or barriers in the work environment

Related to infant receiving supplemental feedings with artificial nipple*

Related to maternal medications (Hale, 2010)

 Author's Note

In managing breastfeeding, nurses strive to reduce or eliminate factors that contribute to *Ineffective Breastfeeding* or factors that can increase vulnerability for a problem using the diagnosis *Risk for Ineffective Breastfeeding*.

In the acute setting after delivery, little time will have elapsed for the nurse to conclude that there is no problem in breastfeeding, unless the mother is experienced. For many mother–infant dyads, *Risk for Ineffective Breastfeeding related to inexperience with the breastfeeding process* would represent a nursing focus on preventing problems in breastfeeding. *Risk* would not be indicated for all mothers.

NOC
Breastfeeding Establishment: Infant, Breastfeeding Establishment: Maternal, Breastfeeding Management, Knowledge: Breastfeeding, Infant Nutritional Status, Fatigue Level

Goals

Mother

The mother will report confidence in establishing satisfying, effective breastfeeding.

The mother will demonstrate effective breastfeeding independently.

Indicators
- Identify factors that deter breastfeeding
- Identify factors that promote breastfeeding
- Demonstrate effective positioning

Infant

Infant will show signs of adequate intake, as evidenced by these indicators: wet diapers, weight gain, relaxed, feeding.

NIC

Breastfeeding Assistance, Lactation Counseling, Emotional Support

Interventions

(Amir & ABM, 2014; Arizona Department of Health Services [AZDHS], 2012; Evans et al., 2014; Lawrence & Lawrence, 2010)

Assess for Causative or Contributing Factors

- Lack of knowledge
- Lack of role model or support (partner, physician, family)
- Discomfort
- Milk leakage from engorgement or over supply
- Engorgement
- Nipple soreness
- Embarrassment
- Attitudes and misconceptions of mother
- Social pressure against breastfeeding
- Change in body image
- Change in sexuality
- Feelings of being tied down
- Stress
- Lack of conviction regarding decision to breastfeed
- Sleepy, unresponsive infant
- Infant with hyperbilirubinemia
- Fatigue
- Separation from infant (premature or sick infant, sick mother)
- Barriers in workplace

Promote Open Dialogue

- Assess knowledge.
  - Has the woman taken a class in breastfeeding?
  - Has the woman attended a breastfeeding support group prior to delivery?
  - Has she read anything on the subject?
  - Does she have friends who are breastfeeding their babies?
  - Did her mother breastfeed?
- Explain myths and misconceptions. Ask the mother to list anticipated difficulties. Common myths include the following:
  - My breasts are too small.
  - My breasts are too large.

- My mother couldn't breastfeed.
- How do I know my milk is good?
- How do I know the baby is getting enough?
- The baby will know that I'm nervous.
- I have to go back to work, so what's the point of breastfeeding for a short time?
- I'll never have any freedom.
- Breastfeeding will cause my breasts to sag.
- My nipples are inverted, so I can't breastfeed.
- My husband won't like my breasts anymore.
- I'll have to stay fat, if I breastfeed.
- I can't breastfeed, if I have a cesarean section.
- You cannot get pregnant when breastfeeding.

- Build on the mother's knowledge.
  - Clarify misconceptions.
  - Explain process of breastfeeding.
  - Offer literature.
  - Show video.
  - Discuss advantages and disadvantages.
  - Bring breastfeeding mothers together to talk about breastfeeding and their concerns.
  - Discuss contraindications to breastfeeding.
- Support mother's decision to breastfeed or bottle-feed.

Assist Mother During First Feedings

- Promote relaxation.
  - Position comfortably, using pillows (especially cesarean-section mothers). The use of breastfeeding support pillows will also promote comfort in bringing the infant up to her to feed.
  - Use a footstool or phone book to bring knees up while sitting.
  - Use relaxation breathing techniques. Encourage relaxing and opening/pulling shoulders back to promote oxygenation and blood flow to the breast tissue (physical therapy).
- Demonstrate different positions and rooting reflex.
  - Sitting
  - Lying
  - Football hold
  - Skin-to-skin
- Instruct the mother to place a supporting hand on the baby's bottom and turn the body toward her (promotes security in infant).
- Show the mother how she can help the infant latch on. Tell her to look at where the infant's nose and chin are on her breast and to compress her breast with her thumb and middle finger behind these contact points.

- Skin-to-skin
  - Use of skin-to-skin contact for a minimum of 60 minutes per session 1 to 2 times per day has been shown to bring the mother's milk in an average of 18 hours faster.
  - Skin-to-skin allows infant vital signs to be regulated.
  - It allows for infant to be colonized by beneficial bacteria from the mother.
  - Infants will cry less; breasts will warm or cool depending on the needs of baby's body temperature.

Promote Successful Breastfeeding

- Advise the mother to increase feeding times gradually.
  - Allow infant to finish the first breast before moving to the second.
  - Allow the infant unrestricted, unlimited access to the breast.
  - Average feeding time may be 5 to 45 minutes on each side (*Walker, 2006).
- Instruct the mother to offer both breasts at each feeding.
- Discuss burping.
  - Inform the mother that burping may be unnecessary with breastfed infants but to always attempt.
  - If the infant grunts and seems full between breasts, the mother should attempt to burp the infant, and then continue feeding.

Provide Follow-Up Support During Hospital Stay

- During the hospital stay, develop a care plan so other health team members are aware of any problems or needs. Tell the mother to be flexible as the plan of care may change throughout the day and over the next few days and weeks as the infant's feeding behaviors change.
- Allow for flexibility of feeding schedule; avoid scheduling feedings. Strive for 10 to 12 feedings every 24 hours according to the infant's size and need (frequent feedings help prevent or reduce breast engorgement). Feeding on demand will aid in milk supply increasing. Allow the infant unlimited, unrestricted access to the breasts.
- Ensure that the mother has resources for breastfeeding assistance when leaving the hospital.
- Heating and massaging prior to each feeding throughout the engorgement phase will help to reduce painful engorgement (AZDHS, 2010).

Teach Ways to Control Specific Nursing Problems (May Need Assistance of Lactation Consultant)

- Engorgement
- Sore nipples
- For stasis, mastitis
  - If one area of the breast is sore or tender, apply moist heat before each breastfeeding session.
  - Gently massage the breast from the base toward the nipple before beginning to breastfeed and during feeding.
  - Breastfeed frequently and change the infant's position during feeding.
  - Rest frequently.
  - Monitor for and teach mother signs and symptoms of mastitis: chills, body aches, fatigue, and fever above 100.4° F.
  - Consult obstetrician if painful area accompanied by signs and symptoms of mastitis do not resolve within 24 to 48 hours. Observe for signs of abscess.

Assist the Family With the Following

- Sibling reaction
  - Explore feelings and anticipation of problems. An older child may be jealous of contact with the baby. Mother can use this time to read to the older child.
  - The older child may want to be breastfed. Allow him or her to try; usually, the child will not like it.
  - Stress the older child's attributes: freedom, movement, and choices.
- Fatigue and stress
  - Encourage her to limit visitors for the first 2 weeks to allow optimum bonding and learning to breastfeed for mother and baby.
  - Emphasize that the mother will need support and assistance during the first 4 weeks. Encourage the support person to help as much as possible.

Initiate Referrals, as Indicated

- Refer to lactation consultant if indicated by
  - Lack of confidence
  - Ambivalence
  - Problems with infant suck and latch-on
  - Infant weight drop or lack of urination
  - Barriers in the workplace
  - Prolonged soreness
  - Hot, tender spots on the breast

- Refer to La Leche League or other community agencies.
- Refer to childbirth educator and childbirth class members.
- Refer to other breastfeeding mothers.

INTERRUPTED BREASTFEEDING

NANDA-I Definition

Break in the continuity of the breastfeeding process as a result of inability or inadvisability to put baby to breast for feeding

Defining Characteristics*

Infant receives no nourishment at the breast for some or all
   feedings
Maternal desire to eventually provide breast milk for child's
   nutritional needs
Maternal desire to maintain breastfeeding for child's nutritional
   needs

Related Factors*

Maternal or infant illness
Prematurity
Maternal employment

Contraindications (e.g., drugs, true
   breast milk, jaundice)
Need to wean infant abruptly

 Author's Note

This diagnosis represents a situation, not a response. Nursing interventions do not treat the interruption but, instead, its effects. When the situation is interrupted breastfeeding, the responses can vary. For example, if continued breastfeeding or use of a breast pump is contraindicated, the nurse focuses on the loss of this breastfeeding experience using the nursing diagnosis *Grieving*.

   If breastfeeding continues with expression and storage of breast milk, teaching, and support, the diagnosis will be *Risk for Ineffective Breastfeeding related to continuity problems secondary to (specify)* (e.g., maternal employment). If difficulty is experienced, the diagnosis would be *Ineffective Breastfeeding related to interruption secondary to (specify) and lack of knowledge*.

INSUFFICIENT BREAST MILK

NANDA-I Definition

Low production of maternal breast milk

Defining Characteristics*

Infant
Constipation
Does not seemed satisfied after
   sucking
Frequent crying
Voids small amounts of
   concentrated urine (less than
   4 to 6 times a day)

Long breastfeeding time
Wants to suck very
   frequently
Refuses to suck
Weight gain is lower than
   500 g in a month (com-
   paring two measures)

Related Factors

Infant
Ineffective latching on
Rejection of breast

Ineffective sucking

Short sucking time
Insufficient opportunity
   to suckle

Mother
Alcohol intake
Medication side effects (e.g.,
   contraceptives, diuretics)
Malnutrition
Tobacco smoking/use

Pregnancy
Fluid volume depletion (e.g.,
   dehydration, hemorrhage)
Insufficient education

 Author's Note

In managing breastfeeding, nurses strive to reduce or eliminate factors that contribute to *Ineffective Breastfeeding* or factors that can increase vulnerability for a problem using the diagnosis *Risk for Ineffective Breastfeeding*.

In the acute setting after delivery, too little time will have lapsed for the nurse to conclude that there is no problem in breastfeeding, unless the mother is experienced. For many mother–infant dyads, *Risk for Ineffective Breastfeeding related to inexperience with the breastfeeding process* would represent a nursing focus on preventing problems in breastfeeding. Risk would not be indicated for all inexperienced mothers.

Insufficient Breast Milk is a new NANDA-I accepted diagnosis that represents a more specific diagnosis under *Ineffective Breastfeeding*. When this specific etiology can be identified with *Ineffective Breastfeeding*, the nurse can use either one.

Goals/Interventions

Refer to *Ineffective Breastfeeding*.

DECREASED CARDIAC OUTPUT

See also *Risk for Complications of Decreased Cardiac Output* in Section 3.

NANDA-I Definition

Inadequate blood pumped by the heart to meet metabolic demands of the body

Defining Characteristics*

Altered heart rate/rhythm (e.g., arrhythmias, bradycardia, EKG changes, palpitations, tachycardia)
Altered preload (e.g., edema, decreased central venous pressure, decreased pulmonary artery wedge pressure [PAWP])
Altered contractility
Altered afterload
Behavioral/Emotional (anxiety, restlessness)

Related Factors*

Altered heart rate   Altered afterload
Altered rhythm   Altered contractility
Altered stroke volume   Altered preload

Author's Note

This nursing diagnosis represents a situation in which nurses have multiple responsibilities. People experiencing decreased cardiac output may display various responses that disrupt functioning (e.g., activity intolerance, disturbed sleep–rest, anxiety, fear). Or they may be at risk for developing such physiologic complications as dysrhythmias, cardiogenic shock, and congestive heart failure.

When *Decreased Cardiac Output* is used clinically, associated goals usually are written as follows:

* Systolic blood pressure is greater than 100 mm Hg.
* Urine output is greater than 30 mL/h.
* Cardiac output is greater than 5.0 L/min.
* Cardiac rate and rhythm are within normal limits.

These goals do not represent parameters for evaluating nursing care, but for evaluating the individual's status. Because they are monitoring criteria that the nurse uses to guide implementation of nurse-prescribed and physician-prescribed interventions, students consult with faculty to determine which diagnosis to use: *Decreased Cardiac Output* or *Risk for Complications of Decreased Cardiac Output*. Refer to *Activity Intolerance related to insufficient knowledge of adaptive techniques needed secondary to impaired cardiac function* and *RC of Cardiac/Vascular Dysfunction* in Section 3.

CAREGIVER ROLE STRAIN

Caregiver Role Strain

Risk for Caregiver Role Strain

Definition

Difficulty in performing family/significant other caregiver role (NANDA-I)

A state in which a person is experiencing physical, emotional, social, and/or financial burden(s) in the process of giving care to a significant other.[3]

---

[3] This definition has been added by Lynda Juall Carpenito, the author, for clarity and usefulness.

Defining Characteristics

Expressed or Observed
Insufficient time or physical energy
Difficulty performing required caregiving activities
Conflicts between caregiving responsibilities and other important roles (e.g., work, relationships)
Apprehension about the future for the care receiver's health and ability to provide care
Apprehension about the care receiver's care when caregiver is ill or deceased
Feelings of depression or anger
Feelings of exhaustion and resentment

Related Factors

Pathophysiologic

Related to unrelenting or complex care requirements secondary to:

Addiction*
Chronic mental illness
Cognitive problems*
Debilitating conditions
(acute, progressive)

Disability
Progressive dementia
Unpredictability of illness
course*

Treatment Related

*Related to 24-hour care responsibilities**

Related to time-consuming activities (e.g., dialysis, transportation)

*Related to complexity of activities**

*Related to increasing care needs**

Situational (Personal, Environmental)

*Related to years of caregiving**

*Related to unpredictability of care situation or illness course**

*Related to inadequate informal support**

*Related to unrealistic expectations of caregiver by care receiver, self, or others**

Related to pattern of impaired individual coping (e.g., abuse, violence, addiction) *

Related to compromised physical or mental health of caregiver *

Related to history of poor relationship or family dysfunction* *

Related to history of marginal family coping *

Related to duration of caregiving required

Related to isolation

Related to insufficient respite

Related to insufficient finances *

Related to inadequate community resources *

Related to no or unavailable support

Related to insufficient resources

Related to inexperience with caregiving *

Related to deficient knowledge about community resources *

Maturational

Infant, Child, and Adolescent
Related to unrelenting care requirements secondary to:
Developmental delay
Mental disabilities (specify)
Physical disabilities (specify)

 Author's Note

"Health care policies that rely on caregiver sacrifice can be made to appear cost-effective only if the emotional, social, physical, and financial costs incurred by the caregiver are ignored" (*Winslow & Carter, 1999, p. 285). Worldwide, family caregivers provide the most care for dependent persons of all ages whether living in developing countries or developed countries (AARP, 2009). The care receivers have physical and/or mental disabilities, which can be temporary or permanent. Some disabilities are permanent but stable (e.g., blindness); others signal progressive deterioration (e.g., Alzheimer's disease).

Caring and caregiving are intrinsic to all close relationships. They are "found in the context of established roles such as wife–husband, child–parent" (*Pearlin, Mullan, Semple, & Skaff, 1990, p. 583). Under some circumstances, caregiving is "transformed from the ordinary exchange of assistance among people standing in close relationship to one another to an extraordinary and unequally distributed burden" (*Pearlin et al., 1990, p. 583). It becomes a dominant, overriding component occupying the entire situation (*Pearlin et al., 1990).

Caregiver Role Strain represents the burden of caregiving on the physical and emotional health of the caregiver and its effects on the family and social system of the caregiver and care receiver. *Risk for Caregiver Role Strain* can be a very significant nursing diagnosis because nurses can identify those at high risk and assist them to prevent this grave situation.

Chronic sorrow has been associated with caregivers of people with mental illness and children with chronic illness. See *Chronic Sorrow* for more information.

NOC

Caregiver Well-Being, Caregiver Lifestyle Disruption, Caregiver Emotional Health, Caregiver Role Endurance Potential, Family Coping, Family Integrity

Goals

The caregiver will report a plan to decrease the caregiver's burden:

- Share frustrations regarding caregiving responsibilities
- Identify one source of support
- Identify two changes that would improve daily life, if implemented

The family will establish a plan for weekly support or help:

- Relate two strategies to increase support
- Convey empathy to caregiver regarding daily responsibilities

NIC

Caregiver Support, Respite Care, Coping Enhancement, Family Mobilization, Mutual Goal Setting, Support System Enhancement, Anticipatory Guidance

Interventions

Assess for Causative or Contributing Factors

- Refer to Related Factors

Provide Empathy and Promote a Sense of Competency

- Allow caregiver to share feelings.
- Emphasize the difficulties of the caregiving responsibilities.
- Convey admiration of the caregiver's competency.
- Evaluate effects of caregiving periodically (depression, burnout).

Promote Realistic Appraisal of the Situation

- Determine how long the caregiving has taken place (Winslow & Carter, 1999).
- Ask the caregiver to describe future life in 3 months, 6 months, and 1 year.
- Discuss the effects of present schedule and responsibilities on physical health, emotional status, and relationships.
- Discuss positive outcomes of caregiving responsibilities (for self, care receiver, family).
- Evaluate if behavior is getting worse.

Promote Insight Into the Situation

- Ask the caregiver to describe "a typical day":
  - Caregiving and household tasks
  - Work outside the home
  - Role responsibilities
- Ask the caregiver to describe:
  - At-home leisure activities (daily, weekly)
  - Outside-the-home social activities (weekly)
- Engage other family members in discussion, as appropriate.
- Caution the caregiver about the danger of viewing helpers as less competent or less essential.
- Explain that dementia causes memory loss, which results in the following (Miller et al., 2001):
  - Repetitive questions
  - Denial of memory loss
  - Forgetting
  - Fluctuations in memory

Assist Caregiver to Identify Activities for Which He or She Desires Assistance

- Care receiver's needs (hygiene, food, treatments, mobility; refer to *Self-Care Deficits*)
  - Laundry
  - House cleaning
  - Meals
  - Shopping, errands
  - Transportation
  - Appointments (doctor, hairdresser)
  - Yard work
  - House repairs
  - Respite (hours per week)
  - Money management

Stress Importance of Health Promotion

- Rest–exercise balance
- Effective stress management (e.g., yoga, relaxation training, creative arts)
- Low-fat, high–complex-carbohydrate diet
- Supportive social networks
- Appropriate screening practices for age
- Maintain a good sense of humor; associate with others who laugh.
- Advise caregivers to initiate phone contacts or visits with friends or relatives rather than waiting for others to do it.

Engage Family to Appraise Situation (Apart from Caregiver) (*Shields, 1992)

- Allow the family to share frustrations.
- Share the need for the caregiver to feel appreciated.
- Discuss the importance of regularly acknowledging the burden of the situation for the caregiver.
- Discuss the benefits of listening without giving advice.
- Differentiate the types of social support (emotional, appraisal, informational, instrumental).
- Emphasize the importance of emotional and appraisal support, and identify sources of this support.
- Regular phone calls
- Cards, letters
- Visits
- Stress "that in many situations, there are no problems to be solved, only pain to be shared" (*Shields, 1992).
- Discuss the need to give the caregiver "permission" to enjoy self (e.g., vacations, day trips).
- Allow caregiver opportunities to respond to "How can I help you?"

Assist With Accessing Informational and Instrumental Support

- Provide information that is needed with problem-solving strategies.
- Provide information that is needed for skill-building.

Role-Play How to Ask for Help With Activities

- For example: "I have three appointments this week, could you drive me to one?" "I could watch your children once or twice a week in exchange for you watching my husband."
- Identify all possible sources of volunteer help: family (siblings, cousins), friends, neighbors, church, and community groups.
- Discuss how most people feel good when they provide a "little help."

Advise Caregivers About Sources of More Information

- National Center for Women's Health Information (www .womenshealth.gov)
- National Health Statistics (www.cdc.gov/)
- If appropriate, discuss whether and when an alternative source of care (e.g., nursing home) may be indicated.
- Evaluate factors that reduce the stress of deciding on nursing home placement (Hagen, 2001):
  - Low level of guilt
  - Independence in the relationship
  - Availability of support from others
  - Low fear of loneliness
  - Positive or neutral nursing home attitudes
  - Positive sense of life without care burden

Initiate Health Teaching and Referrals, if Indicated

- Explain the benefits of sharing with other caregivers:
  - Support group
  - Individual and group counseling
  - Telephone buddy system with another caregiver
- Identify community resources available (e.g., counseling, social service, day care).
- Arrange a home visit by a professional nurse or a physical therapist to provide strategies to improve communication, time management, and caregiving.
- Engage others to work actively to increase state, federal, and private agencies' financial support for resources to enhance caregiving in the home.

Pediatric Interventions

- Determine parents' understanding of and concerns about child's illness, course, prognosis, and related care needs.
- Elicit the effects of caregiving responsibility on
  - Personal life (work, rest, leisure)
  - Marriage (time alone, communication, decisions, attention)
- Assist parents to meet the well siblings' needs for
  - Knowledge of sibling's illness and relationship to own health
  - Sharing feelings of anger, unfairness, and embarrassment
  - Discussions of future of ill sibling and self (e.g., family planning, care responsibilities)
- Discuss strategies to help siblings adapt.
  - Include in family decisions when appropriate.
  - Keep informed about ill child's condition.
  - Maintain routines (e.g., meals, vacations).
  - Prepare for changes in home life.

- • Promote activities with peers.
- • Avoid making the ill child the center of the family.
- • Determine what daily assistance in caregiving is realistic.
- • Plan for time alone.
- Advise teachers of home situation.
- Address developmental needs. See *Delayed Growth and Development*.
- Advise that caregiving activities produce fatigue that can increase over time (Gambert, 2013).
- Discuss strategies to reduce caregiver fatigue (Gambert, 2013).
  - • Partner support
  - • Household help
  - • Child care for siblings
  - • Provisions to ensure adequacy of caregiver's sleep

Risk for Caregiver Role Strain

NANDA-I Definition

At risk for caregiver vulnerability for felt difficulty in performing the family caregiver role

Risk Factors

Primary caregiver responsibilities for a recipient who requires regular assistance with self-care or supervision because of physical or mental disabilities in addition to one or more of the related factors for *Caregiver Role Strain*

 Author's Note

Refer to *Caregiver Role Strain*.

Refer to *Caregiver Role Strain*.

Goals

The individual will relate a plan for how to continue social activities despite caregiving responsibilities, as evidenced by the following indicators:

- Identify activities that are important for self
- Relate intent to enlist the help of at least two people weekly

Refer to *Caregiver Role Strain*.

Interventions

Explain Causes of Caregiver Role Strain

- Refer to Related Factors for *Caregiver Role Strain*.

Teach Caregiver and Significant Others to Be Alert for Danger Signals (*Murray, Zentner, & Yakimo, 2009)

- No matter what you do, it is never enough.
- You believe you are the only individual in the world doing this.
- You have no time or place to be alone for a brief respite.
- Family relationships are breaking down because of the care-giving pressures.
- Your caregiving duties are interfering with your work and social life.
- You are in a "no-win situation" and will not admit difficulty.
- You are alone because you have alienated everyone who could help.
- You are overeating, undereating, abusing drugs or alcohol, or being harsh and abusive with others.
- There are no more happy times. Love and care have given way to exhaustion and resentment. You no longer feel good about yourself or take pride in what you are doing.

Explain the Four Types of Social Support to All Involved

- Emotional (e.g., concern, trust)
- Appraisal (e.g., affirms self-worth)
- Informational (e.g., useful advice, information for problem solving)
- Instrumental assistance (e.g., caregiving) or tangible assistance (e.g., money, help with chores)

Discuss the Implications of Daily Responsibilities With the Primary Caregiver

- Encourage caregiver to set realistic goals for self and care recipient.
- Discuss the need for respite and short-term relief.
- Encourage caregiver to accept offers of help.
- Practice asking for help; avoid "they should know I need help" thinking and martyrdom behavior.

- Caution on viewing others as not "competent enough."
- Discuss that past conflicts will not disappear. Try to work on resolution and emphasize today.

Stress Importance of Daily Health Promotion

- Rest–exercise balance
- Effective stress management
- Low-fat, high–complex-carbohydrate diet
- Supportive social networks
- Appropriate screening practices for age
- Maintain a good sense of humor; associate with others who laugh.
- Advise caregivers to initiate phone contacts or visits with friends or relatives rather than waiting for others to do it.

Assist Those Involved to Appraise the Situation

- What is at stake? What are the choices?
- Provide accurate information and answers to encourage a realistic perspective.
- Initiate discussions concerning stressors of home care (e.g., physical, emotional, environmental, financial).
- Emphasize the importance of respites to prevent isolating behaviors that foster depression.
- Discuss with nonprimary caregivers their responsibilities in caring for the primary caregiver.
- Where is their help? Direct the family to community agencies, home health-care organizations, and sources of financial assistance as needed. (Refer to *Impaired Home Maintenance*.)

Discuss With All Household Members the Implications of Caring for an Ill Family Member

- Available resources (e.g., finances, environmental)
- 24-hour responsibility
- Effects on other household members
- Likelihood of progressive deterioration
- Sharing of responsibilities with other household members, siblings, and neighbors
- Likelihood of exacerbation of long-standing conflicts
- Effects on lifestyle
- Alternative or assistive options (e.g., community-based providers, group living, nursing home)

Assist Caregiver to Identify Activities for Which He or She Desires Assistance

- Refer to *Caregiver Role Strain*.

Assist With Accessing Informational and Instrumental Support

- Refer to *Caregiver Role Strain*.

Initiate Health Teaching and Referrals, If Indicated

- Refer to *Caregiver Role Strain*.

INEFFECTIVE CHILDBEARING PROCESS

Ineffective Childbearing Process
Risk for Ineffective Childbearing Process

NANDA-I Definition

Pregnancy and childbirth process and care of the newborn that does not match the environmental context, norms, and expectations

Defining Characteristics*

During Pregnancy
Does not access support systems appropriately
Does report appropriate physical preparations
Does not report appropriate prenatal lifestyle (e.g., nutrition, elimination, sleep, bodily movement, exercise, personal hygiene)
Does not report availability of support systems
Does not report managing unpleasant symptoms in pregnancy
Does not report realistic birth plan
Does not seek necessary knowledge (e.g., labor and delivery, newborn care)
Failure to prepare necessary newborn care items
Inconsistent prenatal health visits
Lack of prenatal visits
Lack of respect for unborn baby

During Labor and Delivery
Does not access support systems appropriately
Does not report lifestyle (e.g., diet, elimination, sleep, bodily

movement, personal hygiene) that is appropriate for the stage of labor

Does not report availability of support systems

Does not demonstrate attachment behavior to the newborn

Does not respond appropriately to onset of labor

Lacks proactivity during labor and delivery

After Birth

Does not access support systems appropriately

Does not demonstrate appropriate baby feeding techniques

Does not demonstrate appropriate breast care

Does not demonstrate attachment behavior to the newborn

Does not demonstrate basic baby care techniques

Does not provide safe environment for the baby

Does not report appropriate postpartum lifestyle (e.g., diet, elimination, sleep, bodily movement, exercise, personal hygiene)

Does not report availability of support systems

Related Factors

Deficient knowledge (e.g., of labor and delivery, newborn care)

Domestic violence

Inconsistent prenatal health visits

Lack of appropriate role models for parenthood

Lack of cognitive readiness for parenthood

Lack of maternal confidence

Lack of a realistic birth plan

Lack of sufficient support systems

Maternal powerlessness

Suboptimal maternal nutrition

Substance abuse

Unplanned pregnancy

Unsafe environment

 Author's Note

This new NANDA-I diagnosis represents numerous situations and factors that can compromise the well-being of a mother and her relationship with her infant during labor and delivery and after birth. It can be used to organize a standard of care for all pregnant women during the process of labor and delivery and after birth.

Imbedded in this broad diagnosis is a multitude of specific actual or risk problematic responses; some examples are as follows:

Risk for Dysfunctional Family Processes

Interrupted Family Processes

Altered Nutrition
Risk-Prone Health Behavior
Ineffective Coping
Powerlessness
Ineffective Self-Health Management
Risk for Ineffective Childbearing Process would be the standard of care on the appropriate units.

If *Ineffective Childbearing Process* is validated, it may be more clinically useful to use a more specific nursing diagnosis. However, if there are multiple related factors complicating the childbearing process, this diagnosis would be useful.

Due to the extensive art and science of nursing that is related to this specialty diagnosis, the author refers the reader to *Maternal–Child Nursing* literature for goals, interventions, and rationale.

Risk for Ineffective Childbearing Process

NANDA-I Definition

Vulnerable for a pregnancy and childbirth process and care of the newborn that does not match the environmental context, norms, and expectations, which can compromise health

Risk Factors*

Deficient knowledge (e.g., of labor and delivery, newborn care)
Domestic violence
Inconsistent prenatal health visits
Lack of appropriate role models for parenthood
Lack of cognitive readiness for parenthood
Lack of maternal confidence
Lack of prenatal health visits
Lack of a realistic birth plan
Lack of sufficient support systems
Maternal powerlessness
Maternal psychological distress
Suboptimal maternal; nutrition
Substance abuse
Unsafe environment
Unplanned pregnancy

Author's Note

Refer to Author's Note under *Ineffective Childbearing Process*.

IMPAIRED COMFORT[4]

Impaired Comfort

Acute Pain

Chronic Pain

Chronic Pain Syndrome

Labor Pain

Nausea

NANDA-I Definition

Perceived lack of ease, relief, and transcendence in physical, psychospiritual, environmental, cultural, and social dimensions

Defining Characteristics

Reports or demonstrates discomfort

Autonomic response in
  acute pain
  Increased blood pressure
  Increased pulse
  Increased respirations
  Diaphoresis
  Dilated pupils
Guarded position
Facial mask of pain
Crying, moaning
Inability to relax*
Irritability*

Reports*
  Abdominal heaviness
  Anxiety
  Being cold or hot
  Being uncomfortable
  Lack of privacy
  Malaise
  Nausea
  Pruritus
  Treatment-related side effects
    (medications, radiation)
  Disturbed sleep pattern
  Itching
  Vomiting

---

[4] This diagnosis was developed by Lynda Juall Carpenito.

Related Factors

Any factor can contribute to impaired comfort. The most common are listed below.

Biopathophysiologic

Related to uterine contractions during labor

Related to trauma to perineum during labor and delivery

Related to involution of uterus and engorged breasts

Related to tissue trauma and reflex muscle spasms secondary to:

Musculoskeletal Disorders
Fractures   Arthritis
Contractures   Spinal cord disorders
Spasms   Fibromyalgia

Visceral Disorders
Cardiac   Intestinal
Renal   Pulmonary
Hepatic

Cancer

Vascular Disorders
Vasospasm   Phlebitis
Occlusion   Vasodilation (headache)

Related to inflammation of, or injury to:
Nerve   Joint
Tendon   Muscle
Bursa   Juxta-articular structures

Related to fatigue, malaise, or pruritus secondary to contagious diseases:
Rubella   Chicken pox
Hepatitis   Mononucleosis
Pancreatitis

Related to effects of cancer on (specify)

Related to abdominal cramps, diarrhea, and vomiting secondary to:
Gastroenteritis   Influenza
Gastric ulcers

Related to inflammation and smooth muscle spasms secondary to:
Gastrointestinal infections   Renal calculi

Treatment Related

Related to tissue trauma and reflex muscle spasms secondary to:

Accidents	Diagnostic tests (venipuncture, invasive scanning, biopsy)
Burns	Surgery

Related to nausea and vomiting secondary to:

Anesthesia	Side effects of (specify)
Chemotherapy	

Situational (Personal, Environmental)

Related to fever

Related to immobility/improper positioning

Related to overactivity

Related to pressure points (tight cast, elastic bandages)

Related to allergic response

Related to chemical irritants

Related to unmet dependency needs

Related to severe repressed anxiety

Maturational

Related to tissue trauma and reflex muscle spasms secondary to:
Infancy: Colic
Infancy and early childhood: Teething, ear pain
Middle childhood: Recurrent abdominal pain, growing pains
Adolescence: Headaches, chest pain, dysmenorrhea

 Author's Note

A diagnosis not on the current NANDA-I list, *Impaired Comfort* can represent various uncomfortable sensations (e.g., pruritus, immobility, NPO status). For an individual experiencing nausea and vomiting, the nurse should assess whether *Impaired Comfort*, *Risk for Impaired Comfort*, or *Risk for Imbalanced Nutrition: Less Than Body Requirements* is appropriate. Short-lived episodes of nausea, vomiting, or both (e.g., postoperatively) is best described with *Impaired Comfort* related to effects of anesthesia or analgesics. When nausea/vomiting may compromise nutritional intake, the appropriate diagnosis may be *Risk for Imbalanced Nutrition: Less Than Body Requirements related to nausea and vomiting secondary to (specify)*. *Impaired Comfort* also can be used to describe a cluster of discomforts related to a condition or treatment, such as radiation therapy.

NOC

Symptom Control; Comfort Status

Goals

The individual will report acceptable control of symptoms, as evidenced by the following indicators:

* Describe factors that increase symptoms
* Describe measures to improve comfort

NIC

Pruritus Management, Fever Treatment, Environmental Management: Comfort

Interventions

Assess for Sources of Discomfort

* Pruritus
* Prolonged bed rest (refer to *Disuse Syndrome*)
* Fever (refer to *Risk for Altered Body Temperature*)

Reduce Pruritus and Promote Comfort

Maintain Hygiene Without Producing Dry Skin
* Encourage frequent baths:
  * Use cool water when acceptable.
  * Use mild soap (Castile, lanolin) or soap substitute (Williams, Svensson, & Diepgen).
  * Blot skin dry; do not rub.

Prevent Excessive Dryness
* Lubricate skin with a moisturizer or emollients, unless contraindicated; pat on with hand or gauze.
  * Apply ointments/lotions with gloved or bare hand, depending on type, to lightly cover skin; rub creams into skin.
  * Use frequent, thin applications of ointment, rather than one thick application.
  * Apply emollient creams or lotions at least two or three times daily and after bathing. Recommended emollient creams include Eucerin or Nivea or lotions such as Lubriderm, Alpha Keri, or Nivea.

- Avoid skin products containing alcohol and menthol.
- Avoid petroleum products on irradiated skin.
- Limit bathing to ½ hour daily or every other day.
- Add oil at the end of a bath or add a colloidal oatmeal treatment early to the bath.
- Avoid topical agents including talcum powders, perfumed powders, bubble baths, and cornstarch.
  - ○ Use cornstarch to areas of irradiated skin following bathing.
  - ○ Avoid underarm deodorants or antiperspirants during radiation therapy.
- Apply lubrication after bath, before skin is dry, to encourage moisture retention.
- Apply wet dressings continuously or intermittently. Provide 20- to 30-minute tub soaks of 32° F to 38° F; water can contain oatmeal powder, Aveeno, cornstarch, or baking soda.
  - Avoid excessive warmth or dryness; create a humid environment (e.g., humidifier)
  - Avoid perfumes, cosmetics, deodorants, rough fabrics, fatigue, stress, and monotony (lack of distractions)

Promote Comfort and Prevent Further Injury

- Advise against scratching; explain the scratch–itch–scratch cycle.
  - Teach to apply a cool washcloth or ice over the site, which may be useful. Firm pressure at the site of itching, at a site contralateral to the site of itching, and at acupressure points may break the neural pathway.
- Use mitts (or cotton socks), if necessary, on children and confused adults.
- Maintain trimmed nails to prevent injury; file after trimming.
- Lubricate skin with a moisturizer or emollients, unless contraindicated; pat on with hand or gauze.
- Apply lubrication after bath, before skin is dry, to encourage moisture retention.
- Apply wet dressings continuously or intermittently. Provide 20- to 30-minute tub soaks of 32° F to 38° F; water can contain oatmeal powder, Aveeno, cornstarch, or baking soda.
- Avoid excessive warmth or dryness, perfumes, cosmetics, deodorants, rough fabrics, fatigue, stress, and monotony (lack of distractions).
- Advise against scratching; explain the scratch–itch–scratch cycle.
- Secure order for topical corticosteroid cream for local inflamed pruritic areas; apply sparingly and occlude area with plastic

wrap at night to increase effectiveness of cream and prevent further scratching.
- Secure an antihistamine order if itching is unrelieved.
- Use mitts (or cotton socks), if necessary, on children and confused adults.
- Maintain trimmed nails to prevent injury; file after trimming.
- Remove particles from bed (food crumbs, caked powder).
- Use old, soft sheets, and avoid wrinkles in bed; if bed protector pads are used, place draw sheet over them to eliminate direct contact with the skin.
- Avoid using perfumes and scented lotions.
- Avoid contact with chemical irritants/solutions.
- Wash clothes in a mild detergent and put through a second rinse cycle to reduce residue; avoid use of fabric softeners.
- Prevent excessive warmth by the use of cool room temperatures and low humidity, light covers with bed cradle; avoid overdressing.
- Apply ointments with gloved or bare hand, depending on type, to lightly cover skin; rub creams into the skin.
- Use frequent, thin applications of ointment, rather than one thick application.

Proceed With Health Teaching, When Indicated
- Explain causes of pruritus and possible prevention methods.
- Explain factors that increase symptoms (e.g., low humidity, heat).
- Wash sheets, clothing, and undergarments in mild soaps for infant clothing (e.g.,Dreft, Purrex). Avoid use of fabric softeners. Double rinse or add 1 teaspoon of white vinegar per quart of water to rinse clothes.
- Teach about medications, such as diuretics, that decrease skin moisture.
- Advise about exposure to sun and heat and protective products.
- Teach the individual to avoid fabrics that irritate skin (wool, coarse textures).
- For further interventions, refer to *Ineffective Coping* if pruritus is stress related.

Pediatric Interventions

- Explain to children why they should not scratch.
- Dress child in long sleeves, long pants, or a one-piece outfit to prevent scratching.
- Avoid overdressing child, which will increase warmth.
- Give child a tepid bath before bedtime; add two cups of cornstarch to bath water.

- Apply Caladryl lotion to weeping pruritic lesions; apply with small paintbrush.
- Use cotton blankets or sheets next to skin.
- Remove furry toys that may increase lint and pruritus.
- Teach child to press or (if permitted) put a cool cloth on the area that itches, but not to scratch.

Acute Pain

NANDA-I Definition

Unpleasant sensory and emotional experience arising from actual or potential tissue damage or described in terms of such damage (International Association for the Study of Pain); sudden or slow onset of any intensity from mild to severe with anticipated or predictable end and a duration of <6 months

Defining Characteristics

Appetite changes
Physiologic responses (e.g., mean arterial pressure [MAP], heart rate [HR], respiratory rate [RR], transcutaneous oxygen saturation [SpO$_2$], and end-tidal CO$_2$)
Diaphoresis
Distraction behavior (e.g., pacing, seeking out other people and/ or activities, repetitive activities)
Expressive behavior (e.g., restlessness, moaning, crying)
Facial expressions of pain (e.g., eyes lack luster, beaten look, fixed or scattered movement, grimace)
Guarding behavior
Hopelessness
Narrowed focus (e.g., altered time perception, impaired thought processes, reduced interaction with people and environment)
Narrowed focus (e.g., altered time perception, impaired thought processes, reduced interaction with people and environment)
Observed evidence of pain using standardized pain behavior checklists
For those unable to verbally communicate; refer to the appropriate assessment tool (e.g., Behavioral Pain Scale, Neonatal Infant Pain Scale, Pain Assessment Checklist for Seniors with Limited Ability to Communicate)
Positioning to avoid pain

Protective gestures

Proxy reporting of pain and behavior/activity changes (e.g.,
family members, caregivers)

Pupillary dilation

Self-focused

Self-report of intensity using standardized pain intensity scales
(e.g., Wong-Baker FACES scale, visual analogue scale, numeric rating scale)

Self-report of pain characteristics (e.g., aching, burning, electric
shock, pins and needles, shooting, sore/tender, stabbing,
throbbing) using standardized pain scales (e.g., McGill Pain
Questionnaire, Brief Pain Inventory)

Related Factors

See *Impaired Comfort*.

 Author's Note

Nursing management of pain presents specific challenges. Is acute pain a
response that nurses treat as a nursing diagnosis or collaborative problem? Is acute pain the etiology of another response that better describes
the condition that nurses treat? Does some cluster of nursing diagnoses
represent a pain syndrome or chronic pain syndrome (e.g., *Fear, Risk for
Ineffective Family Coping, Impaired Physical Mobility, Social Isolation, Ineffective Sexuality Patterns, Risk for Colonic Constipation, Fatigue*)? McCaffery
and Beebe (1989) cite 18 nursing diagnoses that can apply to people experiencing pain. Viewing pain as a syndrome diagnosis can provide nurses
with a comprehensive nursing diagnosis for people in pain to whom many
related nursing diagnoses could apply.

 NOC

Comfort Level, Pain Control

Goals

The individual will experience a satisfactory relief measure, as evidenced by (specify):

• Increased participation in activities of recovery
• Reduction in pain behaviors (specify)
• Improvement in mood, coping

NIC
Pain Management, Medication Management, Emotional Support, Teaching: Individual, Hot/Cold Application, Simple Massage

Interventions

Assess for Factors That Decrease Pain Tolerance

- Disbelief from others; uncertainty of prognosis
- Fatigue
- Fear (e.g., of addiction or loss of control)
- Monotony
- Financial and social stressors
- Lack of knowledge

Reduce or Eliminate Factors That Increase Pain

Disbelief from Others
- Establish a supportive accepting relationship:
  - Acknowledge the pain.
  - Listen attentively to the individual's discussion of pain.
  - Convey that you are assessing pain because you want to understand it better (not determine if it really exists).
- Assess the family for any misconceptions about pain or its treatment:
  - Explain the concept of pain as an individual experience.
  - Discuss factors related to increased pain and options to manage.
  - Encourage family members to share their concerns privately (e.g., fear that the individual will use pain for secondary gains if he or she receives too much attention).

Lack of Knowledge/Uncertainty
- Explain the cause of the pain, if known.
- Relate the severity of the pain and how long it will last, if known.
- Explain diagnostic tests and procedures in detail by relating the discomforts and sensations that the individual will feel; approximate the duration.
- Support individual in addressing specific questions regarding diagnosis, risks, benefits of treatment, and prognosis. Consult with the specialist or primary care provider.

Fear
- Provide accurate information to reduce fear of addiction.
  - Explore reasons for the fear.

- Assist in reducing fear of losing control.
  - Provide privacy for the individual's pain experience.
  - Allow the individual to share intensity of pain; express to the individual how well he or she tolerated it.
- Provide information to reduce fear that the medication will gradually lose its effectiveness.
  - Discuss interventions for drug tolerance with the physician/PA/NP (e.g., changing the medication, increasing the dose, decreasing the interval, adding adjunct therapy).
  - Discuss the effect of relaxation techniques on medication effects.

Fatigue

- Determine the cause of fatigue (pain, sedatives, analgesics, sleep deprivation).
- Assess present sleep pattern and the influence of pain on sleep. Refer to *Disturbed Sleep Pattern*.

Provide Optimal Pain Relief With Prescribed Analgesics

- Use oral route when feasible; use intravenous or rectal routes, if needed, with permission.
- Avoid intramuscular routes due to erratic absorption and unnecessary pain.
- Assess vital signs, especially respiratory rate, before administration.
- Consult with pharmacist for possible adverse interactions with other medications (e.g., muscle relaxants, tranquilizers).
- Use the around-the-clock approach, not PRN.
  - Carefully monitor individuals who taking sedating medications and opioid analgesics for respiratory failure every hour for first 12 hours with pulse oximetry, blood pressure, respiratory rate).

Explain to the Individuals and Family the Various Noninvasive Pain-Relief Methods and Why They Are Effective

- Discuss the use of heat applications,* their therapeutic effects, indications, and related precautions.
  - Hot water bottle
  - Warm tub
  - Hot summer sun
  - Electric heating pad
  - Moist heat pack
  - Thin plastic wrap over painful area to retain body heat (e.g., knee, elbow)

- Discuss the use of cold applications,* their therapeutic effects, indications, and related precautions.
  - Cold towels (wrung out)
  - Cold water immersion for small body parts
  - Ice bag
  - Cold gel pack
  - Ice massage
- Explain the therapeutic uses of menthol preparations, massage, and vibration.
- Teach the individual to avoid negative thoughts about ability to cope with pain.
- Practice distraction (e.g., guided imagery, music).
- Practice relaxation techniques.

Reduce or Eliminate Common Side Effects of Opioids

- Refer to *Chronic Pain Syndrome* for interventions

Minimize Procedural and Diagnostic Pain

- Anticipate pain and premedicate the individual prior to painful procedures (e.g., sedation).
- Consider the use of either intradermal 0.9% sodium chloride next to the vein or a topical anesthetic per protocol prior to intravenous starts.
- Encourage the use of relaxation or guided imagery during procedures.

Initiate Health Teaching, as Indicated

- Discuss with the individual and family noninvasive pain-relief measures (e.g., relaxation, distraction, massage, music).
- Teach the techniques of choice to the individual and family.
- Explain the expected course of the pain (resolution) if known (e.g., fractured arm, surgical incision).
- Provide the individual with written guidelines for weaning from pain medications when the acute event is relieved.

Pediatric Interventions

Assess the Child's Pain Experience

- Ask the child to point to the area that hurts. See Focus Assessment Criteria under *Impaired Comfort*.
- Determine the intensity of the pain at its worst and best. Use a pain scale appropriate for the child's developmental age. Use the same scale the same way each time and encourage its use by parents and other health-care professionals. Indicate on the care plan which scale to use and how (introduction of scale, language specific for child); attach copy if visual scale.

- Ask the child what makes the pain better and what makes it worse.
- With infants, assess crying, facial expressions, body postures, and movements. Infants exhibit distress from environmental stimuli (light, sound) as well as from touch and treatments.
- Use tactile and vocal stimuli to comfort infants while assessing the effects of comfort measures and individualized interventions.
- Explain the pain source to the child, as developmentally appropriate, using verbal and sensory (visual, tactile) explanations (e.g., perform treatment on doll, allow the child to handle equipment). Explicitly explain and reinforce to the child that he or she is not being punished.

Assess the Child and Family for Misconceptions About Pain or Its Treatment

- Explain to the parents the necessity of good explanations to promote trust.
- Do not lie to parents or especially child that something will not hurt if there is possibility that it likely will for the sake of easing the child's anxiety about pain. Doing this breeds mistrust between family/patient and the medical team.
- Explain to the parents that the child may cry more openly when they are present, but that their presence is important for promoting trust.

Promote Security With Honest Explanations and Opportunities for Choice

Promote Open, Honest Communication
- Tell the truth; explain:
  - How much it will hurt.
  - How long it will last.
  - What will help with the pain.
- Do not threaten (e.g., do not tell the child, "If you don't hold still, you won't go home.")
- Explain to the child that the procedure is necessary so he or she can get better and that holding still is important so it can be done quickly *and possibly with less pain.*
- Discuss with parents the importance of truth-telling. Instruct them to
  - Tell the child when they are leaving and when they will return.
  - Relate to the child that they cannot take away pain, but that they will be with him or her (except in circumstances when parents are not permitted to remain).

- Allow parents opportunities to share their feelings about witnessing their child's pain and their helplessness.

Prepare the Child for a Painful Procedure

- Discuss the procedure with the parents; determine what they have told the child.
- Explain the procedure in words suited to the child's age and developmental level (see *Delayed Growth and Development* for age-appropriate needs).
- Relate the likely discomforts (e.g., what the child will feel, taste, see, or smell). "You will get an injection that will hurt for a little while and then it will stop."
- Be sure to explain when an injection will cause two discomforts: The prick of the needle and the injection of the drug.
- Encourage the child to ask questions before and during the procedure; ask the child to share what he or she thinks will happen and why.
- Share with the older child that
  - You expect them to hold still and that it will please you if he or she can.
  - It is all right to cry or squeeze someone's hand if it hurts.
- Find something to praise after the procedure, even if the child could not hold still.
- Arrange to have the parents present for procedures (especially for young children) and explain to them what to expect before the procedure. Give them a role during the procedure such as holding child's hand or talking to them.

Reduce the Pain During Treatments When Possible

- If restraints must be used, have sufficient staff available so the procedure is not delayed and so restraints are applied smoothly as not to increase anxiety/discomfort.
- If injections are ordered, try to obtain an order for oral or IV analgesics instead. If injections must be used:
  - Have the child participate by holding the Band-Aid for you.
  - Tell the child how pleased you are that he or she helped.
  - Comfort the child after the procedure, or leave room so that parents can comfort child in the event that staff's presence continues to upset child.
- Offer the child, as age appropriate, the option of learning distraction techniques for use during procedure. (The use of distraction without the child's knowledge of the impending discomfort is not advocated because the child will learn to mistrust):
  - Tell a story with a puppet.
  - Use of cell phone, hand-held gaming device, or electronic tablet.

- Blow a party noisemaker, pinwheels, or bubbles.
- Ask the child to name or count objects in a picture.
- Ask the child to look at the picture and to locate certain objects (e.g., "Where is the dog?")
- Ask the child to tell you a story or about something from their lives.
- Ask the child to count your blinks.
- Avoid rectal thermometers in preschoolers; if possible, use other methods such as tympanic, temporal, or oral (if tolerated) as allowed by the medical institution's guidelines and protocols.
- Provide the child with privacy during the painful procedure; use a treatment room rather than the child's bed.

Provide the Child Optimal Pain Relief With Prescribed Analgesics

- Medicate child before painful procedure or activity (e.g., dressing change, obtaining X-ray of fractured limb, ambulation, injection/PIV placement).
- Consult with physician/NP/PA for change of the IM route to the PO, topical, or IV route when appropriate.
- Along with using pain assessment scales, observe for behavioral signs of pain (because the child may deny pain); if possible, identify specific behaviors that indicate pain in an individual child.
- Assess the potential for use of patient-controlled analgesia (PCA), which provides intermittent controlled doses of IV analgesia (with or without continuous infusion) as determined by the child's need. Children as young as 5 years can use PCA. Parents of children physically unable can administer it to them. PCA has been found safe and to provide superior pain relief compared with conventional-demand analgesia.

Reduce or Eliminate the Common Side Effects of Opioids

Sedation

- Assess whether the cause is the opioid, fatigue, sleep deprivation, or other drugs (sedatives, antiemetics).
- If drowsiness is excessive, consult with physician about reducing dose.

Constipation

- Explain to older children why pain medications cause constipation.
- Increase fiber-containing foods and water in diet.
- Instruct the child to keep a record of exercises (e.g., make a chart with a star sticker placed on it whenever the exercises are done).
- Refer to *Constipation* for additional interventions.

Dry Mouth
- Explain to older children that narcotics decrease saliva production.
- Instruct the child to rinse mouth often, suck on sugarless sour candies, eat pineapple chunks and watermelon, and drink liquids often.
- Explain the necessity of brushing teeth after every meal.
- Discontinue medications/treatments that are causing symptoms as soon as appropriate.

Assist Child With the Aftermath of Pain

- Tell the child when the painful procedure is over. Allow the child to have contact with parent or person whom they find comforting.
- Encourage the child to discuss pain experience (draw or act out with dolls).
- Encourage the child to perform the painful procedure using the same equipment on a doll under supervision.
- Praise the child for his or her endurance and convey that he or she handled the pain well regardless of actual behavior (unless the child was violent to others).
- Reward for good behavior such as sticker, ice pop, or other prize.
- Teach the child to keep a record of painful experiences and to plan a reward each time he or she achieves a behavioral goal, such as a sticker (reward) for each time the child holds still (goal) during an injection. Encourage achievable goals; holding still during an injection may not be possible for every child, but counting or taking deep breaths may be.
- Consult with child life specialists for assistance in teaching coping techniques, providing distraction, and modifying behavior in cases where child is receiving repetitive, unpleasant treatments (e.g., child who has difficulty with frequent, routine blood draws).

Collaborate With Child to Initiate Appropriate Noninvasive Pain-Relief Modalities

- Encourage mobility as much as indicated, especially when pain is lowest.
- Discuss with the child and parents activities that they like and incorporate them in daily schedule (e.g., clay modeling, drawing/coloring).

Assist Family to Respond Optimally to Child's Pain Experience

- Assess family's knowledge of and response to pain (e.g., Do parents support the child who has pain?)

- Assure parents that they can touch or hold their child, if feasible (e.g., demonstrate that touching is possible even with tubes and equipment).
- Give accurate information to correct misconceptions (e.g., the necessity of the treatment even though it causes pain).

Initiate Health Teaching and Referrals, if Indicated

- Provide child and family with ongoing explanations.
- Use available mental health professionals, if needed, for assistance with guided imagery, progressive relaxations, and hypnosis.
- Use available pain service (pain team) at pediatric health-care centers for an interdisciplinary and comprehensive approach to pain management in children.

Chronic Pain

NANDA-I Definition

Unpleasant sensory and emotional experience arising from actual or potential tissue damage or described in terms of such damage (International Association for the Study of Pain); sudden or slow onset of any intensity from mild to severe constant or reoccurring with anticipated or predictable end and a duration of >3 months

Defining Characteristics

The individual reports that pain has existed for more than 3 months (may be the only assessment data present).

Evidence of pain using standardized pain behavior checklist for those unable to communicate verbally (e.g., Neonatal Infant Pain Scale, Pain Assessment Checklist for Those with Limited Ability to Communicate):

Discomfort
Anger, frustration, depression because of situation
Facial mask of pain
Anorexia, weight loss
Insomnia
Guarded movement
Muscle spasms
Redness, swelling, heat
Color changes in the affected area
Reflex abnormalities

Related Factors

See *Impaired Comfort*.

 Author's Note

In the United States, at least 116 million adults in 2011 report living with chronic pain (Institute of Medicine, 2011). "No matter what the cause or pattern of the pain, its chronicity causes physiologic and psychological stress that wears on the patient (and their loved ones) physically and emotionally" (*D'Arcy, 2008).

The real tragedy of experiencing chronic pain is the failure of health-care professionals to understand the lived experience or perhaps worse project disbelief or commendation toward those who suffer. "Thus pain and psychological illness should be viewed as having a reciprocal psychological and behavioral effects involving both processes of illness expression and adaption, as well as pain having specific effects on emotional state and behavioral function" (*Von Korff & Simon, 1996).

NOC

Pain Control, Pain Level, Pain: Disruptive Effects, Pain Control, Depression Control, Pain: Adverse Psychological Response

Goals

The individual will relate improvement of pain and increased daily activities, as evidenced by the following indicators:

- Relate that others validate that their pain exists
- Practice selected noninvasive pain-relief measures

The child will demonstrate coping mechanism for pain, methods to control pain and the pain cause/disease, as evidenced by increased play and usual activities of childhood and the following indicators:

- Communicate improvement in pain verbally, by pain assessment scale, or by behavior (specify).
- Maintain usual family role and relationships throughout pain experience, as evidenced by (specify).

NIC

Pain Management, Medication Management, Exercise Promotion, Mood Management, Coping Enhancement

Interventions

Assess the Individual's Pain Experience

Assess for Factors that Decrease Pain Tolerance

- See *Acute Pain*.

Reduce or Eliminate Factors that Increase Pain

- See *Acute Pain*.

Explore the Individual's/Families' Pain Experience and the Influences of Their Culture

- Language and interpretation problems.
- Reluctance to share personal complaints.

R: *Some cultural groups tend to instill in their members' self-efficacy— a sense of control over life, including how to respond to and manage pain.*

- Believe they can exert little influence over the future (e.g., fatalistic).
- Pain is viewed as something to be tolerated or deserved as a punishment.
- Confusion over nonverbal behaviors
- Reluctance to use pain medications (e.g., fears of misuse, cultural taboos)

Determine With the Individual and Family the Effects of Chronic Pain on the Individual's

- Physical well-being (fatigue, strength, appetite, sleep, function, constipation, nausea)
- Psychologic well-being (anxiety, depression, coping, control, concentration, sense of usefulness, fear, enjoyment)
- Spiritual well-being (religiosity, uncertainty, positive changes, sense of purpose, hopefulness, suffering, meaning of pain, transcendence)
- Social well-being (family support, family distress, sexuality, affection, employment, isolation, financial burden, appearance, roles, relationships)

Assist the Individual and Family to Cope With the Mood Effects of Persistent Pain

- Explain the relationship between chronic pain and mood disorders (e.g., anger, anxiety, depression).
- Encourage verbalization concerning difficult situations.

- Listen carefully.
- See *Ineffective Coping* for additional interventions.

Collaborate With the Individual About Possible Methods to Reduce Pain Intensity

- See *Acute Pain*.

Collaborate With the Individual to Initiate Appropriate Nonpharmaceutical Pain-Relief Measures[5]

- See *Acute Pain*.

Discuss Fears (Individual, Family) of Addiction and Under Treatment of Pain

- Explain tolerance versus addiction. Refer to *Acute Pain* for interventions.

Reduce or Eliminate Common Side Effects of Opioids

Constipation
- For individuals with predisposing factors (advanced age, immobility, poor diet, intra-abdominal pathology, on other constipating medications):
  - Consider prophylactic laxative therapy (e.g., senna 2 tablets at bedtime with or without a stool softener).
  - Encourage the individual to consume increased fiber with increased fluids.

Nausea and Vomiting (Refer to *Nausea*)
Dry Mouth (Refer also to *Impaired oral mucous membranes*)
- Explain that opioids decrease saliva production.
- Instruct the individual to rinse mouth often, suck on sugarless sour candies, eat pineapple chunks or watermelon (if permissible), and drink liquids often.
- Explain the necessity of good oral hygiene and dental care.

Explain to the Individual and Family the Various Noninvasive Pain-Relief Methods and Why They Are Effective

- Explain the therapeutic uses of menthol preparations, massage, and vibration.
- Train them in mindfulness meditation.
  - Relaxation (e.g., yoga, breathing exercises, guided imagery)
  - Music

---

[5] May require a primary care provider's order.

- Discuss the use of heat applications,* the therapeutic effects, indications, and related precautions. Apply dry heat to the area for 20 to 30 minutes every 2 hours for as many days as directed.
  - Hot water bottle
  - Warm tub
  - Hot summer sun
  - Electric heating pad
  - Moist heat pack
  - Thin plastic wrap over painful area to retain body heat (e.g., knee, elbow)
- Discuss the use of cold applications, the therapeutic effects, indications, and related precautions. Use an ice pack or put crushed ice in a plastic bag. Cover it with a towel and place it on the area for 15 to 20 minutes every hour as directed.
  - Cold towels (wrung out)
  - Ice bag
  - Ice massage
  - Cold water immersion for small body parts
  - Cold gel pack
- Ice pack should be soft (e.g., gel to conform to painful site). Homemade gel packs are made with 1 cup of water to ¼ cup rubbing alcohol (can double or triple the quantities for larger ice packs) and poured into a ziploc bag sealed and placed in another bag to prevent leaking. Place in freezer.

Initiate Health Teaching and Referrals as Indicated

- Encourage family to seek assistance if needed for specific problems, such as coping with chronic pain: family counselor; financial and service agencies (e.g., American Cancer Society).

Geriatric Interventions

- Assess cognitive status (e.g., dementia, delirium), mental state (e.g., anxiety, agitation, depression), and functional status.
- Explore the impact of chronic pain on the functionality of the individual within the community, including shopping, home chores, and socialization, as well as the ability to perform activities of daily living (ADLs).
- Plan daily activities when pain is at its lowest level.
- Assessment of chronic pain in older adults can be particularly challenging due to comorbidities, polypharmacy, and possible effects of increased sensitivities to pain medication (*Dewar, 2006).
- Special attention must be paid to the beliefs of the individual and the past experiences that they have had with pain and pain treatments (*Dewar, 2006).

- Exploration of chronic pain should include its impact on the functionality of the individual within the community, including shopping, home chores, and socialization, as well as the ability to perform ADLs (*Dewar, 2006).

🌿 Pediatric Interventions

- Assess pain experiences by using developmentally appropriate assessment scales and by assessing behavior. Incorporate child and family in ongoing assessment. Identify potential for secondary gain for reporting pain (e.g., companionship, attention, concern, caring, distraction); include strategies for meeting identified needs in plan of care.
- Set short-term and long-term goals for pain management with child and family and evaluate regularly (e.g., totally or partially relieve pain, control behavior, or anxiety associated with pain).
- Promote normal growth and development; involve family and available resources, such as occupational, physical, and child life therapists.
- Promote the "normal" aspects of the child's life: play, school, family relationships, physical activity.
- Promote a trusting environment for child and family.
- Believe the child's pain.
- Encourage child's perception that interventions are attempts to help.
- Provide continuity of care and pain management by health-care providers (nurse, physician, pain team) and in different settings (inpatient, outpatient, emergency department, home).
- Use interdisciplinary team for pain management as necessary (e.g., nurse, physician, child life therapist, mental health therapist, occupational therapist, physical therapist, nutritionist).
- Identify myths and misconceptions about pediatric pain management (e.g., IM analgesia, narcotic use and dosing, assessment) in attitudes of health-care professionals, child, and family; provide accurate information and opportunities for effective communication.
- Provide opportunities for parents and siblings to share their experiences and fears.

Chronic Pain Syndrome

Definition

Unpleasant sensory and emotional experience associated with acute or potential tissue damage, or described in terms of such damage (International Association for the Study of Pain); sudden or slow onset of any intensity from mild to severe, constant or recurring without an anticipated or predictable end and a duration of >3 months.

NANDA-I Defining Characteristics

Alteration in ability to continue previous activities
Alteration in sleep pattern
Anorexia
Evidence of pain using standardized pain behavior checklist for those unable to communicate verbally (e.g., Neonatal Infant Pain Scale, Pain Assessment Checklist for Seniors with Limited Ability to Communicate)
Facial expression of pain (e.g., eyes lack luster, beaten look, fixed or scattered movement, grimace)
Proxy report of pain behavior/activity changes (e.g., family member caregiver)
Self-focused
Self-report of intensity using standardized pain scale (e.g., Wong-Baker FACES scale, visual analogue scale, numeric rating scale)
Self-report of pain characteristics using standardized pain instrument (e.g., McGill Pain Questionnaire, Brief Pain Inventory)

NANDA-I Related Factors

Age >50
Alteration in sleep pattern
Chronic musculoskeletal condition
Contusion
Crush injury
Damage to the nervous system
Emotional distress
Fatigue
Female gender
Fracture
Genetic disorder
History of abuse (e.g., physical, psychological, sexual)
History of genital mutilation
History of over-indebtedness
History of static work postures
History of substance abuse
History of vigorous exercise

Imbalance of neurotransmitters, neuromodulators, and receptors
Immune disorder (e.g., HIV-associated neuropathy,
 varicella-zoster virus)
Impaired metabolic functioning
Increase in body mass index
Ineffective sexuality pattern
Injury agent*
Ischemic condition
Malnutrition
Muscle injury
Nerve compression
Post-trauma-related condition (e.g., infection, inflammation)
Prolonged increase in cortisol level
Repeated handling of heavy loads
Social isolation
Rheumatoid arthritis
Tumor infiltration
Whole-body vibration

 Author's Note

Chronic Pain Syndrome is a newly accepted NANDA-I nursing diagnosis. This "syndrome" is problematic as approved as a nursing diagnosis. As one reviews the defining characteristic, they represent *Chronic Pain*. As one reviews the list of "related factors," they represent causative or contributing factors for *Chronic Pain*.

"It is important to distinguish between *Chronic Pain* and *Chronic Pain Syndrome*. The pathophysiology of chronic pain syndrome (CPS) is multifactorial and complex and is still poorly understood. CPS differs from chronic pain in that people with CPS, over time, develop a number of related life problems beyond the sensation of pain itself. It is important to distinguish between the two because they respond to different types of treatment" (Singh, 2014; Grossman & Porth, 2014).

Treatment of CPS must be tailored for each individual patient. The treatment should be aimed at interruption of reinforcement of the pain behavior and modulation of the pain response. The goals of treatment must be realistic and should be focused on restoration of normal function (minimal disability), better quality of life, reduction of use of medication, and prevention of relapse of chronic symptoms.

A self-directed or therapist-directed physical therapy (PT) program, individualized to the patient's needs and goals and provided in association with occupational therapy (OT), has an important role in functional restoration for patients with CPS.

The goal of a PT program is to increase strength and flexibility gradually, beginning with gentle gliding exercises. Patients usually are reluctant to participate in PT because of intense pain.

PT techniques include hot or cold applications, positioning, stretching exercises, traction, massage, ultrasonographic therapy, transcutaneous electrical nerve stimulation (TENS), and manipulations.

NOC

Pain Control, Pain Level, Pain: Disruptive Effects, Pain Control, Depression Control, Pain: Adverse Psychological Response, Coping, Stress Level

Goals

The individual will experience a satisfactory relief measure, as evidenced by (specify):

- Increased participation in activities of recovery
- Reduction in pain behaviors (specify)
- Improvement in mood, coping

NIC

Pain Management, Medication Management, Exercise Promotion, Mood Management, Coping Enhancement, Acupressure, Heat/Cold Application, Distraction

Interventions

Refer to *Chronic Pain* for interventions related to the individual's pain management.

The Interventions to Follow Are Strategies, Utilizing Basic-Level Principles of Cognitive-Behavioral Therapy That a Professional Nurse Can Utilize to:

- Create a therapeutic relationship with the individual
- Promote positive self-esteem
- Reward nonillness-related behaviors

Carefully Evaluate Your Beliefs or Biases Which Can Be Barriers to Providing Empathetic, Ethical, Professional Nursing Care to this Individual

- Individuals with this syndrome are not faking, they do experience the symptoms. Refer to Key Concepts for the differentiation of *Factious Disorder* and *Malingering*.

Do You Believe?

- *Somatic Symptom Disorder* is not valid for this person?
- You can correctly differentiate between "deserving pain patients" and "undeserving addicts"?
- This person is faking?
- This person is drug-seeking?
- This person is wasting your time?
- Most people who chronically take opioids are addictive.

As One Examines One's Biases, Keep in Mind "There Are No Such Thing as Bad Thoughts, Only Bad Actions."

- Attempt to limit the number of nurses assigned to person.
- Specifically validate that you believe his or her symptoms are real. Share this with other staff.
- Specifically explore what makes her or him feel less stressed or anxious.
- "Listen to understand rather than listening to respond" (Procter, Hamer, McGarry, Wilson, & Froggatt, 2014, p. 93), especially in non–illness-related discussions.
- Stop by his or her room when the person has not called with a request or comfort.

Reduce His or Her Anxiety About Illness (Boyd, 2012)

- Explain diagnostic tests that have been ordered.
- Do not advise that specific diagnostic testing may be needed.

Explain to the Individual and Family the Various Noninvasive Stress-Relief Methods and Why They are Effective

- Explain the therapeutic uses of menthol preparations, massage, and vibration.
- Train them in mindfulness meditation.
  - Relaxation (e.g., yoga, breathing exercises, guided imagery)
  - Music

Initiate Health Teaching and Referrals as Indicated

- Clarify with the individual/family what follow-up has been recommended.

Labor Pain

NANDA-I Definition

Sensory and emotional experience that varies from cramping to severe pain and intense pressure which can be highly variable, associated with labor and childbirth (Personal Communication, T Wilson).

Defining Characteristics

Altered muscle tension
Altered neuroendocrine
  function
Altered urinary function
Change in blood pressure
Change in heart rate
Change in respiratory rate
Diaphoresis
Distraction behavior
Expressive behavior
Facial mask
Increased appetite
Lack of appetite
Narrowed focus

Nausea
Noted evidence of contractions
Observed evidence of
  contractions
Perineum pressure sensation
Positioning to avoid pain
Protective gesture
Pupillary dilation
Reports pressure[6]
Reports pain
Requests pain relief inter-
  ventions[4]
Self-focused
Sleep pattern disturbance
Vomiting

Related Factors

Physiologic

Related to dilation period (uterine contractions, cervical stretching, and dilation and distention of lower uterine segment)

Related to transition and expulsion period (uterine contractions and distension of pelvic floor, vagina and perineum, pressure on pelvic nerves)

Situational (Personal, Environmental)

Related to:

Fear
Anxiety
Emotional stress
Anticipation of pain
No prenatal education
Absent labor support
Fatigue
Anemia
Previous experience with
  pain
History of perinatal loss

History of neonatal death
History of neonatal health
  problems
Fetal position
Prior surgical procedures
Language barriers
Substance abuse (history,
  present)
History of abuse
History of sexual abuse/violence
History of trauma
Sexual orientation

---

[6] Added by T. Wilson, contributor.

Maturational

Adolescent
Developmental delay

 Author's Note

This new NANDA-I nursing diagnosis contains the etiology of the pain in the diagnostic statement. What is problematic are what are the related factors when a woman is experiencing normal labor pain. The experience of labor can be complicated when the mother is 14 years old, drug addicted, or there is a history of perinatal loss. Labor pain is complicated by fear and anxiety; thus, this nursing diagnosis should be added with the related factors that reflect why this labor experience may be more difficult and necessitates additional nursing individuals.

Labor Pain may be more clinically useful as Labor Syndrome, which would include Acute Pain, Impaired Comfort, Fear, Anxiety, and Interrupted Family Processes.

NOC
Refer to Acute Pain.

Goals

The mother will report or exhibit satisfactory pain level, as evidenced by

- Reduction in pain behaviors (specify)
- Increased relaxation between contractions
- Improved coping skills

NIC
Refer to Acute Pain.

Interventions

Refer to nursing diagnosis *Acute Pain* for basic pain management interventions.

Assess Progress in Labor

- Uterine contraction pattern
- Cervical dilation
- Fetal position and station

R: *Location and intensity of pain varies with phase or stage of labor.*

Assess Support Person's Readiness to Participate

Determine effect of
- Age and developmental status
- Culture and religion on expectations

R: *Perception and expression of pain is influenced by life experience, developmental stage, and cultural or religious norms.*

Provide comfort measures
- Gown and linen changes as needed
- Frequent pericare
- Cool damp cloth to forehead, neck, or upper back

Provide labor support

R: *Women who are provided with continuously available support during labor have improved outcomes compared with women who do not have one-to-one continuously available support. The element that best predicts a woman's experience of labor pain is her level of confidence in her ability to cope with labor (*Simkin & Bolding, 2004).*

- Labor support ideally is continuous and provided by a variety of individuals.
- Labor support should begin in early labor and continued through delivery.
- Assist the woman to cope with pain, build her self-confidence, and maintain a sense of mastery and well-being.
- Be supportive of patient's choices and wishes for her birth experience.
- Provide acceptance of her coping style.
- Reinforce positive coping mechanisms.
- Introduce and demonstrate new methods for coping with pain.

R: *For women in labor, continuous support can result in the following:*

- *Shorter labor*
- *Decreased use of analgesia/anesthesia*
- *Decreased operative vaginal births or cesarean births*
- *Decreased need for oxytocin/uterotonics*
- *Increased likelihood of breastfeeding*
- *Increased satisfaction with childbirth experience*
- *Many of the mother's childbirth outcomes listed above also benefit the neonate (*AWHONN, 2011)*

Encourage Adequate Intake of Oral Fluids by Monitoring Oral and IV Intake and by Offering the Following

- Ice chips
- Popsicles
- Jell-O
- Suckers
- Wet washcloths

Encourage Woman to Void at Least Every 2 Hours If No Urinary Catheter

- Catheterize patient as indicated.

R: *Bladder distention can interfere with fetal descent and increase uterine contraction pain.*

Guide and Support Woman and Her Support Person in Using Self-Comforting Techniques

Demonstrate and Encourage Support Person to Assist With Supportive Techniques as Needed

R: *Qualitative research has demonstrated that one of the most significant aspects of the experience of labor for women is the presence of one or more support persons. Postpartum women report that one of the things contributing to a positive labor experience was the presence of a family member or friend in the room (Burke, 2014).*

Encourage Rest and Promote Relaxation Between Contractions

Encourage and Support Nonpharmacologic Pain Relief Measures

R: *Achieving a state of relaxation is the basis of all nonpharmacologic interventions during labor. Relaxation enhances the effectiveness of nonpharmacologic and pharmacologic pain-management strategies (Burke, 2014).*

- Relaxation techniques
- Patterned breathing techniques

R: *Breathing techniques are used as a distraction during labor to decrease pain and promote relaxation (Burke, 2014).*

- Discourage supine position to prevent supine hypotension or vena cava syndrome.
- Encourage patterned physical movement, frequent position changes, and ambulation.

R: *Women naturally choose positions of comfort and are more likely to change positions in early labor (Burke, 2014).*

- Leaning or leaning forward with support
- Sitting, standing
- Side lying
- Pillows to help with positioning
- Squatting: hands and knees
- Rocking chair
- Birthing ball

R: *The birthing ball provides support for the woman's body as she assumes a variety of positions during labor. This may enhance maternal comfort. A birthing ball helps the woman use pelvic rocking, promotes mobility, and helps to provide support for the woman in the upright position (*AWHONN, 2008 a, b).*

- Biofeedback
- Hypnosis
- Attention focusing—focal point or imagery
- Music
- Aromatherapy
- Hydrotherapy
  - Shower, pool, or tub

R: *With appropriate attention to water temperature, duration of the bath, and safety considerations, baths in labor are effective in reducing pain and suffering during labor (*Simkin & Bolding, 2004).*

- Touch
  - Massage, effleurage, and counterpressure
  - Application of heat or cold
  - Therapeutic touch and healing touch

R: *Various forms of touch can convey to the woman a sense of caring, reassurance, understanding, or nonverbal support (Simkin & Ancheta, 2011). Purposeful use of massage is employed during labor as a relaxation and stress-reduction technique that functions as a distraction, may stimulate cutaneous nerve fibers that block painful impulses, and stimulates the local release of endorphins (Burke, 2014).*

- TENS decreases pain perception by providing alternate sensation.

R: *TENS provides modest pain relief benefits and is a satisfying option for most women who use it (*Simkin & Bolding, 2004).*

- Acupuncture/Acupressure

R: *Acupuncture provides an effective alternative to pharmacologic pain relief (*Simkin & Bolding, 2004).*

- Intradermal injections of sterile water

R: *Intradermal injections of sterile water decrease lower back pain in most laboring women without any identified side effects on the fetus or mother (*Simkin & Bolding, 2004).*

Offer/Encourage Pharmacologic Pain-Relief Measures (Burke, 2014)

Sedatives and hypnotics
- Provide sedation or sleep
- Depress the central nervous system
- Decrease anxiety
- Rarely used in modern-day obstetrics because of long half-life
- Historically, women experiencing prolonged latent labor were thought to benefit from the brief period of therapeutic rest or sleep following administration of barbiturates.

R: *H_1-receptor antagonists may be administered with narcotics during labor to*

- *Decrease anxiety*
- *Increase sedation*
- *Decrease nausea and vomiting*

- Analgesics

R: *Analgesics allow women to relax and rest between contractions by*

- *Blunting effect with increase in pain threshold*
- *Decreased perception of pain*
- *Somnolence*

Consult With OB Provider for

- Neuraxial analgesia

R: *Neuraxial analgesia in labor*

- *Provides superior pain relief*
- *Provides sufficient analgesia effect with as little motor block as possible*
- *Is flexible and effective method of pain relief*
- *Results in less central nervous system depression of mother and neonate than other pharmacologic methods*

- Regional anesthesia (rarely used in modern obstetrics)
  - Pudendal block—provides vaginal, vulvar, and perineal anesthesia via injection of anesthetic agent through lateral walls into area of pudendal nerve
  - Paracervical block—injection of anesthetic agent around the cervix

Monitor and Evaluate Effects of Pain Management Interventions on Mother and Fetus

- Assess comfort level before and after pain management interventions.
- Monitor fetal heart rate for nonreassuring characteristics (refer to Nonreassuring Fetal Status in *Risk for Complications of Reproductive Dysfunction*).

CLINICAL ALERT Notify the anesthesia provider if any of the following occurs:

- Hypotension
- High sensory level block
- Bradycardia
- Respiratory compromise
- Apnea
- Arm/hand numbness or paralysis
- Nausea
- Anxiety
- Decreasing level of consciousness

Initiate Health Teaching as Indicated

- Instruct mother and her family on labor process.
- Explain physiology of pain in labor.
- Provide information about analgesia/anesthesia measures, side effects, and potential complications.
- Provide information about procedures to the mother and her family.

Nausea

NANDA-I Definition

A subjective phenomenon of an unpleasant feeling in the back of the throat and stomach that may or may not result in vomiting

Defining Characteristics*

Aversion toward food	Reports nausea
Increased swallowing	Increased salivation
Gagging sensation	Reports sour taste in mouth

Related Factors

Biopathophysiologic

Related to tissue trauma and reflex muscle spasms secondary to:

Acute gastroenteritis
Peptic ulcer disease
Irritable bowel syndrome
Pancreatitis
Infections (e.g., food poisoning)

Drug overdose
Renal calculi
Uterine cramps associated
  with menses
Motion sickness

Treatment Related

Related to effects of chemotherapy, theophylline, digitalis, antibiotics, iron supplements

Related to effects of anesthesia

Situational (Personal, Environmental)*

Anxiety
Noxious odors, taste
Fear
Pain

Psychologic factors
Unpleasant visual stimulation

NOC

Comfort Level, Nutrition Status, Hydration

Goals

The individual will report decreased nausea, as evidenced by the following indicators:

- Name foods or beverages that do not increase nausea
- Describe factors that increase nausea

NIC

Medication Management, Nausea Management, Fluid/Electrolyte Management, Nutrition Management, Relaxation Therapy, Vomiting Management

Interventions

Take Measures to Prevent Treatment-Related Nausea

- Aggressive management before, during, and after chemotherapy can prevent nausea (Yarbro, Wujcik, & Gobel, 2013).

- Aggressively prevent nausea and vomiting in those with risk factors (Pasero & McCaffery, 2011):
  - Female gender
  - Nonsmoker
  - History of motion sickness/postoperative nausea/vomiting
  - Use of volatile anesthetics within 0 to 2 hours, nitrous oxide and/or intraoperative and postoperative opioids.
  - Duration of surgery
  - Type of surgery (e.g., laparoscopic, ENT, neurosurgery, breast, plastic surgery)
- Consult with specialist to prevent postoperative nausea and vomiting intraoperatively and postoperatively (Pasero & McCaffery, 2011).
- Use multimodal analgesics to reduce the dose of opioids to lowest possible.
- Use multimodal antiemetics preinduction and at the end of surgery

Promote Comfort During Nausea and Vomiting

- Protect those at risk for aspiration (immobile, children).
- Address the cleanliness of the individual and environment.
- Provide an opportunity for oral care after each episode.
- Apply a cool, damp cloth to the individual's forehead, neck, and wrists.
- Offer muscle relaxation and distraction techniques (e.g., music).

Reduce or Eliminate Noxious Stimuli

Pain
- Plan care to avoid unpleasant or painful procedures before meals.
- Medicate individuals for pain 30 minutes before meals according to physician/NP's orders.
- Provide a pleasant, relaxed atmosphere for eating (no bedpans in sight, do not rush); try a "surprise" (e.g., flowers with meal).
- Arrange the plan of care to decrease or eliminate nauseating odors or procedures near mealtimes.

Fatigue
- Teach or assist the individual to rest before meals.
- Teach the individual to spend minimal energy preparing food (cook large quantities and freeze several meals at a time, request assistance from others).

Odor of Food

- Teach the individual to avoid cooking odors—frying food, brewing coffee—if possible (take a walk; select foods that can be eaten cold).
- Suggest using foods that require little cooking during periods of nausea.
- Suggest trying sour foods.

Decrease Stimulation of the Vomiting Center

- Reduce unpleasant sights and odors. Restrict activity.
- Provide good mouth care after vomiting.
- Teach the individual to practice deep breathing and voluntary swallowing to suppress the vomiting reflex.
- Instruct the individual to sit down after eating, but not to lie down.
- Encourage the individual to eat smaller meals and to eat slowly.
- Restrict liquids with meals to avoid overdistending the stomach; also, avoid fluids 1 hour before and after meals.
- Loosen clothing.
- Encourage the individual to sit in fresh air or use a fan to circulate air.
- Advise the individual to avoid lying flat for at least 2 hours after eating. (An individual who must rest should sit or recline so that the head is at least 4 inches higher than the feet.)
- Advise the individual to listen to music.
- Offer small amounts of clear fluids and foods and beverages with ginger.
- Offer muscle relaxation and distraction techniques to adult cancer patients.
- If qualified, use acupressure at pressure points postoperatively.

🏃 Maternal Interventions

Teach That Various Interventions Have Been Reported to Help Control Nausea During Pregnancy

- Assure her that nausea is common during pregnancy (Pillitteri, 2014).
- Avoid fatigue and sudden movements.
- Avoid greasy, high-fat foods and strong odors.
- Eat high-protein meals and a snack before retiring.
- Chew gum or suck hard candies.
- Eat carbohydrates (e.g., crackers, toast, sour ball candy) on arising; delay eating breakfast until nausea passes.
- Eat immediately when hungry.
- Do not go longer than 12 hours without eating.

- If nauseated, sip/consume carbonated beverages (e.g., Coke syrup, orange juice, ginger ale, and herbal teas such as ginger).
- Try deep breaths of fresh air.
- Lie down to relieve symptoms.
- Use acupressure (refer to description under general interventions for nausea).
- Explain ginger as an effective treatment for nausea/vomiting during pregnancy. Consult with OB provider if small amounts of ginger ale (real ginger) are permissible.

Advised to Notify Health-Care Provider If Person

- Vomits more than once daily
- Is losing weight
- Is not eating enough during the day
- Has decreased urine or a darker yellow colored urine
- Must alter her lifestyle (e.g., work schedule) (Pillitteri, 2014)

IMPAIRED COMMUNICATION[7]

Impaired Communication

Impaired Verbal Communication

Definition

The state in which a person experiences, or is at risk to experience, difficulty exchanging thoughts, ideas, wants, or needs with others

Defining Characteristics

Major (Must Be Present)

Inappropriate or absent speech or response
Impaired ability to speak or hear

---

[7] This diagnosis is not presently on the NANDA-I list but has been added for clarity and usefulness.

Minor (May Be Present)

Incongruence between verbal and nonverbal messages
Stuttering
Slurring
Word-finding problems
Weak or absent voice
Statements of being misunderstood or not understanding
Dysarthria
Aphasia
Language barrier

Related Factors

Pathophysiologic

Related to disordered, unrealistic thinking secondary to:
Schizophrenic disorder   Delusional disorder
Psychotic disorder   Paranoid disorder

Related to impaired motor function of muscles of speech secondary to:
Cerebrovascular accident ("brain attack")
Oral or facial trauma
Brain damage (e.g., birth/head trauma)
Central nervous system (CNS) depression/increased intracranial
  pressure
Tumor (of the head, neck, or spinal cord)
Chronic hypoxia/decreased cerebral blood flow
Nervous system diseases (e.g., myasthenia gravis, multiple sclero-
  sis, muscular dystrophy, Alzheimer's disease)
Vocal cord paralysis/quadriplegia

Related to impaired ability to produce speech secondary to:
Respiratory impairment (e.g., shortness of breath)
Laryngeal edema/infection
Oral deformities
  Cleft lip or palate
  Missing teeth
  Malocclusion or fractured jaw
  Dysarthria

Related to auditory impairment

Treatment Related

Related to impaired ability to produce speech secondary to:

  Endotracheal intubation   Tracheostomy/tracheotomy/
                                 laryngectomy

Surgery of the head, face, neck, or mouth
CNS depressants

Pain (especially of the mouth or throat)

Situational (Personal, Environmental)

Related to decreased attention secondary to fatigue, anger, anxiety, or pain

Related to no access to or malfunction of hearing aid

Related to psychologic barrier (e.g., fear, shyness)

Related to lack of privacy

Related to unavailable interpreter

Maturational

Infant/Child
Related to inadequate sensory stimulation

Older Adult (Auditory Losses)
Related to hearing impairment

Related to cognitive impairments secondary to (specify)

 Author's Note

Impaired Communication is clinically useful with individuals with communication-receptive deficits and language barriers.

Impaired Communication may not be useful to describe communication problems that are a manifestation of psychiatric illness or coping problems. If nursing interventions focus on reducing hallucinations, fear, or anxiety, *Confusion; Fear*, or *Anxiety* would be more appropriate.

NOC
Communication

Goals

The person will report improved satisfaction with ability to communicate, as evidenced by the following indicators:

- Demonstrate increased ability to understand
- Demonstrate improved ability to express self
- Use alternative methods of communication, as indicated

NIC

Communication Enhancement: Speech, Communication Enhancement: Hearing Active Listening, Socialization Enhancement

Interventions

Identify a Method to Communicate Basic Needs

- Assess ability to comprehend, speak, read, and write.
- Provide alternative methods of communication.
  - Use a computer, pad and pencil, hand signals, eye blinks, head nods, and bell signals.
  - Make flash cards with pictures or words depicting frequently used phrases (e.g., "Wet my lips," "Move my foot," "I need a glass of water," or "I need a bedpan").
  - Encourage the person to point, use gestures, and pantomime.
- Practice "listening to understand rather than listening to respond" by quieting your mind (Procter, Hamer, McGarry, Wilson, & Froggatt., 2014, p. 93).

Identify Factors That Promote Communication

- Create atmosphere of acceptance and privacy.
- Provide a nonrushed environment.
- Use techniques to increase understanding.
  - Face the individual and establish eye contact if possible. Avoid standing over person, sit down.
  - Use uncomplicated one-step commands and directives.
  - Match words with actions; use pictures.
  - Validate that the individual understands the message.
  - Give information in writing to reinforce.

If the Person Can Speech-Read, Do Not Call it Lipreading (Bauman & Gell, 2000; Office of Student Disabilities Services, 2014)

- Look directly at the person, even a slight turn of your head can obscure the speech reading view, and
  - Speak slowly and clearly.
  - Do not yell, exaggerate, or over enunciate.
  - Try to enunciate each word without force or tension. Short sentences are easier to understand than long ones.
  - Do not place anything in your mouth when speaking.
  - Mustaches that obscure the lips and putting your hands in front of your face can make lip reading difficult.
  - Avoid standing in front of light—have the light on your face so the person can see your lips.
  - If the person looks surprised/perplexed/bemused, stop and clarify.

- Use open-ended questions, which must be answered by more than "yes", or "no."
- Reinforce important communications by writing them down.

Assess Ability to Communicate in English, Determine Language the Individual Speaks Best

- Do not evaluate understanding based on "yes" or "no" responses.
- Assess the individual's ability to read, write, speak, and comprehend English and for red flags for lack of comprehension (De Walt et al., 2010).
- Use a *fluent* translator when discussing important matters (e.g., taking a health history, signing an operation permit). Reinforce communications through the translator with written information. (Many hospitals require a "Certified Translator" to be used at least once per day. This should be documented in the medical record per hospital policy.)
- If possible, allow the translator to spend as much time as the person wishes (be flexible with visitors' rules and regulations).
- If a translator is unavailable, plan a daily visit from someone who has some knowledge of the person's language. (Many hospitals and social welfare offices keep a language bank with names and phone numbers of people who are willing to translate.)
- Use a telephone translating system when necessary.

Initiate Health Teaching and Referrals, If Needed

- Seek consultation with a speech or audiology specialist.

Pediatric Interventions

- Use age-appropriate words and gestures.
- Initially talk to parent and allow the child to observe. Gradually include the child.
  - Approach the child slowly and speak in a quiet, unhurried, confident voice.
  - Assume an eye-level position.
  - Use simple words and short sentences.
  - Talk about something not related to the present situation (e.g., school, toy, hair, clothes).
- Offer choices as much as possible.
- Encourage the child to share concerns and fears.
- Allow the child an opportunity to touch and use articles (e.g., stethoscope, tongue blade).

Geriatric Interventions

- If the person can hear with a hearing aid, make sure that it is on and functioning.

- If the person can hear with one ear, speak slowly and clearly into the good ear. It is more important to speak distinctly than to speak loudly.
- If the person can read and write, provide pad and pencil at all times (even when going to another department).
- If the person can understand only sign language, have an interpreter with him or her as much as possible.
- Write and speak all important messages.
- Validate the person's understanding by asking questions that require more than "yes" or "no" answers. Avoid asking, "Do you understand?"
- Assess if cerumen impaction is impairing hearing.

Impaired Verbal Communication

NANDA-I Definition

Decreased, delayed, or absent ability to receive, process, transmit, and/or use a system of symbols

Defining Characteristics

Difficulty or inability to speak words but can understand others
Articulation or motor planning deficits

Related Factors

See *Impaired Communication*.

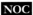
Communication: Expressive Ability

Goals

The person will demonstrate improved ability to express self, as evidenced by the following indicators:

- Relate decreased frustration with communication
- Use alternative methods as indicated

Active Listening, Communication Enhancement: Speech Deficit

Interventions

Identify a Method for Communicating Basic Needs

- See *Impaired Communication* for general interventions.

Identify Factors That Promote Communication

For Individuals With Dysarthria (Slurred or Slow Speech)
- Do not alter your speech or messages, because the individual's comprehension is not affected; speak on an adult level.
- Encourage the individual to make a conscious effort to slow down speech and to speak louder (e.g., "Take a deep breath between sentences.").
- Ask the individual to repeat unclear words; observe for non-verbal cues to help understanding.
- If the individual is tired, ask questions that require only short answers.
- If speech is unintelligible, teach use of gestures, written messages, and communication cards.

For Those Who Cannot Speak (e.g., Endotracheal Intubation, Tracheostomy)
- Reassure that speech will return, if it will. If not, explain available alternatives (e.g., esophageal speech, sign language).
- Do not alter your speech, tone, or type of message; speak on an adult level.
- Use gestures, head nods, mouthing of words, writing, use of letter/picture boards and common words or phrases tailored to meet individualized patients' needs (Grossbach, Stranberg, & Chlan, 2011).
- Utilize stress-reducing and comfort intervention with every encounter.
  - Touch
  - "It must be frightening to be in your situation. Is there anything I can do to make you feel better, safer?
  - Ensure the call bell system is always visible and available.

Promote Continuity of Care to Reduce Frustration

Observe for Signs of Frustration or Withdrawal
- Verbally address frustration over inability to communicate. Explain that both nurse and individual must use patience.
- Maintain a calm, positive attitude (e.g., "I can understand you if we work at it.").
- Use reassurance (e.g., "I know it's difficult, but you'll get it.").
- Maintain a sense of humor.

- Allow tears (e.g., "It's OK. I know it's frustrating. Crying can let it all out.").
- For the individual with limited speaking ability (e.g., can make simple requests, but not lengthy statements), encourage letter writing or keeping a diary to express feelings and share concerns.
- Anticipate needs and ask questions that need a simple "yes" or "no" answer.

Maintain a Specific Care Plan

- Document the method of communication that is used (e.g., "Uses word cards," "Points for bedpan," alphabet board, picture board writing materials).
- Record directions for specific measures (e.g., allow him to keep a urinal in bed).

Pediatric Interventions

- Establish a method of communication appropriate for age.
- If a young child is deprived of vocalization, teach basic language gestures (time, food, family relationships, emotions, animals, numbers, frequent requests).
- Ensure that the family and child are connected to services for hearing impaired.
- Consult with a speech pathologist for ongoing assistance.

ACUTE CONFUSION

Acute Confusion

Risk for Acute Confusion

NANDA-I Definition

Abrupt onset of reversible disturbances of consciousness, attention, cognition, and perception that develop over a short period of time

Defining Characteristics

Major (Must be Present)

Abrupt onset of:
Fluctuation in cognition*
Fluctuation in level of consciousness*

Fluctuation in psychomotor activity
Increased agitation*   Incoherence
Reduced ability to focus   Fear
Disorientation   Anxiety
Increased restlessness*   Excitement
Hypervigilance

Symptoms are worse at night or when fatigued or in new situations.

Minor (May Be Present)

Illusions   Delusions
Hallucinations*   Misperceptions*

Related Factors

Factors that increase the risk for delirium and confusional states can be classified into those that increase baseline vulnerability (e.g., underlying brain diseases such as dementia, stroke, or Parkinson's disease) and those that precipitate the disturbance (e.g., infection, sedatives, immobility; Francis & Young, 2014).

Related to abrupt onset of cerebral hypoxia or disturbance in cerebral metabolism secondary to (Miller, 2015):

Fluid and Electrolyte Disturbances
Dehydration   Hypokalemia
Acidosis/alkalosis   Hyponatremia/hypernatremia
Hypercalcemia/hypocalcemia   Hypoglycemia/hyperglycemia

Nutritional Deficiencies
Folate or vitamin B_{12} deficiency   Niacin deficiency
Anemia   Magnesium deficiency

Cardiovascular Disturbances
Myocardial infarction
Congestive heart failure   Heart block
Dysrhythmias   Temporal arteritis
                               Subdural hematoma

Respiratory Disorders
Chronic obstructive pulmonary disease: tuberculosis and
    pneumonia
Pulmonary embolism

Infections
Sepsis
Meningitis, encephalitis
Urinary tract infection (especially elderly)
Metabolic and endocrine disorders
Hypothyroidism/hyperthyroidism: hypoadrenocorticism/
    hyperadrenocorticism
Hypopituitarism/hyperpituitarism: postural hypotension,
    hypothermia/hyperthermia
Parathyroid disorders: hepatic or renal failure

Central Nervous System (CNS) Disorders
Cerebrovascular accident
Multiple infarctions
Tumors
Normal-pressure hydrocephalus
Head trauma
Seizures and postconvulsive states

Treatment Related

Related to a disturbance in cerebral metabolism secondary to:

Surgery
Therapeutic drug intoxication
    Neuroleptics: opioids
    General anesthesia

Side effects of medication:

Diuretics	Barbiturates	Sulfa drugs
Digitalis	Methyldopa	Ciprofloxacin
Propranolol	Disulfiram	Metronidazole
Atropine	Lithium	Acyclovir
Oral hypoglycemic	Phenytoin	H_2-receptor
Anti-inflammatories	Over-the-counter	antagonists
Antianxiety agents	cold, cough, and	Anticholinergics
Phenothiazines	sleeping	
Benzodiazepines	preparations	

Situational (Personal, Environmental)

Related to disturbance in cerebral metabolism secondary to:
Withdrawal from alcohol, opioids, sedatives, hypnotics
Heavy metal or carbon monoxide intoxication

Related to:

Pain	Depression
Bowel impaction	Unfamiliar situations
Immobility	

Related to chemical intoxications or medications (specify):

Alcohol	Methamphetamines
Cocaine	PCP
Methadone	Opioids (e.g., heroin)

 Author's Note

"Confusion" is a term nurses use frequently to describe an array of cognitive impairments. "Identifying a person as confused is just an initial step" (*Rasin, 1990; *Roberts, 2001). Confusion is a behavior that indicates a disturbance in cerebral metabolism.

Acute confusion (delirium) can occur in any age group, which can develop over a period of hours to days (Grossman & Porth, 2014). Factors that increase the risk for delirium and confusional states can be classified into those that increase baseline vulnerability (e.g., underlying brain diseases such as dementia, stroke, or Parkinson's disease) and those that precipitate the disturbance (e.g. infection, sedatives, immobility). The disturbance is typically caused by a medical condition, substance intoxication, or medication side effect (Francis & Young, 2014).

"Chronic Confusion (dementia) is a syndrome of acquired, persistent, impairment in several domains of intellectual function, including memory, language, visuospatial ability, and cognition" (Grossman & Porth, 2014, p. 65).

Individuals with dementia can experience acute confusion (delirium). Nurses need to determine prehospital function and confer with family to observe for deterioration.

NOC

Cognition, Cognitive Orientation, Distorted Thought Self-Control

Goals

The person will have diminished episodes of delirium, as evidenced by the following indicators:

- Be less agitated
- Participate in ADLs
- Be less combative

NIC
Delirium Management, Calming Technique, Reality Orientation, Environmental Management: Safety

Interventions

Promote the Individual's Sense of Integrity

- Educate family, significant others, and caregivers about the situation and cause and coping methods (Young, 2001):
  - Explain the cause of the confusion.
  - Explain that the individual does not realize the situation.
  - Explain the need to remain patient, flexible, and calm.
  - Stress the need to respond to the individual as an adult.
  - Explain that the behavior is part of a disorder and is not voluntary.
- Maintain standards of empathic, respectful care:
  - Expect empathic, respectful care, and monitor its administration.
  - Attempt to obtain information for conversation (likes, dislikes; interests, hobbies; work history). Interview early in the day.
  - Encourage significant others and caregivers to speak slowly with a low voice pitch and at an average volume (unless hearing deficits are present), with eye contact, and as if expecting the individual to understand.
- Provide respect and promote sharing.
  - Pay attention to what the individual says.
  - Pick out meaningful comments and continue talking.
  - Call the individual by name and introduce yourself each time you make contact; use touch if welcomed.
  - Use the name the individual prefers; avoid "Pops" or "Mom," which can increase confusion and is unacceptable.
  - Convey to the individual that you are concerned and friendly (through smiles, an unhurried pace, gentle touch, humor, and praise; do not argue).
  - Focus on the feeling behind the spoken word or action.

Provide Sufficient and Meaningful Sensory Input

- Reduce abrupt changes in schedule or relocation.
  - Keep oriented to time and place.
  - Refer to time of day and place each morning.
  - Provide the individual with a clock and calendar large enough to see.
  - Ensure corrective lenses are available and used.
  - Use nightlights or dim lights at night.
  - Use indirect lighting and turn on lights before dark.
  - Provide with the opportunity to see daylight and dark through a window, or take the individual outdoors.
  - Single out holidays with cards or pins (e.g., wear a red heart for Valentine's Day).
- Encourage the family to bring in familiar objects from home (e.g., photographs with nonglare glass, afghan).
  - Ask the individual to tell you about the picture.
  - Focus on familiar topics.
- In teaching a task or activity—such as eating—break it into small, brief steps by giving only one instruction at a time.

Discuss Current and Seasonal Events (Snow, Water Activities);
Share Your Interests (Travel, Crafts)

Do Not Endorse Confusion

- Do not argue with the individual.
- Determine the best response to confused statements.
- Sometimes the confused individual may be comforted by a response that reduces his or her fear; for example, "I want to see my mother," when his or her mother has been dead for 20 years. The nurse may respond with, "I know that your mother loved you."
- Direct the individual back to reality; do not allow him or her to ramble.
- Avoid talking to coworkers about other topics in the individual's presence.
- Remember to acknowledge your entrance with a greeting and your exit with a closure ("I will be back in 10 minutes").

Prevent Injury to the Individual

- Refer to *Risk for Injury* for strategies for assessing and manipulating the environment for hazards.

Initiate Referrals, as Needed

- Refer caregivers to appropriate community resources.

Risk for Acute Confusion

NANDA-I Definition

Vulnerable to reversible disturbances of consciousness, attention, cognition, and perception that develop over a short period of time

Risk Factors

Refer to Related Factors under *Acute Confusion*.

 NOC
Refer to *Acute Confusion*.

Goal

The individual will demonstrate continued level of orientation, attention, and cognition.

Interventions

 NOC
Refer to *Acute Confusion*.

CHRONIC CONFUSION

NANDA-I Definition

Irreversible, long-standing, and/or progressive deterioration of intellect and personality characterized by decreased ability to interpret environmental stimuli; decreased capacity for intellectual thought processes; and manifested by disturbances of memory, orientation, and behavior

Defining Characteristics

Normal level of consciousness

Irreversible, long-standing, and/or progressive:
    Alteration in interpretation; Chronic cognitive impairment
    Alteration in long-term memory; Impaired social functioning
    Alteration in personality; Organic brain disorder
    Alteration in short-term memory; Alteration in response to
        stimuli
    Alteration in cognitive functioning

Related Factors

Pathophysiologic

Alzheimer's disease*
Multi-infarct dementia (MID)*
Vascular dementia (damaged areas of brain) because of reduced
    blood flow (e.g., from chronic high blood pressure, uncon-
    trolled diabetes mellitus)
Cumulative damage to the brain (e.g., chronic alcoholism or
    repeated head injuries [e.g., former professional boxers or
    football players])
Frontotemporal dementia (formerly called Pick's disease)
Inflammatory and autoimmune diseases (e.g., multiple sclerosis,
    systemic lupus erythematosus, encephalitis)
Toxic substance injection
Brain tumors
Infectious diseases (e.g., HIV-associated neurocognitive disorder
    [HAND], herpes encephalitis, neurosyphilis)
End-stage diseases(AIDS, cirrhosis, cancer, renal failure, cardiac
    failure, chronic obstructive pulmonary disease)
Creutzfeldt–Jakob disease
Degenerative neurologic disease
Huntington's chorea
Psychiatric disorders
Dementia with Lewy bodies is a form of dementia caused by
    abnormal protein structures called Lewy bodies

 Author's Note

Refer to *Acute Confusion*.

NOC

Cognitive Ability, Cognitive Orientation, Distorted Thought Self-Control, Surveillance:
Safety, Emotional Support, Environmental Management, Fall Prevention, Calming
Technique

Goals

The person will participate to the maximum level of independence in a therapeutic milieu, as evidenced by the following indicators:

- Decreased frustration
- Diminished episodes of combativeness
- Increased hours of sleep at night
- Stabilized or increased weight

NIC

Dementia Management: Multisensory Therapy, Cognitive Stimulation, Calming Technique, Reality Orientation, Environmental Management: Safety

Interventions

Determine If Prediagnostic Counseling Was Done

Explore Who the Person Was Before the Onset of Confusion With Significant Others

- Educational level, career
- Hobbies, lifestyle
- Coping styles

Observe to Determine Baseline Behaviors

- Best time of day
- Response time to a simple question
- Amount of distraction tolerated
- Judgment
- Insight into disability
- Signs and symptoms of depression
- Routine

Promote the Individual's Sense of Integrity (Miller, 2015)

- Adapt communication to the individual's level:
  - Avoid "baby talk" and a condescending tone of voice.
  - Use simple sentences and present one idea at a time.
- Unless a safety issue is involved, do not argue.
- Avoid general questions, such as, "What would you like to do?" Instead, ask, "Do you want to go for a walk or work on your rug?"
- Avoid questions you know the individual cannot answer.
- Use light touch to gain attention or show concern unless a negative response is elicited.

Promote the Individual's Safety (Miller, 2015)

- Refer to *Risks for Falls* for additional interventions.
- Ensure the appropriateness and safety of invasive therapies (e.g., IV equipment, urinary catheters, gastrointestinal tubes).

If Combative, Determine the Source of the Fear and Frustration

- Fatigue
- Misleading or inappropriate stimuli
- Change in routine, environment, caregiver
- Pressure to exceed functional capacity
- Physical stress, pain, infection, acute illness, discomfort
- Give the person something to hold (e.g., stuffed animal).

If a Dysfunctional Episode or Sudden Functional Loss Has Occurred

- Address by surname.
- Assume a dependent position to the individual.
- Distract the individual with cues that require automatic social behavior (e.g., "Mrs. Smith, would you like some juice now?").
- After the episode has passed, discuss the episode with the individual.

Provide Reality Orientation and Support Remotivation Therapy Per Occupational Therapist Recommendations

Provide Modalities Involving the Five Senses (Hearing, Sight, Smell, Taste, and Touch) That Provide Favorable Stimuli for the Individual

- Stimulate vision (with brightly colored items of different shape, pictures, colored decorations, kaleidoscopes).
- Stimulate smell (with flowers, soothing aromas from lavender or scented lotion).
- Stimulate hearing (play music with soothing sounds such as ocean or rain).
- Stimulate touch (massage, vibrating recliner, fuzzy objects, velvet, silk, stuffed animals).
- Stimulate taste (spices, salt, sugar, sour substances).

Techniques to Lower the Stress Threshold (Hall & Buckwalter, 1987; Miller, 2015)

Address Sundowners Syndrome
- Observe individuals with dementia showing increased agitation, restlessness, and confusion in late afternoon, evening, or night. Consult with prescribing professional if an underlying

condition is suspected, such as a urinary tract infection or sleep apnea, might be worsening sundowning behavior.
- Reduce factors that may aggravate late-day confusion, including
  - Fatigue
  - Low lighting
  - Increased shadows
  - Disruption of the body's "internal clock"
  - Difficulty separating reality from dream

Provide Interventions to Reduce Sundowning (Khachiyants, Trinkle, Son, & Kim)

- Try to maintain a predictable routine for bedtime, waking, meals, and activities.
- Allow for light exposure in the early morning to help set internal clock.
- Discourage daytime napping to regulate sleep cycle.
- Plan for activities and exposure to light during the day to encourage nighttime sleepiness.
- Limit daytime napping.
- Limit caffeine and sugar to morning hours.
- Among many factors, Smith (2010) reported that low lighting and increased shadows may aggravate late-day confusion and sundowning.
- Keep a night light on to reduce agitation that occurs when surroundings are dark or unfamiliar.
- In the evening, try to reduce background noise and stimulating activities, including TV viewing, which can sometimes be upsetting.
- In a strange or unfamiliar setting, bring familiar items—such as photographs—to create a more relaxed, familiar setting.
- Play familiar gentle music in the evening or relaxing sounds of nature, such as the sound of waves.

Initiate Health Teaching and Referrals, as Needed

- Support groups
- Community-based programs (e.g., day care, respite care)
- Alzheimer's association (www.alz.org)
- Assisted living, long-term care facilities

INDIVIDUAL CONTAMINATION

Individual Contamination

Risk for Individual Contamination

NANDA-I Definition

Exposure to environmental contaminants in doses sufficient to cause adverse health effects

Defining Characteristics

Defining characteristics are dependent on the causative agent. Causative agents include pesticides*, chemicals*, biologics*, waste*, radiation*, and pollution*.

Pesticide Exposure Effects

Pulmonary

Anaphylactic reaction
Asthma
Irritation to nose and throat
Burning sensation in throat and chest
Pulmonary edema
Shortness of breath
Pneumonia
Upper airway irritation

Dyspnea
Bronchitis
Pulmonary fibrosis
Chronic obstructive pulmonary disease
Bronchiolitis
Airway hyperreactivity
Damage to the mucous membranes of the respiratory tract

Neurologic

Reye's-like syndrome
Confusion
Anxiety
Seizures
Decreased level of consciousness
Coma
Muscle fasciculation
Skeletal muscle myotonia

Peripheral neuropathy
Pinpoint pupils
Blurred vision
Headache
Dizziness
CNS excitation
Depression
Paresthesia

Gastrointestinal
Nausea, vomiting, diarrhea, and flu-like symptoms

Dermatologic
Chloracne

Cardiac
Cardiac dysrhythmia, tachycardia, bradycardia, conduction block, and hypotension

Hepatic
Liver dysfunction

Chemical Exposure Effects

Pulmonary
Irritation of nose and throat, dyspnea, bronchitis, pulmonary edema, and cough

Neurologic

Headache	Mood changes	Memory changes
Ataxia	Delirium	Encephalopathy
Confusion	Hallucinations	Hearing Loss
Seizures	Nystagmus	Parkinson's-like
Lethargy	Diplopia	syndrome
Unconsciousness	Psychosis	Euphoria
Coma	CNS depression	Narcosis
Lacrimation	Tremors	Syncope
Ataxia	Weakness	Hyperthermia
Vertigo	Paralysis	

Renal
Acetonuria and renal failure

Gastrointestinal

Nausea	Ulceration of the gastrointestinal tract
Vomiting	Metabolic acidosis

Endocrine
Hyperglycemia, hypoglycemia   Dermatologic

Dermatitis

Irritation of the skin and mucous membranes	Dermal burns
Mucosal burns of eyes, nose, pharynx, and larynx	Immunologic
Conjunctivitis	Altered blood clotting and bone marrow depression
Hyperpigmentation of skin and nails	

Reproductive
Shortening of menstrual cycle

Cardiac
Hypotension and chest pain

Ophthalmic
Pupil changes, blurred vision, severe eye pain, corneal irritation, temporary or permanent blindness

Hepatic

| Jaundice | Hepatitis |
| Hepatomegaly | Pancreatitis |

Biologic Exposure Effects

Bacteria
Anthrax (*Bacillus anthracis*): fever, chills, drenching sweats, profound fatigue, minimally productive cough, nausea and vomiting, and chest discomfort
Cholera (*Vibrio cholerae*): profuse watery diarrhea, vomiting, leg cramps, dehydration, and shock
Salmonella (*Salmonellosis*): fever, abdominal cramps, diarrhea (sometimes bloody), localized infection, and sepsis
E. coli (*Escherichia coli* 0157:H7): severe, bloody diarrhea, and abdominal cramps; mild or no fever

Viruses
Smallpox (Variola virus): high fever, head and body aches, vomiting, and skin rash with bumps and raised pustules that crust, scab, and form a pitted scar
Ebola hemorrhagic fever (Ebola filovirus): headache, fever, joint and muscle aches, sore throat, and weaknesses followed by diarrhea, vomiting, stomachache, rash, red eyes, and skin rash
Lassa fever (Lassa virus): fever, retrosternal pain, sore throat, back pain, cough, abdominal pain, vomiting, diarrhea, conjunctivitis, facial swelling, proteinuria, and mucosal bleeding

Toxins
Ricin: respiratory distress, fever, cough, nausea, tightness in chest, heavy sweating, pulmonary edema, cyanosis, hypotension, respiratory failure, hallucinations, seizures, and blood in urine
Staphylococcal enterotoxin B: fever, headache, myalgia, malaise, diarrhea, sore throat, sinus congestion, rhinorrhea, hoarseness, and conjunctivitis

Radiation Exposure Effects

Oncologic
Skin cancer, thyroid cancer, and leukemia

Immunologic
Impaired response to immunizations, bone marrow suppression, autoimmune diseases

Genetic
DNA mutations, teratogenic effect including smaller head or brain size, poorly formed eyes, abnormally slow growth, and mental retardation

Neurologic
CNS damage, malfunctions of the peripheral nervous system, neuro autoimmune changes, and disturbances in neuro-endocrine control

Dermatologic
Burns, skin irritation, dryness, inflammation, erythema, dry or moist desquamation, itching, blistering, and ulceration

Systemic Radiation Poisoning
Nausea, fatigue, weakness, hair loss, changes in blood chemistries, hemorrhage, diminished organ function, and death

Ophthalmic
Cataracts, degeneration of the macula

Cardiovascular
Changes in cardiovascular control, irregular heartbeat, changes in the electrocardiogram, development of atherosclerosis, hypertension, and ischemia

Pulmonary
Disturbances in respiratory volume, increase in the number of allergic illnesses, atypical cells in the bronchial mucosa

Gastrointestinal
Pathologic changes in the digestive system, inflammation of the duodenum, spontaneously hyperplasic mucous membranes

Waste Exposure Effects

Coliform bacteria: diarrhea and abdominal cramps
Giardia lamblia (protozoa): diarrhea, abdominal cramps, nausea, and weight loss
Cryptosporidium (protozoa): diarrhea, headache, abdominal cramps, nausea, vomiting, and low fever

Hepatitis A (enteric virus): lassitude, anorexia, weakness, nausea, fever, and jaundice

Helminths (parasitic worms): diarrhea, vomiting, gas, stomach pain, and loss of appetite

Fever

Pollution Exposure Effects

Pulmonary: coughing, wheezing, labored breathing, pulmonary and nasal congestion, exacerbated allergies, asthma exacerbation, pain when breathing, and lung cancer

Cardiac: chest pain

Neurologic: headaches, developmental delay

Reproductive: reduced fertility

Ophthalmic: eye irritation

Related Factors

Pathophysiologic

Presence of bacteria, viruses, and toxins

Nutritional factors (obesity, vitamin, and mineral deficiencies)

Preexisting disease states

Gender (females have greater proportion of body fat, which increases the chance of accumulating more lipid-soluble toxins than men; pregnancy)

History of smoking

Treatment Related

Recent vaccinations

Insufficient or absent use of decontamination protocol

Inappropriate or no use of protective clothing

Situational (Personal, Environmental)

Flooding, earthquakes, or other natural disasters

Sewer-line leaks

Industrial plant emissions; intentional or accidental discharge of contaminants by industries or businesses

Physical factors: climactic conditions such as temperature, wind; geographic area

Social factors: crowding, sanitation, poverty, personal and household hygiene practices, and lack of access to health care

Biologic factors: presence of vectors (mosquitoes, ticks, rodents)

Bioterrorism
Occupation
Dietary practices

Environmental

Contamination of aquifers by septic tanks
Intentional/accidental contamination of food and water supply
Concomitant or previous exposures
Exposure to heavy metals or chemicals, atmospheric pollutants,
  radiation, bioterrorism, and disaster
Use of environmental contaminants in the home (pesticides,
  chemicals, radon, tobacco smoke)
Playing in outdoor areas where environmental contaminants are
  used
Type of flooring surface

Maturational

Developmental characteristics of children
Children younger than 5 years of age
Older adults
Gestational age during exposure

NOC

Anxiety Level, Fear Level, Grief Resolution, Health Beliefs: Perceived Threat, Immunization Behavior, Infection Control, Knowledge: Health Resources, Personal Safety Behavior, Community Risk Control, Safe Home Environment

Goal

Individual adverse health effects of contamination will be minimized.

NIC

Community Disaster Preparedness, Environmental Management, Anger Control Assistance, Anxiety Reduction, Grief Work Facilitation, Crisis Intervention, Counseling, Health Education, Health Screening, Immunization/Vaccination Management, Infection Control, Resiliency Promotion, Risk Identification

Interventions

General Interventions

Help Individuals Cope With Contamination Incident; Use Groups That Have Survived Terrorist Attacks as a Useful Resource for Victims

- Provide accurate information on risks involved, preventive measures, use of antibiotics, and vaccines.
- Assist victims in dealing with feelings of fear, vulnerability, and grief.
- Encourage victims to talk to others about their fears.
- Assist victims in thinking positively and moving to the future.

Specific Interventions

- Employ skin decontamination with dermal exposures.
- Clinical effects on body systems vary with exposure to specific agents. Monitor carefully and provide supportive care.
- Employ appropriate isolation precautions: universal, airborne, droplet, and contact isolation.

Monitor the Individual for Therapeutic Effects, Side Effects, and Compliance With Postexposure Drug Therapy

Decontamination Procedure
- Primary decontamination of exposed personnel is agent specific.
  - Remove contaminated clothing.
  - Use copious amounts of water and soap or diluted (0.5%) sodium hypochlorite.
- For secondary decontamination from clothing or equipment of those exposed, use proper physical protection.

Risk for Individual Contamination

NANDA-I Definition

Vulnerable to exposure to environmental contaminants in doses sufficient to cause adverse health effects

Risk Factors

See Related Factors under *Individual Contamination*.

NOC
Community Risk Control, Community Health Status, Health Beliefs: Perceived Threat, Knowledge: Health Resources, Knowledge: Health Behavior

Goal

The individual will remain free of the adverse effects of contamination.

NIC
Community Disaster Preparedness Environmental Risk Protection, Environmental Management: Safety, Health Education, Health Screening, Immunization/Vaccination Management, Risk Identification, Surveillance: Safety

Interventions

General Interventions

Provide Accurate Information About Risks Involved and Preventive Measures

- Assist to deal with feelings of fear and vulnerability.
- Encourage them to talk to others about their fears.

Specific Interventions

Conduct Surveillance for Environmental Contamination

- Notify agencies authorized to protect the environment of contaminants in the area.
- Assist individuals in relocating to safer environment.
- Modify the environment to minimize risk.

FAMILY CONTAMINATION

Family Contamination

Risk for Family Contamination

NANDA-I Definition

Exposure to environmental contaminants in doses sufficient to cause adverse health effects

Defining Characteristics

Refer to Defining Characteristics for *Individual Contamination* and *Community Contamination*.

Related Factors

Refer to Defining Characteristics for *Individual Contamination* and *Community Contamination*.

NOC
Refer to *Individual Contamination* and *Community Contamination* for possible NOC outcomes.

Goal

Family adverse health effects of contamination will be minimized.

NIC
Refer to *Individual Contamination* and *Community Contamination* for possible NOC outcomes. Also refer to appropriate NIC interventions based on family's defining characteristics.

Interventions

Refer to *Individual Contamination* and *Community Contamination* for possible interventions.

Risk for Community Contamination

NANDA-I Definition

For exposure to environmental contaminants in doses sufficient to cause adverse health effects

Risk Factors

Refer to Related Factors under *Community Contamination*.

NOC
Community Disaster Readiness, Community Health Status, Community Risk Control: Communicable Disease; see *Community Contamination* for other possible NOC outcomes

Goals

- Community will use health surveillance data system to monitor for contamination incidents.
- Community will participate in mass casualty and disaster readiness drills.
- Community will remain free of contamination-related health effects.

NIC
Environmental Management, Environmental Risk Protection, Community Health Development, Bioterrorism Preparedness, Communicable Disease Management, Community Disaster Preparedness, Health Education, Health Policy Monitoring, Surveillance: Community

Interventions

Monitor for Contamination Incidents Using Health Surveillance Data

Provide Accurate Information About Risks Involved and Preventive Measures

- Encourage community members to talk to others about their fears.

Specific Interventions

Identify Community Risk Factors and Develop Programs to Prevent Disasters From Occurring

- Notify agencies authorized to protect the environment from contaminants in the area.
- Modify the environment to minimize risk.

INEFFECTIVE COPING

Ineffective Coping

Defensive Coping

Ineffective Impulse Control

Ineffective Denial

Labile Emotional Control

Impaired Mood Regulation

NANDA-I Definition

Inability to form a valid appraisal of the stressors, inadequate choices of practiced responses, and/or inability to use available resources

Defining Characteristics

Verbalization of inability to cope or ask for help*

Inappropriate use of defense mechanisms

Inability to meet role expectations*

Chronic worry, anxiety

Sleep disturbance*

Fatigue*

High illness rate*

Reported difficulty with life stressors

Poor concentration*

Difficulty organizing information*

Decreased use of social support*

Inadequate problem solving*

Impaired social participation

Use of forms of coping that impede adaptive behavior*

Risk taking*

Lack of goal-directed behavior*

Destructive behavior toward self or others*

Change in usual communication patterns*

High incidence of accidents

Substance abuse*

Related Factors

Pathophysiologic

Related to chronicity of condition

Related to biochemical changes in brain secondary to:
Bipolar disorder   Personality disorder
Chemical dependency   Attention-deficient disorders
Schizophrenia

Related to complex self-care regimens

Related to neurologic changes in brain secondary to:
Stroke   Multiple sclerosis
Alzheimer's disease   End-stage diseases

Related to changes in body integrity secondary to:
Loss of body part   Disfigurement secondary to trauma

Related to altered affect caused by changes secondary to:
Body chemistry   Intake of mood-altering substance
Tumor (brain)   Mental retardation

Treatment Related

Related to separation from family and home (e.g., hospitalization, nursing home)

Related to disfigurement caused by surgery

Related to altered appearance from drugs, radiation, or other treatment

Situational (Personal, Environmental)

Related to poor impulse control and frustration tolerance

Related to disturbed relationship with parent/caregiver

Related to disorganized family system

Related to ineffective problem-solving skills

Related to increased food consumption in response to stressors

Related to changes in physical environment secondary to:
War   Poverty   Natural disaster
Homelessness   Relocation   Inadequate finances
Seasonal work

Related to disruption of emotional bonds secondary to:
Death   Institutionalization   Relocation
Desertion   Separation or divorce   Orphanage/foster care
Jail   Educational institution

Related to unsatisfactory support system

Related to sensory overload secondary to:
Factory environment
Urbanization: crowding, noise pollution, excessive activity

Related to inadequate psychological resources secondary to:

Poor self-esteem

Excessive negative beliefs about self

Negative role modeling

Helplessness

Lack of motivation to respond

Related to culturally related conflicts with (specify):
Premarital sex
Abortion

Maturational

Child/Adolescent
Related to:

Poor impulse control

Parental substance abuse

Inconsistent methods of discipline

Repressed anxiety

Panic

Childhood trauma

Poor social skills

Peer rejection

Parental rejection

Fear of failure

Adolescent
Related to inadequate psychological resources to adapt to:

Physical and emotional changes

Educational demands

Sexual awareness

Sexual relationships

Independence from family

Career choices

Young Adult
Related to inadequate psychological resources to adapt to:

Career choices

Parenthood

Marriage

Leaving home

Educational demands

Middle Adult
Related to inadequate psychological resources to adapt to:

Physical signs of aging

Social status needs

Problems with relatives

Child-rearing problems

Career pressures

Aging parents

Older Adult
Related to inadequate psychological resources to adapt to:

Physical changes

Retirement

Changes in residence

Changes in financial status

Author's Note

Margaret O's son Nicholas, age 26, diagnosed with schizophrenia died on a psychiatric unit of mixed drug toxicity. Margaret wrote to students in mental health "To care for people with mental illness in times of crisis with insight and compassion . . . these are my hopes for you" (Procter, Hamer, McGarry, Wilson, & Froggatt, 2014, p vii).

World Health Organization (WHO, 2014) defines mental health "as a state of well-being in which every individual realizes his or her own potential, can cope with the normal stresses of life, can work productively and fruitfully, and is able to make a contribution to her or his community." In addition, WHO has described mental health and illness as follows:

- Mental health is an integral part of health; indeed, there is no health without mental health.
- Mental health is more than the absence of mental disorders.
- Mental and substance use disorders are the leading cause of disability worldwide. Mental disorders increase the risk of getting ill from other diseases such as HIV, cardiovascular disease, diabetes, and vice versa.
- Stigma and discrimination against patients and families prevent people from seeking mental health care.

Ineffective Coping describes a person who is experiencing difficulty adapting to stressful event(s). *Ineffective Coping* can be a recent, episodic problem or a chronic problem. Usual effective coping mechanisms may be inappropriate or ineffective, or the person may have a poor history of coping with stressors.

If the event is recent, *Ineffective Coping* may be a premature judgment. For example, a person may respond to overwhelming stress with a grief response such as denial, anger, or sadness, making a *Grieving* diagnosis appropriate.

Impaired Adjustment may be more useful than *Ineffective Coping* in the initial period after a stressful event. *Ineffective Coping* and its related diagnoses may be more applicable to prolonged or chronic coping problems, such as *Defensive Coping* for a person with a long-standing pattern of ineffective coping.

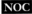 **NOC**
Coping, Self-Esteem, Social Interaction Skills

Goals

The person will make decisions and follow through with appropriate actions to change provocative situations in the personal environment, as evidenced by the following indicators:

- Verbalize feelings related to emotional state
- Focus on the present
- Identify personal strengths, and accept support through the nursing relationship

The child/adolescent will comply "with requests and limits on behavior in absence of arguments, tantrums, or other acting-out behaviors," as evidenced by the following indicators (Varcarolis, 2011):

- Demonstrate increased impulse control within (specify time)
- Demonstrate the ability to tolerate frustration and delay gratification within (specify time)
- Demonstrate an absence of tantrums, rage reactions, or other acting-out behaviors within (specify time)
- Describe the behavior limits and rationale to an authority figure
- Acknowledge the responsibility for misbehaviors and increased impulse control within (specify time)

NIC

Coping Enhancement, Counseling, Emotional Support, Active Listening, Assertiveness Training, Behavior Modification

Interventions

Assess Causative and Contributing Factors

- Refer to Related Factors.

Establish Rapport

- Spend time with the individual. Provide supportive companionship.
- Avoid being overly cheerful and cliché such as, "Things will get better."
- Convey honesty and empathy.
- Offer support. Encourage expression of feelings. Let the individual know you understand his or her feelings. Do not argue with expressions of worthlessness by saying things such as, "How can you say that? Look at all you accomplished in life."
- Offer matter-of-fact appraisals. Be realistic.
- Allow extra time for the individual to respond.

Assess Present Coping Status

- Determine the onset of feelings and symptoms and their correlation with events and life changes.

- Listen carefully as the individual speaks; observe facial expressions, gestures, eye contact, body positioning, and tone and intensity of voice.
- Determine the risk of the individual's inflicting self-harm; intervene appropriately.
- Assess for signs of potential suicide:
  - History of previous attempts or threats (overt and covert)
  - Changes in personality, behavior, sex life, appetite, and sleep habits
  - Preparations for death (putting things in order, making a will, giving away personal possessions, acquiring a weapon)
  - Sudden elevation in mood
- See *Risk for Suicide* for additional information on suicide prevention.

Assist the Individual in Developing Appropriate Problem-Solving Strategies

- Ask the individual to describe previous encounters with conflict and how he or she resolved them.
- Evaluate whether his or her stress response is "fight or flight" or "tend and befriend."
- Encourage the individual to evaluate his or her behavior. "Did that work for you?" "How did it help?" "What did you learn from that experience?"
- Discuss possible alternatives (i.e., talk over the problem with those involved, try to change the situation, or do nothing and accept the consequences).
- Assist the individual in identifying problems that he or she cannot control directly; help the individual to practice stress-reducing activities for control (e.g., exercise, yoga).
- Be supportive of functional coping behaviors. (e.g., "The way you handled this situation 2 years ago worked well then. Can you do it now?")
- Mobilize the individual to gradually increase activity:
  - Identify activities that were previously gratifying but have been neglected: personal grooming or dress habits, shopping, hobbies, athletic endeavors, and arts and crafts.
  - Encourage to include these activities in the daily routine for a set time span (e.g., "I will play the piano for 30 minutes every afternoon").
- Explore outlets that foster feelings of personal achievement and self-esteem:
  - Make time for relaxing activities (e.g., dancing, exercising, sewing, woodworking).
  - Find a helper to take over responsibilities occasionally (e.g., sitter).

- Learn to compartmentalize (do not carry problems around with you always; enjoy free time).
- Encourage longer vacations (not just a few days here and there).
- Provide opportunities to learn and use stress management techniques (e.g., jogging, yoga).
- Teach self-monitoring tools (*Finkelman, 2000):
  - Develop a daily schedule to monitor for signs of improvement or worsening.
  - Discuss reasonable goals for present relationships.
  - Write down what is done when in control, depressed, confused, angry, and happy.
  - Identify activities tried, would like to try, or should do more.
  - Create a warning sign checklist that indicates worsening and how to access help.

Differentiate Possible Problem-Solving Techniques

- Goal setting is consciously setting time limits on behaviors, which is useful when goals are attainable and manageable. It may become stress-inducing if unrealistic or short-sighted.
- Information seeking is learning about all aspects of a problem, which provides perspective and, in some cases, reinforces self-control.
- Mastery is learning new procedures or skills, which facilitates self-esteem and self-control (e.g., self-care of colostomies, insulin injection, or catheter care).

Initiate Health Teaching and Referrals, as Indicated

- Prepare for problems that may occur after transition and constructive responses:
  - Medications—schedule, cost, misuse, side effects
  - Increased anxiety
  - Sleep problems
  - Family/significant other conflicts
  - Follow-up—forgetting, access, difficulty organizing time
- Instruct in relaxation techniques; emphasize the importance of setting 15 to 20 minutes aside each day to practice relaxation:
  - Find a comfortable position in a chair or on the floor.
  - Close the eyes.
  - Keep the noise to a minimum (only very soft music, if desired).
  - Concentrate on breathing slowly and deeply.
  - Feel the heaviness of all extremities.
  - If muscles are tense, tighten, then relax each one from toes to scalp.

⚛ Pediatric Interventions

Assess for Attention Difficulties With Parent and Child (AAP, 2015)

- Daydream a lot
- Forget or lose things a lot
- Squirm or fidget
- Talk too much
- Make careless mistakes or take unnecessary risks
- Have a hard time resisting temptation
- Have trouble taking turns
- Have difficulty getting along with others

Provide Consistency in Interactions, Expectations, and Consequences

- Establish eye contact before giving instructions.
- Set firm, responsible limits; do not lecture. Avoid power struggles and no-win situation. Look for a compromise.
- Monitor for rising levels of frustration. Intervene early to calm child.
- Reinforce appropriate behavior with a positive reinforcer (e.g., praise, hug).
- Advise parents to avoid disagreeing with each other in child's presence.
- If hyperactive, provide for periods of activity using large muscles.
- Provide immediate and constant feedback.
- Advise parents to consult with educational professionals for educational programming.

Teach Parents/Caregivers of Hyperactive Children to (CDC, 2015)

- Create a routine: Try to follow the same schedule every day, from wake-up time to bedtime.
- Get organized: Put schoolbags, clothing, and toys in the same place every day so your child will be less likely to lose them.
- Avoid distractions: Turn off the TV, radio, and computer, especially when your child is doing homework.
- Limit choices: Offer a choice between two things (this outfit, meal, toy, etc. or that one) so that your child is not overwhelmed and overstimulated.
- Change your interactions with your child: Instead of long-winded explanations and cajoling, use clear, brief directions to remind your child of responsibilities.
- Use goals and rewards: Use a chart to list goals and track positive behaviors, then reward your child's efforts. Be sure the goals are realistic—baby steps are important!

- Discipline effectively: Instead of yelling or spanking, use time-outs or removal of privileges as consequences for inappropriate behavior.
- Help your child discover a talent: All kids need to experience success to feel good about themselves. Finding out what your child does well—whether it is sports, art, or music—can boost social skills and self-esteem.

Provide Information About Medication Therapy if Indicated

- Refer to specialists as needed (e.g., psychological, learning specialists).

Geriatric Interventions

Assess for Risk Factors for Ineffective Coping in Older Adults (Miller, 2015)

- Inadequate economic resources
- Immature developmental level
- Unanticipated stressful events
- Several major events in short period
- Unrealistic goals

Evaluate Coping Resources Available (Miller, 2015)

- Social supports, especially religious support
- Instrumental support (meals, transportation, personal care)
- Emotional support that he or she is valued, loved, and respected
- Information support regarding resources available

Specifically Address Daily Stressors (Food Preparation, Medication Schedule, Self-Care, and Housekeeping)

- Review possible options to reduce daily stress (e.g., weekly pill boxes, frozen complete meals).

Defensive Coping

NANDA-I Definition

Repeated projection of falsely positive self-evaluation based on a self-protective pattern that defends against underlying perceived threats to positive self-regard.

Defining Characteristics*

Delays seeking health care
Denies fear of death
Denies fear of invalidism
Displaces fear of impact of the condition
Displaces sources of symptoms
Does not admit impact of disease on life
Does not perceive relevance of danger
Does not perceive relevance of symptoms
Inappropriate affect
Minimizes symptoms
Refusal of health care
Use of dismissive gestures when speaking of distressing events
Use of treatment not advised by health-care professional

Related Factors*

Related to:

Conflict between self-
    perception and value system
Deficient support system
Fear of failure
Fear of humiliation
Fear of repercussions

Low level of confidence in
    others
Low level of self-confidence
Uncertainty
Unrealistic expectations of
    self

 Author's Note

In selecting this diagnosis, it is important to consider the potentially related diagnoses of *Chronic Low Self-Esteem, Powerlessness,* and *Impaired Social Interaction.* They may express how the person established, or why he or she maintains, the defensive pattern.

Defensive Coping is the "repeated projection of falsely-positive self-evaluation based on a self-protection pattern that defends against perceived threats to positive self-regard" (Halter, 2014; Varcarolis, 2011). When a defensive pattern is a barrier to effective relationships, *Defensive Coping* is a useful diagnosis.

NOC

Acceptance: Health Status, Coping, Self-Esteem, Social Interaction Skills

Goals

The individual will demonstrate appropriate interactions with others and report that they feel safe and are more in control, as evidenced by the following indicators:

- Adhere to treatment, for example, medications, therapy, and goals
- Use newly learned constructive methods to deal with stress and promote feelings of control
- Remove self from situations that increase their anxiety

The child/adolescent will comply "with requests and limits on behavior in absence of arguments, tantrums, or other acting-out behaviors", as evidenced by the following indicators (Varcarolis, 2011):

- Demonstrate increased impulse control within (specify time)
- Demonstrate ability to tolerate frustration and delay gratification within (specify time)
- Demonstrate an absence of tantrums, rage reactions, or other acting-out behaviors within (specify time)
- Describe the behavior limits and rationale to an authority figure
- Acknowledge responsibility for misbehaviors and increased impulse control within (specify time)

NIC

Coping Enhancement, Emotional Support, Self-Awareness Enhancement, Environment Management, Presence, Active Listening

Interventions

Reduce Demands on the Individual If Stress Levels Increase

- Modify the level of or remove environmental stimuli (e.g., noise, activity).
- Decrease (or limit) contacts with others (e.g., visitors, other individuals, staff) as required.
- Clearly articulate minimal expectations for activities. Decrease or increase as tolerated.
- Identify stressors placing demands on the individual's coping resources; develop plans to deal with them. The general goal is to freeze, reduce, or eliminate stress; more specifically, it is to target and deal with those stressors most exacerbating the defensive pattern.

Establish a Therapeutic Relationship

- Maintain a neutral, matter-of-fact tone with a consistent positive regard. Ensure that all staff relate in a consistent fashion, with consistent expectations.
- Focus on simple, here-and-now, goal-directed topics when encountering the individual's defenses.
- Do not react to, defend, or dwell on the individual's negative projections or displacements; also do not challenge distortions or unrealistic/grandiose self-expressions. Try instead to shift to more neutral, positive, or goal-directed topics.
- Avoid control issues; attempt to present positive options to the individual, which allows a measure of choice.
- To promote learning from the individual's own actions (i.e., "natural consequences"), identify those actions that have interfered with the achievement of established goals.
- Reinforce more adaptive coping patterns (e.g., formal problem solving, rationalization) that assist the person in achieving established goals.
- Evaluate interactions, progress, and approach with other team members to ensure consistency within the treatment milieu.

Promote Dialogue to Decrease Paranoia and Permit a More Direct Addressing of Underlying Related Factors (see also Chronic Low Self-Esteem)

- Validate the individual's reluctance to trust in the beginning. Over time, reinforce the consistency of your statements, responses, and actions. Give special attention to your meeting of (reasonable) requests or your following through with plans and agreements.
- Use clear, simple language. Explain activities before you do them.
- Be honest, nonjudgmental, and nondefensive; take a neutral approach.
- Do not whisper, laugh, or engage in behavior that can be misinterpreted.
- Engage the individual in diversional, non–goal-directed, noncompetitive activities (e.g., relaxation therapy, games, and outings).
  - Initially, provide solitary, noncompetitive activities (Varcarolis, 2011).
  - Encourage self-expression of neutral themes, positive reminiscences, and so forth.
  - Encourage other means for self-expression (e.g., writing, art) if verbal interaction is difficult or if this is an area of personal strength.

- Listen passively to *some* grandiose or negative self-expression to reinforce your positive regard. If this does not lead to more positive self-expression or activity, then such listening may prove counterproductive.

Ineffective Impulse Control

NANDA-I Definition

A pattern of performing rapid, unplanned reactions to internal or external stimuli without regard to negative consequences of these reactions to the impulsive individual or to others

Defining Characteristics*

Acting without thinking
Gambling addiction
Asking questions of others despite their discomfort
Sensation seeking
Bulimia

Sexual promiscuity
Inability to save money or regulate finances
Inappropriate sharing of personal details
Temper outbursts
Too familiar with strangers

Related Factors

Alcohol dependence
Disorder of cognition*
Anger*
Disorder of development*
Codependency*
Disorder of mood*
Compunction*
Disorder of personality*
Delusion*
Disorder of body image
Denial*
Substance abuse (drugs)
Disorder of brain function

Environment that might cause irritation or frustration*
Fatigue*
Hopelessness*
Ineffective coping*
Insomnia*
Low self-esteem
Poor
Smoker*
Social isolation*
Stress vulnerability*
Suicidal feelings*
Unpleasant physical symptoms*

Author's Note

Ineffective Impulse Control is a new NANDA-I nursing diagnosis that represents a behavior that can cause a variety of problems in the individual or to others such as substance abuse, violence, sexual promiscuity, and so on. It is a component of the *DSM-5* diagnoses *Personality Disorders*, *Oppositional Defiant Disorder*, *Intermittent Explosive Disorder*, and *Conduct Disorder*.

It may be more clinically useful to view *Ineffective Impulse Control* as behavior that contributes to a nursing diagnosis and/or a manifestation rather than as the response or nursing diagnosis. For example, *Risk for Other-Directed Violence*, *Ineffective Coping*, *Dysfunctional Family Processes*, *Defensive Coping*, *Self-Mutilation*, *Impaired Social Interactions*, *Loneliness*, *Noncompliance*, *Ineffective Health Maintenance*, and *Stress Overload* all can have a component of poor impulse control that contributes to the diagnosis.

The clinician can choose to use *Ineffective Impulse Control* as a nursing diagnosis or can use a more specific nursing diagnosis as discussed in this Author's Note. The following interventions can also be used with the aforementioned diagnoses.

NOC

Impulse Self-Control, Suicide Self-Restraint

Goals

The individual will consistently demonstrate the use of effective coping responses, as evidenced by the following indicators:

- Identify consequences of impulsive behavior
- Identify feelings that precede impulsive behavior
- Control impulsive behavior

NIC

Self-Awareness Enhancement, Presence, Counseling, Behavioral Modification, Anger Control, Coping Enhancement, Milieu Therapy, Limit Setting

Interventions

"In a Respectful, Neutral Manner, Explain Expected Individual Behaviors, Limits, and Responsibilities" (Varcarolis, 2011)

Explain a Behavioral Contract and Its Components (Videbeck, 2013)

- The individual identifies
  - Their problematic behavior and how it affects others

- An alternative to the problematic behavior
- A reward (the reward may be that communication focuses on making a positive choice and the feeling of success)
- The consequences of a poor choice, which results in a negative response from others
- If written, sign and date (both individual and clinician).
- When a positive choice is observed or related, specifically address how the individual feels.
- When a problematic choice is observed or related, specifically address how the individual feels about the situational response. Focus on to continue the process of trying.

Encourage Participation in Group Therapy

- Avoid
  - Giving attention to inappropriate behaviors
  - Showing own frustration
  - Accepting gift giving, flattery, seductive behaviors, and instilling guilt by individuals (Varcarolis, 2011)

Initiate Referrals as Indicated

- Social services
- Vocational rehabilitation
- Legal services

Ineffective Denial

NANDA-I Definition

Conscious or unconscious attempt to disavow the knowledge or meaning of an event to reduce anxiety and/or fear, leading to the detriment of health

Defining Characteristics[8]

Major* (Must Be Present)

Delays seeking or refuses health-care attention
Does not perceive personal relevance of symptoms or danger

---

[8] *Source*: Lynch, C. S., & Phillips, M. W. (1989). Nursing diagnosis: Ineffective denial. In R. M. Carroll-Johnson (Ed.), *Classification of nursing diagnosis: Proceedings of the eighth conference*. Philadelphia, PA: J. B. Lippincott.

Minor (May Be Present)

Uses home remedies (self-treatment) to relieve symptoms
Does not admit fear of death or invalidism*
Minimizes symptoms*
Displaces the source of symptoms to other areas of the body
Cannot admit the effects of the disease on life pattern
Makes dismissive gestures when speaking of distressing events*
Displaces the fear of effects of the condition
Displays inappropriate affect*

Related Factors

Pathophysiologic

Related to inability to tolerate consciously the consequences of (any chronic or terminal illness) secondary to:

AIDS	HIV infection
Cancer	Progressive debilitating disorders (e.g., multiple sclerosis, myasthenia gravis)

Treatment Related

Related to prolonged treatment with no positive results

Psychological

Related to inability to tolerate consciously the consequences of (Halter, 2014; Varcarolis, 2011):

Loss of a job	Obesity
Financial crisis	Loss of spouse/ significant other
Negative self-concept, inadequacy, guilt, loneliness, despair, sense of failure	Domestic abuse
Smoking	

Related to inability to tolerate consciously physical or/and emotional dependence on (Halter, 2014; Varcarolis, 2011):

Alcohol	Cannabis
Cocaine, crack	Barbiturates/sedatives
Stimulants	Hallucinogens
Opiates	

Related to long-term self-destructive patterns of behavior and lifestyle (Varcarolis, 2011)

Related to feelings of increased anxiety/stress, need to escape personal problems, anger, and frustration

Related to feelings of omnipotence

Related to genetic origins of alcoholism

 Author's Note

Ineffective Denial differs from denial in response to loss. Denial in response to illness or loss is necessary and beneficial to maintain psychological equilibrium. *Ineffective Denial* is not beneficial when the person will not participate in regimens to improve health or the situation (e.g., denies substance abuse). If the cause is not known, *Ineffective Denial related to unknown etiology* can be used, such as *Ineffective Denial related to unknown etiology as evidenced by repetitive refusal to admit barbiturate use is a problem*.

NOC

Acceptance: Health Status, Anxiety Self-Control, Fear Self-Control, Health Beliefs: Perceived Threat

Goals

The individual will use alternative coping mechanism in response to stressor instead of denial, as evidenced by the following indicators:

- Acknowledge the source of anxiety or stress
- Use problem-focused coping skills

OR

The individual will maintain abstinence from alcohol/drug use and state recognition of the need for continued treatment, as evidenced by the following indicators (Halter, 2014; Varcarolis, 2011):

Immediate
- Acknowledge an addiction problem and responsibility for own behavior
- Express a sense of hope
- Identify three areas of one's life that drugs have negatively affected*
- State recognition of the need for continued treatment
- Agree to contact a support person when feeling the need to abuse*
- Abstain from substance or behavior addiction

Postacute
- Acknowledge when using denial rationalization and projection in relation to their addiction
- Participate in a support group at least three times a week by (specify)*
- Identify three alternative strategies to cope with stressors*
- Have a plan for high-risk situations for relapse

NIC
Teaching: Disease Process, Anxiety Reduction, Counseling, Active Listening

Interventions

Initiate a Therapeutic Relationship

- Assess effectiveness of denial.
- Avoid confronting the individual that he or she is using denial.
- Approach the individual directly, matter-of-factly, and nonjudgmentally.

Encourage the Individual to Share Perceptions of the Situation (e.g., Fears, Anxieties)

- Focus on the feelings shared.
- Use reflection to encourage more sharing.

When Appropriate, Help the Individual With Problem Solving

- Attempt to elicit from the individual a description of the problem.

Assist the Individual to Understand Addictions

- Be nonjudgmental.
- Assist the individual to gain an intellectual understanding that this is an illness, not a moral problem.
- Provide opportunities to perform successfully; gradually increase responsibility.
- Provide educational information about the progressive nature of substance abuse and its effects on the body and interpersonal relationships.
- Explain that "addiction does not cure itself" and that it requires abstinence and treatment of the underlying issues (Varcarolis, 2011, p. 336).
- Provide opportunities to share fears and anxieties.
- Focus on present response.
- Assist in lowering anxiety level (see *Anxiety* for additional interventions).

- Avoid confronting person on use of denial.
- Carefully explore with person his or her interpretation of the situation:
  - Reflect self-reported cues used to minimize the situation (e.g., "a little," "only").
  - Identify recent detrimental behavior and discuss the effects of this behavior on health.
- Emphasize strengths and past successful coping.
- Provide positive reinforcement for any expressions of insight.
- Do not accept rationalization or projection. Be polite, caring, but firm.
- If substance abuse is present:
  - Review observations and findings with individual and family.
  - Present evidence of damage (e.g., physical, social, financial, spiritual, familial).
  - Establish goals.
  - Provide self-help manuals or other pamphlets.
  - Acquire commitment to keep daily log of alcohol/drug use.
- At next visit:
  - Review log.
  - Review progress.
  - Refer those who are dependent and desire to continue abstinence.
  - Explain why women are more affected by alcohol than are men.

Initiate Health Teaching and Referrals

- Explain the probability of genetic predisposition, the addiction, and the importance of prevention.
- Encourage a discussion on addictions, substances, and behavioral with family.
- Monitor for early signs in children (e.g., impulsivity, unable to delay gratification).
- Seek out appropriate assistance: primary care provider, pediatrician, support groups suggesting a possible shared genetic vulnerability between pathological gambling and other addictions (Grant, 2011; *Shah, Potenza, & Eisen, 2004).
- Advise the individual to consult with primary care provider regarding pharmaceutical treatment if indicated (e.g., opioid antagonists [naltrexone, nalmefene], selective serotonin reuptake inhibitors [SSRIs]).
- Refer to Alcoholics Anonymous, Al-Anon, or Alateen.
- Refer to a treatment facility for a structured treatment program.
- Reinforce healthy living choices (e.g., balanced diet, exercise, recreation, rest).

Labile Emotional Control

NANDA-I Definition

Uncontrollable outbursts of exaggerated and involuntary emotional expression

Defining Characteristics

Absence of eye contact
Difficulty in use of facial
expressions
Embarrassment regarding
emotional expression
Excessive crying without feeling
sadness
Excessive laughing without
feeling happiness
Expression of emotional incongruent with triggering factor
Involuntary crying
Involuntary laughing

Tearfulness
Uncontrollable crying
Uncontrollable laughing
Withdrawal from
occupational situation
Withdrawal from social
situation
Mood swings[9]
Angry outbursts[9]
Behavior outbursts,
threats, throwing
objects[9]

Related Factors

Alternation in self-esteem
Brain injury[10] (e.g., traumatic,
stroke, tumors)
Emotional disturbance
Fatigue
Functional impairment
Insufficient knowledge about
symptom control
Insufficient knowledge of disease
Insufficient muscle strength

Mood disorder
Musculoskeletal
impairment
Pharmaceutical agent
Physical disability
Psychiatric disorder
Social distress
Stressors
Substance abuse

---

[9]Added by Lynda Juall Carpenito for clarity and usefulness.
[10]Neurological disorders, e.g., Parkinson's disease, amyotrophic lateral sclerosis, extrapyramidal and cerebellar disorders, multiple sclerosis, Alzheimer's disease.

Author's Note

Labile Emotional Control, as approved by NANDA-I, represents two different responses, with two distinct origins. One is represented in a neurologic disorder [pseudobulbar affect (PBA)] "of emotional expression characterized clinically by frequent, involuntary, and uncontrollable outbursts of laughing and/or crying that are incongruous with or disproportionate to the patient's emotional state" (Ahmed & Simmons, 2013).

The other is emotional dysregulation. "Emotional dysregulation (ED) is a term used in the mental health community to refer to an emotional response that is poorly modulated, and does not fall within the conventionally accepted range of emotive response. ED may be referred to as labile mood (marked fluctuation of mood) or mood swings" (Beauchaine, Gatzke-KoppL, & Mead, 2007).

Labile emotional responses, which are mood swings, disrupt relationships. Smoking, self-harm, eating disorders, and addiction have all been associated with ED. A functional health assessment would be indicated to validate how these mood swings are negatively affecting the individual/ family lives. Thus labile emotions would then be related factors or sign/ symptoms of a nursing diagnosis (e.g., *Risk for Violence, Disabled Family Coping, Fear*).

Labile Emotional Control, defined as uncontrollable outbursts of exaggerated and involuntary emotional expression, would represent involuntary crying and/or laughing related to neurologic etiology.

NOC

Coping: Self-Esteem, Knowledge: Stress Management

Goals

The person will report improved satisfaction with the response of others to his or her behavior, as evidenced by the following indicators:

- Describe responses of others as respectful
- Report privacy is maintained

NIC

Family Integrity Promotion, Coping Enhancement, Emotional Support, Caregiver Support

Interventions

Explain the Cause of Labile Emotions

- The frontal lobe of our brain normally keeps our emotions under control. The cerebellum and brain stem are where our reflexes are mediated. In PBA, there is a disconnect between the frontal lobe of the brain and the cerebellum and brain stem.
- The response is often a normal reaction in standard contexts but is combined with evidence of impaired ability to regulate an excessive or prolonged emotional response (e.g., laughs at a joke; Wortzel et al., 2008).

Explain the Possibility That Emotional Lability Is Often Worse Soon After the Stroke Happens, But Usually Lessens or Goes Away With Time as the Person Recovers (Olney, Goodkind, & Lomen-Hoerth, 2011)

- Gently explore his or her feelings.
- If appropriate, ask the person affected how they would like to be treated when they have an episode of crying.

Observe for Triggers (Acquired Brain Injury Outreach Service, 2011)

- Fatigue
- Increased stress
- Excessive stimuli (e.g., loud music, multiple conversations)
- Discussions of sensitive topics (e.g., finances, work, speaking in a group)

Provide a Rest Period Before an Activity (e.g., Physical Therapy, Mealtime, Visiting Time)

In Response to Uncontrolled Crying or Laughing, It May be Helpful to (Acquired Brain Injury Outreach Service, 2011)

- Try and change the subject
- Redirect the person to a different activity (e.g., short walk)
- Instruct to take deep breaths
- Avoid tell the person to control themselves
- Be matter of fact
- Touch their arm, if appropriate
- Ask if they want you to stay or leave

Provide Information and Education to Those Who Witness the Uncontrolled Outburst. Advise Them Not to Laugh

Initiate Health Teaching and Referral as Needed

- Provide counseling and support (e.g., individual, family).
- Advise to pursue strategies to reduce stress (e.g., exercise, relaxation breathing).
- Refer to community agencies if indicated (e.g., home health care, social services).

Impaired Mood Regulation

Definition

A mental state characterized by shifts in mood or affect and which is comprised of a constellation of affective, cognitive, somatic, and/or psychological manifestations varying from mild to severe.

Defining Characteristics

Changes in verbal behavior
Disinhibition
Dysphoria
Excessive guilt
Excessive self-awareness
Excessive self-blame
Flight of thoughts
Hopelessness

Impaired concentration
Influenced self-esteem
Irritability
Psychomotor agitation
Psychomotor retardation
Sad effect
Withdrawal

Related Factors

Alteration in sleep pattern
Anxiety
Appetite change
Chronic illness
Functional impairment
Hypervigilance
Impaired social functioning
Loneliness

Pain
Psychosis
Recurrent thoughts of death
Recurrent thoughts of suicide
Social isolation
Substance misuse
Weight change

Author's Note

The top five mental illnesses listed as the primary diagnosis for hospitalization are mood disorders, substance-related disorders, delirium/dementia, anxiety disorders, and schizophrenia (Halter, 2014). Mood disorders include bipolar disorders and major depressive disorders (APA, 2014). *Impaired Mood Regulation*, as approved by NANDA-I above, represents manifestations of individuals with bipolar or major depressive disorders. Some of related factors represent signs and symptoms of mood disorders (e.g., alteration in sleep pattern, appetite changes, hypervigilance); some are individual's responses to *Impaired Mood Regulation* as social isolation, weight change, loneliness substance abuse, recurrent thoughts of death, recurrent thoughts of suicide, impaired social functioning, anxiety. The principle treatment for bipolar or major depressive disorders are medications, which can stabilize the individual's mood fluctuations.

Impaired Mood Regulation is not the focus of nursing interventions. Using a Functional Health Assessment, the nurse, the individual, and the family will determine which patterns are disrupted by the individual's mood disorder. Some related nursing diagnoses are *Risk for Self-Harm*, *Insomnia*, *Ineffective Coping*, *Compromised Family Coping*, *Defensive Coping*, *Impaired Social Interactions*, *Risk for Violence to Others*, and *Ineffective Denial*. Refer to the specific nursing diagnoses throughout this book.

INEFFECTIVE COMMUNITY COPING

NANDA-I Definition

Pattern of community activities for adaptation and problem solving that is unsatisfactory for meeting the demands or needs of the community

Defining Characteristics*

Community does not meet its own expectations
Deficits in community participation
Excessive community conflicts
Reports of community powerlessness
Reports of community vulnerability
High rates of illness

Increased social problems (e.g., homicides, vandalism, arson,
    terrorism, robbery, infanticide, abuse, divorce, unemployment,
    poverty, militancy, mental illness)
Stressors perceived as excessive

Risk Factors

Presence of risk factors (see Related Factors)

Related Factors

Situational

*Related to ineffective or nonexistent community systems (e.g., lack of
emergency medical system, transportation system, disaster planning
system)*[11]

Related to lack of knowledge of resources

Related to inadequate communication patterns

Related to inadequate community cohesiveness

Related to inadequate resources for problem solving[11]

Related to natural disasters[11] *secondary to:*
Flood   Epidemic
Hurricane   Avalanche
Earthquake

Related to traumatic effects of[11]:
Airplane crash   Environmental accident
Industrial disaster   Earthquake
Large fire

*Related to threat to community safety (e.g., murder, rape, kidnapping,
robberies)*[11]

Related to sudden rise in community unemployment

Maturational

Related to inadequate resources for:
Children   Adolescents
Working parents   Older adults

---

[11]These represent risk factors for *Risk for Ineffective Community Coping*. Refer to
    Author's Note for additional clarification.

Author's Note

Ineffective Community Coping is a diagnosis of a community that does not have a constructive system in place to cope with events or changes that occur. The focus of interventions is to improve community dialogue, planning, and resource identification.

When a community has experienced a natural disaster (e.g., hurricane, flood), a threat to safety (e.g., murder, violence, rape), or a man-made disaster (e.g., airplane crash, large fire), the focus should be on preventive strategies. The diagnosis *Risk for Ineffective Community Coping* is more appropriate when the community has been a victim of a disaster or a violent crime.

NOC

Community Competence, Community Health Status, Community Risk Control

Goals

The community will engage in effective problem solving, as evidenced by the following indicators:

- Identify problem
- Access information to improve coping
- Use communication channels to access assistance

NIC

Community Health Development, Environmental Risk Protection, Program Development, Risk Identification

Interventions

Assess for Causative or Contributing Factors

- Refer to Related Factors.

Provide Opportunities for Community Members (e.g., Schools, Churches, Synagogues, Town Hall) to Meet and Discuss the Situation

- Demonstrate acceptance of community members' anger, withdrawal, or denial.
- Correct misinformation as needed.
- Discourage blaming.

Provide for Effective Communication (Allender, Rector, & Warner, 2010)

- Allow for and address questions.
- Convey the facts.

- Convey seriousness.
- Be clear, simple, and repetitive.
- Present solutions and suggestions.
- Address real and perceived needs.

Promote Community Competence in Coping

- Focus on community goals, not individuals' goals.
- Engage subgroups in group discussions and planning.
- Ensure access to resources for all members (e.g., flexible hours for working members).
- Devise a method for formal disagreements.
- Evaluate each decision's impact on all community members.

Establish a Community Information Center at the Local Library to Access Information and Support (e.g., Telephone, Online)

Identify the Collaborative Resources That Can Be Accessed in the Health Department, Faith-Based Organization, Social Services, and Health-Care Provider Agencies

Use the Community Information Center (e.g., Local Library) to Inform Residents of Ongoing Activities and Progress

COMPROMISED FAMILY COPING

NANDA-I Definition

A usually supportive primary person (family member, significant other, or close friend) provides insufficient, ineffective, or compromised support, comfort, assistance, or encouragement that may be needed by the individual to manage or master adaptive tasks related to his or her health challenge

Defining Characteristics*

Subjective Data

Individual reports a concern about significant person's response to health problem.
Significant person reports preoccupation with personal reaction (e.g., fear, anticipatory grief, guilt, anxiety) to individual's need.
Significant person reports inadequate understanding, which interferes with effective supportive behaviors

Objective Data

Significant person attempts assistive or supportive behaviors with unsatisfactory results.

Significant person enters into limited personal communication with the individual.

Significant person displays protective behavior disproportionate to individual's need for autonomy.

Related Factors

Refer to *Interrupted Family Processes*.

 Author's Note

This nursing diagnosis describes situations similar to the diagnosis *Interrupted Family Processes* or *Risk for Interrupted Family Processes*. Until clinical research differentiates this diagnosis from the aforementioned diagnosis, use *Interrupted Family Processes*.

DISABLED FAMILY COPING

Definition

Behavior of primary person (family member, significant other, or close friend) that disables his or her capacities and the individual's capacities to effectively address tasks essential to either person's adaptation to the health challenge (NANDA-I)

The state in which a family demonstrates, or is at risk to demonstrate, destructive behavior in response to an inability to manage internal or external stressors due to inadequate resources (physical, psychological, cognitive)[12]

Defining Characteristics

Decisions/actions that are detrimental to family well-being[12]
Neglectful care of individual in regard to basic human needs*

---

[12] This definition and characteristic have been added by the author for clarity and usefulness.

Neglectful care of individual in regard to illness treatment*
Neglectful relationships with other family members
Family behaviors that are detrimental to well-being*
Distortion of reality regarding the individual's health problem*
Rejection*
Agitation*
Aggression*
Impaired restructuring of a family unit
Intolerance*
Abandonment*
Depression*
Hostility*

Related Factors

Biopathophysiologic

Related to impaired ability to fulfill role responsibilities secondary to:
Any acute or chronic illness

Situational (Personal, Environmental)

Related to impaired ability to constructively manage stressors secondary to:

Substance abuse (e.g., alcoholism)
Negative role modeling

History of ineffective relationship with own parents
History of abusive relationship with parents

Related to unrealistic expectations of child by parent

Related to unrealistic expectations of parent by child

Related to unmet psychosocial needs of child by parent

Related to unmet psychosocial needs of parent by child

Related to marital stressors secondary to:
Financial difficulties
Separation
Infidelities

Problematic children
Problematic relatives

Author's Note

Disabled Family Coping describes a family with a history of overt or covert destructive behavior or responses to stressors. This diagnosis necessitates long-term care from a nurse therapist with advanced specialization in family systems and abuse.

The use of this diagnosis in this book focuses on nursing interventions appropriate for a nurse generalist in a short-term relationship (e.g., emergency unit, nonpsychiatric in-house unit) and for any nurse in the position to prevent *Disabled Family Coping* through teaching, counseling, or referrals.

NOC

Caregiver Emotional Health, Caregiver Stressors, Family Coping, Family Normalization

Goals

Each family member will set short- and long-term goals for change, as evidenced by the following indicators:

- Appraise unhealthy coping behaviors of family members
- Relate expectations for self and family
- Relate community resources available

NIC

Caregiver Support, Referral, Emotional Support, Family Therapy, Family Involvement Promotion

Interventions

Identify With Each Family Member Their Strengths

Identify With Each Family Member Their Stressors

Assist Members to Appraise Family Behaviors (Effective, Ineffective, Destructive)

Discuss the Effects of Behaviors on Individuals and Family Unit

- Emotions
- Roles
- Support
- Performance

Assist Family to Set Short-Term and Long-Term Goals

Promote Family Resilience

- Ask each family member to identify one activity he or she would like to add to their family.

Promote Adaption to Stressors and Crises (Kaakinen, Gedaly-Duff, Coehlo, & Hanson, 2010)

- Identify stressors that can be reduced or eliminated.
- Engage the family members to discuss the situation.
- Allow each member to share their thoughts and suggestions for improving the situation.
- Negotiate necessary changes.
- Identify available resources.
- Ask each family member to identify one behavior he or she could control. Begin to help members to work through resentments of the past.

Improve Family Cohesiveness

- Determine family recreational activities that include all members and are enjoyable.

Provide Anticipatory Guidance (Kaakinen et al., 2010)

- Identify relevant life changes that will occur in this family (e.g., birth of child, relocation, empty nest). Discuss necessary adjustments in the family routines.
- Identify family member's responsibilities. Evaluate the balance of responsibilities.
- Initiate referrals, as needed.
- Support groups, family therapy, economic support.

Encourage Decision Making If Domestic Abuse Is Suspected

- Provide an opportunity to validate abuse, and talk about feelings; if the acutely injured individual is accompanied by a spouse/caregiver who is persistent about staying, make an attempt to see the individual alone (e.g., tell her that you need a urine specimen and accompany her to the bathroom).
- Be direct and nonjudgmental:
  - How do you handle stress?
  - How does your partner or caregiver handle stress?
  - How do you and your partner argue?
  - Are you afraid of him?
  - Have you ever been hit, pushed, or injured by your partner?
- Provide options but allow individual to make a decision at her own pace.
- Encourage a realistic appraisal of the situation; dispel guilt and myths.

- Violence is not normal for most families.
- Violence may stop, but it usually becomes increasingly worse.
- The victim is not responsible for the violence.

Provide Legal and Referral Information

- Discreetly inform of community agencies available to victim and abuser (emergency and long-term).
  - Hotlines
  - Legal services
  - Shelters
  - Counseling agencies
- Discuss mandatory reporting.
- Discuss the availability of the social service department for assistance.
- Consult with legal resources in the community and familiarize the victim with state laws regarding:
  - Abuse
  - Eviction of abuser
  - Counseling
  - Temporary support
  - Protection orders
  - Criminal law
  - Types of police interventions
- Document findings and dialogue (*Carlson & Smith-DiJulio, 2006).
- Refer for individual, group, or couples counseling.
- Explore strategies to reduce stress and more constructively manage stressors (e.g., relaxation exercises, walking, and assertiveness training).

░ Pediatric Interventions

Report Suspected Cases of Child Abuse

- Know your state's child abuse laws and procedures for reporting child abuse (e.g., Bureau of Child Welfare, Department of Social Services, and Child Protective Services).
- Maintain an objective record (*Cowen, 1999):
  - Health history, including accidental or environmental injuries
  - Detailed description of physical examination (nutritional status, hygiene, growth and development, cognitive and functional status)
  - Environmental assessment of home (if in community)

- Description of injuries
- Verbal conversations with parents and child in quotes
- Description of behaviors, not interpretation (e.g., avoid "angry father," instead, "Father screamed at child, 'If you weren't so bad this wouldn't have happened.'")
- Description of parent–child's interactions (e.g., "shies away from mother's touch")

Promote a Therapeutic Environment

Provide the Child With Acceptance and Affection

- Show child attention without reinforcing inappropriate behavior.
- Use play therapy to allow child's self-expression.
- Provide consistent caregivers and reasonable limits on behavior; avoid pity.
- Avoid asking too many questions and criticizing parent's actions.
- Ensure that play and educational needs are met.
- Explain in detail all routines and procedures in age-appropriate language.

Assist Child With Grieving If Placement in Foster Home Is Necessary

- Acknowledge that child will not want to leave parents despite severity of abuse.
- Allow opportunities for child to express feelings.
- Explain reasons for not allowing child to return home; dispel belief it is a punishment.
- Encourage foster parents to visit child in hospital.

Provide Interventions That Promote Parent's Self-Esteem and Sense of Trust

- Tell them it was good that they brought the child to the hospital.
- Welcome parents to the unit and orient them to activities.
- Promote their confidence by presenting a warm, helpful attitude and acknowledging any competent parenting activities.
- Provide opportunities for parents to participate in child's care (e.g., feeding, bathing).

Initiate Health Teaching and Referrals, as Indicated

- Provide anticipatory guidance for families at risk.
- Disseminate information to the community about child abuse (e.g., parent–school organizations, radio, television, newspaper).

✤ Geriatric Interventions

Identify Suspected Cases of Elder Abuse (*Fulmer & Paveza, 1998)

- Signs include the following:
  - Failure to adhere to therapeutic regimens, which can pose threats to life (e.g., insulin administration, ulcerated conditions)
  - Evidence of malnutrition, dehydration, elimination problems
  - Bruises, swelling, lacerations, burns, bites
  - Pressure ulcers
  - Caregiver not allowing nurse to be alone with elder

Report Suspected Cases

- Consult with supervisor for procedures for reporting suspected cases of abuse.
- Maintain an objective record, including the following:
  - Description of injuries
  - Conversations with elder and caregiver(s)
  - Description of behaviors
  - Nutritional, hydration status
- Consider the elder's right to choose to live at risk of harm, providing he or she is capable of making that choice.
- Do not initiate an action that could increase the elder's risk of harm or antagonize the abuser.
- Respect the elder's right to secrecy and the right for self-determination.

Initiate Health Teaching and Referrals, as Indicated

- Refer high-risk families to a home health agency for an comprehensive assessment
- Refer elder for counseling to explore choices. Reassure him or her that they did nothing wrong to deserve maltreatment (Varcarolis, 2011).
- Explore support services (e.g., respite, home health aide, homemaker services).
- Disseminate information to community regarding prevention.

DECISIONAL CONFLICT

NANDA-I Definition

Uncertainty about course of action to be taken when choice among competing actions involves risk, loss, or challenge to values and beliefs

Defining Characteristics*

Verbalized uncertainty about choices
Verbalizes undesired consequences of alternatives being considered
Vacillation among alternative choices
Delayed decision making
Self-focusing
Verbalizes feeling of distress while attempting a decision
Physical signs of distress or tension (e.g., increased heart rate, increased muscle tension, restlessness)
Questioning of personal values and/or beliefs while attempting to make a decision
Questioning moral values while attempting a decision
Questioning moral rules while attempting a decision
Questioning moral principles while attempting a decision

Related Factors

Many situations can contribute to decisional conflict, particularly those that involve complex medical interventions of great risk. Any decisional situation can precipitate conflict for an individual; thus, the following examples are not exhaustive, but reflect situations that may be problematic and possess factors that increase the difficulty.

Treatment Related

Related to lack of relevant information

Related to risks versus the benefits of (specify test, treatment):

Surgery
  Tumor removal
  Cosmetic
    surgery
  Cosmetic
  surgery
  Amputation
  Transplant
  Orchiectomy
  Prostatectomy
  Hysterectomy
  Laminectomy

Mastectomy
Joint replacement
Cataract
  removal
Cataract removal
Cesarean section
Diagnostics
  Amniocentesis
  X-rays
  Ultrasound
Chemotherapy
Radiation
Dialysis

Mechanical
  ventilation
Mechanical
  ventilation
Enteral feedings
Intravenous
  hydration
Use of preterm
  labor medications
Participation in
  treatment study
  trials
HIV antiviral
  therapy

Situational (Personal, Environmental)

Related to perceived threat to value system

Related to risks versus the benefits of:

Personal
  Marriage
  Breastfeeding versus
    bottle-feeding
  Parenthood
  Sterilization
  In vitro fertilization
  Transport from rural
    facilities
  Circumcision
  Divorce
  Abortion
  Artificial insemination

Adoption
Institutionalization
  (child, parent)
Contraception
Nursing home placement
Foster home placement
Separation
Work/task
  Career change
  Professional ethics
  Business investments
  Relocation

Related to:
Lack of relevant information*
Confusing information

Related to:
Disagreement within support systems
Inexperience with decision making
Unclear personal values/beliefs*
Conflict with personal values/beliefs
Family history of poor prognosis
Hospital paternalism—loss of control

Ethical or moral dilemmas of:

Quality of life

Cessation of life-support systems

"Do not resuscitate" orders

Termination of pregnancy

Organ transplant

Selective termination with
multiple-gestation
pregnancies

Maturational

Related to risks versus benefits of:

Adolescent

Peer pressure

Alcohol/drug use

Career choice

Use of birth control

Adult

College

Whether to continue a relationship

Career change

Relocation

Retirement

Sexual activity

Illegal/dangerous
situations

Older Adult

Retirement

Out of home (relative's home, assisted
living, skilled care)

 Author's Note

The nurse has an important role in assisting individuals and families with making decisions. Because nurses usually do not benefit financially from decisions made regarding treatments and transfers, they are in an ideal position to assist with decisions. Although, according to Davis (*1989), "Nursing or medical expertise does not enable health care professionals to know the values of patients or what patients think is best for themselves," nursing expertise enables nurses to facilitate systematic decision making that considers all possible alternatives and possible outcomes, as well as individual beliefs and values. The focus is on assisting with logical decision making, not on promoting a certain decision.

When people are making a treatment decision of considerable risk, they do not necessarily experience conflict. In situations where the treatment option is "choosing life," individual perception may be one of submitting to fate and be relatively unconflicted. Because of this, nurses must be cautious in labeling patients with the nursing diagnosis of *Decisional Conflict* without sufficient validating cues (*Soholt, 1990).

NOC

Decision-Making, Information Processing, Participation: Health Care Decisions

Goals

The individual/group will make an informed choice, as evidenced by the following indicators:

- Relate the advantages and disadvantages of choices
- Share fears and concerns regarding choices and responses of others
- Define what would be most helpful to support the decision-making process

NIC

Decision-Making Support, Mutual Goal Setting, Learning Facilitation, Health System Guidance, Anticipatory Guidance, Patient Right Protection, Values Clarification, Anxiety Reduction

Interventions

Address Each Element to Ensure Shared Decision Making
(Lilley et al., 2010)

- Clarify the decision to be made.
- Explore what is important to the individual.
- Clarify options available, perceived/actual barriers.
- Communicate risks and benefits of the treatment options.

Assess Causative/Contributing Factors

- Refer to Related Factors.

Reduce or Eliminate Causative or Contributing Factors

Internal
Lack of Experience With Decision Making or Ineffective Decision Making
- Facilitate logical decision making:
  - Assist in recognizing the problem and clearly identifying the needed decision.
  - Generate a list of all possible alternatives or options.
  - Help identify the probable outcomes of the various alternatives.
  - Aid in evaluating the alternatives based on actual or potential threats to beliefs/values.
  - Encourage to make a decision.
- Encourage significant others to be involved in the entire decision-making process.

- Suggest the individual use significant others as a sounding board when considering alternatives.
- Respect and support the role that the individual desires in the decision, whether it is active, collaborative, or passive.
- Be available to review the needed decision and the various alternatives.

Value Conflict (Also Refer to *Spiritual Distress*)
- Explore what is important to the individual (Lilley et al., 2010).

Insufficient or Inconsistent Information
- Clarify options available in accordance with individual values.
- Communicate risks and benefits of the treatment options.

Fear of Outcome/Response of Others (Also Refer to *Fear*)
- Provide clarification regarding potential outcomes and correct misconceptions.
- Explore what the risks of not deciding would be. Encourage the individual to face fears.
- Actively reassure the individual that the decision is his or hers to make and that he or she has the right to do so.

External

Controversy with Support System
- Reassure that he or she does not have to give in to pressure from others, whether family, friends, or health professionals.
- Advocate for the individual's wishes if others attempt to undermine his or her ability to make the decision personally.
- Identify those within the support system who support the person's decision; discuss with the individual, who has power of attorney or is their designated decision maker if indicated.
  Recognize that the individual may become ambivalent about "choosing" when putting the needs of the support system above his or her own. Stress the risks of not choosing.

Pediatric Interventions

- Include children and adolescents in decision-making process.

Geriatric Interventions

- Ensure that older adult is involved in decisions.
- Facilitate communication among the elder, family, and professionals.
- If needed, use simple explanations and provide the pros and cons of the decision.

DIARRHEA

NANDA-I Definition

Passage of loose, unformed stools

Defining Characteristics*

At least three loose, liquid stools per day
Urgency
Cramping/abdominal pain
Hyperactive bowel sounds

Related Factors

Pathophysiologic

Related to malabsorption or inflammation* secondary to:*

Colon cancer	Celiac disease (sprue)
Diverticulitis	Gastritis
Irritable bowel	Spastic colon
Crohn's disease	Ulcerative colitis
Peptic ulcer	

Related to lactose deficiency, dumping syndrome

Related to increased peristalsis secondary to increased metabolic rate (hyperthyroidism)

Related to infectious processes secondary to:*

Trichinosis	Shigellosis	Dysentery
Typhoid fever	Cholera	Infectious hepatitis
Malaria	Microsporidia	Cryptosporidium

Related to excessive secretion of fats in stool secondary to liver dysfunction

Related to inflammation and ulceration of gastrointestinal mucosa secondary to high levels of nitrogenous wastes (renal failure)

Treatment Related

Related to malabsorption or inflammation secondary to surgical intervention of the bowel

Related to adverse effects of pharmaceutical agents of (specify):*

Thyroid agents	Chemotherapy	Antacids
Analgesics	Laxatives	Cimetidine
Stool softeners	Iron sulfate	Antibiotics

Related to tube feedings

Situational (Personal, Environmental)

*Related to stress or anxiety**

Related to irritating foods (fruits, bran cereals) or increase in caffeine consumption

*Related to changes in water and food, secondary to travel**

Related to change in bacteria in water

Related to bacteria, virus, or parasite to which no immunity is present

 Author's Note

See *Constipation*.

NOC
Bowel Elimination, Electrolyte & Acid–Base Balance, Fluid Balance, Hydration, Symptom Control

Goal

The individual/parent will report less diarrhea, as evidenced by the following indicator:

• Describe contributing factors when known

NIC
Bowel Management, Diarrhea Management, Fluid/Electrolyte Management, Nutrition Management, Enteral Tube Feeding

Interventions

Assess Causative Contributing Factors

• Tube feedings
• Dietetic foods
• Foreign travel
• Dietary indiscretions/contaminated foods
• Food allergies
• Medications

Eliminate or Reduce Contributing Factors

Side Effects of Tube Feeding (Fuhrman, 1999)
- Control the infusion rate (depending on delivery set).
- Administer smaller, more frequent feedings.
- Change to continuous-drip tube feedings.
- Administer more slowly if signs of gastrointestinal intolerance occur.
- Control temperature.
- If formula has been refrigerated, warm it in hot water to room temperature.
- Dilute the strength of feeding temporarily.
- Follow the standard procedure for administration of tube feeding.
- Follow tube feeding with the specified amount of water to ensure hydration.
- Be careful of contamination/spoilage (unused but opened formula should not be used after 24 hours; keep unused portion refrigerated).

Contaminated Foods (Possible Sources)
- Raw seafood
- Raw milk
- Shellfish
- Restaurants
- Excess milk consumption
- Improperly cooked/stored food

Dietetic Foods: Eliminate Foods Containing Large Amounts of the Hexitol, Sorbitol, and Mannitol That Are Used as Sugar Substitutes in Dietetic Foods, Candy, and Chewing Gum

Reduce Diarrhea

- Advise not to stop eating or from withholding food from children.
- Avoid milk (lactose) products, fat, whole grains, fried and spicy foods, and fresh fruits and vegetables.
- Gradually add semisolids and solids (crackers, yogurt, rice, bananas, applesauce).
- Instruct the individual to seek medical care if blood and mucous are in stool and fever greater than 101° F.

Replace Fluids and Electrolytes

- Increase oral intake to maintain a normal urine specific gravity (light yellow in color).

- Encourage liquids (tea, water, apple juice, flat ginger ale).
- When diarrhea is severe, use an over-the-counter oral rehydration solution.
- Teach the individual to monitor the color of urine to determine hydration needs. Increase fluids if urine color is amber or dark yellow.
- Caution against the use of very hot or cold liquids.
- See *Deficient Fluid Volume* for additional interventions.

Conduct Health Teaching as Indicated

- Explain safe food handling (e.g., required temperature storage, washing of food preparation objects after use with raw food, frequent hand washing).
- Explain the interventions required to prevent future episodes and effects of diarrhea on hydration.
- Consult with primary health-care provider for prophylactic use of bismuth subsalicylate (e.g., Pepto-Bismol) 30 to 60 mL or 2 tablets qid during travel and 2 days after return; or antimicrobials for prevention of traveler's diarrhea.
- Advise not to treat traveler's diarrhea with antimotility agents (e.g., Lomotil, Imodium).
- Teach precautions to take when traveling to foreign lands (Connor, 2015):
  - Avoid salads, milk, fresh cheese, cold cuts, and salsa.
  - Drink carbonated or bottled beverages; avoid ice.
  - Peel fresh fruits and vegetables.
  - Avoid foods not stored at proper temperature.
  - Advise not to treat traveler's diarrhea with antimotility agents (e.g., Lomotil, Imodium), which can delay the clearance of organisms and thus can increase the severity of traveler's diarrhea with complications (e.g., sepsis, toxic megacolon).
- Explain how to prevent food-borne diseases at home:
  - Refrigerate all perishable foods.
  - Cook all food at high temperature or boil (212° F) for at least 15 minutes before serving.
  - Avoid allowing food to stand at warm temperatures for several hours.
  - Caution about foods at picnics in hot summer.
- Thoroughly clean kitchen equipment after contact with perishable foods (e.g., meats, dairy, fish).
- Explain that a diet primarily made up of dietetic foods containing sugar substitutes (hexitol, sorbitol, and mannitol) can cause diarrhea.
- Teach the individual to gently clean the anal area after bowel movements; lubricants (e.g., petroleum jelly) can protect skin.

⁙ Pediatric Interventions

Monitor Fluid and Electrolyte Losses

- Fluid volume lost
- Urine color and output
- Skin color
- Mucous membranes
- Capillary refill time

Consult With Primary Care Provider If

- Diarrhea persists.
- Blood or mucus is in stools.
- Child is lethargic.
- Urine output is scanty.
- Stools suddenly increase.
- Child is vomiting.

Reduce Diarrhea

- Avoid milk (lactose) products, fat, whole grains, and fresh fruits and vegetables.
- Avoid high-carbohydrate fluids (e.g., soft drinks), gelatin, fruit juices, caffeinated drinks, and chicken or beef broths.

Provide Oral Rehydration

- Use oral rehydration solutions (e.g., Pedialyte, Lytren, Ricelyte, Resol [Larson, 2000]).
- Determine fluid loss by body weight loss. If less than 5% of total weight is lost, 50 mL/kg of fluids will be needed during the next 3 to 6 hours (Pillitteri, 2014).
- For more than a 5% weight loss, consult with the primary care provider for fluid replacement.
- Fluids must be given to replace losses and continuing losses until diarrhea improves (Pillitteri, 2014).

Reintroduce Food

- Begin with bananas, rice, cereal, and crackers in small quantities.
- Gradually return to regular diet (except milk products) after 36 to 48 hours; after 3 to 5 days, gradually add milk products (half-strength skim milk to skim milk to half-strength milk [whole or 1%]).
- Gradually introduce formula (half-strength formula to full-strength formula).

For Breastfed Infants

- Continue breastfeeding.
- Use oral rehydration therapy if needed.

Protect Skin From Irritation With Non–Water-Soluble Cream (e.g., Petroleum Jelly)

Initiate Health Teaching as Needed

Teach Parents Signs to Report
- Sunken eyes
- Dry mucous membranes
- Rapid, thready pulse
- Rapid breathing
- Lethargy
- Diarrhea increases

Geriatric Interventions

- Determine if impaction is present; if so, remove it (refer to *Constipation* for specific interventions).
- Monitor closely for hypovolemia and electrolyte imbalances (e.g., potassium, sodium).
- Advise individual to seek medical care if diarrhea continues over 24 hours.

RISK FOR DISUSE SYNDROME

NANDA-I Definition

At risk for deterioration of body systems as the result of prescribed or unavoidable musculoskeletal inactivity

Defining Characteristics

Presence of a cluster of actual- or risk-nursing diagnoses related to inactivity:

Risk for Impaired Skin Integrity
Risk for Constipation
Risk for Altered Respiratory Function
Risk for Ineffective Peripheral Tissue Perfusion
Risk for Infection
Risk for Activity Intolerance
Risk for Impaired Physical Mobility
Risk for Injury
Powerlessness
Disturbed Body Image

Related Factors

(Optional) Refer to Author's Notes

Pathophysiologic

Related to:
Decreased sensorium   Unconsciousness

Neuromuscular impairment secondary to:
Multiple sclerosis   Partial/total paralysis
Muscular dystrophy   Guillain–Barré syndrome
Parkinsonism   Spinal cord injury

Musculoskeletal impairment secondary to:
Fractures   Rheumatic diseases

End-stage disease
AIDS   Renal cancer
Cardiac

Psychiatric/Mental health disorders
Major depression   Severe phobias
Catatonic state

Treatment Related

Related to:
Surgery (amputation, skeletal)   Invasive vascular lines
Mechanical ventilation   Prescribed immobility
Traction/casts/splints

Situational (Personal, Environmental)

Related to:
Depression   Fatigue
Debilitated state   Pain

Maturational

Newborn/Infant/Child/Adolescent
Related to:
Down syndrome   Mental/physical disability
Juvenile arthritis   Legg–Calvé–Perthes disease
Cerebral palsy   Autism
Risser-Turnbuckle jacket   Spina bifida
Osteogenesis imperfecta

Older Adult
Related to:
Decreased motor agility   Presenile dementia
Muscle weakness

 Author's Note

Risk for Disuse Syndrome describes an individual at risk for the adverse effects of immobility (Table I.2). *Risk for Disuse Syndrome* identifies vulnerability to certain complications and also altered functioning in a health pattern. As a syndrome diagnosis, its etiology or contributing factor is within the diagnostic label (*Disuse*); a "related to" statement is not necessary. As discussed in Chapter 2, a syndrome diagnosis comprises a cluster of predicted actual- or risk-nursing diagnoses because of the situation. Eleven risk- or actual-nursing diagnoses are clustered under *Disuse Syndrome* (see Defining Characteristics).

The nurse no longer needs to use separate diagnoses, such as *Risk for Ineffective Respiratory Function* or *Risk for Impaired Skin Integrity*, because they are incorporated into the syndrome category. If an immobile individual manifests signs or symptoms of impaired skin integrity or another diagnosis, however, the nurse should use the specific diagnosis. He or she should continue to use *Risk for Disuse Syndrome* so other body systems do not deteriorate.

NOC

Endurance, Immobility Consequences: Physiologic, Immobility Consequences: Psycho-Cognitive, Mobility Level Joint Movement

Goals

The individual will not experience complications of immobility, as evidenced by the following indicators:

- Have intact skin/tissue integrity
- Show maximum pulmonary function
- Show maximum peripheral blood flow
- Exhibit full range of motion
- Have bowel, bladder, and renal functioning within normal limits
- Use social contacts and activities when possible
- Explain rationale for treatments
- Make decisions regarding care when possible
- Share feelings regarding immobile state

NIC

Activity Therapy, Energy Management, Mutual Goal Settings, Exercise Therapy, Fall Prevention, Pressure Ulcer Prevention, Body Mechanics Correction, Skin Surveillance, Positioning, Coping Enhancement, Decision-Making, Support Therapeutic Play

Table 1.2	ADVERSE EFFECTS OF IMMOBILITY ON BODY SYSTEMS
System	**Effect**
Cardiac	Decreased myocardial performance
	Decreased aerobic capacity
	Decreased stroke volume
	Increased heart rate at rest and with increased activity
	Decreased oxygen uptake
	Reduction in plasma volume reduces cardiac preload, stroke volume, cardiac output
Circulatory	Venous stasis
	Orthostatic intolerance
	Dependent edema
	Decreased resting heart rate
	Reduced venous return
Respiratory	Increased intravascular pressure
	Stasis of secretions
	Impaired cilia
	Drying of sections of mucous membranes
	Decreased chest expansion
	Slower, more shallow respirations
Musculoskeletal	Muscle atrophy
	Decreased skeletal muscle volume, most pronounced in the antigravity muscles
	Shortening of muscle fiber (contracture)
	Decreased strength/tone (e.g., back)
	Decreased bone density
	Joint degeneration
	Fibrosis of collagen fibers (joints)
Metabolic/hemopoietic	Increased bone resorption leads to a negative calcium balance (hypercalcemia) and eventually decreased bone mass
	Decreased nitrogen excretion
	Decreased tissue heat conduction
	Decreased glucose tolerance
	Insulin resistance
	Decreased red blood cells
	Decreased phagocytosis
	Change in circadian release of hormones (e.g., insulin, epinephrine)

System	Effect
	Anorexia
	Decreased metabolic rate
	Elevated creatine levels
Gastrointestinal	Constipation
	Anorexia
Genitourinary	Urinary stasis
	Urinary calculi
	Urinary retention
	Inadequate gravitational force
Integumentary	Decreased capillary flow
	Tissue acidosis to necrosis
Neurosensory	Reduced innervation of nerves
	Decreased near vision
	Increased auditory sensitivity
	Increased sensitivity to thermal stimuli
	Altered circadian rhythm

Sources: Hockenberry, M. J., & Wilson, D. (2015). *Wong's essentials of pediatric nursing* (10th ed.). New York: Elsevier; Grossman, S., & Porth, C. A. (2014). *Porth's pathophysiology: Concepts of altered health states* (9th ed.). Philadelphia: Wolters Kluwer; Stuempfle, K. J., & Drury, D. G. (2003). Comparison of 3 methods to assess urine specific gravity in collegiate wrestlers. *Journal of Athletic Training, 38*, 315–319 .

Interventions

Identify Causative and Contributing Factors

- Pain (refer also to *Impaired Comfort*)
- Fatigue (refer also to *Fatigue*)
- Decreased motivation (refer also to *Activity Intolerance*)
- Depression (refer also to *Ineffective Coping*)

Initiate a Mobility Ambulation Protocol for Hemodynamically Stable Individual

- Refer to *Impaired Physical Mobility*

For Individuals Unable to Ambulate, Aggressively Reposition (Hourly If Possible) as Follows (Zomorodi, Topley, & McAnaw, 2012)

- Position upright as soon as possible
- Turning frequently from side-to-side, partial side-to-side
- Raising and lowering head of bed
- Bed in chair position

Promote Optimal Mobility

- Refer to *Impaired Mobility* for a progressive mobility program.

Promote Optimal Respiratory Function

- Encourage deep breathing and controlled coughing exercises five times every hour.
- Teach to use a blow bottle or incentive spirometer every hour when awake (with severe neuromuscular impairment; the individual also may have to be awakened at night).
- For a child, use colored water in the blow bottle; have him or her blow up balloons, soap bubbles, or cotton balls with straw.
- Auscultate lung fields every 8 hours; increase frequency if breath sounds are altered.
- Encourage small, frequent feedings to prevent abdominal distention.

Maintain Usual Pattern of Bowel Elimination

- Refer to *Constipation* for specific interventions.

Prevent Pressure Ulcers

- Refer to *Risk for Pressure Ulcer* for specific interventions.

Promote Factors That Improve Venous Blood Flow

- Elevate extremity above the level of the heart (may be contraindicated if the individual is hemodynamically unstable).
- Ensure the individual avoids standing or sitting with legs dependent for long periods.
- Reduce or remove external venous compression, which impedes venous flow.
- Avoid pillows behind the knees or suggest a bed that is elevated at the knees.
- Tell the individual to avoid crossing the legs.
- Remind to change positions, move extremities, or wiggle fingers and toes every hour.
- Monitor legs for edema, tissue warmth, and redness daily.

Maintain Limb Mobility and Prevent Contractures
(Maher, Salmond, & Pellino, 2006)

Increase Limb Mobility
- Perform range-of-motion exercises (frequency to be determined on condition).
- Support extremity with pillows to prevent or reduce swelling.
- Encourage the individual to perform exercise regimens for specific joints as prescribed by physician/PA/NP or physical therapist.

Position the Individual in Alignment to Prevent Complications

- Point toes and knees toward ceiling when the individual is supine. Keep them flat when in a chair.
- Use footboard.
- Instruct the individual to wiggle toes, point them up and downward, and rotate their ankles inward and outward every hour.
- Avoid placing pillows under the knee; support calf instead.
- Avoid prolonged periods of hip flexion (i.e., sitting position).
- To position hips, place rolled towel lateral to the hip to prevent external rotation.
- Keep arms abducted from the body with pillows.
- Keep elbows in slight flexion.
- Keep wrist neutral, with fingers slightly flexed and thumb abducted and slightly flexed.
- Change position of shoulder joints during the day (e.g., abduction, adduction, range of circular motion).

Reduce and Monitor Bone Demineralization

- Monitor serum levels.
- Monitor for nausea/vomiting, polydipsia, polyuria, and lethargy.
- Maintain vigorous hydration (adults: 2,000 mL/day; adolescents: 3,000 to 4,000 mL/day) unless contraindicated (e.g., renal failure, heart failure).

Promote Sharing and a Sense of Well-Being

- Encourage the individual to share feelings and fears regarding restricted movement.
- Encourage the individual to wear own clothes, rather than pajamas, and unique adornments (e.g., baseball caps, colorful socks) to express individuality.

Reduce the Monotony of Immobility

- Vary daily routine when possible (e.g., give a bath in the afternoon so the individual can watch a special show or talk with a visitor during the morning).

Include the Individual in Planning Daily Schedule

Be Creative; Vary the Physical Environment and Daily Routine When Possible

- Update bulletin boards, change pictures on the walls, and move furniture within the room.
- Maintain a pleasant, cheerful environment (e.g., plenty of light, flowers).
- Place the individual near a window, if possible.
- Provide reading material (print or audio), radio, and television.

- Plan an activity daily to give the individual something to look forward to; always keep promises.
- Discourage the use of television as the primary source of recreation unless it is highly desired.
- Consider using a volunteer to spend time reading to the individual or helping with an activity.
- Encourage suggestions and new ideas (e.g., "Can you think of things you might like to do?").

⚜ Pediatric Interventions

Explain Types of Play in the Health-Care Setting

- Exercise/Energy-releasing play: promotes use of large upper/lower extremities (e.g., throwing a ball, playing in water)
- Diversional/recreational play: provides enjoyable activities to combat boredom
- Developmentally supportive play: selected age-appropriate activities to challenge the infant/child
- Therapeutic play: provides the child with activities that with interactions with a health-care professional, facilitates expression of feeling and fears about the health-care experience. This dialogue clarifies misunderstandings and reasons for certain treatments.

Explain to Parents/Caregiver That Play Can

- Relieve the stress caused by immobility.
- Allow for continued growth and development physically, mentally, and emotionally.
- Allow the parent and child to dialogue about concerns or misunderstandings about their care, procedures, and others.
- Encourage sharing of feelings.
- Provide choices for the child, to increase his feeling of control.
- Provide "well role," as child sees he can still succeed.
- Provide for family support and involvement.
- Provide an escape from pain, boredom, and sadness.
- Help to minimize any possible physical side effects due to decreased activity.

Source: Arkansas Children's Hospital, *A Parent's Guide . . . Play and Your Immobilized Child*. Retrieved from www.archildrens.org/documents/child_life/PlayImmoblizedChild.pdf

Plan Appropriate Activities for Children

- Provide an environment with accessible toys that suit the child's developmental age; ensure they are well within reach.

- Encourage the family to bring in the child's favorite toys, including items from nature that will keep the "real world" alive (e.g., goldfish, leaves in fall).
- Limit TV watching to a few favorite programs.

Use Play Therapy (Pillitteri, 2014)

- As an energy release:
  - Pound pegs.
  - Cut wood with pretend saw.
  - Pound clay.
  - Punch a balloon.
- As dramatic play:
  - Provide health-care equipment as dolls, doll beds, play stethoscopes, IV equipment, syringes, masks, and gowns.
  - Allow the child to choose the objects.
  - Allow the child opportunities to play and express their feelings.
  - Use opportunities to ask the child questions.
  - Reflect only what the child expresses.
  - Do not criticize.
- As creative play:
  - Provide opportunities to draw pictures.
  - Ask the child to describe the picture.
- Vary the environment.
- Transport child outside the room as much as possible.

Access Information for Managing Prolonged Immobility

- Refer to the Arkansas Children's Hospital publication, "A Parent's Guide: Play and Your Immobilized Child," and to the Children's Hospital of Philadelphia's web page, "Play and Recreation During Hospitalization."

DEFICIENT DIVERSIONAL ACTIVITY

NANDA-I Definition

Decreased stimulation from (or interest or engagement in) recreational or leisure activities

Defining Characteristics

Observed and/or statements of boredom due to inactivity

Related Factors

Pathophysiologic

Related to difficulty accessing or participating in usual activities secondary to:

Communicable disease   Pain

Situational (Personal, Environmental)

Related to unsatisfactory social behaviors

Related to no peers or friends

Related to monotonous environment

Related to long-term hospitalization or confinement

Related to lack of motivation

Related to difficulty accessing or participating in usual activities secondary to:

Excessive stressful work	Immobility
No time for leisure activities	Decreased sensory
Career changes (e.g., new job,	perception
retirement)	Multiple role
Children leaving home ("empty nest")	responsibilities

Maturational

Infant/Child
Related to lack of appropriate stimulation toys/peers

Older Adult
Related to difficulty accessing or participating in usual activities secondary to:

Sensory/motor deficits	Lack of peer group
Lack of transportation	Limited finances
Fear of crime	Confusion

Author's Note

Only the individual can express a deficit in diversional activities based on his or her determination that types and amounts of activities are desired. Miller (2015) writes that activities associated with various roles affirm an individual's self-concept.

To validate *Deficient Diversional Activity*, explore the etiology of factors amenable to nursing interventions, keeping your main focus on improving the quality of leisure activities. For an individual with personality problems that hinder relationships and decrease social activities, *Impaired Social Interactions* is more valid. In this case, focus on helping the individual identify behavior that imposes barriers to socialization.

NOC

Leisure Participation, Social Involvement

Goals

The individual will rate that he or she is more satisfied with current activity level, as evidenced by the following indicators:

- Relate methods of coping with anger or depression resulting from boredom
- Report participation in one enjoyable activity each day

NIC

Recreation Therapy, Socialization Enhancement, Self-Esteem Enhancement, Therapeutic Play

Interventions

Assess Causative Factors

- Refer to Related Factors.

Reduce or Eliminate Causative Factors

Monotony
- Refer to Interventions, "Reduce the monotony of immobility," under *Disuse Syndrome*.
- Provide opportunities for reminiscence individually or in groups (e.g., past trips, hobbies).
- Provide music therapy with audiocassette players with lightweight headphones. For group music therapy (*Rantz, 1991), the following is recommended:
  - Introduce a topic.

- Play related music.
- Develop the topic with discussion.
- Discuss responses.
- Consider using holistic and complementary therapies (e.g., aromatherapy, pet therapy, therapeutic touch). For pet therapy (*Rantz, 1991), the following is recommended:
  - Animals must be well groomed, healthy, and clean.
  - Animals should be relaxed with strangers.
  - Animals should eliminate before entering the facility.
  - Sponsors always should ask the individual if he or she likes the type of animal before approaching the individual.

Lack of Motivation

- Stimulate motivation by showing interest and encouraging sharing of feelings and experiences.
- Explore fears and concerns about participating in activities.
- Discuss likes and dislikes.
- Encourage sharing of feelings of present and past experiences.
- Spend time with the individual purposefully talking about other topics (e.g., "I just got back from the shore. Have you ever gone there?").
- Point out the need to "get going" and try something new.
- Help the individual work through feelings of anger and grief:
  - Allow him or her to express feelings.
  - Take the time to be a good listener.
  - See *Anxiety* for additional interventions.
- Encourage the individual to join a group of possible interest or help. (He or she may have to participate by way of intercom or special arrangement.)
- Consider the use of music therapy or reminiscence therapy.

Inability to Concentrate

- Plan a simple daily routine with concrete activities (e.g., walking, drawing, folding linens).
- If the individual is anxious, suggest solitary, noncompetitive activities (e.g., puzzles, photography).

Identify Factors That Promote Activity and Socialization

Encourage Socialization With Peers and All Age Groups (Frequently Very Young and Very Old Individuals Mutually Benefit From Interactions)

Acquire Assistance to Increase the Individual's Ability to Travel

- Arrange transportation to activities if necessary.
- Acquire aids for safety (e.g., wheelchair for shopping, walker for ambulating in hallways).

Increase the Individual's Feelings of Productivity and Self-Worth

- Encourage the individual to use strengths to help others and self (e.g., assign him or her tasks to perform in a general project). Acknowledge these efforts (e.g., "Thank you for helping Mr. Jones with his dinner").
- Encourage open communication; value the individual's opinion ("Mr. Jones, what do you think about _____?").
- Encourage the individual to challenge himself or herself to learn a new skill or pursue a new interest.
- Provide opportunities to interact with nature and animals.

Refer to *Social Isolation* for Additional Interventions

Pediatric Interventions

- Provide an environment with accessible toys that suit the child's developmental age; ensure that they are well within reach.
- Keep toys in all waiting areas.
- Encourage the family to bring in the child's favorite toys, including items from nature that will help to keep the "real world" alive (e.g., goldfish, leaves in fall).
- Consult a child life specialist as indicated.
- Refer to the Pediatric Interventions in the nursing diagnosis *Disuse Syndrome* for specifics on how to engage in therapeutic play.

Geriatric Interventions

- Explore interests and the feasibility of trying a new activity (e.g., mobility).
- Arrange for someone to accompany or orient the individual during initial encounters.
- Explore possible volunteer opportunities (e.g., Red Cross, hospitals).

Initiate Referrals, If Indicated

- Suggest joining the American Association of Retired Persons (AARP).
- Write local health and welfare council or agencies.
- Provide a list of associations/clubs with senior citizen activities (i.e., YMCA), such as Sixty Plus Club, Churches, XYZ Group (Extra Years of Zest), Golden Age Club, Young at Heart Club, SOS (Senior Outreach Services), Encore Club, Leisure Hour Group, MORA (Men of Retirement Age), Gray Panthers.

AUTONOMIC DYSREFLEXIA

Autonomic Dysreflexia

Risk for Autonomic Dysreflexia

NANDA-I Definition

Life-threatening, uninhibited sympathetic response of the nervous system to a noxious stimulus after a spinal cord injury at T7 or above

Defining Characteristics

The individual with spinal cord injury (T6 or above) with the following:

Paroxysmal hypertension* (sudden periodic elevated blood pressure in which systolic pressure is above 140 mm Hg and diastolic above 90 mm Hg)

Bradycardia or tachycardia* (pulse rate less than 60 beats/min or more than 100 beats/min)

Diaphoresis (above the injury)*

Red splotches on skin (above the injury)*

Pallor (below the injury)*

Headache (a diffuse pain in different portions of the head and not confined to any nerve distribution area)*

Apprehension

Dilated pupils

Chilling*

Conjunctival congestion*

Horner's syndrome* (pupillary contraction; partial ptosis of the eyelid; enophthalmos; sometimes, loss of sweating over the affected side of the face)

Paresthesia*

Pilomotor reflex* (gooseflesh)

Blurred vision*

Chest pain*

Metallic taste in mouth*

Nasal congestion*

Penile erection and semen emission

Related Factors

Pathophysiologic

Related to visceral stretching and irritation secondary to:

Gastrointestinal
Gallstones
Gastric ulcers
Hemorrhoids
Gastrocolic irritation
Anal fissure
Gastric distention

Constipation
Fecal impaction
Hemorrhoids
Acute abdominal condition,
    infection, trauma
Anal fissure

Urologic
Bladder distension*
Urinary calculi

Urinary tract infection
Epididymitis or scrotal compression

Skin Irritation*
Pressure ulcers
Insect bites
Burns
Ingrown toenails

Sunburn
Blister
Insect bites
Contact with hard or sharp objects

Reproductive
Menstruation
Epididymitis
Ejaculation
Sexual intercourse

Pregnancy or delivery
Uterine contraction
Vaginal infection
Vaginal dilation

Related to fracture

Related to stimulation of skin (abdominal, thigh)

Related to spastic sphincter

Related to deep vein thrombosis

Related to pulmonary embolism

Related to pain

Related to fractures or other skeletal trauma

Related to surgical or diagnostic procedures

Treatment Related

Related to visceral stretching secondary to:
Removal of fecal impaction
Clogged or nonpatent catheter
Visceral stretching and irritation secondary to surgical incision
    and enemas

Catheterization and enema
Bowel instrumentation/colonoscopy
Cystoscopy/instrumentation
Urodynamic study

Situational (Personal, Environmental)

Related to deficient individual knowledge* of prevention or treatment

Related to visceral stretching secondary to:
"Boosting" (binding legs and distending bladder to boost nor-
  epinephrine production for competitive wheelchair sports;
  *McClain, Shields, & Sixsmith, 1999).
Sexual activity

Related to neural stimulation secondary to immersion in cold water

Related to temperature fluctuations

Related to constrictive clothing, shoes, or appliances

 Author's Note

Autonomic Dysreflexia represents a life-threatening situation that nurse-prescribed interventions can prevent or treat. Prevention involves teaching the individual to reduce sympathetic nervous system stimulation and not using interventions that can cause such stimulation. Treatment focuses on reducing or eliminating noxious stimuli (e.g., fecal impaction, urinary retention). If nursing actions do not resolve symptoms, initiation of medical intervention is critical. When an individual requires medical treatment for all or most episodes of dysreflexia, the situation can be labeled a collaborative problem: *RC of Dysreflexia.*

 NOC

Neurologic Status, Neurologic Status: Autonomic, Vital Signs Status

Goals

The individual/family will respond to early signs and symptoms.
The individual/family will take action to prevent dysreflexia, evidenced by the following indicators:

- State factors that cause dysreflexia
- Describe the treatment for dysreflexia
- Relate indications for emergency treatment

NIC

Dysreflexia Management, Vital Signs Monitoring, Emergency Care, Medication Administration

Interventions

Assess for Causative or Contributing Factors

- See Related Factors.

Proceed as Follows If Signs of Dysreflexia Occur

- Stand or sit the individual up.
- Lower the individual's legs.
- Loosen all the individual's constrictive clothing or appliances.

Check for Distended Bladder

If the Individual Is Catheterized
- Check the catheter for kinks or compression.
- Irrigate the catheter with only 30 mL of saline, very slowly.
- Replace the catheter if it will not drain.

If the Individual Is Not Catheterized
- Insert the catheter using dibucaine hydrochloride ointment (Nupercainal).
- Remove 500 mL, then clamp for 15 minutes.
- Repeat the cycle until the bladder is drained.

Check for Fecal Impaction

- First apply hydrochloride ointment (Nupercainal) to the anus and into the rectum for 1 inch (2.54 cm).
- Gently check the rectum with a well-lubricated glove using your index finger.
- Insert rectal suppository or gently remove impaction.

Check for Skin Irritation

- Spray the skin lesion that is triggering the dysreflexia with a topical anesthetic agent.
- Remove support hose.

Continue to Monitor Blood Pressure Every 3 to 5 Minutes

Immediately Consult Physician/NP/PA for Pharmacologic Treatment If Hypertension Is Double Baseline or Noxious Stimuli Are Unable to Be Eliminated

Initiate Health Teaching and Referrals as Indicated

- Teach the signs, symptoms, and treatment of dysreflexia to the individual and family.
- Teach the indications that warrant immediate medical intervention.

- Explain situations that trigger dysreflexia (menstrual cycle, sexual activity, elimination).
- Teach the individual to watch for early signs and to intervene immediately.
- Teach the individual to observe for early signs of bladder infections and skin lesions (pressure ulcers, ingrown toenails).
- Advise consultation with a physician for long-term pharmacologic management if the individual is very vulnerable.
- Document the frequency of episodes and precipitating factor(s).

Risk for Autonomic Dysreflexia

NANDA-I Definition

Vulnerable to a life-threatening, uninhibited sympathetic response of the nervous system to a noxious stimulus after a spinal cord injury at T7 or above, which can compromise health.
Refer to *Autonomic Dysreflexia*.

Risk Factors

Refer to *Autonomic Dysreflexia*—Related Factors.

Goals

Refer to *Autonomic Dysreflexia*.

Interventions

Refer to *Autonomic Dysreflexia*.

RISK FOR ELECTROLYTE IMBALANCE

See also *Risk for Complications of Electrolyte Imbalance* in Section 3, Collaborative Problems.

NANDA-I Definition

Vulnerable for a change in serum electrolyte levels, which may compromise health

Risk Factors*

Endocrine dysfunction
Diarrhea
Fluid imbalance (e.g., dehydration, water intoxication)
Impaired regulatory mechanisms (e.g., diabetes insipidus, syndrome of inappropriate secretion of antidiuretic hormones)
Renal dysfunction
Treatment-related side effects (e.g., medications, drains)
Vomiting

 Author's Note

This NANDA-I diagnosis is a collaborative problem. Refer to Section 3, Collaborative Problems, for *Risk for Complications of Electrolyte Imbalances.*

INTERRUPTED FAMILY PROCESSES

Interrupted Family Processes

Dysfunctional Family Processes

Definition

Change in family relationships and/or functioning (NANDA-I)
    State in which a usually supportive family experiences, or is at risk to experience, a stressor that challenges its previously effective functioning[11]

---

[13]This definition has been added by the author for clarity and usefulness.

Defining Characteristics

Major (Must Be Present)

Family system cannot or does not:
Adapt constructively to crisis
Communicate openly and effectively between family members

Minor (May Be Present)

Family system cannot or does not:
Meet physical needs of all its members
Meet emotional needs of all its members
Meet spiritual needs of all its members
Express or accept a wide range of feelings
Seek or accept help appropriately

Related Factors

Any factor can contribute to *Interrupted Family Processes*. Common factors are as follows.

Treatment Related

Related to:
Disruption of family routines because of time-consuming treatments (e.g., home dialysis)
Physical changes because of treatments of ill family member
Emotional changes in all family members because of treatments of ill family member
Financial burden of treatments for ill family member
Hospitalization of ill family member

Situational (Personal, Environmental)

Related to loss of home (e.g., homeless, living with relative)

Related to loss of family member:

Death	Separation
Incarceration	Hospitalization
Going away to school	Divorce
Desertion	

Related to addition of new family member:

Birth	Adoption
Marriage	Elderly relative

Related to losses associated with:

Poverty

Economic crisis

Change in family roles
  (e.g., retirement)

Birth of child with defect

Relocation

Disaster

Related to conflict (moral, goal, cultural)

Related to breach of trust between members

Related to social deviance by family member (e.g., crime)

 Author's Note

This nursing diagnosis describes situations similar to the diagnosis *Compromised Family Coping*. Until clinical research differentiates this diagnosis from the aforementioned diagnosis, use *Compromised Family Coping*.

Interrupted Family Processes describes a family that reports usual constructive function but is experiencing an alteration from a current stress-related challenge. The family is viewed as a system, with interdependence among members. Thus, life challenges for individual members also challenge the family system. Certain situations may negatively influence family functioning; examples include illness, an older relative moving in homeless, separation, and divorce. *Risk for Interrupted Family Processes* can represent such a situation.

Interrupted Family Processes differs from *Caregiver Role Strain*. Certain situations require one or more family members to assume a caregiver role for a relative. Caregiver role responsibilities can vary from ensuring an older parent has three balanced meals daily to providing all hygiene and self-care activities for an adult or child. *Caregiver Role Strain* describes the mental and physical burden that the caregiver role places on individuals, which influences all their concurrent relationships and role responsibilities. It focuses specifically on the individual or individuals with multiple direct caregiver responsibilities.

NOC

Family Coping, Family Functioning, parenting, Family Normalization

NIC

Coping Enhancements, Referral, Family Process Maintenance, Family Integrity Promotion, Limit Setting, Support Group

Interventions

Assess the Composition of the "Family" (Pillitteri, 2014)

- Dyad—two people living together (e.g., married, unmarried, gay, lesbian)

- Nuclear—traditional family of a husband, wife, and children
- Multigenerational—a nuclear family with other family members such as grandparents, cousins, grandchildren
- Cohabitation—unmarried couples with children living together
- Polygamous—although illegal in the United States, a family of one man with several wives may immigrate to the United States.
- Blended—remarriage or reconstituted family with children (e.g., divorced, widowed)
- Single-parent—55% of families are single-parent (US Census Bureau, 2013)
- Communal—groups of people who chose to live together
- Same gender—about one in five families have same-gender parents.

Assess Causative and Contributing Factors

Illness-Related Factors
- Sudden, unexpected nature of illness
- Burdensome, chronic problems
- Potentially disabling nature of illness
- Symptoms creating disfiguring change in physical appearance
- Social stigma associated with illness
- Financial burden

Factors Related to Behavior of a Family Member
- Refuses to cooperate with necessary interventions
- Engages in socially deviant behavior associated with illness (e.g., suicide attempts, violence, substance abuse)
- Isolates himself or herself from family
- Acts out or is verbally abusive to health-care professionals and family members

Factors Related to Overall Family Functioning
- Loss of home (e.g., homeless, living with relative)
- Negative change in financial income
- Inability to solve problems
- Ineffective communication patterns among members
- Changes in role expectations and resulting tension

Promote Cohesiveness

- Approach the family with warmth, respect, and support.
- Keep family members abreast of changes in ill family member's condition when appropriate.
- Avoid discussing what caused the problem or blaming.
- Encourage verbalization of guilt, anger, blame, and hostility and subsequent recognition of own feelings in family members.
- Explain the importance of functional communications, which uses verbal and nonverbal communication to teach

behavior, share feelings and values, and evolve decisions about family health practices (Kaakinen, Gedaly-Duff, Hanson, & Padgett, 2010).

Assist Family to Appraise the Situation

- What is at stake? Encourage family to have a realistic perspective by providing accurate information and answers to questions. Ensure all family members have input.
- What are the choices? Assist family to reorganize roles at home and set priorities to maintain family integrity and reduce stress.
- Initiate discussions regarding stressors of home care (physical, emotional, environmental, and financial).
- "Family-oriented approaches that include helping a family gain insight and make behavioral changes are most successful" (Varcarolis, Carson, & Shoemaker, 2010).

Promote Clear Boundaries Between Individuals in Family

- Ensure that all family members share their concerns.
- Elicit the responsibilities of each member.
- Acknowledge the differences.

Initiate Health Teaching and Referrals, as Necessary

- Include family members in group education sessions.
- Refer families to lay support and self-help groups.
  - Al-Anon
  - Lupus Foundation of America
  - Syn-Anon
  - Arthritis Foundation
  - Alcoholics Anonymous
  - National Multiple Sclerosis Society
  - Sharing and Caring
  - American Cancer Society
  - American Hospital Association
  - American Heart Association
  - American Diabetes Association
  - Ostomy Association
  - American Lung Association
  - Reach for Recovery
  - Alzheimer's Disease and Related Disorders Association
- Facilitate family involvement with social supports.
- Assist family members to identify reliable friends (e.g., clergy, significant others); encourage seeking help (emotional, technical) when appropriate.
- Enlist help of other professionals (social work, therapist, psychiatrist, school nurse).

Dysfunctional Family Processes

NANDA-I Definition

Psychosocial, spiritual, and physiologic functions of the family unit are chronically disorganized, which leads to conflict, denial of problems, resistance to change, ineffective problem-solving, and a series of self-perpetuating crises

Defining Characteristics
(*Lindeman, Hokanson, & Batek, 1994)

Major (Must Be Present)

Behaviors
Inappropriate expression of anger*
Inadequate understanding or knowledge of alcoholism
Manipulation*
Denial of problems*
Dependency*
Loss of control of drinking
Refusal to get help*
Impaired communication*

Alcohol abuse
Rationalization*
Enabling behaviors
Blaming*
Ineffective problem solving*
Inability to meet emotional needs
Broken promises*
Criticizing*

Feelings*
Hopelessness
Anger
Guilt
Powerlessness
Emotional isolation
Worthlessness
Vulnerability
Suppressed rage

Repressed emotions
Anxiety
Shame
Mistrust
Loneliness
Responsible for alcoholic's behavior
Embarrassment

Roles and Relationships
Deteriorated family relationships
Inconsistent parenting
Disturbed family dynamics
Closed communication systems
Family denial

Marital problems
Ineffective spouse communication
Intimacy dysfunction
Disruption of family roles

Minor (May Be Present)

Behaviors

Inability to accept a wide range of feelings*

Inability to get or receive help appropriately*

Orientation toward tension relief rather than goal achievement*

Ineffective decision making

Failure to deal with conflict

Contradictory, paradoxical communication*

Family's special occasions are alcohol centered*

Harsh self-judgment*

Escalating conflict*

Isolation

Lying*

Failure to send clear messages

Difficulty having fun*

Immaturity*

Disturbances in concentration*

Chaos*

Inability to adapt to change*

Power struggles*

Substance abuse other than alcohol

Difficulty with life-cycle transitions*

Verbal abuse of spouse or parent*

Stress-related physical illnesses*

Failure to accomplish current or past developmental tasks*

Lack of reliability*

Disturbances in academic performance in children*

Feelings

Being different from other people*

Lack of identity*

Unresolved grief

Feelings misunderstood

Loss*

Depression*

Fear*

Hostility*

Abandonment*

Moodiness*

Confused love and pity

Emotional control by others*

Dissatisfaction*

Confusion*

Failure*

Being unloved*

Self-blaming

Roles and Relationships

Triangulating family relationships*

Inability to meet spiritual needs of members

Reduced ability to relate to one another for mutual growth and maturation*

Lack of skills necessary for relationships*

Lack of cohesiveness*

Disrupted family rituals or no family rituals*

Inability to meet security needs of members

Does not demonstrate respect for individuality of its members
Decreased sexual communication and individuality of its
members
Low perception of parental support*
Pattern of rejection
Neglected obligations*

Related Factors

*Related to inadequate coping skills and/or inadequate problem-solving
skills secondary to:*

Change in financial status (e.g., foreclosure, unemployment)
Homeless status (specify)
Transition (e.g., separation, divorce)
Situation crisis*
Shifts in family roles*

Addition of new family members (e.g., blended family, aging relative)
Alcohol abuse of (specify)
Substance abuse*(specify)
Mental illness of (specify)
Compromised cognitive function of (specify)

 Author's Note

Disabled Family Coping can represent the consequences of the disturbed family dynamics related to chronic mental illness, progressive cognitive decline, substance abuse, alcohol abuse by a family member. Alcoholism is a family disease. This nursing diagnosis can represent the effects of alcohol abuse on each family member. In addition, the individual with substance abuse will also have a specific nursing diagnosis of *Ineffective Coping* or *Ineffective Denial.*

 NOC

Family Coping, Family Functioning, Substance Abuse and Mental Illness

Goals

The family will acknowledge the alcoholism in the family and will set short- and long-term goals, as evidenced by the following indicators:

• Relate the effects of alcoholism on the family unit and individuals
• Identify destructive response patterns
• Describe resources available for individual and family therapy

Coping Enhancements, Referral, Family Process Maintenance, Substance Use Treatment, Family Integrity Promotion, Limit Setting, Support Group

Interventions

Assess the Composition of the "Family" (Pillitteri, 2014)

- Dyad—two people living together (e.g., married, unmarried, gay, lesbian)
- Nuclear—traditional family of a husband, wife, and children
- Multigenerational—a nuclear family with other family members such as grandparents, cousins, grandchildren
- Cohabitation—unmarried couples with children living together
- Polygamous—although illegal in the United States, a family of one man with several wives may immigrate to the United States.
- Blended—remarriage or reconstituted family with children (e.g., divorced, widowed)
- Single-parent—55% of families are single-parent (US Census Bureau, 2013)
- Communal—groups of people who chose to live together
- Same gender—about one in five families have same-gender parents.

Explore the Family's Beliefs About Situation and Goals

- Discuss characteristics of alcoholism; review a screening test (e.g., MAST, CAGE) that outlines characteristics of alcoholism.
- Discuss causes and correct misinformation.
- Acknowledge that relapses are expected.
- Assist to establish short- and long-term goals.

Assist the Family to Gain Insight Into Behavior; Discuss Ineffective Methods Families Use

- Hiding alcohol or car keys
- Anger, silence, threats, crying
- Making excuses for work, family, or friends
- Bailing the individual out of jail
- Does not stop drinking
- Increases family anger
- Removes the responsibility for drinking from the individual
- Prevents the individual from suffering the consequences of his or her drinking behavior

Emphasize to Family That Helping the Alcoholic Means First Helping Themselves

- Focus on changing their response.
- Allow the individual to be responsible for his or her drinking behavior.
- Describe activities that will improve their lives, as individuals and a family.
- Initiate one stress management technique (e.g., aerobic exercise, assertiveness course, meditation).
- Plan time as a family together outside the home (e.g., museum, zoos, and picnic). If the alcoholic is included, he or she must contract not to drink during the activity and agree on a consequence if he or she does.

Discuss With Family That Recovery Will Dramatically Change Usual Family Dynamics

- The alcoholic is removed from the center of attention.
- All family roles will be challenged.
- Family members will have to focus on themselves instead of the alcoholic individual.
- Family members will have to assume responsibility for their behavior, rather than blaming others.
- Behavioral problems of children serve a purpose for the family.

Initiate Health Teaching Regarding Community Resources and Referrals, as Indicated

- Al-Anon
- Alcoholics Anonymous family therapy
- Individual therapy
- Self-help groups
- National Association for Children of Alcoholics (NACoA)

FEAR

NANDA-I Definition

Response to perceived threat that is consciously recognized as a danger

Defining Characteristics

Verbal Reports of Panic*
Alarm*
Aggression
Apprehension*
Avoidance behaviors*
Being scared*
Decreased self-assurance*
Dread*

Excitement*
Impulsiveness*
Increased alertness*/tension
Narrowed focus on source of
  the fear*
Panic
Terror*

Visceral–Somatic Activity
Musculoskeletal
Shortness of breath
Fatigue*/limb weakness
Muscle tightness*
Respiratory
Increased rate*
Trembling
Cardiovascular
Palpitations
Rapid pulse*
Increased systolic blood
  pressure*
Skin
Flush/pallor*
Increased perspiration*
Paresthesia

Gastrointestinal
Anorexia*
Nausea/vomiting
Diarrhea*/urge to defecate
Dry mouth*/throat
Central Nervous System
  (CNS)/Perceptual
Syncope
Irritability
Insomnia
Absentmindedness
Lack of concentration
Nightmares
Pupil dilation*
Diminished problem-solving
  ability*
Genitourinary
Urinary frequency/urgency

Related Factors

Fear can be a response to various health problems, situations, or conflicts. Some common sources are indicated in the following:

Pathophysiologic

Related to perceived immediate and long-term effects of:
Cognitive impairment
Disabling illness
Long-term disability

Loss of body function or part
Sensory impairment
Terminal disease

Treatment Related

Related to loss of control and unpredictable outcome secondary to:

Hospitalization
Invasive procedures
Surgery and its outcome
Radiation
Anesthesia

Situational (Personal, Environmental)

Related to loss of control and unpredictable outcome secondary to:

Change or loss of significant
  other
Pain
New environment
New people
Success
Divorce
Lack of knowledge
Failure
Related to potential loss of
  income

Maturational

Preschool (2 to 5 years)
Related to:

Age-related fears
Animals
Being alone
Bodily harm
Dark, strangers, ghosts
Not being liked
Separation from parents, peers
Strangers

School-Age (6 to 12 years)
Related to:

Being lost
Being in trouble
Thunder, lightning
Bad dreams
Weapons

Adolescent (13 to 18 years)
Related to uncertainty of:

Appearance
Scholastic success
Peer support

Adult
Related to uncertainty of:

Marriage
Job security
Pregnancy
Effects of aging
Parenthood

Older Adult
Related to anticipated dependence:

Prolonged suffering
Financial insecurity
Vulnerability to crime
Abandonment

Author's Note

See Anxiety.

 NOC

Anxiety Self-Control, Fear Self-Control

Goals

The adult will relate increased psychological and physiologic comfort, as evidenced by the following indicators:

* Show decreased visceral response (pulse, respirations)
* Differentiate real from imagined situations
* Describe effective and ineffective coping patterns
* Identify own coping responses

The child will exhibit or relate increased psychological and physiologic comfort, as evidenced by the following indicators:

* Discuss fears
* Exhibit less crying

 NIC

Anxiety Reduction, Coping Enhancement; Presence, Counseling, Relaxation Therapy

Interventions

Nursing interventions for *Fear* represent interventions for any individual with fear, regardless of the etiologic or contributing factors.

Assess Possible Contributing Factors

* Refer to Related Factors

Reduce or Eliminate Contributing Factors

Unfamiliar Environment
* Orient individual to environment using simple explanations.
* Speak slowly and calmly.
* Avoid surprises and painful stimuli.
* Use soft lights and music.
* Remove threatening stimulus.
* Plan one-day-at-a-time, familiar routine.
* Encourage gradual mastery of a situation.

- Provide a transitional object with symbolic safeness (security blanket, religious medal).

Intrusion on Personal Space
- Allow personal space.
- Move the individual away from the stimulus.
- Remain with the individual until fear subsides (listen, use silence).
- Later, establish frequent and consistent contacts; use family members and significant others to stay with the individual.
- Use touch as tolerated. Offer a hug.

Threat to Self-Esteem
- Support preferred coping style when individual uses adaptive mechanisms.
- Initially, decrease the individual's number of choices.
- Use simple, direct statements (avoid detail).
- Give direct suggestions to manage everyday events (some prefer details; others like general explanations).
- Encourage expression of feelings (helplessness, anger).
- Give feedback about expressed feelings (support realistic assessments).
- Refocus interaction on areas of capability rather than dysfunction.
- Encourage normal coping mechanisms.
- Encourage sharing common problems with others.
- Give feedback of effect the individual's behavior has on others.
- Encourage the individual to face the fear.

When Intensity of Feelings Has Decreased, Assist With Insight and Controlling Response

- Ask to write their fears in narrative form.
- Ask to write their fears in narrative form.
- Teach how to solve problems.
  - What is the problem?
  - Who or what is responsible?
  - What are the options?
  - What are the advantages and disadvantages of each option?

Initiate Health Teaching and Referrals as Indicated

- Progressive relaxation technique
- Reading, music, breathing exercises
- Desensitization, self-coaching

- Thought stopping, guided fantasy
- Yoga, hypnosis, assertiveness training

⚏ Pediatric Interventions

Participate in Community Functions to Teach Parents Age-Related Fears and Constructive Interventions (e.g., Parent–School Organizations, Newsletters, Civic Groups)

- Provide child opportunities to talk and write about fears and to learn healthy outlets for anger or sadness, such as play therapy.
- Acknowledge illness, death, and pain as real; refrain from protecting children from the reality of existence; encourage open, honest sharing that is age-appropriate.
- Never make fun of the child. Share with child that these fears are okay.
- Fear of imaginary animals and intruders (e.g., "I don't see a lion in your room, but I will leave the light on for you, and if you need me again, please call.")
- Fear of parent being late (establish a contingency plan [e.g., "If you come home from school and Mommy is not here, go to Mrs. S next door."])
- Fear of vanishing down a toilet or bathtub drain:
  - Wait until child is out of the tub before releasing the drain.
  - Wait until child is off the toilet before flushing.
  - Leave toys in bathtub and demonstrate how they do not go down the drain.
- Fear of dogs and cats:
  - Allow child to watch a child and a dog playing from a distance.
  - Do not force child to touch the animal.
- Fear of death
- Fear of pain (see Pediatric Interventions for *Pain*)
- Refusal to go to sleep:
  - Establish a realistic hour for retiring.
  - Contract for a reward if the child is successful.
  - Do not sleep with the child or take the child to the parent's room.
- Provide opportunities for expectant father to share his concerns and fears.

DEFICIENT FLUID VOLUME

Deficient Fluid Volume

Risk for Deficient Fluid Volume

NANDA-I Definition

Decreased intravascular, interstitial, and/or intracellular fluid. This refers to dehydration, water loss alone without change in sodium.

Defining Characteristics

Major (Must Be Present, One or More)

Insufficient oral fluid intake
Dry skin*/mucous membranes*
Negative balance of intake and output
Weight loss

Minor (May Be Present)

Increased serum sodium
Thirst*/nausea/anorexia
Concentrated urine or urinary frequency
Decreased urine output* or excessive urine output

Related Factors

Pathophysiologic

Related to excessive urinary output:
Uncontrolled diabetes
Diabetes insipidus (inadequate antidiuretic hormone)

Related to increased capillary permeability and evaporative loss from burn wound (nonacute)

Related to losses secondary to:

Abnormal drainage	Fever or increased metabolic rate
Diarrhea	Peritonitis
Excessive menses	Wound

Situational (Personal, Environmental)

Related to vomiting/nausea

Related to decreased motivation to drink liquids secondary to:
Depression
Fatigue

Related to fad diets/fasting

Related to high-solute tube feedings

Related to difficulty swallowing or feeding self secondary to:
Oral or throat pain
Fatigue

Related to extreme heat/sun/dryness

Related to excessive loss through:
Indwelling catheters
Drains

Related to insufficient fluids for exercise effort or weather conditions

Related to excessive use of:
Laxatives or enemas
Diuretics, alcohol, or caffeine

Maturational

Infant/Child
Related to increased vulnerability secondary to:
Decreased fluid reserve and decreased ability to concentrate
  urine

Older Adult
Related to increased vulnerability secondary to:
Decreased fluid reserve and decreased sensation of thirst

 Author's Note

Deficient Fluid Volume frequently is used to describe people who are NPO, in hypovolemic shock, or experiencing bleeding. This author recommends its use only when an individual can drink but has an insufficient intake for metabolic needs. If the individual cannot drink or needs intravenous therapy, refer to the collaborative problems *Risk for Complications of Hypovolemia* and *Risk for Complications of Electrolyte Imbalances* in Section 3 Collaborative Problems.

Should *Deficient Fluid Volume* be used to represent such clinical situations as shock, renal failure, or thermal injury? Most nurses would agree that these are collaborative problems to report to the physician for collaborative treatments.

 NOC

Electrolyte and Acid/Base Balance, Fluid Balance, Hydration

Goals

The individual will maintain urine specific gravity within normal range, as evidenced by the following indicators:

- Increase fluid intake to a specified amount according to age and metabolic needs
- Identify risk factors for fluid deficit and relate need for increased fluid intake as indicated
- Demonstrate no signs and symptoms of dehydration

NIC

Fluid/Electrolyte Management, Fluid Monitoring

Interventions

Assess Causative Factors

Prevent Dehydration in High-Risk Individuals

- Monitor output; ensure at least 5 mg/kg/hr.
- Monitor intake; ensure at least 2,000 mL of oral fluids every 24 hours unless contraindicated. Offer fluids that are desired hourly.
- Teach the individual to avoid coffee, tea, grapefruit juice, sugared drinks, and alcohol.
- Weigh daily in the same clothes, at the same time. A 2% to 4% weight loss indicates mild dehydration; 5% to 9% weight loss indicates moderate dehydration.
- For older people scheduled to fast before diagnostic studies, advise them to increase fluid intake 8 hours before fasting. Remind them that when fasting for blood tests, water is permissible.
- Review the individual's medications. Do they contribute to dehydration (e.g., diuretics)? Do they require increased fluid intake (e.g., lithium)?

Initiate Health Teaching, as Indicated

- Give verbal and written directions for desired fluids and amounts.
- Explain to the individual, the need to drink fluids and to use a system for reminding himself or herself not to rely on thirst.
- Incorporate strategies to prompt fluid intake:
  - Fill a large pitcher of water in the morning to monitor intake.
  - Drink an extra glass of water with medications.
  - In care facilities, structure a schedule with a beverage cart with choices.
- Explain the need to increase fluids during exercise, fever, infection, and hot weather.
- Teach the individual/family how to observe for dehydration (especially in infants, elderly) and to intervene by increasing fluid intake (see Subjective and Objective Data for signs of dehydration).
- For athletes, stress the need to hydrate before and during exercise, preferably with a high–sodium-content beverage. (Refer to *Hyperthermia* for additional interventions.)

Pediatric Interventions

To Increase Fluid Intake

- Offer appealing fluids (popsicles, frozen juice bars, snow cones, water, milk, Jell-O); let the child help make them.
- Use unusual containers (colorful cups, straws).
- Conduct a game or activity.
  - On a chart, have the child cross out the number of cups he or she drank each day.
  - Read a book to the child and have him or her drink a sip when turning a page, or have a tea party.
  - Have the child take a drink when it is his or her turn in a game.
  - Set a schedule for supplementary liquids to promote the habit of in-between–meal fluids (e.g., juice or Kool-Aid at 10 AM and 2 PM each day).
  - Decorate straws.
  - Let the child fill small cups with a syringe.
- Make a progress poster; use stickers or stars to indicate fluid goals met. Older children usually respond to the challenge of meeting a specific intake goal.
- Rewards and contracts are also effective (e.g., a sticker for drinking a certain amount).
- Young children usually respond to games that integrate drinking fluids.

Prevention of Exertional Heat Illness

Teach Risk Factors to Children/Adolescents and Parents
- Hot and/or humid weather
- Poor preparation
- Not heat-acclimatized
- Inadequate prehydration
- Excessive physical exertion
- Insufficient rest/recovery time between repeated bouts of high-intensity exercise (e.g., repeat sprints)
- Insufficient access to fluids and opportunities to rehydrate
- Insufficient rest/recovery time between practices, games, or matches
- Overweight/obese (BMI 85th percentile for age)
- Clinical conditions (e.g., diabetes) or medications (e.g., attention-deficit/hyperactivity disorder medications)
- Current or recent illness (especially if it involves/involved gastrointestinal distress or fever) (American Academy of Pediatrics, 2011)

Preventive Interventions
- Provide and promote consumption of readily accessible fluids at regular intervals before, during, and after activity.
- Allow gradual introduction and adaptation to the climate, intensity, and duration of activities and uniform/protective gear.
- Ensure that personnel and facilities for effectively treating heat illness are readily available on site. In response to an affected (moderate or severe heat stress) child or adolescent, promptly activate emergency medical services and rapidly cool the victim.

Teach to Closely Monitor All Children and Adolescents at All Times During Sports and Other Physical Activity in the Heat for Signs and Symptoms of Developing Heat Illness
- Any significant deterioration in performance with notable signs of struggling
- Negative changes in personality or mental status
- Other concerning clinical markers of well-being, including pallor, bright-red flushing, dizziness, headache, excessive fatigue, vomiting
- Complaints of feeling cold or extremely hot

Advise to Initiate Immediate Treatment
- Move the victim to the shade, immediately removing protective equipment and clothing.
- When feasible, rectal temperature should be promptly checked by trained personnel, and if indicated (rectal temperature 40° C

[104° F]), on-site whole-body rapid cooling using proven techniques should be initiated without delay.

- If rectal temperature cannot be assessed in a child or adolescent with clinical signs or symptoms suggestive of moderate or severe heat stress, appropriate treatment should not be delayed.
- Initiate cooling by cold- or ice-water immersion (preferred, most effective method) or by applying ice packs to the neck, axillae, and groin and rotating ice-water– soaked towels to all other areas of the body until rectal temperature reaches just under 39° C (approximately 102° F) or the victim shows clinical improvement.
- Prompt rapid cooling for 10 to 15 minutes, and if the child or adolescent is alert enough to ingest fluid, hydration should be initiated by attending staff while awaiting the arrival of medical assistance.

Risk for Deficient Fluid Volume

NANDA-I Definition

Vulnerable for experiencing decreased intravascular, interstitial, and/or intracellular fluid. This refers to dehydration, water loss alone without change in sodium, which can compromise health

Risk Factors*

Deviations affecting access to fluids
Deviations affecting intake of fluids
Deviations affecting absorption of fluids
Excessive losses through normal routes (e.g., diarrhea)
Extremes of age
Extremes of weight
Factors influencing fluid needs (e.g., hypermetabolic state)
Loss of fluid through abnormal routes (e.g., indwelling tubes)
Deficient knowledge
Pharmaceutical agents (e.g., diuretics)

Author's Note

If the individual is NPO, refer to the collaborative problem *Risk for Complications of Hypovolemia in Section 3*. If the person can drink, refer to *Deficient Fluid Volume* for interventions.

EXCESS FLUID VOLUME

NANDA-I Definition

Increased isotonic fluid retention

Defining Characteristics

Major (Must Be Present, One or More)

Edema (peripheral, sacral)
Taut, shiny skin

Minor (May Be Present)

Intake greater than output
Weight gain

Related Factors

Pathophysiologic

Related to compromised regulatory mechanisms secondary to:
Renal failure (acute or chronic)   Endocrine dysfunction
Systemic and metabolic abnormalities   Lipedema

Related to portal hypertension, lower plasma colloidal osmotic pressure, and sodium retention secondary to:
Liver disease   Ascites
Cirrhosis   Cancer

Related to venous and arterial abnormalities secondary to:
Varicose veins   Trauma
Phlebitis   Thrombus

Infection

Peripheral vascular disease

Immobility

Lymphedema

Neoplasms

Treatment Related

Related to sodium and water retention secondary to corticosteroid therapy

Related to inadequate lymphatic drainage secondary to mastectomy

Situational (Personal, Environmental)

Related to impaired venous return secondary to increased peripheral resistance and decreased efficiency of valves related to excess body weight

Related to excessive sodium intake/fluid intake

Related to low protein intake:
Fad diets
Malnutrition

Related to dependent venous pooling/venostasis secondary to:
Standing or sitting for long
periods   Tight cast or bandage
Immobility

Related to venous compression from pregnant uterus

Maturational

Older Adult

Related to impaired venous return secondary to increased peripheral resistance and decreased efficiency of valves

 Author's Note

Excess Fluid Volume is frequently used to describe pulmonary edema, ascites, or renal insufficiency or failure. These are all collaborative problems that should not be renamed as *Excess Fluid Volume*. Refer to Section 3 for collaborative problems. This diagnosis represents a situation for which nurses can prescribe if the focus is on peripheral edema. Nursing interventions center on teaching the individual or family how to minimize edema and protect tissue from injury.

NOC

Electrolyte Balance, Fluid Balance, Hydration

Goals

The individual will exhibit decreased edema (specify site), as evidenced by the following indicators:

- Relate causative factors
- Relate methods of preventing edema

NIC

Electrolyte Management, Fluid Management, Fluid Monitoring, Skin Surveillance

Interventions

Identify Contributing and Causative Factors

- Refer to Related Factors.

Reduce or Eliminate Causative and Contributing Factors

Excess Salt in Diet
- Assess dietary intake and habits that may contribute to fluid retention.
- Be specific; record daily and weekly intake of food and fluids.
- Assess weekly diet for inadequate protein or excessive sodium intake.
  - Discuss likes and dislikes of foods that provide protein.
  - Teach the individual to plan a weekly menu that provides protein at an affordable price.
  - Teach the individual to decrease salt intake.
  - Read labels for sodium content.
  - Avoid convenience and canned and frozen foods.
  - Cook without salt; use spices (lemon, basil, tarragon, mint) to add flavor.
  - Use vinegar in place of salt to flavor soups, stews, and others (e.g., 2 to 3 teaspoons of vinegar per 4 to 6 quarts, according to taste).
  - Ascertain whether the individual may use salt substitute (caution that he or she must use the exact substitute prescribed).

Dependent Venous Pooling
- Assess for evidence of dependent venous pooling or venous stasis.
- Encourage alternating periods of horizontal rest (legs elevated) with vertical activity (standing); this may be contraindicated in congestive heart failure.
  - Keep the edematous extremity elevated above the level of the heart whenever possible (unless contraindicated by heart failure).
  - Keep the edematous arms elevated on two pillows or with IV pole sling.
  - Elevate the legs whenever possible, using pillows under them (avoid pressure points, especially behind the knees).
  - Discourage leg and ankle crossing.
- Reduce constriction of vessels.
  - Assess clothing for proper fit and constrictive areas.
  - Instruct to avoid panty girdles/garters, knee-high stockings, and leg crossing and to practice elevating the legs when possible.
- Consider using anti-embolism stockings or ACE bandages; measure the legs carefully for stockings/support hose.*
- Apply stockings while lying down (e.g., in the morning before arising).
- Check extremities frequently for adequate circulation and evidence of constrictive areas.

Venous Pressure Points
- Assess for venous pressure points associated with casts, bandages, and tight stockings.
  - Observe circulation at edges of casts, bandages, and stockings.
  - For casts, insert soft material to cushion pressure points at the edges.
- Check circulation frequently.
- Shift body weight in the cast to redistribute weight within (unless contraindicated).
  - Encourage individual to do this every 15 to 30 minutes while awake to prevent venostasis.
  - Encourage wiggling of fingers or toes and isometric exercise of unaffected muscles within the cast.
  - If the individual cannot do this alone, assist him or her at least hourly to shift body weight.

Inadequate Lymphatic Drainage
- Keep the extremity elevated on pillows.
  - If the edema is marked, the arm should be elevated *but not in adduction* (this position may constrict the axilla).

- • The elbow should be higher than the shoulder.
- • The hand should be higher than the elbow.
- Measure blood pressure in the unaffected arm.
- Do not give injections or start IV fluids in the affected arm.
- Protect the affected limb from injury.
- Encourage the individual to wear a Medic-Alert tag engraved with "Caution: lymphedema arm—no tests/no needle injections."
- Caution the individual to visit a physician if the arm becomes red, swollen, or unusually hard.
- After a mastectomy, encourage range-of-motion (ROM) exercises and use of the affected arm to facilitate development of a collateral lymphatic drainage system (explain that lymphedema often decreases within 1 month, but that the individual should continue massaging, exercising, and elevating the arm for 3 to 4 months after surgery).

Protect Edematous Skin From Injury

- Refer to *Risk for Pressure Ulcer* for additional information about preventing injury.

Initiate Health Teaching and Referrals, as Indicated

- Give clear verbal and written instructions for all medications: what, when, how often, why, side effects; pay special attention to drugs that directly influence fluid balance (e.g., diuretics, steroids).
- Write down instructions for diet, activity, and use of ACE bandages, stockings, and so forth.
- Have the individual demonstrate the instructions.
- With severe fluctuations in edema, have the individual weigh himself or herself every morning and before bedtime daily; instruct the individual to keep a written record of weights. For less severe illness, the individual may need to weigh himself or herself only once daily and record the weight.
- Caution the individual to call a physician for excessive edema/weight gain (greater than 2 lb/day) or increased shortness of breath at night or upon exertion. Explain that these signs may indicate early heart problems and may require medication to prevent them from worsening.
- Consider home care or visiting nurses referral to follow at home.
- Provide literature concerning low-salt diets; consult with a dietitian if necessary.

Maternal Interventions

- Explain the cause of edema of ankles and fingers.
- Advise the individual to limit salt intake moderately (e.g., eliminate processed meats, chips) and to maintain water intake of 8 to 10 glasses daily unless contraindicated.
- Advise to consult with an OB specialist or primary care provider for facial puffiness, sacral or pitting edema, or weight gain of more than 2 lb in 1 week.

RISK FOR IMBALANCED FLUID VOLUME

NANDA-I Definition

Vulnerable for a decrease, increase, or rapid shift from one to the other of intravascular, interstitial, and/or intracellular fluid that may compromise health, which may compromise health. This refers to body fluid loss, gain, or both.

Risk Factors*

Abdominal surgery	Pancreatitis
Ascites	Receiving apheresis
Burns	Sepsis
Intestinal obstruction	Traumatic injury (e.g., fractured hip)

Author's Note

This diagnosis can represent several clinical conditions, such as edema, hemorrhage, dehydration, and compartmental syndrome. If the nurse is monitoring an individual for imbalanced fluid volume, labeling the specific imbalance as a collaborative problem, such as hypovolemia, compartment syndrome, increased intracranial pressure, gastrointestinal bleeding, or postpartum hemorrhage, would be more useful clinically. For example, most intraoperative individuals would be monitored for hypovolemia. If the procedure was neurosurgery, then cranial pressure would also be monitored. If the procedure were orthopedic, compartment syndrome would be addressed. Refer to Section 3 for specific collaborative problems and interventions.

DYSFUNCTIONAL GASTROINTESTINAL MOTILITY

Dysfunctional Gastrointestinal Motility

Risk for Dysfunctional Gastrointestinal Motility

See also Risk for Complications of Paralytic Ileus in Section 3.

NANDA-I Definition

Increased, decreased, ineffective, or lack of peristaltic activity within the gastrointestinal system

Defining Characteristics*

Absence of flatus
Abdominal cramping or pain
Abdominal distention
Accelerated gastric emptying
Bile-colored gastric residual
Change in bowel sounds
(e.g., absent, hypoactive,
hyperactive)

Diarrhea
Dry stool difficulty passing
stools
Hard stools
Increased gastric residual
Nausea
Regurgitation, vomiting

Related Factors*

Aging
Anxiety
Enteral feedings
Food intolerance (e.g., glu-
ten lactose)
Immobility Ingestion of
contaminates (e.g., food,
water)

Ingestion of contaminates
(e.g., food, water)
Malnutrition
Pharmaceutical agents
(e.g., narcotics/opiates, anti-
biotics, laxatives, anesthesia)
Prematurity, sedentary lifestyle
Surgery

 Author's Note

This NANDA-I diagnosis is too broad for clinical usefulness. It represents collaborative problems and some nursing diagnoses such as *Diarrhea, Constipation.* Refer to Section 3, Collaborative Problems, for more

specific collaborative problems as *Risk for Complications of Gastrointestinal Dysfunction*, *Risk for Complications of Paralytic Ileus*, and *Risk for Complications for GI Bleeding*.

Goals/Interventions

The nurse should examine the assessment data to determine the focus.

- To monitor for physiologic complications that require nursing and medical interventions as *Risk for Complications of Paralytic Ileus or GI Bleeding* (collaborative problem), refer to Refer to Section 3.
- To prevent or treat a physiologic dysfunction as constipation, diarrhea, fluid imbalance, compromised nutrition, or complications of immobility, refer to *Risk for Imbalanced Nutrition*, *Deficient Fluid Volume*, *Diarrhea*, *Disuse Syndrome*, or *Risk for Constipation* (nursing diagnoses) in Section 1.

Risk for Dysfunctional Gastrointestinal Motility

See also *Risk for Complications of Gastrointestinal Dysfunction* in Section 3.

NANDA-I Definition

Vulnerable for an increased, decreased, ineffective, or lack of peristaltic activity within the gastrointestinal system, which may compromise health

Risk Factors*

Abdominal surgery
Aging
Anxiety
Change in food or water
Decreased gastrointestinal circulation
Diabetes mellitus

Immobility
Infection (e.g., bacteria parasitic, viral)
Pharmaceutical agents (e.g., antibiotics, laxatives, narcotics/opiates, proton pump inhibitors)
Prematurity

Food intolerance (gluten, lactose)
Gastroesophageal reflux disease (GERD)

Sedentary lifestyle
Stress
Unsanitary food preparation

 Author's Note

This NANDA-I diagnosis is too broad for clinical use. This diagnosis represents some collaborative problems such as *Risk for Complications of Gastrointestinal Dysfunction*, *Risk for Complications of GI Bleeding*, *Risk for Complications of Paralytic Ileus*, and nursing diagnoses such as *Risk for Diarrhea*, *Risk for Constipation*, and *Risk for Infection*. Refer to Section 3, Collaborative Problems.

Examine the risk factors in the individual and determine if the focus of nursing interventions is prevention; if yes, use *Risk for Infection*, *Risk for Diarrhea*, or *Risk for Constipation*. If the focus is to monitor gastrointestinal function for complications that require medical and nursing interventions, use a collaborative problem as *Risk for Complications of (specify)*.

GRIEVING

Grieving

Anticipatory Grieving

Complicated Grieving

Risk for Complicated Grieving

NANDA-I Definition

A normal complex process that includes emotional, physical, spiritual, social, and intellectual responses and behaviors by which individuals, families, and communities, incorporate an actual, anticipated, or perceived loss into their daily lives

Defining Characteristics

Major (Must Be Present)

The individual reports an actual or perceived loss (person, pet, object, function, status, or relationship) with varied responses such as the following:

Denial	In sleep patterns*
Suicidal thoughts	Blame*
Guilt	Detachment*
Crying	Anergia
Anger*	Disorganization*
Sorrow	Feelings of worthlessness
Despair*	Numbness
Longing/searching behaviors	Disbelief
Inability to concentrate	Anxiety
Alterations	Helplessness

Related Factors

Many situations can contribute to feelings of loss. Some common situations follow.

Pathophysiologic

Related to loss of function or independence secondary to:

Neurologic	Sensory
Digestive	Renal
Cardiovascular	Musculoskeletal
Respiratory	Trauma

Treatment Related

Related to losses associated with:
Long-term dialysis
Surgery (e.g., mastectomy)

Situational (Personal, Environmental)

Related to loss of health

Related to losing a job

Related to loss of financial stability

Related to death of a pet

Related to loss of a cherished dream

Related to a loved one's serious illness

Related to loss of a friendship

Related to loss of home

Related to the negative effects and losses secondary to:
Chronic pain   Terminal illness
Death

Related to losses in lifestyle associated with:

Childbirth	Divorce
Child leaving home	Separation
Marriage	Role function

Related to loss of normalcy secondary to:

Handicap	Scars
Illness	

Maturational

Related to losses and/or changes attributed to aging:

Independence (loss of driving license, own home, meal preparation)	Occupation
	Sexual performance
Friends, siblings	

Related to loss of hope, dreams

 Author's Note

Grieving, Anticipatory Grieving, and *Complicated Grieving* represent three types of responses of individuals or families experiencing a loss. *Grieving* describes normal grieving after a loss and participation in grief work. *Anticipatory Grieving* describes engaging in grief work before an expected loss. *Complicated Grieving* represents a maladaptive process in which grief work is suppressed or absent or an individual exhibits prolonged exaggerated responses. For all three diagnoses, the goal of nursing is to promote grief work. In addition, for *Complicated Grieving,* the nurse directs interventions to reduce excessive, prolonged, problematic responses.

In many clinical situations, the nurse expects a grief response (e.g., loss of body part, death of significant other). Other situations that evoke strong grief responses are sometimes ignored or minimized (e.g., abortion, newborn death, death of one twin or triplet, death of secreted lover, suicide, loss of children to foster homes, or adoption).

NOC
Coping, Family Coping, Grief Resolution, Psychosocial Adjustment, Life Change

Goals

The individual will express his or her grief, as evidenced by the following indicators:

- Describe the meaning of the death or loss to him or her
- Share his or her grief with significant others

NIC

Family Support, Grief Work Facilitation, Coping Enhancement, Anticipatory Guidance, Emotional Support

Interventions

Assess for Factors That May Delay Grief Work

- Unavailable or no support system
- Dependency
- Previous emotional illness
- Uncertain loss (e.g., missing child)
- Inability to grieve
- Early object loss
- Failure to grieve for past loss
- Personality structure
- Nature of relationship
- Multiple losses

Reduce or Eliminate Factors, If Possible

Promote a Trust Relationship

- Promote feelings of self-worth through one-on-one or group sessions.
- Allow for established time to meet and discuss feelings.
- Communicate clearly, simply, and to the point.
- Never try to lessen the loss (e.g., "She didn't suffer long"; or "You can have another baby").
- Use feedback to assess what the individual and the family are learning.
- Offer support and reassurance.
- Create a therapeutic milieu (convey that you care).
- Establish a safe, secure, and private environment.
- Demonstrate respect for the individual's culture, religion, race, and values.
- Provide privacy but be careful not to isolate the individual or family inadvertently.
- Provide a presence of simply "being" with the bereaved.

Support Grief Reactions
- Explain grief reactions: shock and disbelief, developing awareness, and resolution.
- Describe varied acceptable expressions:
  - Elated or manic behavior as a defense against depression
  - Elation and hyperactivity as a reaction of love and protection from depression
  - Various states of depression
  - Various somatic manifestations (weight loss or gain, indigestion, dizziness)
- Assess for past experiences with loss (e.g., losses in childhood and later life).

Determine Whether Family Has Special Requests Regarding Viewing the Deceased (*Vanezis & McGee, 1999)
- Prepare them for possible body changes.
- Remove all equipment; change soiled linen.
- Support their request (e.g., holding, washing, touching, kissing).

Promote Family Cohesiveness
- Support the family at its level of functioning.
- Encourage self-exploration of feelings with family members.
- Explain the need to discuss behaviors that interfere with relationships.
- Recognize and reinforce the strengths of each family member.
- Encourage family members to evaluate their feelings and support one another.

Promote Grief Work with Each Response
Denial
- Recognize that response is useful and necessary.
- Explain the use of denial by one family member to the other members.
- Do not push individual to move past denial without emotional readiness.

Isolation
- Convey acceptance by acknowledging grief.
- Create open, honest communication to promote sharing.
- Encourage individual/family to increase social activities (e.g., support groups, church groups) gradually.
- Encourage individual/family to let significant others know their needs (e.g., support, privacy, permission to share their experience).

Depression
- Reinforce the individual's self-esteem.

- Identify the level of depression and develop the approach accordingly.
- Use empathic sharing; acknowledge grief ("It must be very difficult").
- Identify any indications of suicidal behavior (frequent statements of intent, revealed plan).
- See *Risk for Self-Harm* for additional information.

Anger
- Acknowledge the individual's anger as a coping mechanism.
- Explain to the family that anger serves to try to control one's environment more closely because of an inability to control loss.
- Stress that the illness or death did not result from being bad or because the well child wished it.

Identify Individuals at High Risk for Complicated Grieving Reactions
- Length of relationship: more than 55 years, less than 5 years; consider significance and quality of relationship to the survivor
- Medical issues: pending treatments or surgeries; history of acute or chronic illness
- Mental health history or treatment: outpatient counseling/ follow-up; psychiatric medications (depression, anxiety, sleep, etc.); psychiatric hospitalizations; suicide attempts; suicidal ideations
- Substance abuse: alcohol or drug abuse treatment
- Suicidality: in family history, suicidal ideation or potential for it
- Family dynamics: alliances, conflicts
- Children: 17 years or younger, either in home or with significant relationship to deceased (e.g., grandparent who lived in the same home)
- Multiple losses: deaths, moves, retirement, divorce
- Traumatic death: circumstances of death, sudden or unexpected, as perceived by bereaved
- Isolation: geographical, social, emotional

Encourage Family Members to Share Their Feelings and Support One Another
- Specifically, dialogue with the "strong" family members about their feelings.

Teach the Individual/Family Signs of Pathologic Grieving, Especially Those at Risk
- Continued searching for the deceased (frequent moves/ relocations)
- Delusions

- Isolation
- Egocentricity
- Overt hostility (usually toward a family member)

Provide Health Teaching and Referrals, as Indicated

- Identify agencies that may be helpful (e.g., community agencies, religious groups).

Pediatric Interventions

When a Child is Dying (Ball, Bindler, & Cowen, 2015)

- Cultural differences should be observed and respected as this aspect can be pivotal in the dying process for the family as well as the child who is about to die.
- Some examples of traditions involving the dying process based on religion:
  - Catholicism: commonly buried; sacrament of the sick performed
  - Judaism: seven-day mourning period; body to ritually washed; buried as soon as possible
  - Islam: deathbed should be turned to face Mecca; autopsy only for medical or legal reasons; body is washed only by Muslim of the same gender
  - Jehovah's Witness: organ donation is forbidden; autopsy only for legal reasons
- Sometimes the child is aware they are dying before being formally told. If the parents decide to keep the prognosis from the child for fear of causing child to lose hope, they can actually be causing child to feel isolated.
- Consult a bereavement specialist or counselor for suggestions and as a resource for the child as well as the parents/family.
- Listen to the child. Each child will cope differently. Allow the child to speak openly and answer their questions honestly.
- Allow the children to develop friendships with other children with similar interests or problems.

When Someone the Child Knows Dies, Explain What Caused the Death

- Clarify child's perceptions.
- Openly clarify that the child did not cause the death.

Openly Discuss Possible Responses (*Hooyman & Kramer, 2006)

- "Sometimes when someone dies we feel bad if we said or did something bad to them."

- "Sometimes we feel glad we didn't die and then feel bad because _____ did."
- "When someone dies, we can become afraid that we may die also."
- "I remember when _____ said or did _____. What do you remember?"

Explain Rituals (e.g., Read Children's Book About Death)

Assist Family With the Decision About the Child Attending the Funeral and Determine If the Following Are Present (*Hooyman & Kramer, 2006; Boyd, 2012)

- Child has a basic understanding of death and good coping skills.
- Child is not afraid of adults' emotional responses.
- The ethnic group approaches death openly (e.g., children commonly attend funerals).
- A familiar adult who is coping well with his or her own grief is available to monitor the child's needs.
- Child expresses a desire to attend and has a basic understanding of what will happen.

Explore the Child's Modified Involvement in Funeral Activities (e.g., Visit Funeral Home Before Guests Come, Attend After-Service Gathering)

Allow Child to Grieve at Own Pace. Give Adolescents Permission to Grieve Openly. Consider a Sibling Support Group, If Indicated

🕯 Maternal Interventions

Assist Parents of a Deceased Infant, Newborn, or Fetus With Grief Work (*Mina, 1985; Hockenberry & Wilson, 2015)

Promote Grieving
- Use baby's name when discussing the loss.
- Allow parents to share the hopes and dreams they had for the child.
- Provide parents with access to a hospital chaplain or religious leader of their choice.
- Encourage parents to see and to hold their infant to validate the reality of the loss.
- Design a method to communicate to auxiliary departments that the parents are in mourning (e.g., rose sticker on door, chart).
- Prepare a memory packet wrapped in a clean baby blanket (photograph [Polaroid], ID bracelet, footprints with birth

certificate, lock of hair, crib card, fetal monitor strip, infant's blanket). Encourage them to take the memory packet home. If they prefer not to, keep the packet on file in case they change their minds later.

- Encourage parents to share the experience with their other children at home (refer to pertinent literature for consumers).
- Provide for follow-up support and referral services (e.g., support group) after discharge.

Assist Others to Comfort Grieving Parents

- Stress the importance of openly acknowledging the death.
- If the baby or fetus was named, use the name in discussions.
- Never try to lessen the loss with discussions of future pregnancies or other healthy siblings.
- Send sympathy cards. Create a remembrance (e.g., plant a tree).
- Be sensitive to the gravity of the loss for both the mother and the father.

Anticipatory Grieving[14]

Definition

State in which an individual or a group experience reactions in response to an expected significant loss

Defining Characteristics

Major (Must Be Present)

Expressed distress at potential loss

Minor (May Be Present)

Anger   Guilt
Change in communication patterns, eating   Sorrow
  habits, sleep patterns, and/or social patterns   Withdrawal
Decreased libido
Denial

---

[14]This diagnosis is not presently on the NANDA-I list but has been added for clarity and usefulness.

Related Factors

See *Grieving*.

 Author's Note

Anticipatory Grieving is thought to begin when an individual is forewarned of an impending death. Anticipatory grieving may take the form of sadness, anxiety, attempts to reconcile unresolved relationship issues, and efforts to reconstitute or strengthen family bonds. Caretaking behavior may be a form of anticipatory grieving, as the caretaker expresses affection, respect, and attachment through the physical acts of providing care. Anticipation and an opportunity to prepare psychologically for death is thought to ease the adaptation of the grieving individual after death (Block, 2013).

NOC
See also *Grieving*.

Goals

The individual will identify expected loss, and grief reactions will be freely expressed, as evidenced by the following indicators:

- Participate in decision making for the future
- Share concerns with significant others

NIC
See also *Grieving*.

Interventions

Assess for Causative and Contributing Factors of Anticipated or Potential Loss

- Aging
- Body image, self-esteem, or role changes
- Impending retirement
- Terminal illness
- Separation (divorce, hospitalization, marriage, relocation, job)
- Socioeconomic status

Encourage to Share Concerns

- Use open-ended questions and reflection ("What are your thoughts today?" "How do you feel?").

- Acknowledge the value of the individual and his or her grief by using touch, sitting with him or her, and verbalizing your concern ("This must be very difficult," "What is most important to you now?").
- Recognize that some people may choose not to share their concerns, but convey that you are available if they desire to do so later ("What do you hope for?").

Assist the Individual and the Family to Identify Strengths

- "What do you do well?"
- "What are you willing to do to address this issue?"
- "Is religion/spirituality a source of strength for you?"
- "Do you have close friends?"
- "Whom do you turn to in times of need?"
- "What does this person do for you?"
- "What sources of strength have you called upon successfully in the past?"

Promote Integrity of the Individual and the Family by Acknowledging Strengths

- "Your brother looks forward to your visit."
- "Your family is so concerned for you."

Explore With Loved Ones for Factors That Can Hinder Grieving (Worden, 2009)

- History of an ambivalent, hostile, overly dependent relationship
- Uncertainty of death (e.g., missing inaction)
- Multiple losses at the same time (e.g., 9/11, entire family killed in accident)
- History of complicated or delayed grieving
- Family member designated as the "strong one" is not allowed to grieve

Promote Family Cohesiveness

Identify Availability of a Support System
- Meet consistently with family members.
- Identify family member roles, strengths, and weaknesses.

Identify Communication Patterns Within the Family Unit
- Assess positive and negative feedback, verbal and nonverbal communication, and body language.
- Listen and clarify messages being sent.

Provide for the Concept of Hope
- Supply accurate information.
- Resist the temptation to give false hope.
- Help the family reframe hope (i.e., for a peaceful death).

Promote Group Decision Making to Enhance Group Autonomy
- Establish consistent times to meet with the individual and the family.
- Encourage members to talk directly with and to listen to one another.

Provide for Expression of Grief

- Encourage emotional expressions of grieving.
- Caution the individual about use of sedatives and tranquilizers, which may prevent or delay expressions.
- Encourage verbalization by individuals of all age groups and families.
  - Support family cohesiveness.
  - Promote and verbalize strengths of the family group.
- Encourage the individual and the family to engage in life review.
  - Focus and support the social network relationships.
  - Reevaluate past life experiences and integrate them into a new meaning.
  - Convey empathic understanding.
  - Explore unfinished business.

Identify Potential Complicated Grieving Reactions

- Suicidal indications
- Delusions
- Hallucinations
- Difficulty crying
- Difficulty controlling crying
- Phobias
- Obsessions
- Isolation
- Conversion hysteria
- Agitated depression
- Restrictions of pleasure
- Delay in grief work
- Intense longing or pining (longer than 12 to 18 months with few signs of relief)
- Loss of control of environment, leading to hopelessness/helplessness

Provide Health Teaching and Referrals, as Indicated

Refer the Individual With Potential for Dysfunctional Grieving Responses for Counseling (Psychiatrist, Nurse Therapist, Counselor, Psychologist)
- Explain what to expect:
  - Anger
  - Fear
  - Feelings of aloneness
  - Feeling of "going crazy"
  - Guilt
  - Labile emotions
  - Sadness
  - Rejection

Teach the Individual and the Family Signs of Integration of the Loss Into Their Lives
- Grieving individual no longer lives in the past but is future oriented and is establishing new goals.
- Grieving individual redefines the relationship with the lost object/person.
- Grieving individual begins to resocialize; seeks new relationships and experiences.

Identify Agencies That May Be Helpful
- Support groups
- Mental health agencies
- Psychotherapists
- Grief specialists
- Faith communities

Complicated Grieving

NANDA-I Definition

A disorder that occurs after the death of a significant other, in which the experience of distress accompanying bereavement fails to follow normative expectations and manifests in functional impairment

Defining Characteristics

Major (Must Be Present, One or More)

Unsuccessful adaptation to loss
Prolonged denial, depression
Delayed emotional reaction
Inability to assume normal patterns of living
Grief avoidance*
Yearning*

Minor (May Be Present)

Social isolation or withdrawal
Inability to develop new relationships/interests
Inability to restructure life after loss
Rumination*
Self-blame*
Verbalizes persistent painful memories*

Related Factors

See *Grieving*.

 Author's Note

How one responds to loss is highly individual. Responses to acute loss should not be labeled dysfunctional, regardless of the severity. *Complicated Grieving* is characterized by its sustained or prolonged detrimental response in the grieving person. The validation of *Complicated Grieving* cannot occur until several months or 1 to 2 years after the death. Careful assessment with the grieving person can help to determine if the grieving process is being integrated into his or her life or if it is damaging his or her life. In many clinical settings, the diagnosis of *Risk for Complicated Grieving* for individuals at risk for unsuccessful reintegration after a loss may be more useful.

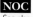 **NOC**

See also *Grieving*.

Goals

The individual will verbalize intent to seek professional assistance, as evidenced by the following indicators:

- Acknowledge the loss
- Acknowledge an unresolved grief process

See also *Grieving.*

Interventions

Assess for Causative and Contributing Factors

- Unavailable (or lack of) support system
- History of dependency on deceased
- History of a difficult relationship with the lost person or object
- Multiple past losses
- Ineffective coping strategies
- Unexpected or traumatic death
- Expectations to "be strong"

Promote a Trust Relationship

- Implement the General Interventions under *Grieving.*

Support the Individual's and the Family's Grief Reactions

- Implement the General Interventions under *Grieving.*

Promote Family Cohesiveness

- Implement the General Interventions under *Grieving.*
- Slowly and carefully identify the reality of the situation (e.g., "After your husband died, who helped you most?").

Promote Grief Work With Each Response

- Explain the use of denial by one family member to the other members.
- Do not force the individual to move past denial without emotional readiness.

Isolation
- Convey a feeling of acceptance by allowing grief.
- Create open, honest communication to promote sharing.
- Reinforce the individual's self-worth by allowing privacy.

- Encourage the individual/family gradually to increase social activities (e.g., support or church groups).

Depression
- Implement the General Interventions under *Grieving*.

Anger
- Understand that this feeling usually replaces denial.
- Explain to the family that anger serves to try to control one's environment more closely because of the inability to control loss.
- Encourage verbalization of the anger.
- See *Anxiety* for additional information for anger.

Guilt/Ambivalence
- Acknowledge the individual's expressed self-view.
- Role-play to allow the individual to "express" to dead person what he or she wants to say or how he or she feels.
- Encourage the individual to identify positive contributions/aspects of the relationship.
- Avoid arguing and participating in the individual's system of shoulds and should nots.
- Discuss the individual's preoccupation with dead person, and attempt to move verbally beyond the present.

Fear
- Focus on the present and maintain a safe and secure environment.
- Help the individual to explore reasons for a meaning of the behavior.
- Consider alternative ways of expressing his or her feelings.

Provide Health Teaching and Referrals, as Indicated

Teach the Individual and the Family Signs of Integration of the Loss Into Their Lives
- Grieving individual no longer lives in the past, but is future oriented and is establishing new goals.
- Grieving individual redefines the relationship with the lost object/person.
- Grieving individual begins to resocialize; seeks new relationships and experiences.

Teach the Individual/Family to Recognize Signs of Complicated Grieving, Especially for People Who Are at Risk, and to Seek Professional Counseling
- Continued searching for deceased
- Prolonged depression
- Denial

- Living in past
- Prolonged hallucinations
- Delusions
- Isolation
- Egocentricity
- Overthostility

Identify Agencies That May Be Helpful
- Support groups
- Mental health agencies
- Psychotherapists
- Grief specialists
- Faith communities

Risk for Complicated Grieving

NANDA-I Definition

Vulnerable for a disorder that occurs after the death of a significant other, in which the experience or distress accompanying bereavement fails to follow normative expectations and manifests in functional impairment, which may compromise health

Risk Factors*

Death of significant other
Lack of support
Significant loss or losses (e.g., divorce, termination, natural disaster, war)

Goals

Refer to *Grieving*.

Interventions

- Identify individuals at high risk for complicated grieving response:
  - Length of relationship: more than 55 years, less than 5 years

- Medical issues: pending treatments, surgeries, history of acute or chronic illness
- Significant mental health issues of deceased or grieving person
- Substance abuse
- Suicide in family history, potential for suicide
- Family conflicts
- Refer also to *Complicated Grieving*.

DEFICIENT COMMUNITY HEALTH

NANDA-I Definition

Presence of one or more health problems or factors that deter wellness or increase the risk of health problems experienced by an aggregate

Defining Characteristics*

Incidence of risks relating to hospitalization experienced by aggregates or populations

Incidence of risks relating to physiologic states experienced by aggregates or populations

Incidence of risks relating to psychological states experienced by aggregates or populations

Incidence of health problems experienced by aggregates or populations

No program available to enhance wellness for aggregates or populations[15]

No program available to prevent one or more health problems for aggregates or populations[15]

No program available to reduce one or more health problems for aggregates or populations[15]

No program available to eliminate one or more health problems for aggregates or populations[15]

---

[15]These four defining characteristics do not define community health but instead are related factors that contribute to *Deficient Community Health*.

Related Factors*

Lack of access to public health-care providers
Lack of community experts
Limited resources
Program has inadequate budget
Program has inadequate community support
Program has inadequate consumer satisfaction
Program has inadequate evaluation
Program has inadequate outcome data
Program partly addresses health problem

 Author's Note

This NANDA-I nursing diagnosis describes a community that has health problems that need assessment and program development. The programs must be accessible, affordable, available, and realistic for optimal outcomes to be achieved.

This diagnosis, although different from *Ineffective Self-health Management*, shares the same focus of community assessment and program development.

NOC
Refer to *Ineffective Community Health Management*.

Goals

Refer to *Ineffective Community Health Management*.

NIC
Refer to *Ineffective Community Health Management*.

Interventions

Refer to *Ineffective Community Health Management*.

RISK-PRONE HEALTH BEHAVIOR

Definition

Impaired ability to modify lifestyle/behaviors in a manner that improves health status (NANDA-I)

State in which a person has an inability to modify lifestyle/behavior in a manner consistent with a change in health status[16]

Defining Characteristics*

Demonstrates nonacceptance of health status change
Failure to achieve optimal sense of control
Minimizes health status change
Failure to take action that prevents health problems

Related Factors

Situational (Personal, Environmental)

Related to:
Low self-efficacy*   Inadequate resources
Negative attitude toward health   Inadequate finances
  care*   Multiple responsibilities
Multiple stressors
Inadequate social support*

Related to unhealthy lifestyle choices (e.g., tobacco use, excessive alcohol use, overweight)

Related to impaired ability to understand secondary to:
Low literacy
Language barriers

 Author's Note

This nursing diagnosis replaces the NANDA-I diagnosis Impaired Adjustment. *Risk-Prone Health Behavior* has some commonalities with *Ineffective*

---

[16]This definition has been added by Lynda Juall Carpenito, the author, for clarity and usefulness.

Health Maintenance and *Compromised Engagement*. This author recommends that *Ineffective Health Maintenance* be used to describe a person with an unhealthy lifestyle that puts him or her at risk for a chronic health problem or disease. *Risk-Prone Health Behavior* is useful to focus on one's behavior for tobacco use, recreational drug use, high-risk sexual activity. *Compromised Engagement* applies to a person who wants to comply, but factors are present that deter participation.

NOC

Adherence Behavior, Symptom Control, Health Beliefs, Treatment Behavior, Illness/Injury

Goals

The individual will verbalize the intent to modify one behavior to manage health problem, as evidenced by the following indicators:

- Describe the health problem
- Describe the relationship of present practices/behavior to decreased health
- Engage in goal setting

NIC

Health Education, Mutual Goal Setting, Self responsibility, Teaching: Disease Process, Decision Making Process

Interventions

Assess for Barriers

- What do you think is causing your blood pressure (blood sugar or weight) to remain high?
- What could you do to decrease your blood pressure (weight, blood sugar)?
- Would you like to stop smoking (or drinking alcohol)?
- What is preventing you?

If Low Literacy Is Suspected, Start With What the Individual Is Most Stressed

- Refer to Appendix A.

Engage in Collaborative Negotiation (Tyler & Horner, 2008)

- Ask the individual: "How can you be healthier?" Focus on the area they choose.

- Do not provide unsolicited advice.
- Accept that only the individual can make the change.
- Accept resistance.
- If individual is at high risk for diabetes mellitus, review the following:
  - Activity levels
  - Sample intake for 2 days: snacks, types of drinks
  - Body mass index (weight to height)
- Use Teach-Back method. Refer to Index for more information about this method.

Ask the Individual to Repeat the Goal, Behavior, or Activity

Assess Readiness to Change

- Determine how important the individual thinks the behavior change is. For example:
  - How important is it to you to increase your activity? Rate from 0 to 10 (0 = not important, 10 = important).

Determine How Confident the Individual Is to Make the Change

- For example:
  - How confident are you that you can get more exercise? Rate from 0 to 10.
  - Determine if the individual is ready for change.
  - If the importance level is 7 or above, assess confidence level. If the importance level is low, provide more information regarding the risks of not changing behavior.
  - If the level of confidence is 4 or less, ask the individual why it is not 1.
  - Ask individual what is needed to change the low score to 8.

Collaboratively, Set a Realistic Goal and Action Plan

- For example:
  - How often each week could you walk around the block two times?

Establish a Follow-Up Plan. Ask the Individual If You Can Call Him or Her in 2 Weeks to See How He or She Is Doing. Gradually Extend the Time to Monthly Calls

▒ Pediatric Interventions

- "Selected results from the 2013 national YRBS indicated that many high school students are engaged in priority health-risk behaviors associated with the leading causes of death among persons aged 10–24 years in the United States" (Kann et al., 2014).

To Initiate Discussions of Health-Risk Behaviors, The Nurse Needs to Know The High-Risk Behaviors and The Age of Onset (Kann et al., 2014)

Behaviors That Contribute to Unintentional Injuries and Violence
- Of 73.9% of students nationwide who dated or went out with someone during the 12 months before the survey, 10.3% had been hit, slammed into something, or injured with an object or weapon on purpose by someone they were dating or going out with one or more times during the 12 months before the survey.

Suicide
- 17.0% of students had seriously considered attempting suicide during the 12 months before the survey.
- 13.6% of students nationwide had made a plan about how they would attempt suicide during the 12 months before the survey.

Tobacco Use
- 9.3% of students had smoked a whole cigarette for the first time before age 13 years.
- 15.7% of students had smoked cigarettes on at least 1 day during the 30 days before the survey (i.e., current cigarette use).
- 8.8% of students had used smokeless tobacco (e.g., chewing tobacco, snuff, or DIP) on at least 1 day during the 30 days before the survey.

Alcohol and Other Drug Use
- 18.6% of students had drunk alcohol (other than a few sips) for the first time before age 13 years.
- 20.8% of students had had five or more drinks of alcohol in a row (i.e., within a couple of hours) on at least 1 day during the 30 days.
- 40.7% of students had used marijuana one or more times during their life (i.e., ever used marijuana).
- 8.6% of students had tried marijuana for the first time before age 13 years.
- 23.4% of students had used marijuana one or more times during the 30 days before the survey.

Sexual Behaviors That Contribute to Unintended Pregnancy and Sexually Transmitted Infections (STIs), Including Human Immunodeficiency Virus (HIV) Infection
- 46.8% of students had ever had sexual intercourse.
- 5.6% of students had had sexual intercourse for the first time before age 13 years.

- 15.0% of students had had sexual intercourse with four or more persons during their life.
- 34.0% of students are currently sexually active nationwide.
- 13.7% reported that neither they nor their partner had used any method to prevent pregnancy during last sexual intercourse.

Unhealthy Dietary Behaviors

- 19.4% of students had two or more times and 11.2% of students had three or more times drank a can, bottle, or glass of soda or pop (not counting diet soda or diet pop) during the 7 days.
- 13.7% of students had not eaten breakfast during the 7 days before the survey.
- 38.1% of students had eaten breakfast on all 7 days before the survey.
- 13.7% of students were obese.
- 16.6% of students were overweight.
- 31.1% of students described themselves as slightly or very overweight.
- 47.7% of students were trying to lose weight.

Physical Inactivity

- 15.2% of students had not participated in at least 60 minutes of any kind of physical activity that increased their heart rate and made them breathe hard some of the time on at least 1 day during the 7 days before the survey.

Engage in Collaborative Negotiation (Tyler & Horner, 2008)

- Ask the adolescent: "How can you be healthier?" Focus on the area they choose.
- Do not provide unsolicited advice.
- Accept that only the individual can make the change.
- Accept resistance.

If Indicated Explore Risk Behaviors by Asking the Following Questions

- Are you doing something that you would like to stop doing?
- Why do you want to stop?
- What can you do?

Validate Their Concerns of the Dangers of the Behavior and Add Other Relevant Facts. Examples Are as Follows

- Your partner could have no "bumps" and you still can get genial herpes.

- How would getting pregnant change your life?
- If your friends use drug, how difficult would it be to stop using with them?
- Is anyone hurting you? Have you told anyone?

INEFFECTIVE HEALTH MAINTENANCE

Ineffective Health Maintenance

Ineffective Health Management

Definition

Inability to identify, manage, and/or seek out help to maintain health (NANDA-I)

State in which a person experiences or is at risk of experiencing a disruption in health because of lack of knowledge to manage a condition or basic health requirements[17]

Defining Characteristics*

Lack of adaptive behaviors to environmental changes
Lack of knowledge about basic health practices
Lack of expressed interest in improving health behaviors
History of lack of health-seeking behaviors
Inability to take responsibility for meeting basic health practices
Impairment of personal support systems

Related Factors

Various factors can produce *Ineffective Health Maintenance*. Common causes are listed in the following.

---

[17]This definition has been added by Lynda Juall Carpenito, the author, for clarity and usefulness.

Situational (Personal, Environmental)

Related to:

Misinterpretation of information
Insufficient resources*
Lack of motivation
Lack of education or readiness
Deficient communication skills*

Lack of access to adequate
   health-care services
Cognitive impairments*
Perceptual impairment*

Maturational

Related to insufficient knowledge of age-related risk factors. Examples include the following:

Child
Sexuality and sexual development
Inactivity
Substance abuse
Poor nutrition
Safety hazards
Adolescent
Same as children practices
Vehicle safety

Adult
Parenthood
Safety practices
Sexual function
Older Adult
Effects of aging
Sensory deficits

 Author's Note

Ineffective Health Maintenance differs from *Ineffective Health Management*. *Ineffective Health Maintenance* focuses on promoting a healthier lifestyle in individuals; *Ineffective Health Management* focuses on teaching an individual with a medical condition or postsurgical intervention how to manage the treatments (e.g., medications, diet) and to monitor for complications.

Ineffective Health Maintenance applies to both well and ill populations. Health is a dynamic, ever-changing state defined by the individual based on his or her perception of highest level of functioning (e.g., a marathon runner's definition of health will differ from that of a paraplegic). Because individuals are responsible for their own health, an important associated nursing responsibility involves raising individual consciousness that better health is possible.

As focus shifts from an illness/treatment-oriented to a health-oriented health-care system, *Ineffective Health Maintenance* and *Readiness for Enhanced Diagnoses* are becoming increasingly significant. The increasingly high acuity and shortened lengths of stay in hospitals require nurses to be creative in addressing health promotion (e.g., by using printed materials, television instruction, and community-based programs).

NOC

Health Promoting Behavior, Health-Seeking Behaviors, Knowledge: Health Promotion, Knowledge: Health Resources, Participation: Health Care Decisions, Risk Detection

Goal

The individual or caregiver will verbalize intent to engage in health maintenance behaviors, as evidenced by the following indicator:

- Identify barriers to health maintenance

NIC

Health Education, Self-Responsibility Facilitation, Health Screening, Risk Identification, Family Involvement Promotion, Nutrition Counseling, Weight Reduction Assistance

Interventions

Assist Individual and Family to Identify Behaviors That Are Detrimental to Their Health

- Tobacco use (refer to *Refer to index for additional interventions*)
- High-fat, high-carbohydrate, high-calorie diets (refer to *Imbalanced Nutrition*)
- Sedentary life styles (refer to *Sedentary Lifestyle*)
- Inadequate immunizations (refer to *Ineffective Health Maintenance*)
- Excessive stress (refer to *Stress Overload*)

Assess for Barriers to Health Maintenance

- Refer to Related Factors.

Provide Specific Information Concerning Age-Related Health Promotion (see Table I.3)

Discuss Individual's Food Choices and Assist as He or She Identifies New Goals for Health Promotion

- Refer to *Imbalanced Nutrition* for specific interventions to improve nutrition and food insecurity.

Discuss the Benefits of a Regular Exercise Program

Discuss the Elements of Constructive Stress Management

- Assertiveness training
- Problem solving
- Relaxation techniques

Table 1.3 PRIMARY AND SECONDARY PREVENTION FOR AGE-RELATED CONDITIONS (1,4,5)

Developmental Level	Primary Prevention	Secondary Prevention

Infancy (0–1 year)	Parent education
	Infant safety
	Nutrition
	Breast feeding
	Sensory stimulation
	Infant massage and touch
	Visual stimulation
	  Activity
	  Colors
	Auditory stimulation
	  Verbal
	  Music
	Immunizations
	DPT or DTaP
	IPV, Hib
	Hepatitis B (3-dose series)
	Hepatitis A (2)
	Rotavirus (RV)
	Pneumococcal (PCV)
	Meningococcal
	Influenza (yearly)
		Complete physical examination every 2–3 months
		Screening at birth
		  Congenital hip dysplasia
		  PKU
		  G-6-PD deficiency in blacks, Mediterranean, and Far Eastern origin children
		  Sickle cell
		  Hemoglobin or hematocrit (for anemia)
		  Cystic fibrosis
		  Vision (startle reflex)
		  Hearing (response to and localization of sounds)
		  TB test at 12 months
		Developmental assessments
		Screen and intervene for high risk
		  Low birth weight
		  Maternal substance abuse during pregnancy
		  Alcohol: fetal alcohol syndrome
		  Cigarettes: SIDS
		  Drugs: addicted neonate, AIDS
		  Maternal infections during pregnancy

(continued)

267

Table I.3 PRIMARY AND SECONDARY PREVENTION FOR AGE-RELATED CONDITIONS (1,4,5) *(continued)*

Developmental Level	Primary Prevention	Secondary Prevention

Preschool (1–5 years)	Oral hygiene
	  Teething biscuits
	  Fluoride (if needed >6 months)
	  Avoid sugared food and drink
	Parent education
	  Teething
	  Discipline
	  Nutrition
	  Accident prevention
	  Normal growth and development
	Child education
	  Dental self-care
	  Dressing
	  Bathing with assistance
	  Feeding self-care
	Immunizations
	  DTaP
	  IPV
	  MMR
	  HIB
	  H. Influenzae (yearly)
	  Varicella
	  Hepatitis A (2)(two-dose series)
		Complete physical examination between 2 and 3 years and preschool (UA, CBC)
		TB test at 3 years
		Development assessments (annual)
		  Speech development
		  Hearing
		  Vision
		Screen and intervene
		  Lead poisoning
		  Developmental lag
		  Neglect or abuse
		Strong family history of arteriosclerotic diseases (e.g., MI, CVA, peripheral vascular disease), diabetes, hypertension, gout, or hyperlipidemia—fasting serum cholesterol at age 2 years, then every 3–5 years if normal
		  Strabismus
		  Hearing deficit
		  Vision deficit
		  Autism

School age (6–11 years)	Pneumococcal Hepatitis B (3-dose series) Dental/oral hygiene Fluoride treatments Fluoridated water Health education of child "Basic 4" nutrition Accident prevention Outdoor safety Substance abuse counsel Anticipatory guidance for physical changes at puberty Immunizations DTaP age 11–12 MMR (two lifetime doses) OPV/IPV (four lifetime doses) Hepatitis B three-dose series if needed Hepatitis A (2) Pneumococcal (3) Varicella (at age 11–12 if no history of infection)	Complete physical examination TB test every 3 years (at ages 6 and 9) Developmental assessment Language Vision: Snellen charts at school 6–8 years, use "E" chart Older than 8 years, use alphabet chart Hearing: audiogram Cholesterol profile, if high risk, every 3–5 years Serum cholesterol one time (not high risk)

(continued)

Table 1.3 PRIMARY AND SECONDARY PREVENTION FOR AGE-RELATED CONDITIONS (1,4,5) *(continued)*

Developmental Level	Primary Prevention	Secondary Prevention
Adolescence (12–19 years)	Gardisil (HPV) series of three for girls 9–26 years, for boys age 9–18 years Dental hygiene every 6–12 months Continue fluoridation Complete physical examination Health education Proper nutrition and healthful diets Calcium 100mg & Vitamin D 400 units daily Sex education Choices Risks Precautions Sexually transmitted diseases Safe driving skills Adult challenges Seeking employment and career choices Dating and marriage Confrontation with substance abuse Safety in athletics, water	Complete physical exam yearly Blood pressure Cholesterol profile PPD test at 12 years and yearly if high risk RPR, CBC, U/A Female: Breast self-examination (BSE) Male: Testicular self-examination (TSE) Female, Pap and pelvic exam yearly after 3 years of onset of sexual activity or at age 21 Urine gonorrhea and chlamydia tests with yearly PE's Screening Depression Suicide Tobacco use Eating disorders Substance abuse

Skin care
Dental hygiene every 6–12 months
Immunizations
  Tdap if not received then Td every
    10 years thereafter
  Hepatitis B three-dose series if
    needed,
  Hepatitis A series (2) two-dose series
  TOPV (if needed to complete four-
    dose series)
  Gardasil (HPV) (series of three for girls
    ages 11–26, for boys ages 9–18)
  Pneumococcal (3)

Pregnancy
Family history of alcoholism or domestic violence
Sexually transmitted infections

Young adult (20–39 years)

Health education
  Weight management with good
    nutrition as BMR changes
  Low-cholesterol diet
  Calcium 100 mg daily (females)
  Vitamin D 400 units daily (females)
Lifestyle counseling
  Stress management skills
  Safe driving
  Family planning
  Divorce
  Sexual practices

Complete physical exam at about 20 years, then every
  5–6 years
Female: BSE monthly, Pap 1–2 years unless high risk
Male: TSE monthly
Parents-to-be: high-risk screening for Down syndrome,
  Tay-Sachs
Female pregnant: RPR, rubella titer, Rh factor, amniocen-
  tesis for women 35 years or older (if desired)
All females: baseline mammography between ages 35
  and 40

(continued)

271

Table I.3 PRIMARY AND SECONDARY PREVENTION FOR AGE-RELATED CONDITIONS (1,4,5) *(continued)*

Developmental Level	Primary Prevention	Secondary Prevention
	Parenting skills Regular exercise Environmental health choices Alcohol, drug use Use of hearing protection devices Dental hygiene every 6–12 months Immunizations If needed one time dose of Tdap, then Td every 10 years thereafter Influenza yearly Pneumovax (3) Varicella (two-dose series for those with no evidence of immunity) Female: rubella, if serum negative for antibodies Hepatitis B three-dose series Hepatitis A (2) Gardasil (three-dose series for females from age 11–26) MMR (if born in 1957 or later, one or more doses) Pneumococcal Diabetes mellitus	If high risk, female with previous breast cancer: annual mammography at 35 years and yearly after, a female with mother or sister who has had breast cancer, same as above Family history colorectal cancer or high risk: annual stool guaiac, digital rectal, and colonoscopy at intervals de- termined after baseline colonoscopy; PPD if high risk Glaucoma screening at 35 years and along with routine physical exams Cholesterol profile every 5 years, if normal Cholesterol profile every year if borderline Screening (Refer to Adolescent section)

Middle-aged adult (40–59 years)	Health education: continue with young adult Calcium 1,000–1,500 mg daily Vitamin D 400 units daily Midlife changes, male and female counseling (see also Young adult) "Empty nest syndrome" Anticipatory guidance for retirement Menopause Grandparenting Dental hygiene every 6–12 months Immunizations Hepatitis B three-dose series Hepatitis A (2) If needed one time dose of Tdap, then Td every 10 years thereafter Influenza—yearly Pneumococcal (3) at age 65 for all those who were not high risk for vaccine prior	Complete physical exam ≥every 5–6 years with complete laboratory evaluation (serum/urine tests, X-ray, ECG) DEXA scan (screening for high-risk men and women for osteoporosis) once then as needed Female: BSE monthly Male: TSE monthly PSA yearly after age 40 for African Americans and Hispanics and after age 50 for others All females: mammogram every 1–2 years (40–49 years) then annual mammography 50 years and older Screening (Refer to Adolescent section) Schiotz's tonometry (glaucoma) every 3–5 years Colonoscopy at 50 and 51, then at intervals determined after baseline colonoscopy. Stool guaiac annually at 50 and yearly after
Older adult (60–74 years)	Health education: continue with previous counseling Home safety Retirement Loss of spouse, relatives, friends	Complete physical exam every 2 years with laboratory assessments Blood pressure annually Female: BSE monthly, Pap every 1–3 years annual mammogram Male: TSE monthly, PSA yearly

(continued)

Table 1.3 PRIMARY AND SECONDARY PREVENTION FOR AGE-RELATED CONDITIONS (1,4,5) *(continued)*

Developmental Level	Primary Prevention	Secondary Prevention

	Special health needs
	  Calcium 1,000–1,500 mg daily
	  Vitamin D 400 units daily
	  Changes in hearing or vision
	  Dental/oral hygiene every
	    6–12 months
	Immunizations
	  Tdap one dose then Td every
	    10 years
	  Influenza—annual
	  Hepatitis B 3-dose series
	  Hepatitis A (2)
	  Pneumococcal (3)
	  Herpes Zoster 60 years or older
	    unless a live vaccine is
	    contraindicated
		Annual stool guaiac
		Colonoscopy (interval determined by baseline results)
		Complete eye exam yearly
		DEXA scan once and as needed
		Screen for high-risk
		  Depression
		  Suicide
		  Alcohol/drug abuse
		  "Elder abuse"

Old-age adult (75 years and older)	Dental/oral hygiene
	  every 6–12 months
	Immunizations
	  Tetanus every 10 years
	  Influenza—annual
	  Pneumococcal—if not already
	    received	

Promote Engagement in the Individual Who Is Seeking to Promote Health

Assess Knowledge of Primary Prevention

- Safety—accident prevention (e.g., car, machinery, outdoor safety, occupational)
- Weight control
- Avoidance of substance abuse (e.g., alcohol, drugs, tobacco)
- Avoidance of sexually transmitted diseases
- Dental/oral hygiene (e.g., daily, dentist)
- Immunizations

Determine If Referrals Are Indicated (e.g., Social Services, Housekeeping Services, Home Health)

Identify Strategies to Improve Access for the Vulnerable Populations (e.g., Uninsured, Displaced, Homeless, Poor)

- Community centers, school-based clinics, planned parenthood, faith-based clinics
- Pharmaceutical companies' assistance programs, generic alternative medications

Older Adults Interventions

Determine With the Individual What They Can Do

Discuss Their Feelings About Their Life

- What do they like about their life?
- What gives meaning to their life?
- Discuss what they would like to do, but don't.
- Discuss if realistic. Modifiable?
- Is there another option that is acceptable?
- Explore if assistance is needed, who or what is the source?

Ineffective Health Management

NANDA-I Definition

Pattern of regulation and integrating into daily living a therapeutic regimen for the treatment of illness and its sequelae that is unsatisfactory for meeting specific health goals

Defining Characteristics

Difficulty with prescribed regimen
Failure to include treatment regimen in daily living
Failure to take action to reduce risk factor(s)
Ineffective choices in daily living for meeting health goal(s)

Related Factors

Treatment Related

Related to:
Complexity treatment regimen
Complexity of health-care system
Insufficient knowledge of therapeutic regimen

Situational (Personal, Environmental)

Related to:

Insufficient social support	Perceived seriousness of condition
Perceived barrier(s)	Perceived susceptibility
Perceived benefit(s)	Powerlessness

Related to barriers to comprehension secondary to:

Cognitive deficits	Motivations
Fatigue	Anxiety
Hearing impairments	Memory problems
Low literacy	

 Author's Note

In 2010, the costs of health care in the United States exceeded $2.7 trillion and accounted for 17.9% of the gross domestic product. Projections indicate health care will account for 20% of the US gross domestic product by 2020. Twenty percent to thirty percent of dollars spent in the US health-care system have been identified as wasteful. Providers and administrators have been challenged to contain costs by reducing waste and by improving the effectiveness of care delivered. Patient nonadherence to prescribed medications is associated with poor therapeutic outcomes, progression of disease, and an estimated burden of billions per year in avoidable direct health-care costs (Iuga & McGuire, 2014).

Some reasons for nonadherence can be low health literacy, finance, and lack of or unsatisfactory teaching strategies. *Ineffective Self-Help*

Management is a very useful diagnosis for nurses in most settings. Individuals and families experiencing various health problems, acute or chronic, usually face treatment programs that require changes in previous functioning or lifestyle. Medication nonadherence is a significant contributor to poor outcomes and health-care costs associated with use of emergency rooms and hospital admissions.

Ineffective Self-Health Management focuses on assisting the person and family to identify barriers in management of the condition and to prevent complications at home.

The nursing diagnosis *Risk for Ineffective Health Maintenance* is useful to describe a person who needs teaching or referrals before discharge from an acute care center to prevent problems with health maintenance at home or in community settings.

Risk-Prone Health Behavior, approved in 2006, is different. This diagnosis focuses on habits or lifestyles which are unhealthy and can aggravate an existing condition or contribute to developing a disease.

NOC

Adherence Behavior, Symptom Control, Health Beliefs Treatment Behavior Illness/Injury

Goals

The person will verbalize intent to modify one behavior to manage health problem, as evidenced by the following indicators:

- Describe the relationship of present lifestyle to his or her health problems
- Identify two resources to access after discharge
- Set a date to initiate change

NIC

Heath Education, Mutual Goal Setting, Self-Responsibility, Teaching: Disease Process, Decision-Making Process

Interventions

On Admission Complete a Medication Reconciliation

- Develop a list of current medications.
- Develop a list of medications to be prescribed.
- Compare the medications on the two lists.
- Make clinical decisions based on the comparison.
- Communicate the new list to the individual and/or appropriate caregivers.

Ask the Following Questions to the Individual/Family Member for Each Medication

- What is the reason you are taking each medication?
- Are you taking the medication as prescribed? Specify once a day, twice a day, and so on.
- Are you skipping any doses? Do you sometimes run out of medications?
- How often are you taking the medication prescribed "if needed as a pain medication"?
- Have you stopped taking any of these medications?
- How much does it cost you to take your medications?
- Are you taking anybody else's medication?

Engage in Collaborative Negotiation

- Ask: How can you be healthier? Focus on the area he or she chooses.
- Evaluate:
  - Primary language, ability to read and write in primary language
  - English as a second language
  - English as primary language, ability to read and write

Identify Red Flags for Low Literacy (DeWalt et al., 2010)

- Frequently missed appointments
- Incomplete registration forms
- Noncompliance with medication
- Unable to name medications and explain purpose or dosing
- Identifies pills by looking at them, not reading label
- Unable to give coherent, sequential history
- Asks fewer questions
- Lack of follow-through on tests or referrals

For Comprehension to Occur, the Nurse Must Accept That There Is Limited Time and That the Use of This Time Is Enhanced by

Using Every Contact Time to Teach Something (DeWalt et al., 2010)
- Create a relaxed encounter.
- Use eye contact.
- Slow down—break it down into short statements.
- Limit content—focus on two or three concepts.
- Use plain language.
- Engage individual/family in discussion.
- Use graphics.
- Explain what you are doing to the individual/family and why.

- Ask them to tell you about what you taught. Tell them to use their own words.
- Avoid information overload with older adults and those with low literacy. Consider a home health nurse assessment visit to evaluate competencies at home.

Using the Teach-Back Method
- Explain/Demonstrate
  - Explain one concept (e.g., medication, condition, when to call PCP).
  - Demonstrate one procedure (e.g., dressing charge, use of inhaler).
- Assess
  - I want to make sure, I explained _____ clearly, can you tell me _____.
  - Tell me what I told you.
  - Show me how to _____.
  - Avoid asking, "Do you understand?"
- Clarify
  - Add more explanation if you are not satisfied the person understands or can perform the activity.
  - If the person cannot report the information, do not repeat the same explanation; rephrase it.

Teach-Back Questions (Examples)

- When should you call your PCP?
- How do you know your incision is healing?
- What foods should you avoid?
- How often should you test your blood sugar?
- What should you do for low blood sugar?
- What weight gain should you report to your PCP?
- Which inhaler is your rescue inhaler?
- Is there something you have been told to do that you do not understand?
- What should you bring to your PCP office?
- Is there something you have a question about?

Teach Self-Care or Care at Home by Addressing

The Condition
Medical Conditions
- What do you know about your condition?
- How do you think this condition will affect you after you leave the hospital?
- What do you want to know about your condition?

Surgical Procedure
- What do you know about the surgery you had?
- Do you have any questions about your surgery?
- How will surgery affect you after you leave the hospital?

Medications
- Renew all the medications that the individual will continue to take at home.
- Explain what OTC not to take.
- Finish all the medications like antibiotics.
- Ask the individual not to take any medications that are at home unless approved by PCP.
- Ask to bring all his or her medications to next visit to PCP (e.g., prescribed, OTC, vitamins, herbal medicines).
- Depending on the literacy level of the individual/family
  - Provide a list of each medication, what used for, times to take, with food or without food.
  - Create a pill card with columns.
    - Pictures of pill
    - Simple terms used
    - Time using symbols with pictures of pills in spaces

Evaluate the Financial Implications of Prescribed Medication

- Does the person have insured medication coverage? If yes, does it cover the medication ordered? If yes, what is the copay? Can the person afford this?
- If there is no insurance or no medication coverage, how will the person access these medications?
- Is there an inexpensive generic available?
- Which medications are critical and need immediately?
- Explain that most pharmaceutical companies provide free branded medications (not generic) through patient-assisted programs. Applications can be accessed via the pharmaceutical website. Social service departments can also assist with this process.
- Some medications can be acquired free (e.g., oral diabetic medications, antibiotics) at supermarkets (e.g., Pathmark, ShopRite) or at low cost (e.g., Target).
- Advise individual/family to call PCP office if they do not want to continue a medication.

Dietary Recommendations
- Ask individual/family to report if there are any dietary limitations.
- Ensure there are written directions.

- Explain why some foods/beverages are to be avoided (e.g., avoid olives, pickles on a low-salt diet).

Activities

- Provide instructions on activities permitted and restricted.
- When they can drive.
- Return to work; what kind of job do they have?

Treatments

- Explain each treatment to be continued at home.
- List equipment needed, frequency of treatment.
- Write down what signs and symptoms should be reported (e.g., decrease in output for catheter).

Competence

- Can this treatment be provided safely by the individual or caregiver?
- If not, consult with the transition specialist in the health-care agency.

Initiate Health Teaching and Referrals as Needed

- Refer to a home health agency for an assessment in the home.
- Provide specific teaching for management of a medical disorder and/or postoperative care and/or postpartum care, signs of complications, activity restrictions, dietary recommendations, medications prescribed, and follow-up care.
- Refer to medical surgical textbooks and specialty textbooks for specific information for each medical disorder associated with the individual's condition.
- Refer to Carpenito-Moyet, L. J. (2014). *Nursing Care Plans: Transitional Patient and Family Centered Care* for specific content to teach the individual? Family for self-care at home for 68 medical and surgical conditions.

IMPAIRED HOME MAINTENANCE

NANDA-I Definition

Inability to independently maintain a safe growth-promoting immediate environment

Defining Characteristics

Major (Must Be Present, One or More)

Expressions or observations of:

Difficulty maintaining home hygiene

Difficulty maintaining a safe home

Inability to keep up home

Lack of sufficient finances

Minor (May Be Present)

Repeated infections

Infestations

Accumulated wastes

Unwashed utensils

Offensive odors

Overcrowding

Related Factors

Pathophysiologic

Related to impaired functional ability* secondary to chronic debilitating disease*

Diabetes mellitus

Arthritis

Chronic obstructive pulmonary disease (COPD)

Multiple sclerosis

Congestive heart failure

Cerebrovascular accident

Parkinson's disease

Muscular dystrophy

Cancer

Situational (Personal, Environmental)

Related to change in functional ability of (specify family member) secondary to:

Injury* (fractured limb, spinal cord injury)

Surgery (amputation, ostomy)

Impaired mental status (memory lapses, depression, anxiety–severe panic)

Substance abuse (alcohol, drugs)

Related to inadequate support system*

Related to loss of family member

Related to deficient knowledge

Related to insufficient finances*

Related to unfamiliarity with neighborhood resources*

Maturational

Infant
Related to multiple care requirements secondary to:
High-risk newborn

Older Adult
Related to multiple care requirements secondary to:
Family member with deficits (cognitive, motor, sensory)

 Author's Note

With rising life expectancy and declining mortality rates, the number of older adults is steadily increasing, with many living alone at home. Eighty percent of people 65 years or older report one or more chronic diseases. Of adults 65 to 74 years of age, 20% report activity limitations, and 15% cannot perform at least one activity of daily living (ADL) independently (Miller, 2015). The shift from health care primarily in hospitals to reduced lengths of stay has resulted in the discharge of many functionally compromised people to their homes. Often a false assumption is that someone will assume the management of household responsibilities until the individual has recovered.

Impaired Home Maintenance describes situations in which an individual or family needs teaching, supervision, or assistance to manage the household. Usually, a community health nurse is the best professional to complete an assessment of the home and the individual's functioning there. Nurses in acute settings can make referrals for home visits for assessment.

A nurse who diagnoses a need for teaching to prevent household problems may use *Risk for Impaired Home Maintenance* related to insufficient knowledge of (specify).

NOC
Family Functioning

Goals

The individual or caretaker will express satisfaction with home situation, as evidenced by the following indicators:

- Identify factors that restrict self-care and home management
- Demonstrate ability to perform skills necessary for care of the home

NIC
Home Maintenance Assistance, Environmental Management: Safety, Environmental
Management

Interventions

The following interventions apply to many with impaired home
maintenance, regardless of etiology.

Assess for Causative or Contributing Factors

- Lack of knowledge
- Insufficient funds
- Lack of necessary equipment or aids
- Inability (illness, sensory deficits, motor deficits) to perform
  household activities
- Impaired cognitive functioning
- Impaired emotional functioning

Reduce or Eliminate Causative or Contributing Factors, If Possible

Lack of Knowledge
- Determine with individual and family the information they
  need to learn:
  - Monitoring skills (pulse, circulation, urine)
  - Medication administration (procedure, side effects,
    precautions)
  - Treatment/procedures
  - Equipment use/maintenance
  - Safety issues (e.g., environmental)
  - Community resources
  - Follow-up care
  - Anticipatory guidance (e.g., emotional and social needs, al-
    ternatives to home care)
  - Initiate teaching; give detailed written instruction.

Insufficient Funds
- Consult with social service department for assistance.
- Consult with service organizations (e.g., American Heart Association, The Lung Association, American Cancer Society) for
  assistance.

Lack of Necessary Equipment or Aids
- Determine type of equipment needed, considering availability,
  cost, and durability.
- Seek assistance from agencies that rent or loan supplies.

- Teach care and maintenance of supplies to increase length of use.
- Consider adapting equipment to reduce cost.

Inability to Perform Household Activities
- Determine type of assistance needed (e.g., meals, housework, transportation); assist individual to obtain it.

Meals
- Discuss with relatives the possibility of freezing complete meals that require only heating (e.g., small containers of soup, stews, casseroles).
- Determine availability of meal services for ill people (e.g., Meals on Wheels, church groups).
- Teach people about nutritious foods that are easily prepared (e.g., hard-boiled eggs, tuna fish, peanut butter).

Housework
- Encourage individual to contract with an adolescent for light housekeeping.
- Refer individual to community agency for assistance.

Transportation
- Determine availability of transportation for shopping and health care.
- Suggest individual to request rides with neighbors to places they drive routinely.

Impaired Cognitive Functioning
- Assess individual's ability to maintain a safe household.
- Refer to *Risk for Injury* related to lack of awareness of hazards.
- Initiate appropriate referrals.

Impaired Emotional Functioning
- Assess severity of the dysfunction.
- Refer to *Ineffective Coping* for additional assessment and interventions.

Initiate Health Teaching and Referrals, as Indicated

- Refer to community nursing agency for a home visit.
- Provide information about how to make the home environment safe and clean (Edelman, Kudzma, & Mandle, 2014). Refer to community agencies (e.g., visitors, meal programs, homemakers, adult day care).
- Refer to support groups (e.g., local Alzheimer's Association, American Cancer Society).

HOPELESSNESS

NANDA-I Definition

Subjective state in which an individual sees limited or no alternatives or personal choices available and is unable to mobilize energy on own behalf

Defining Characteristics

Expresses profound, overwhelming, sustained apathy in response to a situation perceived as impossible

Physiologic
Increased sleep   Decreased response to stimuli*
Lack of energy

Emotional

Person Feels:
As though they do not receive any breaks and there is no reason to believe they will in the future.
Empty or drained
Demoralized
Helpless
Lack of meaning or purpose in life

Person Exhibits:

Passivity* and lack of involvement in care	Decreased verbalization*
Decreased affect*	Lack of ambition, initiative*, and interest
Giving up–given up complex	Fatigue
Isolating behaviors	

Cognitive
Rigidity (e.g., all-or-none thinking)
Lack of imagination and wishing capabilities
Inability to identify or accomplish desired objectives and goals
Inability to plan, organize, make decisions, or problem-solve
Inability to recognize sources of hope
Suicidal thoughts

Related Factors

Pathophysiologic

Any chronic or terminal illness (e.g., heart disease, diabetes, kidney disease, cancer, acquired immunodeficiency syndrome [AIDS]) can cause or contribute to hopelessness.

Related to impaired ability to cope secondary to:
Failing or deteriorating physiologic condition
New and unexpected signs or symptoms of previously diagnosed disease process (i.e., recurrence of cancer) (Brothers & Anderson, 2009)
Prolonged pain, discomfort, and weakness
Impaired functional abilities (walking, elimination, eating, dressing, bathing, speaking, writing)

Treatment Related

Related to:
Prolonged treatments (e.g., chemotherapy, radiation) that cause pain, nausea, and discomfort
Treatments that alter body image (e.g., surgery, chemotherapy)
Prolonged diagnostic studies
Prolonged dependence on equipment for life support (e.g., dialysis, respirator)
Prolonged dependence on equipment for monitoring bodily functions (e.g., telemetry)

Situational (Personal, Environmental)

Related to:
Prolonged activity restriction (e.g., fractures, spinal cord injury, imprisonment)
Prolonged isolation (e.g., infectious diseases, reverse isolation for suppressed immune system)
Abandonment by, separation from, or isolation from significant others (Brothers & Anderson, 2009)
Inability to achieve valued goals in life (marriage, education, children)
Inability to participate in desired activities (walking, sports, work)
Loss of something or someone valued (spouse, children, friend, financial resources)
Prolonged caretaking responsibilities (spouse, child, parent)
Recurrence of breast cancer
Exposure to long-term physiologic or psychological stress

Recurrence of breast cancer (Brothers & Anderson, 2009)
Loss of belief in transcendent values/God
Ongoing, repetitive losses in community related to AIDS
Repetitive natural disasters (hurricanes, tornadoes, flooding, fires)
Prolonged exposure to violence and war

Maturational

Child

Loss of autonomy related to illness (e.g., fracture)
Loss of bodily functions
Loss of caregiver
Loss of trust in significant others
Inability to achieve developmental tasks (trust, autonomy, initiative, industry)
Rejection, abuse, or abandonment by caregivers

Adolescent

Change in body image
Inability to achieve developmental task (role identity)
Loss of bodily functions
Loss of significant others (peer, family)
Rejection by family

Adult

Abortion
Impaired bodily functions, loss of body part
Impaired relationships (separation, divorce)
Inability to achieve developmental tasks (intimacy, commitment, productivity)
Loss of job, career
Loss of significant others (death of spouse, child)
Miscarriage

Older Adult

Cognitive deficits
Inability to achieve developmental tasks
Loss of independence
Loss of significant others, things (in general)
Motor deficits
Sensory deficits

 Author's Note

Hopelessness describes a person who sees no possibility that his or her life will improve and maintains that no one can do anything to help. *Hopelessness* differs from *Powerlessness* in that a hopeless person sees no solution or no way to achieve what is desired, even if he or she feels in control. In contrast, a powerless person may see an alternative or answer, yet be unable to do anything about it because of lack of control or resources. Sustained feelings of powerlessness may lead to hopelessness. Hopelessness is commonly related to grief, depression, and suicide. For a person at risk for suicide, the nurse should also use the diagnosis *Risk for Suicide*. Hopelessness is a distinct concept and not merely a symptom of depression.

Decision-Making, Depression Control, Hope, Quality of Life

Goals

- Demonstrate increased energy, as evidenced by an increase in activities (e.g., self-care, exercise)
- Express desirable expectations for the near future. Describe one's own meaning and purpose in life
- Demonstrate initiative, self-direction, and autonomy in decision making; demonstrate effective problem-solving strategies
- Redefine the future; set realistic goals with expectation to meet them

The individual will strive for the goals listed above, as evidenced by the following indicators:

- Share suffering openly and constructively with others
- Reminisce and review life positively
- Consider values and the meaning of life
- Express optimism about the present
- Practice energy conservation
- Develop, improve, and maintain positive relationships with others
- Participate in a significant role
- Express spiritual beliefs

Hope Instillation, Values Classification, Decision-Making Support, Spiritual Support, Support System Enhancement

Interventions

Assist Individual to Identify and Express Feelings

- Listen actively, treat the individual as an individual, and accept his or her feelings. Convey empathy to promote verbalization of doubts, fears, and concerns.

- Validate and reflect impressions with the person. It is important to realize that individuals with cancer often have their own reality, which may differ from the nurse's.
- Assist the individual in recognizing that hopelessness is part of everyone's life and demands recognition. The individual can use it as a source of energy, imagination, and freedom to consider alternatives. Hopelessness can lead to self-discovery.
- Assist the individual to understand that he or she can deal with the hopeless aspects of life by separating them from the hopeful aspects. Help the individual to distinguish between the possible and impossible.
- The nurse mobilizes an individual's internal and external resources to promote and instill hope. Assist individuals to identify their personal reasons for living that provide meaning and purpose to their lives.

Assess and Mobilize the Individual's Internal Resources (Autonomy, Independence, Rationality, Cognitive Thinking, Flexibility, Spirituality)

- Emphasize strengths, not weaknesses.
- Compliment the individual on appearance or efforts as appropriate.
- Identify areas of success and usefulness; emphasize past accomplishments. Use this information to develop goals with the individual.
- Assist the individual in identifying things he or she has fun doing and perceives as humorous. Such activities can serve as distractions to discomfort and allow the individual to progress to cognitive comfort (*Hinds, Martin, & Vogel, 1987).
- Assist the individual in adjusting and developing realistic short- and long-term goals (progress from simple to more complex; may use a "goals poster" to indicate type and time for achieving specific goals). Attainable expectations promote hope.
- Encourage "means–end" thinking in positive terms (i.e., "If I do this, then I'll be able to. . .").
- Foster lightheartedness and the sharing of uplifting memories.

Assist the Individual With Problem Solving and Decision Making

- Respect the individual as a competent decision-maker; treat his or her decisions and desires with respect.
- Encourage verbalization to determine the individual's perception of choices.
- Clarify the individual's values to determine what is important.
- Correct misinformation.
- Assist the individual in identifying those problems he or she cannot resolve, to advance to problems he or she can. In other

words, assist the individual to move away from dwelling on the impossible and hopeless and to begin to deal with realistic and hopeful matters.

- Assess the individual's perceptions of self and others in relation to size. (People with hopelessness often perceive others as large and difficult to deal with and themselves as small.) If perceptions are unrealistic, assist the individual to reassess them to restore proper scale.
- Promote flexibility. Encourage the individual to try alternatives and take risks.

Encourage to Think Beyond the Moment

- Explain the benefits of distraction from negative events.
- Teach and assist with relaxation techniques before anticipated stressful events.
- Encourage mental imagery to promote positive thought processes.
- Teach the individual to maximize aesthetic experiences (e.g., smell of coffee, back rub, feeling warmth of the sun, or a breeze) that can inspire hope.
- Teach the individual to anticipate experiences he or she delights in daily (e.g., walking, reading favorite book, writing a letter).
- Teach the individual ways to conserve and generate energy through moderate physical exercise.
- Encourage music therapy, aromatherapy, and massage with essential oils to improve the individual's physical and mental status.

Assess and Mobilize the Individual's External Resources

Family or Significant Others

- Involve the family and significant others in plan of care.
- Encourage the individual to spend increased time or thoughts with loved ones in healthy relationships.
- Teach the family members their role in sustaining hope through supportive, positive relationships.
- Discuss the individual's attainable goals with family.
- Empower individuals who have chronic disease by instilling hope through the bolstering of support systems.
- Convey hope, information, and confidence to the family because they will convey their feelings to the individual.
- Use touch and closeness with the individual to demonstrate to the family its acceptability (provide privacy).
- Herth (*1993) found the following strategies to foster hope in caregivers of terminally ill people:
  - *Cognitive reframing*—positive self-talk, praying/meditating, and envisioning hopeful images (this may involve letting go of expectations for things to be different)

- *Time refocusing*—focusing less on the future and more on living one day at a time
- *Belief in a power greater than self*—empowering the caregiver's hope
- *Balancing available energy*—listening to music or other favorite activities to empower the caregiver's hope through uplifting energy

Health-Care Team
- Develop a positive, trusting nurse–individual relationship by
  - Answering questions
  - Respecting individual's feelings
  - Providing consistent care
  - Following through on requests
  - Touching
  - Providing comfort
  - Being honest
  - Conveying positive attitude
- Convey attitude of "We care too much about you to let you just give up," or "I can help you."
- Hold conferences and share the individual's goals with staff.
- Share advances in technology and research for treatment of diseases.
- Have available a list of laughter resources (e.g., books, films).
- Provide nurses and caregivers support in times of disaster.

Support Groups
- Encourage the individual to share concerns with others who have had a similar problem or disease and positive experiences from coping effectively with it.
- Provide information on self-help groups (e.g., "Make today count"—40 chapters in the United States and Canada; "I can cope"—series for individuals with cancer; "We Can Weekend"—for families of individuals with cancer).

God or Higher Powers
- Assess the individual's belief support system (value, past experiences, religious activities, relationship with God, meaning and purpose of prayer; refer to *Spiritual Distress*).
- Create an environment in which the individual feels free to express spirituality.
- Allow the individual time and opportunities to reflect on the meaning of suffering, death, and dying.
- Accept, respect, and support the individual's hope in God.

RISK FOR COMPROMISED HUMAN DIGNITY

NANDA-I Definition

Vulnerable for perceived loss of respect and honor, which can compromise health

Risk Factors

End-of-Life Decisions*

Related to providing treatments that were perceived as futile for terminally ill individual (e.g., blood transfusions, chemotherapy, organ transplants, mechanical ventilation)

Related to conflicting attitudes toward advanced directives

Related to participation of life-saving actions when they only prolong dying

Treatment Decisions

Related to disagreement among health-care professionals, family members, and/or the individual regarding:
Treatments
Transition to home, relative's home, or community nursing care facility
The individual's living will
End-of-life care

Related to the individual's/family's refusal of treatments deemed appropriate by the health-care team

Related to inability of the family to make the decision to stop ventilator treatment of terminally ill individual

Related to a family's wishes to continue life support even though it is not in the best interest of the individual

Related to performing a procedure that increases the individual's suffering

Related to providing care that does not relieve the individual's suffering

Related to conflicts between wanting to disclose poor medical practice and wanting to maintain trust in the physician

Cultural Conflicts

Related to decisions made for women by male family members

Related to cultural conflicts with the American health-care system

 Author's Note

Risk for Compromised Human Dignity was accepted by NANDA-I in 2006.

This nursing diagnosis presents a new application for nursing practice. All individuals are at risk for this diagnosis. Providing respect and honor to all individuals, families, and communities is a critical core element of professional nursing. Prevention of compromised human dignity must be a focus of all nursing interventions. It is the central concept of a caring profession.

This diagnosis can also apply to prisoners, who as part of their penalty will be deprived of some rights, for example, privacy and movement. Prisoners, however, should always be treated with respect and not be tortured or humiliated. Nurses have the obligation to honor and "do no harm" in all settings in which they practice.

This author recommends that this diagnosis be developed and integrated into a Standard Care of the Nursing Department for all individuals and families. The outcomes and interventions apply to all individuals, families, and groups. This Department of Nursing Standards of Practice could also include *Risk for Infection*, *Risk for Infection Transmission*, *Risk for Falls*, and *Risk for Compromised Family Coping*.

NOC

Abuse Protection, Comfort Level, Dignified Dying, Information Processing, Knowledge: Illness Care, Self-Esteem, Spiritual Well-Being

Goals

The individual will report respectful and considerate care, as evidenced by the following indicators:

- Respect for privacy
- Consideration of emotions
- Anticipation of feelings
- Given options and control
- Asked for permission
- Given explanations

- Minimization of body part exposure
- No involvement of unnecessary personnel during stressful procedures

NIC

Patient Rights Protection, Anticipatory Guidance, Counseling, Emotional Support, Preparatory Sensory Information, Family Support, Humor, Mutual Goal Setting, and Teaching: Procedure/Treatment, Touch

Interventions

Determine and Accept Your Own Moral Responsibility

- Can a nurse maintain and defend the dignity of an individual or a group if she or he cannot maintain and defend her or his own dignity.

Determine If the Agency Has a Policy for Prevention of Compromised Human Dignity (Note: This Type of Policy or Standard May be Titled Differently)

- Review the policy. Does it include (*Walsh & Kowanko, 2002) the following:
  - Protection of privacy and private space
  - Acquiring permission continuously
  - Providing time for decision making
  - Advocating for the individual

When or If Appropriate, Request the Individual or Family Members to Provide the Following Information

- Person to contact in the event of emergency
- Person whom the individual trusts with personal decisions, power of attorney
- Signed living will/Desire to sign a living will
- Decision on organ donation

When Providing Care

- Provide care to each individual and family as you would expect or demand for your family, partner, child, friend, or colleague.
- When performing a procedure, engage the individual in a conversation; act as if the situation is a matter-of-fact for you in order to reduce embarrassment; use humor if appropriate; talk to the individual even if he or she is unresponsive.
- Explain the procedure to the individual during painful or embarrassing procedures and explain what he or she will feel.

- Determine if unnecessary personnel are present before a vulnerable or stressful event is initiated (e.g., code or a painful or embarrassing procedure); advise them that they are not needed.
- Allow the individual an opportunity to share his or her feelings after a difficult situation and maintain privacy for the individual's information and emotional responses.
- When extreme measures that are futile are planned for or are being provided for an individual, refer to *Moral Distress*.

DISORGANIZED INFANT BEHAVIOR

Disorganized Infant Behavior
Risk for Disorganized Infant Behavior

NANDA-I Definition

Disintegrated physiologic and neurobehavioral responses of infant to the environment

Defining Characteristics
(Hockenberry & Wilson, 2015; *Vandenberg, 1990)

Autonomic System

Cardiac
Increased rate

Respiration
Pauses   Gasping
Tachypnea

Skin Color Changes*
Paling around nostrils   Cyanosis
Perioral duskiness   Grayness
Mottling   Flushing/ruddiness

Visceral
Hiccuping*   Spitting up
Straining as if producing a bowel   Gagging
movement
Grunting

Motor

Seizures	Twitches*
Sneezing*	Sighing*
Tremors/startles*	Coughing*
Yawning	

Motor System

Fluctuating Tone

Flaccidity of:

Trunk	Extremities
Face	

Hypertonicity

Extending legs	Airplaning
Arching	Extending tongue
Saluting	Sitting on air
Splaying fingers*	Fisting*

Hyperflexions

Trunk	Extremities
Fetal tuck	

Frantic Diffuse Activity

State System (Range)

Difficulty maintaining state control
Difficulty in transitions from one state to another

Sleep

Twitches*	Makes jerky movements
Whimpers	Fusses in sleep
Makes sounds	Has irregular respirations
Grimaces	

Awake

Eyes floating	Irritability*
Panicky, worried*, dull look	Staring*
Glassy eyes	Abrupt state changes
Weak cry	Gaze aversion*
Strain, fussiness	

Attention–Interaction System

Attempts at engaging behaviors elicit stress
Difficulty consoling

Related Factors
(Askin & Wilson, 2007)

Pathophysiologic

Related to immature or altered central nervous system (CNS) secondary to:

Prematurity*	Intraventricular hemorrhage
Perinatal factors	Congenital anomalies
Hyperbilirubinemia	Prenatal exposure to drugs/alcohol
Hypoglycemia	Decreased oxygen saturation
Respiratory distress	Infection

Related to nutritional deficits secondary to:

Reflux	Emesis
Feeding intolerance*	Colic
Swallowing problems	Poor suck/swallow coordination

Related to excess stimulation secondary to:
Oral hypersensitivity
Frequent handling and position changes

Treatment Related

Related to excess stimulation secondary to:

Invasive procedures*	Noise (e.g., prolonged alarm,
Movement	voices, environment)
Lights	Chest physical therapy
Medication administration	Feeding
Restraints	Tubes, tape

Related to inability to see caregivers secondary to eye patches

Situational (Personal, Environmental)

Related to unpredictable interactions secondary to multiple caregivers

Related to imbalance of task touch and consoling touch

Related to decreased ability to self-regulate secondary to (Holditch-Davis & Blackburn, 2007):

Sudden movement	Fatigue
Noise	Stimulation that exceeds the
Prematurity*	infant's tolerance threshold
Disrupted sleep–wake cycles	Environmental demands

Author's Note

Disorganized Infant Behavior describes an infant who has difficulty regulating and adapting to external stimuli due to immature neurobehavioral development and increased environmental stimuli associated with neonatal units. When an infant is overstimulated or stressed, he or she uses energy to adapt; this depletes the supply of energy available for physiologic growth. The goal of nursing care is to assist the infant to conserve energy by reducing environmental stimuli, allowing the infant sufficient time to adapt to handling, and providing sensory input appropriate to the infant's physiologic and neurobehavioral status.

Neurologic Status, Preterm Infant Organization, Sleep, Comfort Level

Goals

The infant will demonstrate increased signs of stability, as evidenced by the following indicators:

- Exhibit smooth, stable respirations; pink, stable color; consistent tone; improved posture; calm, focused alertness; well-modulated sleep; response to visual and social stimuli
- Demonstrate self-regulatory skills as sucking, hand to mouth, grasping, hand holding, hand and foot clasping, tucking

The parent(s)/caregiver(s) will describe techniques to reduce environmental stress in agency, at home, or both.

- Describe situations that stress infant
- Describe signs/symptoms of stress in infant
- Describe ways to support infant's efforts to self-calm (Vandenberg, 2007)

Environmental Management, Neurologic Monitoring, Sleep Enhancement, Newborn Care, Parent Education: Newborn Positioning

Interventions

See Related Factors.

Reduce or Eliminate Contributing Factors, If Possible

- Premature infants must adapt to the extrauterine environment with underdeveloped body systems, usually in a neonatal intensive care unit (NICU) (Kenner & McGrath, 2010; *Merenstein & Gardner, 2002).

Pain
- Observe for responses that are different from baseline and have been associated with neonatal pain responses (*Bozzette, 1993):
  - Facial responses (open mouth, brow bulge, grimace, chin quiver, nasolabial furrow, taut tongue)
  - Motor responses (flinch, muscle rigidity, clenched hands, withdrawal) (*AAP, 2006)
- Provide pharmacologic and/or nonpharmacologic pain relief for all painful procedures, such as gavage tube placement, tape removal, needle insertions, heel sticks, insertion and removal of chest tubes, intubation, prolonged mechanical ventilation, eye examinations, circumcision, and surgery.
- Topical anesthetics can reduce pain for some procedures such as venipuncture, lumbar puncture, and IV insertion.
- Nonpharmacologic interventions:
  - Developmental care that includes attention to behavioral cues and reducing environmental stimuli, has shown to be effective in reducing pain from minor procedures.
  - Facilitated tuck
  - Swaddling
  - Supportive bedding
  - Side-lying position
  - Kangaroo care
  - Nonnutritive suck
  - Oral sucrose solution combined with sucking has proved effective at reducing pain from many minor procedures.

Disrupted 24-Hour Diurnal Cycles
- Evaluate the need for and frequency of each intervention.
- Consider 24-hour caregiving assignment and primary caregiving to provide consistent caregiving throughout the day and night for the infant from the onset of admission. This is important in terms of responding to increasingly more mature sleep cycles, feeding ability, and especially emotional development.
- Consider supporting the infant's transition to and maintenance of sleep by avoiding peaks of frenzy and overexhaustion; continuously maintaining a calm, regular environment and schedule; and establishing a reliable, repeatable pattern of gradual transition into sleep in prone and side-lying positions in the isolette or crib.

Problematic Feeding Experiences
- Observe and record infant's readiness for participation with feeding.

Hunger Cues
- Transitioning to drowsy or alert state
- Mouthing, rooting, or sucking
- Bringing hands to mouth
- Crying that is not relieved with pacifier or nonnutritive sucking alone

Physiologic Stability
- Look for regulated breathing patterns, stable color, and stable digestion.
- Provide comfortable seating (be especially sensitive to the needs of postpartum mothers: e.g., soft cushions, small stool to elevate legs, supportive pillows for nursing).
- Encourage softly swaddling the infant to facilitate flexion and balanced tone during feeding.
- Explore feeding methods that meet the goals of both infant and family (e.g., breastfeeding, bottle-feeding, gavage).

Support the Infant's Self-Regulatory Efforts

- When administering painful or stressful procedures, consider actions to enhance calmness.
- Consider supporting the infant's transition to and maintenance of sleep by avoiding peaks of frenzy and overexhaustion; by continuously maintaining a calm, regular environment and schedule; and by establishing a reliable, repeatable pattern of gradual transition into sleep in prone and side-lying positions in the isolette or crib.
- Consider initiating calming on the caregiver's body and then transferring the baby to the crib as necessary. For other infants, this may be too arousing, and transition is accomplished more easily in the isolette with the provision of steady boundaries and encasing without any stimulation.

Reduce Environmental Stimuli (Kenner & McGrath, 2010; *Merenstein & Gardner, 1998; *Thomas, 1989)

Noise
- Do not tap on incubator.
- Place a folded blanket on top of the incubator if it is the only work surface available.
- Slowly open and close porthole.
- Pad incubator doors to reduce banging.
- Use plastic instead of metal waste cans.
- Remove water from ventilator tubing.
- Speak softly at the bedside and only when necessary.
- Slowly drop the head of the mattress.

- Eliminate radios.
- Close doors slowly.
- Position the infant's bed away from sources of noise (e.g., telephone, intercom, unit equipment).
- Consider the following methods to reduce unnecessary noise in the NICU:
  - Perform rounds away from the bedsides.
  - Adapt large equipment to eliminate noise and clutter.
  - Alert staff when the decibel level in the unit exceeds 60 db (e.g., by a light attached to a sound meter). Institute quiet time for 10 minutes to lower noise.
  - Move more vulnerable infants out of unit traffic patterns.

Lights

- Use full-spectrum instead of white light at bedside. Avoid fluorescent lights.
- Cover cribs, incubators, and radiant warmers completely during sleep and partially during awake periods.
- Install dimmer switches, shades, and curtains. Avoid bright lights.
- Shade infants' eyes with a blanket tent or cutout box.
- Avoid visual stimuli on cribs.
- Shield eyes from bright procedure lights. Avoid patches unless for phototherapy.

Position Infant in Postures That Permit Flexion and Minimize Flailing

- Consider gentle, *unhurried* reorganization and stabilization of infant's regulation by supporting the infant in softly tucked prone position, giving opportunities to hold onto caregiver's finger and suck, encasing trunk and back of head in caregiver's hand, and providing inhibition to soles of feet.
- Use the prone/side-lying position. Avoid the supine position.
- Swaddle baby, if possible, to maintain flexion.
- Create a nest using soft bedding (e.g., natural sheepskin, soft cotton, flannel).

Reduce Disorganized Behavior During Active Interventions and Transport

- Have a plan for transport, with assigned roles for each team member.
- Establish behavior cues of stress on the infant with the primary nurse before transport.
- Minimize sensory input:
  - Use calm, quiet voices.

- Shade the infant's eyes from light.
- Protect infant from unnecessary touch.
- Support the infant's softly tucked postures with your hands and offer something to grasp (your finger or corner of a soft blanket or cloth).
- Swaddle the infant or place him or her in a nest made of blankets.
- Ensure that the transport equipment (e.g., ventilator) is ready. Warm mattress or use sheepskin.
- Carefully and smoothly move the infant. Avoid talking, if possible.
- Consider conducting caregiving routines while parent(s) or designated caregiver hold infant, whenever possible.
- Reposition in 2 to 3 hours or sooner if infant behavior suggests discomfort.

Engage Parents in Planning Care

- Encourage them to share their feelings, fears, and expectations.
- Consider involving parents in creating the family's developmental plan:
  - My strengths are: _____
  - Time-out signals: _____
  - These things stress me: _____
  - How you can help me: _____
- Teach caregivers to continually observe the changing capabilities to determine the appropriate positioning and bedding options, for example, infant may fight containment (Hockenberry & Wilson, 2015).

Initiate Health Teaching and Referrals as Indicated

Review the Following Information Relating to Growth and Development of the Infant and Family in Anticipatory Guidance for Home

Health Concerns
- Feeding
- Hygiene
- Illness
- Infection
- Safety
- Temperature
- Growth and development

State Modulation
- Appropriate stimulation
- Sleep–wake patterns

Parent–Infant Interaction
- Behavior cues
- Signs of stress

Infant's Environment
- Animate, inanimate stimulation
- Playing with infant
- Role of father and siblings

Parental Coping and Support
- Support network
- Challenges
- Problem solving

Discuss Transition to Community Supports (Nursing Respite, Social and Civic Groups, Religious Affiliations)
Refer for Follow-Up Home Visits

Risk for Disorganized Infant Behavior

NANDA-I Definition

At risk for alteration in integrating and modulation of the physiologic and behavioral systems of functioning (i.e., autonomic, motor, state-organization, self-regulatory, and attentional-interactional systems)

Risk Factors

Refer to Related Factors.

Related Factors

Refer to *Disorganized Infant Behavior*.

Interventions

Refer to *Disorganized Infant Behavior*.

RISK FOR INFECTION

NANDA-I Definition

At risk for being invaded by pathogenic organisms

Risk Factors

See Related Factors.

Related Factors

Various health problems and situations can create favorable conditions that would encourage the development of infections. Some common factors follow:

Pathophysiologic

Related to compromised host defenses secondary to:

Cancer	Hepatic disorders
Altered or insufficient leukocytes	Diabetes mellitus*
	Acquired immunodeficiency syndrome (AIDS)
Arthritis	
Respiratory disorders	Alcoholism
Periodontal disease	Immunosuppression*
Renal failure	Immunodeficiency secondary to (specify)
Hematologic disorders	

Related to compromised circulation secondary to:

Lymphedema	Peripheral vascular disease
Obesity*	

Treatment Related

Related to a site for organism invasion secondary to:

Surgery	Intubation
Invasive lines	Total parenteral nutrition
Dialysis	Enteral feedings

Related to compromised host defenses secondary to:

Radiation therapy

Organ transplant

Medication therapy (specify; e.g., chemotherapy, immunosuppressants)

Situational (Personal, Environmental)

Related to compromised host defenses secondary to:

History of infections	Stress
Malnutrition*	Increased hospital stay
Prolonged immobility	Smoking

Related to a site for organism invasion secondary to:

Trauma (accidental, intentional)	Thermal injuries
Postpartum period	Warm, moist, dark environment (skin folds, casts)
Bites (animal, insect, human)	

Related to contact with contagious agents (nosocomial or community acquired)

Maturational

Newborns
Related to increased vulnerability of infant secondary to:

HIV-positive mother	Maternal substance addiction
Lack of maternal antibodies (dependent on maternal exposures)	Open wounds (umbilical, circumcision)
Lack of normal flora	Immature immune system

Infant/Child
Related to lack of immunization

Adolescent
Related to lack of immunization

Related to multiple sex partners

Older Adult
Related to increased vulnerability secondary to:

Diminished immune response	Warm, moist, dark environment (skin folds, casts)
Debilitated condition	Chronic diseases

 Author's Note

All people are at risk for infection. Secretion control, environmental control, and hand washing before and after individual care reduce the risk of transmission of organisms. Included in the population of those at risk for infection is a smaller group who are at high risk for infection. *Risk for Infection* describes a person, whose host defenses are compromised, thus increasing susceptibility to environmental pathogens or his or her own endogenous flora (e.g., a person with chronic liver dysfunction or with an invasive line). Nursing interventions for such a person focus on minimizing introduction of organisms and increasing resistance to infection (e.g., improving nutritional status). For a person with an infection, the situation is best described by the collaborative problem *Risk for Complications of Sepsis*.

Risk for Infection Transmission describes a person at high risk for transferring an infectious agent to others. Some people are at high risk both for acquiring opportunistic agents and for transmitting infecting organisms, warranting the use of both *Risk for Infection* and *Risk for Infection Transmission*.

NOC

Infection Status, Wound Healing: Primary Intention, Immune Status

Goals

The person will report risk factors associated with infection and precautions needed, as evidenced by the following indicators:

- Demonstrate meticulous hand washing technique by the time of discharge
- Describe methods of transmission of infection
- Describe the influence of nutrition on prevention of infection

NIC

Infection Control, Wound Care, Incision Site Care, Health Education ⸲

Interventions

Identify Individuals at High Risk for Health-Care Acquired Infections (HAI)

- Refer to Risk Factors.

Use Appropriate Universal Precautions for Every Individual

Antiseptic Hand Hygiene (Quoted From Diaz & Newman, 2015; Centers for Disease Prevention and Control [CDC], 2015)
- Wash with antiseptic soap and water for at least 15 seconds followed by alcohol-based hand rub. If hands were not in

contact with anyone or thing in the room, use an alcohol-based hand rub and rub until dry (CDC, 2015).
- Plain soap is good at reducing bacterial counts but antimicrobial soap is better, and alcohol-based hand rubs are the best (CDC, 2015).
- Wash hands:
  - Before putting on gloves and after taking them off
  - Before and after touching a patient, before handling an invasive device (foley catheter, peripheral vascular catheter) regardless of whether or not gloves are used
  - After contact with body fluids or excretions, mucous membranes, nonintact skin, or wound dressings
  - If moving from a contaminated body site to another body site during the care of the same individual
  - After contact with inanimate surfaces and objects (including medical equipment) in the immediate vicinity of the patient
  - After removing sterile or nonsterile gloves
  - Before handling medications or preparing food

Consider Individual Factors That Increase the Risk for Delayed Wound Healing

- Refer to *Risk for Delayed Surgical Recovery*.

Personal Protective Equipment (PPE)
- Wear PPE when an interaction indicates that contact with blood/body fluids may occur.

Gloves
- Wear gloves when providing direct care. After removing gloves, wash hands with soap and water.

Masks
- Use PPE (masks, goggles, face shields) to protect the mucous membranes of your eyes, mouth, and nose during procedures and direct-care activities that may generate splashes or sprays of blood, body fluids, secretions, and excretions.

Gowns
- Wear a gown for direct contact with uncontained secretions or excretions.
- Remove gown and perform hand hygiene before leaving the room/cubicle.
- Do not reuse gowns even with the same individual.

When Suctioning Oral Secretion
- Wear gloves and mask/goggles or a face shield—sometimes gown (CDC, 2013).

Educate All Staff, Visitors, and Individuals on the Importance of Preventing Droplet Transmission From Themselves to Others

- Provide a surgical mask to persons who are coughing. Explain why.
- Instruct:
  - To cover the mouth and nose during coughing and sneezing
  - To use tissues to contain respiratory secretions with prompt disposal into a no-touch receptacle and to wash hands with soap and water
  - To turn the head away from others and maintain spatial buffer, ideally more than 3 feet, when coughing
- Immediately report any situation that increases the risk of infection transmission to individuals, visitors, or staff.

Initiate Specific Precautions for the Suspected Agent; Follow Infection Prevention According to Institution or the Center for Disease Control for

- Meningitis: droplet, airborne precautions
- Maculopapular rash with cough, fever
- Rubella: airborne precautions
- Abscess *Clostridium difficile*, hand-to-mouth spores or fecal contamination
- MRSA: contact, droplet precautions
- Cough/fever/pulmonary infiltrate in HIV-infected or someone at high risk of HIV infection
- Tuberculosis: airborne/contact (respirators)

Reduce Entry of Organisms

Surgical Site Infection (SSI)
- Identify individuals at high risk for delayed wound healing (refer to Focus Assessment Criteria).
- Maintain normothermia.
  - Monitor temperature every 4 hours; notify physician/NP if temperature is greater than 100.8° F.
  - Advise smokers that the risk of wound infection is tripled in smokers (Armstrong & Mayr, 2014).
  - Aggressively manage postoperative pain using prevention vs. PRN medication administration.
- Prevent hypovolemia.
  - Assess nutritional status to provide adequate protein and caloric intake for healing.

Catheter-Associated Urinary Tract Infection (CAUTI)

- Insert catheters only for appropriate indications.
- Consider condom catheters or alternatives to indwelling catheter such as intermittent catheterization if possible.
- When a catheter is in place, remind the prescriber every 2 days to reconsider if catheter is still indicated (e.g., use reminder protocols or institute the nursing protocol, which allows reassessment and determination if the catheter can be removed).
- Ensure the following:
  - It is secured to the thigh with a securement device.
  - The indwelling urinary catheter (IUC) drainage bag is below the level of the bladder at all times.
  - The drainage bag is emptied every 8 hours and when the bag is two-thirds full or prior to all transfers. Empty using a separate, clean collecting container for each individual.
- Consult with physician/nurse practitioner to discuss the inappropriate or prolonged use of indwelling catheter in a particular individual.
- Once an IUC is removed, offer the patient a bedside commode if they cannot ambulate safely to the bathroom.

Invasive Access Sites

- Follow protocol for invasive access sites for insertion and maintenance. Some general interventions are (O'Grady et al., 2011) as follows:
  - Evaluate the catheter insertion site daily by palpation through the dressing to discern tenderness and by inspection if a transparent dressing is in use.
  - Remove peripheral venous catheters if the individual develops signs of phlebitis (warmth, tenderness, erythema, or palpable venous cord), infection, or a malfunctioning catheter.
  - Maintain aseptic technique for all invasive devices, changing sites, dressings, tubing, and solutions per policy schedule.
  - Use maximal sterile barrier precautions, including the use of a cap, mask, sterile gown, sterile gloves, and a sterile full body drape, for the insertion of CVCs, PICCs, or guidewire exchange.
  - Use a 2% chlorhexidine wash instead of soap and water for daily skin cleansing.

Respiratory Tract Infections

Practice Protective Measures

- Maintain respiratory hygiene (providing masks, tissues, hand hygiene products, designated hand washing sinks, and no-touch waste receptacles).
- Assess the individual's personal hygiene habits; correct any behavior that increases risk for infection.
- If indicated, use airborne infection isolation rooms.
- Monitor temperature at least every 8 hours and notify physician/NP/PA if greater than 100.8° F.
- Evaluate sputum characteristics for frequency, purulence, blood, and odor.
- Assess lung sounds every 8 hours or PRN.
- Prompt to cough and deep breathe hourly.
- If individual has had anesthesia, monitor for appropriate clearing of secretions in lung fields.
- Evaluate need for suctioning if individual cannot clear secretions adequately.
- Assess for risk of aspiration, keeping head of bed elevated 30° unless otherwise contraindicated.
- Ensure optimal pain management to enhance effective coughing.

Pediatric Interventions

- Monitor for signs of infection (e.g., lethargy, feeding difficulties, vomiting, temperature instability, subtle color changes).

For Newborns

- Provide umbilical cord care. Teach cord care and signs of infection (e.g., increased redness, purulent drainage).
- Teach signs of infection of circumcised area (e.g., bleeding, increased redness, or unusual swelling).

Geriatric Interventions

- Explain that the usual signs of infection may not be present (e.g., fever, chills).
- Assess for anorexia, weakness, change in mental status, or hypothermia.
- Monitor skin and urinary system for signs of fungal, viral, or mycobacterial pathogens.

RISK FOR INFECTION TRANSMISSION[18]

Definition

Vulnerable to transferring an opportunistic or pathogenic agent to others

Risk Factors

Presence of risk factors (see Related Factors)

Related Factors

Pathophysiologic

Related to:
Colonization with highly antibiotic-resistant organism
Airborne transmission exposure (sneezing, coughing, spitting)
Contact transmission exposure (direct, indirect, contact droplet)
Vehicle transmission exposure (food, water, contaminated drugs or blood, contaminated sites [IV, catheter])
Vector-borne transmission exposure (animals, rodents, insects)

Treatment Related

Related to exposure to a contaminated wound

Related to devices with contaminated drainage:
Urinary, chest, endotracheal tubes
Suction equipment

Situational (Personal, Environmental)

Related to:
Unsanitary living conditions (sewage, personal hygiene)
Areas considered high risk for vector-borne diseases (malaria, rabies, bubonic plague)
Areas considered high risk for vehicle-borne disease (hepatitis A, *Shigella*, *Salmonella*)

---

[18]This diagnosis is not currently on the NANDA list but has been included for clarity or usefulness.

Exposures to sources of infection as:

   Intravenous/intranasal/intradermal drug use (sharing of
      needles, drug paraphernalia straws)
   Contaminated sex paraphernalia
   Multiple sex partners
   Natural disaster (e.g., flood, hurricane)
   Disaster with hazardous infectious material

Maturational

Newborn

Related to birth outside hospital setting in uncontrolled environment

Related to exposure during prenatal or perinatal period to communicable disease through mother

 NOC

Infection Status, Risk Control, Risk Detection

Goals

The individual will describe the mode of transmission of disease by the time of discharge, as evidenced by the following indicators:

- Relate the need to be isolated until noninfectious (e.g., TB)
- Relate factors that contribute to the transmission of the infection
- Relate methods to reduce or prevent infection transmission
- Demonstrate meticulous hand washing

 NIC

Teaching: Disease Process, Infection Control Infection Protection

Interventions

Initiate Specific Precautions for the Suspected Agent; Follow Infection Prevention According to Institution or the Center for Disease Control for

- Meningitis: droplet, airborne precautions
- Maculopapular rash with cough, fever
- Rubella: airborne precautions
- Abscess *Clostridium difficile*, hand–to-mouth spores or fecal contamination
- MRSA: contact, droplet precautions
- Cough/fever/pulmonary infiltrate in HIV-infected or someone at high risk of HIV infection
- Tuberculosis: airborne/contact (respirators)

Reduce the Transfer of Pathogens

- Isolate individuals with airborne communicable infections (Table I.4).
- Secure appropriate room assignment depending on the type of infection and hygienic practices of the infected individual.

Table I.4 AIRBORNE COMMUNICABLE DISEASES

Disease	Apply Airborne Precautions for How Long	Comments
Anthrax, inhalation	Duration of illness	Promptly report to infection control office
Chickenpox (varicella)	Until all lesions are crusted	Immune person does not need to wear a mask. Exposed susceptible clients should be placed in a private special airflow room on STOP SIGN alert status beginning 10 d after initial exposure until 21 d after last exposure Report to epidemiology
Diphtheria, pharyngeal	Until two cultures from both nose and throat taken at least 24 h after cessation of antimicrobial therapy are negative for *Corynebacterium diphtheriae*	Promptly report to epidemiology
Epiglottis, due to *Haemophilus influenzae*	For 24 h after cessation of antimicrobial therapy	Report to epidemiology
Erythema infectiosum	For 7 d after onset	Report to epidemiology

Table I.4 AIRBORNE COMMUNICABLE DISEASES
(*continued*)

Disease	Apply Airborne Precautions for How Long	Comments
Hemorrhagic fevers	Duration of illness	Call epidemiology office immediately. May call the State Health Department and Centers for Disease Control and Prevention for advice about management of a suspected case
Herpes zoster (varicella zoster), disseminated	Duration of illness	Localized; does not require STOP SIGN
Lassa fever	Duration of illness	Call epidemiology office immediately
Marburg virus disease		May call the State Health Department and Centers for Disease Control and Prevention for advice about management of a suspected case
Measles (rubeola)	For 4 d after start of rash, except in immunocompromised clients, for whom precautions should be maintained for duration of illness	Immune people do not need to wear a mask. Exposed susceptible clients should be placed in a private special air flow room on STOP SIGN alert status beginning the 5th d after exposure until 21 d after last exposure
Meningitis, *Haemophilus influenzae* known or suspected	For 24 h after start of effective antibiotic therapy	Call epidemiology to report

(continued)

Table I.4 AIRBORNE COMMUNICABLE DISEASES
(*continued*)

Disease	Apply Airborne Precautions for How Long	Comments
Neisseria meningitidis (meningococci) known or suspected	For 24 h after start of effective antibiotic therapy	Promptly report to epidemiology
Meningococcal pneumonia	For 24 h after start of effective antibiotic therapy	Promptly report to epidemiology
Meningococcemia	For 24 h after start of effective antibiotic therapy	Consult with epidemiology
Multiply resistant organisms	Until culture negative or as determined by epidemiology	Consult with epidemiology
Mumps (infectious parotitis)	For 9 d after onset of swelling	People with history do not need to wear a mask. Call epidemiology office to report
Pertussis (whooping cough)	For 7 d after start of effective therapy	Call epidemiology to report
Plague, pneumonic	For 3 d after start of effective therapy	Promptly report to epidemiology
Pneumonia, *Haemophilus* in infants and children any age	For 24 h after start of effective therapy	Call epidemiology
Pneumonia, meningococcal	For 24 h after start of effective antibiotic therapy	Promptly report to epidemiology
Rubella (German measles)	For 7 d after onset of rash	Immune people do not need to wear a mask. Promptly report to epidemiology

	Apply Airborne Precautions for	
Disease	**How Long**	**Comments**
Tuberculosis, bronchial, laryngeal, pulmonary, confirmed or suspect	Clients are not considered infectious if they meet all these criteria: Adequate therapy received for 2–3 weeks Favorable clinical response to therapy Three consecutive negative sputum smear results from sputum collected on different days	Call epidemiology to report; prompt use of effective antituberculosis drugs is the most effective means of limiting transmission
Varicella (chickenpox)	Until all lesions crusted over	See chickenpox

Table I.4 AIRBORNE COMMUNICABLE DISEASES (*continued*)

Source: Centers for Disease Control and Prevention. www.cdc.gov.

- Use universal precautions to prevent transmission to self or other susceptible host. Refer to Infection Control Protocol for institution or the CDC (2012).

Initiate Health Education and Referrals as Indicated and Discuss the Mode of Transmission of Infection With the Individual, Family, and Significant Others

RISK FOR INJURY

Risk for Injury

Risk for Aspiration

Risk for Falls

Risk for Poisoning

Risk for Suffocation

Risk for Thermal Injury

Risk for Trauma

Risk for Perioperative Positioning Injury

Risk for Urinary Tract Injury

NANDA-I Definition

Vulnerable for injury as a result of environmental conditions interacting with the individual's adaptive and defensive resources, which may compromise health

Risk Factors

Presence of risk factor (see Related Factors)

Related Factors

Pathophysiologic

Related to altered cerebral function secondary to hypoxia

Related to syncope

Related to vertigo or dizziness

Related to impaired mobility secondary to:
Post-cerebrovascular accident   Parkinsonism
Arthritis   Artificial limb(s)

Related to impaired vision

Related to hearing impairment

Related to fatigue

Related to orthostatic hypotension

Related to vestibular disorders

Related to lack of awareness of environmental hazards secondary to:
Confusion
Unfamiliar setting

Related to tonic–clonic movements secondary to seizures

Treatment Related

Related to prolonged bed rest

Related to effects of (specify) or sensorium
Examples:

Sedatives	Antispasmodics	Vasodilators
Phenothiazine	Diuretics	Psychotropics
Diabetic medications	Antihypertensives	Muscle relaxants
Antihistamines	Pain medications	

Related to casts/crutches, canes, walkers

Situational (Personal, Environmental)

Related to decrease in or loss of short-term memory

Related to faulty judgment secondary to:

Stress	Dehydration
Drug abuse	Depression
Alcohol abuse	

Related to household hazards (specify):

Unsafe walkways	Improperly stored poisons
Slippery floors	Unsafe toys
Bathrooms (tubs, toilets)	Faulty electric wires
Stairs	Throw Rugs
Inadequate lighting	

Related to automotive hazards:
Lack of use of seat belts or child seats
Mechanically unsafe vehicle

Related to fire hazards

Related to unfamiliar setting (hospital, nursing home)

Related to improper footwear

Related to inattentive caretaker

Related to improper use of aids (crutches, canes, walkers, wheelchairs)

Related to history of accidents

Related to unstable gait

Maturational

Infant/Child
Related to lack of awareness of hazards

Older Adult
Related to faulty judgments, secondary cognitive deficits
Related to sedentary lifestyle and loss of muscle strength

 Author's Note

This diagnosis has six subcategories: *Risk for Aspiration*, *Risk for Poisoning*, *Risk for Suffocation*, *Risk for Thermal Injury*, *Risk for Trauma*, and *Risk for Urinary Tract Trauma*.

Interventions to prevent poisoning, suffocation, falls, and trauma are included under the general category *Risk for Injury*. Should the nurse choose to isolate interventions only for prevention of poisoning, suffocation, or trauma, then the diagnosis *Risk for Poisoning*, *Risk for Suffocation*, *Risk for Falls*, *Risk for Trauma*, or *Risk for Urinary Tract Trauma* would be useful.

Nursing interventions related to *Risk for Injury* focus on protecting an individual from injury and teaching precautions to reduce the risk of injury. When the nurse is teaching an individual or family safety measures to prevent injury but is not providing on-site protection (as in the community or outpatient department, or for discharge planning), the diagnosis *Risk for Injury related to insufficient knowledge of safety precautions* may be more appropriate.

NOC
Risk Control, Safe Home Environment, Falls Occurrence, Fall Prevention Behavior

Goals

The individual will relate fewer or no injuries, as evidenced by the following indicators:

- Identify factors that increase risk for injury
- Relate intent to use safety measures to prevent injury (e.g., remove or anchor throw rugs)
- Relate intent to practice selected prevention measures (e.g., wear sunglasses to reduce glare)
- Increase daily activity, if feasible

NIC
Fall Prevention, Environmental Management: Safety, Health Education, Surveillance: Safety, Risk Identification

Interventions

Refer to Related Factors.

Reduce or Eliminate Causative or Contributing Factors, If Possible

Unfamiliar Surroundings

- Orient to surroundings on admission; explain the call system, and assess individual's ability to use it. Use a night-light.
- Closely supervise during the first few nights to assess safety.
- Encourage the individual to request assistance during the night.
- Teach about side effects of certain drugs (e.g., dizziness, fatigue).
- Keep bed at lowest level during the night.
- Consider use of a movement detection monitor (bed-based alarm or personal alarm), if needed.

Impaired Vision

- Provide safe illumination and teach to
  - Ensure adequate lighting in all rooms, with soft light at night
  - Have a light switch easily accessible, next to the bed
  - Provide background light that is soft
- Teach how to reduce glare:
  - Avoid glossy surfaces (e.g., glass, highly polished floors).
  - Use diffuse rather than direct light; use shades that darken the room.
  - Turn the head away when switching on a bright light.
  - Wear sunglasses or hats with brims, or carry umbrellas, to reduce glare outside.
  - Avoid looking directly at bright lights (e.g., headlights).

Decreased Tactile Sensitivity

- Teach preventive measures:
  - Assess temperature of bath water and heating pads before use.
  - Use bath thermometers.
  - Assess extremities daily for undetected injuries.
  - Keep the feet warm and dry and skin softened with emollient lotion (lanolin, mineral oil). (Note: Use socks with grips after just putting on lotion to prevent slips/falls).

Orthostatic Hypotension

- See *Risk for Injury related to vertigo secondary to orthostatic hypotension* for additional interventions.

Decreased Strength/Flexibility

- Perform strengthening exercises daily (*Schoenfelder, 2000). The Centers for Disease Control and Prevention website outlines a safe beginning exercise program for older adults with warm-up and cool-down (CDC, 2015):

- Squats
- Wall pushups
- Toe stands
- Finger marching
- Perform ankle-strengthening exercises daily (Schoenfelder, 2000). The following is an example of toe stands (CDC, 2015).
  - Instruct to
    - Stand in front of a counter or sturdy chair, stand with feet shoulder-width apart. Use the chair or counter for balance.
    - Count of four, slowly push up as far as you can, onto the balls of your feet and hold for two to four seconds. (e.g., one second equals counting, 1 Mississippi, 2 Mississippi, 3 Mississippi, and so on).
    - Then, to a count of four, slowly lower your heels back to the floor.
  - Repeat 5 to 10 times for one set. Rest for 1 to 2 minutes. Then complete a second set of 5 to 10 repetitions. Increase repetitions as strength increases.
- Walk at least two or three times a week.
  - Use ankle exercises as a warm-up before walking.
  - Begin walking with someone at side, if needed, for 10 minutes.
  - Increase time and speed according to capabilities.
- If cognitively impaired, refer to *Chronic Confusion*.

Initiate Health Teaching and Referrals as Needed

Teach About Safety With Potentially Dangerous Equipment (American Academy of Orthopedic Surgeon, 2012)

- Teach to read directions completely before using a new appliance or piece of the appliance.
- Teach children to stay away from all running lawn mowers.
- Children should not be allowed to play in or near where a lawn mower is being used.
- Never allow a child or another passenger to ride on a mower, even with parents. Doctors commonly see children with severe injuries to their feet caused by riding on the back of a rider mower with a parent or grandparent.
- Children should be at least 12 years of age before operating a push lawn mower, and age 16 to operate a riding lawn mower.
- Remove stones, toys, and other objects from the lawn before you start mowing.
- Unplug and turn off any appliance that is not functioning before examining it (e.g., lawn mower, snow blower, electric mixer).

- Most injuries happen when you try to clear the auger/collector or discharge chute with your hands.
- Do not remove safety devices, shields or guards on switches, and keep hands and feet away from moving parts.
- Add fuel before starting the engine, not when it is running or hot.
- Use a stick or broom handle—not your hands or feet—to remove debris in lawn mowers or snow blowers.
- Do not leave a lawn mower or snow blower unattended when it is running. If you must walk away from the machine, shut off the engine.

Pediatric Interventions

- Teach parents to expect frequent changes in infants' and children's ability and to take precautions (e.g., infant who suddenly rolls over for the first time might be on a changing table unattended).
- Discuss with parents the necessity of constant monitoring of small children.
- Explain that walkers are dangerous and in addition *walker use typically delays motor development and cognitive development*. They allow the child to walk faster which can cause them to roll down the stairs and to reach higher (e.g., spill hot coffee, grab pot handles off the stove, touch radiators, fireplaces, or space heaters; American Academy of Pediatrics, 2015).
- Teach parents to expect children to mimic them and to teach their children what they can do with or without supervision (e.g., seat belts, helmets, safe driving).
- Explain and expect compliance with certain rules (depending on age) concerning:
  - Streets
  - Playground equipment
  - Water (e.g., pools, bathtubs)
  - Bicycles
  - Fire
  - Animals
  - Strangers
  - For an excellent resource for parents/families, refer to the Children's Hospitals and Clinics of Minnesota website for "Making Safe Simple" (2014)
- Refer to local fire department for assistance in staging home fire drills.
- Encourage parents to learn basic life-saving skills (e.g., CPR, Heimlich maneuver).
- Teach children how to dial 911.

⚜ Geriatric Interventions

- Recent medical history of potential volume loss (vomiting, diarrhea, fluid restriction, fever)
- Medical history of congestive heart failure, malignancy, diabetes, alcoholism
- Evidence on neurologic history and examination of parkinsonism, ataxia, peripheral neuropathy, or dysautonomia (e.g., abnormal pupillary response, history of constipation, or erectile dysfunction)
- Cardiovascular disorders (systolic hypertension, heart failure, cerebral infarct, anemia, dysrhythmias)
- Fluid or electrolyte imbalances
- Diabetes
- Certain medications (diuretics, antihypertensives, beta-blockers, alpha-blockers anticholinergics, biturates, vasodilators, antidepressants, antipsychotic drugs: olanzapine, risperidone)
- Antihypertensive drugs, nitrates, monoamine oxidase inhibitors, phenothiazine, narcotics, sedatives, muscle relaxants, vasodilators, antiseizure medications (Perlmuter, 2013)
- Alcohol use
- Age 75 years or older
- Prolonged bed rest
- Surgical sympathectomy
- Valsalva maneuver during voiding or defecating
- Arthritis (spurs on cervical vertebrae)

Assess for Orthostatic Hypotension

- Take bilateral brachial pressures with the individual supine.
- If the brachial pressures are different, use the arm with the higher reading and take the blood pressure immediately after the individual stands up quickly. Report differences to the physician/PA/NP.
- Ask to describe sensations (e.g., light-headed, dizzy).
- Assess skin and vital signs.

Teach Techniques to Reduce Orthostatic Hypotension

- Change positions slowly, especially in the morning when orthostatic tolerance is lowest.
- Move from lying to an upright position in stages:
  - Sit up in bed.
  - Dangle first one leg, then the other, over the side of the bed.
  - Allow a few minutes before going on to each step.
  - Gradually pull oneself from a sitting to a standing position.
  - Place a chair, walker, cane, or other assistive device nearby to use to steady oneself when getting out of bed.

- Sleep with the head of the bed elevated 10° to 20°.
- During day, rest in a recliner rather than in bed.
- Avoid prolonged bed rest.
- Avoid prolonged standing.
- Avoid stooping to pick something up from the floor; use an assistive device available from an orthotics department or a self-help store.
- Avoid straining, coughing, and walking in hot weather; these activities reduce venous return and worsen orthostatic hypotension.
- Maintain hydration and avoid overheating. Drink water before exposure to hot weather.
- Refer to prescribing provider for a discussion about the possible effectiveness of waist-high stockings.
- Assess for orthostatic hypotension. Compare brachial blood pressure (e.g., supine, standing).
- Discuss physiology of orthostatic hypotension with individual.
- Teach techniques to reduce orthostatic hypotension.
  - Change positions slowly.
  - Move from lying to an upright position in stages.
  - During day, rest in a recliner rather than in bed.
  - Avoid prolonged standing.
- Teach to avoid dehydration and vasodilation (e.g., hot tubs).
- Teach exercises to increase strength and flexibility. Refer to interventions earlier in this section.

Risk for Aspiration

NANDA-I Definition

Vulnerable for entry of gastrointestinal secretions, oropharyngeal secretions, solids, or fluids into the tracheobronchial passages, which may compromise health

Risk Factors

Pathophysiologic

Related to reduced level of consciousness secondary to:

Presenile dementia	Alcohol- or drug-induced
Head injury	Coma
Cerebrovascular accident	Seizures
Parkinson's disease	Anesthesia

Related to depressed cough/gag reflexes

Related to increased intragastric pressure secondary to:

Lithotomy position
Ascites

Obesity
Enlarged uterus

Related to impaired swallowing or decreased laryngeal and glottic reflexes secondary to:

Achalasia
Cerebrovascular accident
Myasthenia gravis
Catatonia
Muscular dystrophy
Esophageal strictures

Debilitating conditions
Multiple sclerosis
Scleroderma
Parkinson's disease
Guillain–Barré syndrome

Related to tracheoesophageal fistula

Related to impaired protective reflexes secondary to:

Facial/oral/neck surgery or trauma*
Paraplegia or hemiplegia

Treatment Related

Related to depressed laryngeal and glottic reflexes secondary to:

Tracheostomy/endotracheal tube*   Tube feedings
Sedation

Related to impaired ability to cough secondary to:

Wired jaw*
Imposed prone position

Situational (Personal, Environmental)

Related to inability/impaired ability to elevate upper body

Related to eating when intoxicated

Maturational

Premature
Related to impaired sucking/swallowing reflexes

Neonate
Related to decreased muscle tone of inferior esophageal sphincter

Older Adult
Related to poor dentition

 Author's Note

Risk for Aspiration is a clinically useful diagnosis for people at high risk for aspiration because of reduced level of consciousness, structural deficits, mechanical devices, and neurologic and gastrointestinal disorders. People with swallowing difficulties often are at risk for aspiration; the nursing diagnosis *Impaired Swallowing* should be used to describe an individual with difficulty swallowing who is also at risk for aspiration. *Risk for Aspiration* should be used to describe people who require nursing interventions to prevent aspiration, but do not have a swallowing problem.

NOC

Aspiration Control

Goals

The individual will not experience aspiration, as evidenced by the following indicators:

- Relate measures to prevent aspiration
- Name foods or fluids that are high risk for causing aspiration

The parent will reduce opportunities for aspirations, as evidenced by the following indicators:

- Remove small objects from child's reach
- Inspect toys for removable small objects
- Discourage the child from putting objects in his or her mouth

NIC

Aspiration Precautions, Airway Management, Positioning, Airway Suctioning

Interventions

Assess Causative or Contributing Factors

- Refer to Related Factors.
- Consult with speech-language pathologists (SLPs).

Reduce the Risk of Aspiration in

Individuals with Decreased Strength, Decreased Sensorium, or Autonomic Disorders

- Maintain head-of-bed elevation at an angle of 30° to 45°, unless contraindicated.
- Use sedatives as sparingly as feasible.

Individuals With Gastrointestinal Tubes and Feedings

- Confirm that tube placement has been verified by radiography or aspiration of greenish fluid (check hospital/organizational policy for preferred method).
- Observe for a change in length of the external portion of the feeding tube, as determined by movement of the marked portion of the tube (American Association of Critical Care Nurses, 2011).

- If there is a doubt about the tube's position, request an X-ray.
- Maintain head-of-bed elevation at an angle of 30° to 45°, unless contraindicated.
- Aspirate for residual contents before each feeding for tubes positioned gastrically.
- Measure gastric residual volumes (GRVs) every 4 hours in critically ill person. Delay tube feeding if GRV is greater than 150 mL.
- Regulate gastric feedings using an intermittent schedule, allowing periods for stomach emptying between feeding intervals. Monitor for tolerance to enteral feedings by noting abdominal distention and complaints of abdominal pain, and by observing for passage of flatus and stool at 4-hour intervals (American Association of Critical Care Nurses, 2011).
- Avoid bolus feedings in those at high risk for aspiration.

For an Older Adult With Difficulties Chewing and Swallowing
- See *Impaired Swallowing*.

Initiate Health Teaching and Referrals, as Indicated

- Instruct the individual and family on causes and prevention of aspiration.
- Maintain oral hygiene to prevent pneumonia related to oral bacteria aspiration.
- Have the family demonstrate tube-feeding technique.
- Refer the family to a community nursing agency for assistance at home.
- Teach the individual about the danger of eating when under the influence of alcohol.
- Teach the Heimlich or abdominal thrust maneuver to remove aspirated foreign bodies.

Risk for Falls

NANDA-I Definition

Vulnerable for increased susceptibility to falling that may cause physical harm, which may compromise health

Risk Factors

Pathophysiologic

Related to altered cerebral function secondary to hypoxia

Related to syncope, vertigo, or dizziness

Related to impaired mobility secondary to cerebrovascular accident, arthritis, and Parkinsonism

Related to loss of limb

Related to impaired vision

Related to hearing impairment

Related to fatigue

Related to orthostatic hypotension

Treatment Related

Related to lack of awareness of environmental hazards secondary to confusion

Related to improper use of aids (e.g., crutches, canes, walkers, wheelchairs)

Related to tethering devices (e.g., IV, Foley, compression therapy, telemetry)

Related to prolonged bed rest

Related to side effects of medication(s)

Situational (Personal, Environmental)

Related to history of falls

Related to improper footwear

Related to unstable gait

Older Adult

Related to faulty judgments secondary to cognitive deficits

Related to sedentary lifestyle and loss of muscle strength

Related to fear of falling and the resulting physiologic deconditioning

Author's Note

This nursing diagnosis is very clinically useful to specify an individual at risk for falls. If the individual is at risk for various types of injuries (e.g., a cognitively impaired individual), the broader diagnosis *Risk for Injury* is more useful.

 NOC
Refer to *Risk for Injury.*

Goals

The individual will relate controlled falls or no falls, as evidenced by the following indicators:

- Relate the intent to use safety measures to prevent falls
- Demonstrate selective prevention measures

 NIC
Refer to *Risk for Injury.*

Interventions

Involve All Hospital Personnel on Every Shift in the Fall Prevention Program

- Always glance into the room of a high-risk person when passing his or her room.
- Alert other departments of high-risk individuals when off unit for tests or procedures.
- Address fall prevention and risks with every hand off and transfer.
- Seek to identify reversible risk factors in all individuals. Be aware of changing individual conditions and a change in risk status.
- Identify in a private conference room the number of falls on the unit monthly (e.g., poster).

Identify the Individual's Risk for Falls

- Identify high-risk individuals and initiate the institution's standard and protocol to prevent falls.

Reduce or Eliminate Contributing Factors for Falls

Related to Unfamiliar Environment

- Orient to his or her environment (e.g., location of bathroom, bed controls, call bell). Leave a light on in the bathroom at night. Ensure that path to bathroom is clear.
- Teach him or her to keep the bed in the low position with side rails up at night.
- Make sure that the telephone, eyeglasses, urinal, and frequently used personal belongings are within easy reach.
- Instruct to request assistance whenever needed.
- For individuals with difficulty accessing toilet:
  - If urgency exists, evaluate for a urinary tract infection.
  - Provide an opportunity to use bathroom/urinal/bedpan every 2 hours while awake, at bedtime, and upon awakening.
- Frequently scan floor for wet areas and objects on floor.
- Implement an elimination protocol (e.g., toileting rounds every hour to offer bathroom assistance).

Related to Gait Instability/Balance Problems

- Explain that gait and balance problems are due to underuse and deconditioning, *not aging*.
- Alert individuals that they may not be able to prevent a fall if they trip.
- Seek to include a vitamin D and vitamin B_{12} level in next laboratory tests. Explain that the normal range is 30 to 100 nmol/L.
- Refer to Getting Started for strategies and exercises to improve gait and balance on thePoint at http://thePoint.lww.com/Carpenito6e.
- Instruct the individual to wear slippers with nonskid soles and to avoid shoes with thick, soft soles.

Related to Tethering Devices (IVs, Foley, telemetry, compression devices)

- Evaluate if tethering devices can be discontinued at night.
- Can the IV be converted to a saline port?
- If the individual is competent, teach him or her how to safely ambulate with devices to bathroom or advise to call for assistance.

Related to Medication Side Effects

- Review the person's medication reconciliation completed on admission.
  - Question regarding alcohol use

- Review with pharmacist/physicians/NP the present medications and evaluate those that can contribute to dizziness, and if they should be discontinued, have dose reduced or replaced with an alternative (Kaufman & Kaplan, 2015; *Riefkohl, Bieber, Burlingame, & Lowenthal, 2003).
  - Antidepressants (e.g., SSRIs)
  - Antipsychotics
  - Benzodiazepines
  - Antihistamines (e.g., Benadryl, hydroxyzine)
  - Anticonvulsants
  - Nonsteroidal anti-inflammatory drugs
  - Muscle relaxants
  - Narcotic analgesics
  - Antiarrhythmics (type 1A)
  - Digoxin

If a Person Falls or Reports a Fall

- Call out for help immediately and continue to attend to the individual.
- Implement the following:
  - Do not move initially.
  - If person hit head or if it is not known, immobilize cervical spine.
  - Assess if loss of consciousness was experienced, complains of pain, or the person is confused.
  - Take baseline vital signs, blood glucose.
  - Determine baseline Glasgow Coma Scale.
  - Assess risk for intracranial bleed (anticoagulants, thrombocytopenia, coagulopathy).
  - Assess for lacerations, fractures, contusions, and decreased ROM.

SBAR

Situation: Ask individual and witnesses what happened, at what time? location? who witnessed?

Background: Prior fall risk score? History of falls?

Assessment: Evaluate the following:

Side rails up/down	Fall risk alerts present (placards, wrist band)	
Position of bed	Call light reachable	Sitter present
Nonskid footwear	Use of assistive devices	Visitors present
Presence of clutter	Bed alarm on	Presence of IV, Foley
Staffing ratios		

Recommendation: Communicate identified factors that caused or contributed to the fall.

- Clean and dress any wounds.
- Implement neuro checks q 2 hours for 24 hours.
- Contact the appropriate physician/NP to discuss findings and implications.
- Engage in a postfall huddle within 1 hour of fall. Involve all staff. Avoid all discussions of blaming. Refer institution's protocol for documentation guidelines of postfall huddles.

Risk for Poisoning

NANDA-I Definition

Vulnerable for accidental exposure to or ingestion of drugs or dangerous products in sufficient doses that may compromise health

Risk Factors

Presence of risk factors (see Risk Factors for *Risk for Injury*)

Risk for Suffocation

NANDA-I Definition

Vulnerable of accidental suffocation (inadequate air available for inhalation), which may compromise health

Risk Factors

Presence of risk factors (see Risk Factors for *Risk for Injury*)

Risk for Thermal Injury

NANDA-I Definition

Vulnerable for damage to skin and mucous membranes due to extreme temperatures, which may compromise health

Risk Factors*

Cognitive impairment (e.g., dementia, psychoses)
Developmental level (infants, aged)
Exposure to extreme temperatures
Fatigue
Inadequate supervision
Inattentiveness
Intoxication (alcohol, drug)
Lack of knowledge (individual, caregiver)
Lack of protective clothing (e.g., flame-retardant sleepwear, gloves, ear covering)
Neuromuscular impairment (e.g., stroke, amyotrophic lateral sclerosis, multiple sclerosis)
Neuropathy
Smoking
Treatment-related side effects (e.g., pharmaceutical agents)
Unsafe environment

 Author's Note

Risk for Thermal Injury is a new NANDA-I diagnosis that focuses on thermal injury only. The risk factors listed represent those related to most type of injuries. It is probably more useful to use *Risk for Injury*, to cover all the types of injury including thermal. Individuals who are at risk for thermal injury are also at risk for a multitude of injuries. *Risk for Thermal Injury* could be used in a standard of care to emphasize environmental hazards such as combustibles, fireworks, heaters, fires.

Goals

Refer to *Risk for Injury* related to lack of awareness of environmental hazards.

Interventions

Refer to *Risk for Injury* related to lack of awareness of environmental hazards.

Risk for Trauma

NANDA-I Definition

Vulnerable for accidental tissue injury (e.g., wound, burns, fracture), which may compromise health

Risk Factors

Presence of risk factors (see Risk Factors for *Risk for Injury*)

Risk for Perioperative Positioning Injury

NANDA-I Definition

Vulnerable for inadvertent anatomical and physical changes as a result of posture or equipment used during an invasive/surgical procedure, which may compromise health

Risk Factors

Presence of risk factors (see Related Factors)

Related Factors

Pathophysiologic

Related to increased vulnerability secondary to (Webster, 2012):
Preexisting generalized neuropathy. Structural anomaly/
congenital abnormality (e.g., constriction at thoracic outlet or
condylar groove, or arthritic narrowing of joint space)

Chronic disease	Osteoporosis
Cancer	Compromised immune system
Thin body frame	Renal, hepatic dysfunction
Radiation therapy	Infection

Related to compromised tissue perfusion secondary to:

Diabetes mellitus	Dehydration
Anemia	Peripheral vascular disease
Ascites	History of thrombosis
Cardiovascular disease	Edema*
Hypothermia	

Related to vulnerability of stoma during positioning

Related to preexisting contractures or physical impairments secondary to:
Rheumatoid arthritis
Polio

Treatment Related

Related to position requirements and loss of usual sensory protective responses secondary to anesthesia

Related to surgical procedures of 2 hours or longer

Related to vulnerability of implants or prostheses (e.g., pacemakers) during positioning

Situational (Personal, Environmental)

Related to compromised circulation secondary to:

Obesity*	Pregnancy	Cool operating suite
Tobacco use	Infant status	Elder status

Maturational

Related to increased vulnerability to tissue injury secondary to:

Author's Note

This diagnosis focuses on identifying the vulnerability for tissue, nerve, and joint injury resulting from required positions for surgery. The addition of *perioperative positioning* to *Risk for Injury* adds etiology to the label.

If an individual has no preexisting risk factors that make him or her more vulnerable to injury, this diagnosis could be used with no related factors because they are evident. If related factors are desired, the statement could read *Risk for Perioperative Positioning Injury related to position requirements for surgery and loss of usual sensory protective measures secondary to anesthesia*.

When an individual has preexisting risk factors, the statement should include these—for example, *Risk for Perioperative Positioning Injuries related to compromised tissue perfusion secondary to peripheral arterial disease*.

 NOC

Circulation Status, Neurologic Status, Tissue Perfusion: Peripheral

Goals

The individual will have no neuromuscular damage or injury related to the surgical position, as evidenced by the following indicators:

- Padding is used as indicated for procedure.
- Limbs are secured when at risk.
- Limbs are flexed when indicated.

 NIC

Positioning Intraoperative, Surveillance, Pressure Management

Interventions

Determine Whether the Individual Has Preexisting Risk Factors (Refer to Risk Factors); Communicate Findings to Surgical Team

Before Positioning, Assess and Document

- Range-of-motion ability
- Physical abnormalities (skin, contractions)

- External/internal prostheses or implants
- Neurovascular status
- Circulatory status

Advise If Any Preexisting Factors Exist and Determine If the Position Will Be Arranged Before or After Anesthesia

- Discuss with the surgeon the surgical position desired.
- Move the individual from the transport stretcher to the operating room (OR) bed.
  - Have a minimum of two people with their hands free (e.g., not holding an IV bag).
  - Explain the transfer to the individual. Lock all wheels on the stretcher and bed.
  - Ask the individual to move slowly to the OR bed. Assist during the move. Do not pull or drag the individual.
  - When the individual is on the OR bed, attach a safety belt a few inches above the knees with a space of three fingerbreadths.
  - Check that legs are not crossed and that feet are slightly separated and not over the edge.
  - Do not leave the individual unattended.
- Always ask the anesthesiologist or nurse anesthetist for permission before moving or repositioning an anesthetized. Move the person slowly and gently, watching all tubes, drains, lines, and others.
- Reduce vulnerability to injury (soft tissue, joint, nerves, blood vessels).
  - Align the neck and spine at all times.
  - Gently manipulate the joints. Do not abduct more than 90°.
  - Do not let limbs extend off the OR bed. Reposition slowly and gently.
  - Use a draw sheet above the elbows to tuck in arms at the side, or abduct arm on an arm board with padding.
- Protect eyes and ears from injury.
  - Use padding or a special headrest to protect ears, superficial nerves, and blood vessels of the face if the head is on its side.
  - Ensure that the ear is not bent when positioned.
  - If needed, protect eyes from abrasions with an eye patch or shield.
- Depending on the surgical position used, protect vulnerable areas; document position and protection measures used (Rothrock, 2003).

- Slowly reposition or return the individual to supine position after certain surgical positions (e.g., Trendelenburg, lithotomy, reverse Trendelenburg, jack-knife, lateral).
  - Assess skin condition when surgery is over; document findings; continue to assess and to relieve pressure to vulnerable areas postoperatively.

Risk for Urinary Tract Injury

Definition

Vulnerable to damage of the urinary tract from use of catheters, which may compromise health

Risk Factors

Condition preventing ability to secure catheter (e.g., burn, trauma, amputation)
Long-term use of urinary catheter
Multiple catheterizations
Retention balloon inflated to ≥30 mL
Use of large caliber urinary catheter

 Author's Note

This new NANDA-I nursing diagnosis represents prevention of trauma to the urethra during catheterization and/or with prolonged catheter use. Preventive strategies for reducing or eliminating urethra trauma are part of the protocols for preventing infection. The primary interventions are preventing unnecessary catheterizations, reducing the length of time, and management of the catheter to prevent trauma/infection. Thus this diagnosis is incorporated in *Risk for Infection*.

Goals

Refer to *Risk for Infection*.

Interventions

Note: These interventions are also found with *Risk for Infection*.

Insert Catheters Only for Appropriate Indications

- Presence of acute urinary retention or bladder outlet obstruction
- Need for accurate measurements of urinary output in critically ill individuals
- Perioperative use for selected surgical procedures:
  - Those undergoing urologic surgery or other surgery on contiguous structures of the genitourinary tract
  - Management of hematuria associated with clots
  - Management of patients with neurogenic bladder
  - Anticipated prolonged duration of surgery
  - Need for intraoperative monitoring of urinary output
  - Individuals anticipated to receive large-volume infusions or diuretics during surgery
  - To assist in healing of open sacral or perineal wounds in incontinent individuals
  - Intravesical pharmacologic therapy (e.g., bladder cancer)
  - Prescribed prolonged immobilization (e.g., potentially unstable thoracic or lumbar spine, multiple traumatic injuries such as pelvic fractures)
  - To improve comfort for end-of-life care, if needed
- Consider condom catheters or alternatives to indwelling catheter such as intermittent catheterization, if possible.
- Follow evidence-based procedure for catheter insertion and management.
  - Use a single-use packet of lubricant jelly on the catheter, which is important in the placement of any catheter, and one should use clinical judgment when deciding whether or not to use anesthetic lubricant or plain lubricant.
  - Use the smallest gauge catheter as possible.
  - Maintain unobstructed urine flow; keep tubing free from kinks.
  - Cleanse the patient's genital area with an aseptic cleanser prior to catheter insertion. Do not clean the periurethral area with antiseptics to prevent CAUTI (catheter-associated urinary tract infections) while the catheter is in place. Routine

hygiene (e.g., cleaning of the meatal surface during daily bathing or showering) is appropriate.
- Secure the catheter to the thigh.
- Keep the IUC drainage bag below the level of the bladder at all times.
- Empty the drainage bag every 8 hours, when the bag is two-thirds full, or prior to all patient transfers. Empty using a separate, clean collecting container for each individual.
- Consult with physician/NP/PA to discuss the inappropriate use of indwelling catheter in a particular person.
  - Convenience of nursing staff
  - Person has incontinence
  - Access for obtaining urine for culture or other diagnostic tests when the individual can voluntarily void
  - For prolonged postoperative duration without appropriate indications (e.g., structural repair of urethra or contiguous structures, prolonged effect of epidural anesthesia)
  - If the IUC has been in place for more than 2 days, provide a daily reminder to the health-care provider to evaluate continued need for the device.
  - Once an IUC is removed, if the person does not void within 4 to 6 hours, use a bedside bladder scanner to determine urine volume. In and out catheterize the patient if the volume is greater than 500 mL; avoid replacing an IUC.
  - Once an IUC is removed, offer the individual a bedside commode if he or she cannot ambulate safely to the bathroom.

DECREASED INTRACRANIAL ADAPTIVE CAPACITY

NANDA-I Definition

Intracranial fluid dynamic mechanisms that normally compensate for increases in intracranial volumes are compromised, resulting in repeated disproportionate increases in intracranial pressure (ICP) in response to a variety of noxious and nonnoxious stimuli

Defining Characteristics

Major (Must Be Present)*

Repeated increases of >10 mm Hg for more than 5 minutes following any of a variety of external stimuli

Minor (May Be Present)

Disproportionate increase in ICP following stimulus
Elevated P2 ICP waveform*
Volume–pressure response test variation (volume:pressure ratio 2, pressure–volume index ≥10 mm Hg*)
Wide-amplitude ICP waveform*

 Author's Note

This diagnosis represents increased intracranial pressure (ICP) for an individual at risk for ICP. It is a collaborative problem, because it requires two disciplines to treat—nursing and medicine. In addition, to assess for physiologic changes it requires invasive monitoring for diagnosis. The collaborative problem *Risk for Complications of Increased Intracranial Pressure* represents this clinical situation. Refer to Section 3, Collaborative Problems, for interventions.

NEONATAL JAUNDICE

Neonatal Jaundice

Risk for Neonatal Jaundice

See also *Risk for Complications of Hyperbilirubinemia* in Section 3, Collaborative Problems.

NANDA-I Definition

The yellow-orange tint of the neonate's skin and mucous membranes that occurs after 24 hours of life as a result of unconjugated bilirubin in the circulation

Defining Characteristics*

Abnormal blood profile (hemolysis; total serum bilirubin greater than 2 mg/dL; inherited disorder; total serum bilirubin in high-risk range on age in hour-specific nomogram)
Abnormal skin bruising
Yellow-orange skin
Yellow sclera

Related Factors*

Abnormal weight loss (7% to 8% in breastfeeding newborn; 15% in term infant)
Feeding pattern not well established
Infant experiences difficulty making transition to extrauterine life
Neonate age 1 to 7 days
Stool (meconium) passage delayed

  Author's Note

This NANDA-I diagnosis is a collaborative problem that requires a laboratory test for diagnosis and treatment from medicine and nursing. Refer to *Risk for Complications of Hyperbilirubinemia* in Section 3, Collaborative Problems for neonates at risk for experiencing hyperbilirubinemia.

Risk for Neonatal Jaundice

NANDA-I Definition

Vulnerable for yellow-orange tint of the neonate's skin and mucous membranes that occurs after 24 hours of life as a result of unconjugated bilirubin in the circulation, which may compromise health

Risk Factors*

Abnormal weight loss (7% to 8% in breastfeeding newborn, 15% in term infant)
Feeding pattern not well established
Infant experiences difficulty making the transition to extrauterine life
Neonate aged 1 to 7 days
Prematurity
Stool (meconium) passage delayed

 Author's Note

Refer to Author's Notes under *Neonatal Jaundice*.

DEFICIENT KNOWLEDGE

NANDA-I Definition

Absence or deficiency of cognitive information related to a specific topic

Defining Characteristics

Exaggerated behaviors*
Inappropriate behaviors (e.g., hysterical, hostile, agitated, apathetic)*
Verbalization of a problem
Inaccurate follow-through of instruction*
Inaccurate performance of test*

Related Factors*

Cognitive limitation
Lack of exposure
Information misinterpretation
Lack of interest in learning
Lack of recall
Unfamiliarity with information resources

Author's Note

Deficient Knowledge does not represent a human response, alteration, or pattern of dysfunction; rather, it is an etiologic or contributing factor (Jenny, 1987). Lack of knowledge can contribute to a variety of responses (e.g., anxiety, self-care deficits). All nursing diagnoses have related client/ family teaching as a part of nursing interventions (e.g., *Impaired Bowel Elimination*, *Impaired Verbal Communication*). When the teaching relates directly to a specific nursing diagnosis, incorporate the teaching into the plan. When specific teaching is indicated before a procedure, the diagnosis *Anxiety related to unfamiliar environment or procedure* can be used. When information is given to assist a person or family with self-care at home, the diagnosis *Ineffective Health Management* may be indicated. The new nursing diagnosis added by this author in this edition *Compromised Engagement* and *Risk for Compromised Engagement* focus specifically on strategies to increase motivation and reduce barriers to participation in improving health outcomes.

LATEX ALLERGY RESPONSE

Latex Allergy Response

Risk for Latex Allergy Response

NANDA-I Definition

A hypersensitive reaction to natural latex rubber products

Defining Characteristics

Positive skin or serum test to natural rubber latex (NRL) extract.

After exposure to latex protein:

- Contact dermatitis progressing to generalized symptoms
- Flushing
- Redness
- Eczema
- Wheezing
- Itching
- Edema (e.g., facial, eyelids, tongue)
- Allergic conjunctivitis
- Asthma
- Rhinitis
- Urticaria

Related Factors

Biopathophysiologic

Related to hypersensitivity response to the protein component of NRL

Immune Hypersensitivity Control

Goals

The individual will report no exposure to latex, as evidenced by the following indicators:

- Describe products of NRL
- Describe strategies to avoid exposure

Allergy Management, Latex Precautions, Environmental Risk Protection

Interventions

Assess for Causative and Contributing Factors

Eliminate Exposure to Latex Products

Use Nonlatex Alternative Supplies
- Clear disposable amber bags
- Silicone baby nipples
- 2 × 2 gauze pads with silk tape in place of adhesive bandages
- Clear plastic or Silastic catheters
- Vinyl or neoprene gloves
- Kling-like gauze

For Health-Care Workers and Others Who Regularly Wear Gloves (CDC, 2015)

- Avoid hypoallergenic latex gloves.

Protect From Exposure to Latex
- Cover the skin with cloth before applying the blood pressure cuff.
- Do not allow rubber stethoscope tubing to touch the individual.
- Do not inject through rubber parts (e.g., heparin locks); use syringe and stopcock.

- Change needles after each puncture of rubber stopper.
- Cover rubber parts with tape.

Teach Which Products Are Commonly Made of Latex

Health-Care Equipment
- Natural latex rubber gloves, powdered or unpowdered, including those labeled *hypoallergenic*
- Blood pressure cuffs
- Stethoscopes
- Tourniquets
- Electrode pads
- Airways, endotracheal tubes
- Syringe plunges, bulb syringes
- Masks for anesthesia
- Rubber aprons
- Catheters, wound drains
- Injection ports
- Tops of multidose vials
- Adhesive tape
- Ostomy pouches
- Wheelchair cushions
- Briefs with elastic
- Pads for crutches
- Some prefilled syringes

Office/Household Products
- Erasers
- Rubber bands
- Dishwashing gloves
- Balloons
- Condoms, diaphragms
- Baby bottle nipples, pacifiers
- Rubber balls and toys
- Racquet handles
- Cycle grips
- Tires
- Hot water bottles
- Carpeting
- Shoe soles
- Elastic in underwear
- Rubber cement

Initiate Health Teaching as Indicated

- Explain the importance of completely avoiding direct contact with all NRL products.

- Advise that an individual with a history of a mild skin reaction to latex is at risk for anaphylaxis.
- Instruct the individual to wear a Medic-Alert bracelet stating "Latex Allergy" and to carry auto-injectable epinephrine.
- Instruct the individual to warn all health-care providers (e.g., dental, medical, surgical) of the allergy.
- Refer interested individuals to the CDC publication, "Latex Allergy: A Prevention Guide" at the Centers for Disease Control and Prevention website.
- For a comprehensive list of products containing latex, refer to the website for the American Latex Allergy Association.

Risk for Latex Allergy Response

NANDA-I Definition

Vulnerable to hypersensitivity to natural latex rubber products which may compromise health

Risk Factors

Biopathophysiologic

Related to history of atopic eczema, dermatitis

Related to history of allergic rhinitis

Related to history of asthma*

Treatment Related

Related to multiple surgical procedures, especially beginning in infancy*

Related to frequent urinary catheterizations (e.g., individuals with spina bifida, spinal cord injury, neurogenic bladder)

Related to frequent rectal impaction removal

Related to frequent surgical procedures

Related to barium enema (before 1992)

Situational (Personal, Environmental)

Related to history of allergies*

Related to a history of anaphylaxis of uncertain etiology, especially during past surgeries, hospitalization, or dental visits (American Association of Nurse Anaesthetists, 2014):

History of food allergy to banana, kiwi, avocado, chestnuts, tropical fruits (mango, papaya, passion fruit), poinsettia plants*, tomato, raw potato, peach

History of allergy to gloves, condoms, and so forth

History of greater exposure to latex-containing products due to obstetric procedures, gynecological examinations, and contact with contraceptives (American Association of Nurse Anaesthetists, 2014).

Frequent occupational exposure to NRL*, such as:

Workers making NRL products

Food handlers

Greenhouse workers

Health-care workers

Housekeepers

Hairdressers (American Association of Nurse Anaesthetist, 2014)

 Author's Note

Frequent exposure to airborne latex has contributed to latex allergies. All individuals who do not have latex allergies should use nonpowdered latex gloves (DeJong, Patiwael, de Groot, Burdorf, & Gerth van Wijk, 2011).

 NOC

Immune Hypersensitivity Control

Goals

Refer to *Latex Allergy Response.*

NIC

Allergy Management, Latex Precautions, Environmental Risk Protection

Interventions

Refer to *Latex Allergy Response.*

SEDENTARY LIFESTYLE

NANDA-I Definition

Reports a habit of life that is characterized by a low physical activity level

Defining Characteristics*

Chooses a daily routine lacking physical exercise
Demonstrates physical deconditioning
Verbalizes preference for activities low in physical activity

Related Factors*

Pathophysiologic

Related to decreased endurance secondary to obesity[19]

Situational (Personal, Environment)

Related to inadequate knowledge of health benefits of physical activity

Related to inadequate knowledge of exercise routines[19]

Related to insufficient resources (money, facilities)

Related to perceived lack of time

Related to lack of motivation

Related to lack of interest

Related to lack of training for accomplishment of physical exercise

 Author's Note

This is the first nursing diagnosis submitted by a nurse from another country and accepted by NANDA. Congratulations to J. Adolf Guirao-Goris of Valencia, Spain.

 NOC

Knowledge: Health Behaviors, Physical Fitness

---

[19]Added by author for clarity.

Goals

The individual will verbalize intent to or engage in increased physical activity, as evidenced by the following indicators:

- Set a goal for weekly exercise
- Identify a desired activity or exercise

Exercise Promotion, Exercise Therapy

Interventions

Discuss Benefits of Exercise

- Reduces caloric absorption
- Improves body posture
- Increases metabolic rate
- Preserves lean muscle mass
- Suppresses appetite
- Improves self-esteem
- Reduces depression, anxiety, and stress
- Provides fun, recreation, diversion
- Increases oxygen uptake
- Increases caloric expenditure
- Maintains weight loss
- Increases restful sleep
- Increases resistance to age-related degeneration

Assist Individual to Identify Realistic Exercise Program; Consider:

- Physical limitations (consult nurse or physician)
- Personal preferences
- Lifestyle
- Community resources (e.g., safe places to exercise)
- Individuals must learn to monitor pulse before, during, and after exercise to assist them to achieve target heart rate and not to exceed maximum advisable heart rate for age.

Age (Years)	Maximum Heart Rate (beats/min)	Target Heart Rate (beats/min)
30	190	133 to 162
40	180	126 to 153
50	170	119 to 145
60	160	112 to 136

- A regular exercise program should:
  - Be enjoyable
  - Use a minimum of 400 calories in each session
  - Sustain a heat rate of approximately 120 to 150 beats/min
  - Involve rhythmic, alternating contracting and relaxing of muscles
  - Be integrated into the individual's lifestyle of 4 to 5 days/week for at least 30 to 60 minutes

Discuss Aspects of Starting the Exercise Program

- Start slow and easy; obtain clearance from physician.
- Read, consult experts, and talk with friends/coworkers who exercise.
- Plan a daily walking program:
  - Start at 5 to 10 blocks for 0.5 to 1 mile/day; increase 1 block or 0.1 mile/week.
  - Gradually increase rate and length of walk; remember to progress slowly.
  - Avoid straining or pushing too hard and becoming overly fatigued.
  - Stop immediately if any of the following occur:
    - Lightness or chest pain
    - Dizziness, light-headedness
    - Severe breathlessness
    - Loss of muscle control
    - Nausea
- If pulse is 120 beats/min at 4 minutes or 100 beats/min at 10 minutes after stopping exercise, or if shortness of breath occurs 10 minutes after exercise, slow down either the rate or the distance of walking for 1 week to point before signs appeared and then start to add 1 block/0.1 mile each week.
- Walk at same rate; time with stopwatch or second hand on watch; after reaching 10 blocks (1 mile), try to increase speed.
- Remember, increase only the rate or the distance of walking at one time.
- Establish a regular time for exercise, with the goal of three to five times/week for 15 to 45 minutes and a heart rate of 80% of stress test or gross calculation (170 beats/min for 20 to 29 years of age.) Decrease 10 beats/min for each additional decade (e.g., 160 beats/min for 30 to 39 years of age, 150 beats/min for 40 to 49 years of age).
- Encourage significant others to engage in walking program.
- Add supplemental activity (e.g., parking far from destination, gardening, using stairs, spending weekends at activities that require walking).

- Work up to 1 hour of exercise per day at least 4 days/week.
- Avoid lapses of more than 2 days between exercise sessions.

Assist Individual to Increase Interest and Motivation

- Develop a contract listing realistic short- and long-term goals.
- Keep intake/activity records.
- Increase knowledge by reading and talking with health-conscious friends and coworkers.
- Make new friends who are health conscious.
- Get a friend to follow the program or be a source of support.
- Be aware of rationalization (e.g., a lack of time may be a lack of prioritization).
- Keep a list of positive outcomes.

RISK FOR IMPAIRED LIVER FUNCTION

See also *Risk for Complications of Hepatic Dysfunction* in Section 3, Collaborative Problems.

NANDA-I Definition

Vulnerable for a decrease in liver function that may compromise health

Risk Factors*

Hepatotoxic medications (e.g., acetaminophen, statins)
HIV coinfection
Substance abuse (e.g., alcohol, cocaine)
Viral infection (e.g., hepatitis A, hepatitis B, hepatitis C, Epstein–Barr virus)

 Author's Note

This diagnosis represents a situation that requires collaborative intervention with medicine. This author recommends the collaborative problem *Risk for Complications of Hepatic Dysfunction* be used instead. Refer to

http://thePoint.lww.com/CarpenitoHB14e for interventions. Students should consult with their faculty for advice on the use of *Risk for Impaired Liver Function* or *Risk for Complications of Hepatic Dysfunction*.

RISK FOR DISTURBED MATERNAL/ FETAL DYAD

NANDA-I Definition

At risk for disruption of the symbiotic maternal/fetal dyad as a result of comorbid or pregnancy-related conditions

Risk Factors*

Complications of pregnancy (e.g., premature rupture of membranes, placenta previa or abruption, late prenatal care, multiple gestation)
Compromised oxygen transport (e.g., anemia, cardiac disease, asthma, hypertension, seizures, premature labor, hemorrhage)
Impaired glucose metabolism (e.g., diabetes, steroid use)
Physical abuse
Substance abuse (e.g., tobacco, alcohol, drugs)
Treatment-related side effects (e.g., medications, surgery, chemo-therapy)

 Author's Note

This NANDA-I nursing diagnosis represents numerous situations or fac-tors that can compromise a pregnant woman, her fetus, or both. The primary responsibility of nursing is to monitor the status of the mother, fe-tus, and pregnancy and to collaborate with medicine for monitoring (e.g., electronic fetal monitoring, Doppler, laboratory tests) and treatments.

Refer to Section 3 under *Obstetrics/Gynecologic Conditions* for inter-ventions for this generic collaborative problem or for more specific col-laborative problems such as

* *Risk for Complications of Preterm Labor*
* *Risk for Complications of Nonreassuring Fetal Status*
* *Risk for Complications of Prenatal Bleeding*
* *Risk for Pregnancy-Associated Hypertension*
* *Risk for Complications of Postpartum Hemorrhage*

For example, if a pregnant woman is using cocaine, the collaborative problem *Risk for Complications of* Cocaine Abuse would be valid because cocaine contributes to preterm labor and fetal complications. In another situation such as placenta

IMPAIRED MEMORY

NANDA-I Definition

Inability to remember or recall bits of information or behavioral skills

Defining Characteristics*

Major (Must Be Present, One or More)

Reports experiences of forgetting
Inability to recall if a behavior was performed
Inability to learn or retain new skills or information
Inability to perform a previously learned skill
Inability to recall factual information
Inability to recall events

Related Factors

Pathophysiologic

Related to neurologic disturbances secondary to:*
Degenerative brain disease   Head injury
Lesion   Cerebrovascular accident

Related to reduced quantity and quality of information processed secondary to:
Visual deficits   Learning habits
Hearing deficits   Intellectual skills
Poor physical fitness   Educational level
Fatigue

Related to nutritional deficiencies (e.g., vitamins C and B$_{12}$, folate, niacin, thiamine)

Treatment Related

Related to effects of medication (specify) on memory storage

Situational (Personal, Environmental)

Related to self-fulfilling expectations

Related to excessive self-focus and worry secondary to:

Grieving	Depression
Anxiety	

Related to alcohol consumption

Related to lack of motivation

Related to lack of stimulation

Related to difficulty concentrating secondary to:

Stress	Lack of intellectual stimulation
Pain	Sleep disturbances
Distractions	

 Author's Note

This diagnosis is useful when the individual can be helped to function better because of improved memory. If the individual's memory cannot be improved because of cerebral degeneration, this diagnosis is not appropriate. Instead, the nurse should evaluate the effects of impaired memory on functioning, such as *Self-Care Deficits* or *Risk for Injury*. The focus of interventions for these nursing diagnoses would be improving self-care or protection, not improving memory.

 NOC

Cognitive Orientation, Memory

Goals

The individual will report increased satisfaction with memory, as evidenced by the following indicators:

- Identify three techniques to improve memory
- Relate factors that deter memory

NIC

Reality Orientation, Memory Training, Environmental Management

Interventions

Discuss the Individual's Beliefs About Memory Deficits

- Correct misinformation.
- Explain that negative expectations can result in memory deficits.

Assess for Factors That May Negatively Affect Memory (e.g., Pathophysiologic, Literacy, Stressors)

If the Individual Has Difficulty Concentrating, Explain the Favorable Effects of Relaxation and Imagery

Teach the Individual Two or Three of the Following Methods to Improve Memory Skills (Maier-Lorentz, 2000; Miller, 2015)

- Write things down (e.g., use lists, calendars, notebooks).
- Use auditory cues (e.g., timers, alarm clocks) in conjunction with written cues.
- Use environmental cues (e.g., you might remove something from its usual place, then return it to its normal location after it has served its purpose as a reminder).
- Have specific places for specific items; keep items in their proper place (e.g., keep keys on a hook near the door).
- Rehearse items you want to remember by repeating them aloud or writing them on paper.
- Use self-instruction—say things aloud (e.g., "I'm putting my keys on the counter so I remember to turn off the stove before I leave").
- Use first-letter cues and make associations (e.g., to remember to buy carrots, apples, radishes, pickles, eggs, and tea bags, remember the word *carpet*).
- Search the alphabet while focusing on what you are trying to remember (e.g., to remember that someone's name is Martin, start with names that begin with "A" and continue naming names through the alphabet until your memory is jogged for the correct one).

When Trying to Learn or Remember Something

- Minimize distractions.
- Do not rush.
- Maintain some form of organization of routine tasks.
- Carry a note pad or calendar or use written cues.

IMPAIRED PHYSICAL MOBILITY

Impaired Physical Mobility

Impaired Bed Mobility

Impaired Sitting

Impaired Standing

Impaired Walking

Impaired Wheelchair Mobility

Impaired Transfer Ability

NANDA-I Definition

Limitation in independent, purposeful physical movement of the body or of one or more extremities

Defining Characteristics
(Levin, Krainovitch, Bahrenburg, & Mitchell, 1989)

Compromised ability to move purposefully within the environment (e.g., bed mobility, transfers, ambulation)
Range-of-motion (ROM) limitations

Related Factors

Pathophysiologic

Related to decreased muscle strength* and endurance* secondary to:

Neuromuscular impairment
Autoimmune alterations (e.g., multiple sclerosis, arthritis)
Nervous system diseases (e.g., Parkinson's disease, myasthenia gravis)
Respiratory conditions (e.g., chronic obstructive pulmonary disease [COPD])
Increased intracranial pressure
Sensory deficits
Musculoskeletal impairment
Fractures
Connective tissue disease (systemic lupus erythematosus)

Muscular dystrophy
Partial paralysis (spinal cord injury, stroke)
Central nervous system (CNS) tumor
Trauma
Cancer

Cardiac conditions
Increased intracranial pressure
Sensory deficits
Musculoskeletal impairment

Related to joint stiffness* or contraction* secondary to:
Inflammatory joint disease
Post–joint-replacement or spinal surgery

Degenerative joint disease
Degenerative disc disease

Related to edema

Treatment Related

Related to equipment (e.g., ventilators, enteral therapy, dialysis, total parenteral nutrition)

Related to external devices (casts or splints, braces)

Related to insufficient strength and endurance for ambulation with (specify):
Prosthesis
Crutches

Walker

Situational (Personal, Environmental)

Related to:
Fatigue
Depressive mood state*
Decreased motivation
Pain*

Deconditioning*
Obesity
Dyspnea
Cognitive impairment*

Maturational

Children

Related to abnormal gait secondary to:
Congenital skeletal deficiencies
Congenital hip dysplasia

Legg–Calvé–Perthes disease
Osteomyelitis

Older Adult

Related to decreased motor agility

Related to decreased muscle mass and strength*

Author's Note

Impaired Physical Mobility describes an individual with deconditioning from immobility resulting from a medical or surgical condition. The literature is full of the effects of immobility on body system function. Early progressive mobility programs or progressive mobility activity protocol (PMAP) are designed to prevent these complications, These programs are appropriate for individuals in intensive care units, other hospital units, and skill nursing care facilities.

These programs necessitate continuous nursing attention. Several potential barriers for maintaining PMAP have been identified as lack of mobility education, safety concerns, and lack of interdisciplinary collaboration (King, 2012). Gillis, MacDonald, and MacIssac. (2008) reported that time constraints due to increased acuity and staffing issues have lowered the priority and time available for basic mobility.

Acuity levels on units must address the workload associated of PMAP and factor this into staffing. Several studies have shown the cost effectiveness of PMAP with decreased ICU stays, decreased ventilator use, and decreased hospital stays. In addition, complications of immobility, for example, decreased episodes of deep vein thrombosis, ventilator-associated pneumonia, and delirium.

Nursing interventions for *Impaired Physical Mobility* focus on early mobilization, muscle strengthening and restoring function, and preventing deterioration. *Impaired Physical Mobility* can also be utilized to describe someone with limited use of arm(s) or leg(s) or limited muscle strength.

Impaired Physical Mobility is one of the clusters of diagnoses in *Risk for Disuse Syndrome*. Limitation of physical movement of arms/legs also can be the etiology of other nursing diagnoses, such as *Self-Care Deficit* and *Risk for Injury*. If the individual can exercise but does not, refer to *Sedentary Lifestyle*. If the individual has no limitations in movement but is deconditioned and has reduced endurance, refer to *Activity Intolerance*.

NOC

Ambulation, Joint Movement, Mobility, Fall Prevention Behavior

Goals

The individual will report increased strength and endurance of limbs, as evidenced by the following indicators:

- Demonstrate the use of adaptive devices to increase mobility
- Use safety measures to minimize potential for injury
- Demonstrate measures to increase mobility
- Evaluate pain and quality of management

NIC

Progressive Mobility Protocol[20]: Joint Mobility: Strength Training, Exercise Therapy: Positioning, Teaching: Prescribed Activity/Exercise, Fall Prevention

---

[20]Added by Lynda Juall Carpenito.

Interventions

**Assess for Barriers to Early Mobilization in the Health-Care Setting.
Refer to Box I.1**

> ### BOX I.1   BARRIERS AND FACILITATORS OF PROGRESSIVE MOBILITY ACTIVITY (Winkelman & Pereeboom, 2010)
>
> #### FACILITATORS
> - The presence of a protocol in the institution, which guided decisions about readiness for increased activity
> - Glasgow Coma Score greater than 10
> - Beds that provided a chair position
> - Prescriber's order
> - Expert mentor (nurse, physical therapist)
>
> #### BARRIERS
> - Absence of the above facilitators
> - Nurse's perception of the individual's nonreadiness for increased activity
> - Physical therapist not consulted

Consult With Physical Therapist for Evaluation and Development of a Mobility Plan

Promote Optimal Mobility and Movement in all Health-Care Settings With Stable Individuals Regardless of Ability to Walk

Initiate an In-Bed Mobility Program Within Hours of Admission If Stable (Vollman, 2012)

- Maintain HOB 30°, including individual on ventilators unless contraindicated.
- Initiate a turning schedule within hours of admission, if stable.
- Assess tolerance to position change 5 to 10 minutes after apposition change.
- Initially turn slowly to right side.

Initiate a Progressive Mobility Activity Protocol (PMAP) for Individuals in All Settings as Medical Stability Increases (e.g., Step-Down Unit, Medical and Surgical Units, Skilled Nursing Facilities)

Explain to Individual and Family Why the Staff Are Frequently Moving the Individual

Initiate Early Progressive Mobility Protocol. Consult With Physical Therapy and Prescribing Provider (American Association of Critical Care Nurses [AACN], 2012; American Hospital Association, 2014; Timmerman, 2007; Zomorodi, Topley, & McAnaw, 2012)

Step 1: Safety Screening (American Association of Critical Care Nurses [AACN], 2012)
- M—Myocardial stability
  - No evidence of active myocardial ischemia for 24 hours.
  - No dysrhythmia requiring new antidysrhythmic agent for 24 hours.
- O—Oxygenation adequate on:
  - $FiO_2 < 0.6$
  - $PEEP < 10$ cmH$_2$O
- V—Vasopressor(s) minimal
  - No increase of any vasopressor for 2 hours.
- E—Engages to voice
  - Individuals respond to verbal stimulation.
- Reevaluate in 24 hours.

Prior to Initiating Step 2, Level I
- Evaluate need for analgesics versus risk of increased sedation prior to activity.
- Progress each step to 30 to 60 minutes duration as per individual's tolerance.
- Repeat each step until individual demonstrates hemodynamic and physical tolerance to the activity/position for 60 minutes, then advance to next step at the next activity period.

Step 2: Progressive Mobility
- Level 1
  - Elevate head of bed (HOB) ≥30° TID; progress to 45° plus legs in dependent position (partial chair position).
  - Assess range of motion (ROM) TID.
  - Turn q 2 hours.
  - Passive ROM TID with RN, PCT, PT, OT, or family
  - Turn q 2 hours.
  - Active resistance PT
  - Sitting on edge of bed
  - Sitting position full chair position 20 minutes TID
- Level 2
  - Passive ROM TID
  - Turn q 2 hours.
  - Active resistance PT
  - Sitting position 20 minutes TID
  - Sitting on edge of bed
  - Active transfer to chair 20 min/day

- Level 3
  - Self or assisted turning q 2 hours
  - Passive ROM TID
  - Turn q 2 hours with RN, PCT, PT, OT, or family.
  - Active resistance with PT
  - Elevate HOB to 65° plus legs in full dependent position (full chair position).
  - Consider lower HOB angle if individual's abdomen is large.
  - Sitting position 20 minutes TID
  - Sitting on edge of bed every 2 hours
  - Active transfer to chair 20 to 60 min/day
  - Ambulation (marching in place, walking in halls) (Patient must meet all criteria.)
- Level 4
  - Passive ROM TID
  - Turn q 2 hours.
  - Active resistance PT
  - Sitting position 20 minutes TID
  - Sitting on edge of bed/stand at bedside with RN, PT, OT.
  - Active transfer to chair 20 to 60 min/day (meal time) thrice a day
  - Ambulation (marching in place, walking in halls)
  - Encourage AAROM/AROM thrice a day with RN, PCT, PT, OT, or family.

Assess for Clinical Signs and Symptoms Indicating Terminating a Mobilization Session (Adler & Malone, 2012)

Heart Rate
- >70% age-predicted maximum heart rate
- >20% decrease in resting heart rate
- <40 beats/min; >130 beats/min
- New onset dysrhythmia
- New anti-arrhythmia medication
- New myocardial infarction by ECG or cardiac enzymes

Pulse Oximetry/Saturation of Peripheral Oxygen (SpO_2)
- >4% decrease
- <88% to 90%

Blood Pressure
- Systolic BP > 180 mm Hg
- >20% decrease in systolic/diastolic BP; orthostatic hypotension
- Mean arterial blood pressure <65 mm Hg; >110 mm Hg
- Presence of vasopressor medication; new vasopressor or escalating dose of vasopressor medication

Alertness/Agitation and Patient symptoms
- Patient sedation or coma—Richmond Agitation Sedation Scale, ≤ −3

- Patient agitation requiring addition or escalation of sedative medication—Richmond Agitation Sedation Scale, >2
- Complaints of intolerable dyspnea on exertion

Promote Motivation and Adherence (*Addams & Clough, 1998; Halstead & Stoten, 2010)

- Explain the effects of immobility.
- Explain the purpose of progressive mobility, passive and active ROM exercises.
- Establish short-term goals.
- Ensure that initial exercises are easy and require minimal strength and coordination.
- Progress only if the individual is successful at the present exercise.
- Provide written instructions for prescribed exercises after demonstrating and observing return demonstration.
- Document and discuss improvement specifically (e.g., can lift leg 2 in higher).
- Evaluate the level of motivation and depression. Refer to a specialist as needed.

Increase Limb Mobility and Determine Type of ROM Appropriate for the Individual (Passive, Active Assistive, Active, Active Resistive)

- For passive ROM:
  - Begin exercises slowly, doing only a few movements at first.
  - Support the limb below the joint with one hand.
  - Move joint slowly and smoothly until you feel the stretch.
  - Move the joint to the point of resistance. Stop if the person complaints of discomfort or you observe a facial grimace.
  - Do the exercise 10 times and hold the position for a few seconds.
  - Do all exercises on one side and then repeat them on the opposite side, if indicated.
  - If possible, teach the person or caregiver how to do the passive ROM.
  - Refer to ROM exercises with photos for specific instructions and photos of passive ROM.
- Perform active assistive ROM exercises (frequency determined by individual's condition):
  - If possible, teach the individual/family to perform active ROM exercises on unaffected limbs at least four times a day.
  - Perform ROM on affected limbs. Do the exercises slowly to allow the muscles to relax, and support the extremity above and below the joint to prevent strain on joints and tissues.

- For range of motion exercises (ROM) the rest can stay as ROM, the supine position is most effective. The individual/family member who performs ROM himself or herself can use a supine or sitting position.
- Do ROM daily with bed bath and three daily, if there are specific problem areas. Try to incorporate into activities of daily living.
- Support extremity with pillows to prevent or reduce swelling.
- Medicate for pain as needed, especially before activity.
- Apply heat or cold to reduce pain, inflammation, and hematoma per instructions.
- Encourage the individual to perform exercise regimens for specific joints as prescribed by physical therapist (e.g., isometric, resistive).

Position in Alignment to Prevent Complications

- Use a footboard.
- Avoid prolonged sitting or lying in the same position.
- Change the position of the shoulder joints every 2 to 4 hours.
- Use a small pillow or no pillow when in Fowler's position.
- Support the hand and wrist in natural alignment.
- If supine or prone, place a rolled towel or small pillow under the lumbar curvature or under the end of the rib cage.
- Place a trochanter roll alongside the hips and upper thighs.
- If in the lateral position, place pillow(s) to support the leg from groin to foot, and use a pillow to flex the shoulder and elbow slightly. If needed, support the lower foot in dorsal flexion with a towel roll or special boot.
- For upper extremities:
  - Arms abducted from the body with pillows
  - Elbows in slight flexion
  - Wrist in a neutral position, with fingers slightly flexed and thumb abducted and slightly flexed
  - Position of shoulder joints changed during the day (e.g., adduction, abduction, range of circular motion)

Impaired Bed Mobility

NANDA-I Definition

Limitation of independent movement from one bed position to another

Defining Characteristics*

Impaired ability to turn from side to side
Impaired ability to move from supine to sitting to supine
Impaired ability to reposition self in bed
Impaired ability to move from supine to prone or prone to
    supine
Impaired ability to move from supine to long sitting or long sit-
    ting to supine

Related Factors

Refer to *Impaired Physical Mobility*.

 Author's Note

Impaired Bed Mobility may be a clinically useful diagnosis when an individual is a candidate for rehabilitation to improve strength, ROM, and
movement. The nurse can consult with a physical therapist for a specific
plan. This diagnosis is inappropriate for an unconscious or terminally ill
individual.

NOC
Ambulation Joint Movement, Mobility, Fall Prevention Behavior

Goals

Refer to *Impaired Physical Mobility*.

NIC
Exercise Therapy: Joint Mobility, Exercise Promotion: Strength Training, Exercise
Therapy: Ambulation, Positioning, Teaching: Prescribed Activity/Exercise, Prosthesis
Care

Interventions

Refer to *Impaired Physical Mobility*.

Impaired Sitting

Definition

Limitation of ability to independently and purposefully attain and/or maintain a rest position that is supported by the buttocks and thighs, in which the torso is upright

Defining Characteristics

Impaired ability to adjust position of one or both lower limbs on uneven surface
Impaired ability to attain a balanced position of the torso
Impaired ability to flex or move both hips
Impaired ability to flex or move both knees
Impaired ability to maintain the torso in balanced position
Impaired ability to stress torso with body weight
Insufficient muscle strength

Related Factors

Alteration in cognitive functioning
Impaired metabolic functioning
Insufficient endurance
Insufficient energy
Malnutrition
Neurologic disorder

Orthopedic surgery
Pain
Prescribed posture
Psychological disorder
Sarcopenia
Self-imposed relief posture

 Author's Note

Impaired Sitting (a newly accepted NANDA-I nursing diagnosis) can be a clinically useful diagnosis when an individual is a candidate for rehabilitation to improve strength, ROM, and balance. *Impaired Physical Mobility* addresses impaired sitting. This more specific diagnosis may be clinically useful with rehabilitative specialists as nurses and physical therapists. More specialized interventions are beyond the scope of this book. The nurse can consult with a physical therapist for a specific plan.

Key Concepts

Refer to *Impaired Physical Mobility*.

Focus Assessment Criteria

Refer to *Impaired Physical Mobility*.

Impaired Standing

Definition

Limitation of ability to independently and purposefully attain and/or maintain the body in an upright position from feet to head

Defining Characteristics

Impaired ability to adjust position of one or both lower limbs on uneven surface
Impaired ability to attain a balanced position of the torso
Impaired ability to extend one or both hips
Impaired ability to extend one or both knees
Impaired ability to flex one or both hips
Impaired ability to flex one or both knees
Impaired ability to maintain the torso in balanced position
Impaired ability to stress torso with body weight
Insufficient muscle strength

Related Factors

Circulatory perfusion disorder
Emotional disturbance
Impaired metabolic functioning
Injury to lower extremity
Insufficient endurance

Neurologic disorder
Obesity
Pain
Prescribed posture
Sarcopenia

Insufficient energy
Malnutrition

Self-imposed relief posture
Surgical procedure

 Author's Note

Impaired Standing (a newly accepted NANDA-I nursing diagnosis) can be a clinically useful diagnosis when an individual is a candidate for rehabilitation to improve strength, ROM, and balance. *Impaired Physical Mobility* addresses impaired standing. This more specific diagnosis may be clinically useful with rehabilitative specialists as nurses and physical therapists. More specialized interventions are beyond the scope of this book. The nurse can consult with a physical therapist for a specific plan.

Impaired Walking

NANDA-I Definition

Limitation of independent movement within the environment on foot

Defining Characteristics*

Impaired ability to climb stairs
Impaired ability to walk required distances
Impaired ability to walk on an incline
Impaired ability to walk on uneven surfaces
Impaired ability to navigate curbs

Related Factors

Refer to *Impaired Physical Mobility*.

Refer to *Impaired Physical Mobility*.

Goals

The individual will increase walking distances (specify distance goal), as evidenced by the following indicators:

- Demonstrate safe mobility
- Use mobility aids correctly

Refer to *Impaired Physical Mobility*.

Interventions

Explain That Safe Ambulation Is a Complex Movement Involving the Musculoskeletal, Neurologic, and Cardiovascular Systems and Cognitive Factors Such as Mentation and Orientation

Consult With a Physical Therapist for Evaluation and Planning Prior to Initiation

- To use ambulatory aids (e.g., cane, walker, crutches) correctly and safely), ascertain that individual
  - Wears well-fitting shoes
  - Can ambulate on inclines, uneven surfaces, and up and down stairs
  - Is aware of hazards (e.g., wet floors, throw rugs)

Initiate a Progressive Mobility Activity Protocol

- Refer to *Impaired Physical Mobility*.

Impaired Wheelchair Mobility

NANDA-I Definition

Limitation of independent operation of wheelchair within environment

Defining Characteristics*

Impaired ability to operate manual or power wheelchair on an even or uneven surface

Impaired ability to operate manual or power wheelchair on an incline

Impaired ability to operate manual or power wheelchair on a decline

Impaired ability to operate the wheelchair on curbs

Related Factors

Refer to *Impaired Physical Mobility*.

Ambulation: Wheelchair, Fall Prevention Behavior

Goals

The individual will report satisfactory, safe wheelchair mobility, as evidenced by the following indicators:

- Demonstrate safe use of the wheelchair
- Demonstrate safe transfer to/from the wheelchair
- Demonstrate pressure relief and safety principles

NIC

Exercise Therapy: Ambulation, Exercise Therapy: Balance, Exercise Promotion: Joint Mobility, Exercise Promotion: Strength Training, Muscle Control, Positioning: Wheelchair, Fall Prevention

Interventions

Consult With Physical Therapy for a Collaborative Plan

Monitor Pressure Points of Elbow, Sacrum, Coccyx, Ischial Tuberosities, and Heels of Seated Individuals

Refer to Home Health Nurse and Physical Therapist for Evaluation of Home Environment

For More Specific Information Regarding Wheel Chair Use and Components

- Refer individual/family to the University of Alabama at Birmingham website under "Wheelchair and seating."

Impaired Transfer Ability

NANDA-I Definition

Limitation of independent movement between two nearby surfaces

Defining Characteristics*

Impaired ability to transfer:
From bed to chair and chair to bed
On or off a toilet or commode
In and out of tub or shower
Between uneven levels
From chair to car or car to chair
From chair to floor or floor to chair
From standing to floor or floor to standing
From bed to standing or standing to bed
From chair to standing or standing to chair

Related Factors

Refer to *Impaired Physical Mobility*.

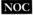

Transfer Performance, Fall Prevention Behavior

Goals

The individual will demonstrate transfer to and from the wheel-chair, as evidenced by the following indicators:

• Identify when assistance is needed
• Demonstrate ability to transfer in varied situations (e.g., toilet, bed, car, chair, uneven levels)

Positioning: Wheelchair, Fall Prevention

Interventions

Consult With and Refer to a Physical Therapist to Evaluate the Individual's Ability to Transfer

- Consider weight, strength, movement ability, tolerance to position changes, balance, motivation, and cognition.
- Use manual transfer or device-assisted lift.
- Consider ratio of staff to individuals.

Proceed With Established Plan to Transfer

- Before transferring the individual, assess the number of personnel needed for assistance.
- The individual should transfer toward the unaffected side.
- Position the individual on the side of the bed. His or her feet should be touching the floor, and he or she should be wearing stable shoes or slippers with nonskid soles.
- For getting in and out of bed, encourage weight-bearing on the uninvolved or stronger side.
- Lock the wheelchair before the transfer. If using a regular chair, be sure it will not move.
- Instruct the individual to use the arm of the chair closer to him or her for support while standing.
- Use a gait belt (preferred) or place your arm around the individual's rib cage and keep the back straight, with knees slightly bent.
- Tell the individual to place his or her arms around your waist or rib cage, *not the neck*.
- Support individual's legs by bracing his or her with yours. (While facing the individual, lock his or her knees with your knees.)
- Instruct individuals with hemiplegia to pivot on the uninvolved foot.

For Individuals With Lower Limb Weakness or Paralysis, a Sliding Board Transfer May Be Used

- The individual should wear pajamas so he or she will not stick to the board.
- The individual needs good upper extremity strength to be able to slide the buttocks from the bed to the chair or wheelchair. (Wheelchairs should have removable arms.)
- When the individual's arms are strong enough, he or she should progress to a sitting transfer without the board if he or she can lift his or her buttocks enough to clear the bed and chair seat.

- If the individual's legs give out, guide him or her gently to the floor and seek additional assistance.
- Consult and refer individual and family to home health nurses for a home evaluation and to access resources for discharge.

MORAL DISTRESS

Moral Distress

Risk for Moral Distress

Definition

Response to the inability to carry out one's chosen ethical/moral decision/action (NANDA-I)

The state in which a person experiences psychological disequilibrium, physical discomforts, anxiety, and/or anguish that result when a person makes a moral decision but does not follow through with the moral behavior[21]

Defining Characteristics*

Expresses anguish (e.g., powerlessness, guilt, frustration, anxiety, self-doubt, fear) over difficulty acting on one's moral choice

Related Factors

When *Moral Distress* is used to describe a response in nurses, as explained in this section, related factors are not useful. These diagnoses are not documented but rather represent a response that requires actions by the nurse, unit, and/or institution.

The related factors listed below represent a variety of situations that can precipitate *Moral Distress*.

---

[21]This definition has been added by Lynda Juall Carpenito, the author, for clarity and clinical usefulness.

Situational (Personal, Environmental)

End-of-Life Decisions*

Related to providing treatments that were perceived as futile for terminally ill individual (e.g., blood transfusions, chemotherapy, organ transplants, mechanical ventilation)

Related to conflicting attitudes toward advanced directives

Related to participation of life-saving actions when they only prolong dying

Treatment Decisions

Related to the individual/family's refusal of treatments deemed appropriate by the health-care team

Related to inability of the family to make the decision to stop ventilator treatment of terminally ill individual

Related to a family's wishes to continue life support even though it is not in the best interest of the individual

Related to performing a procedure that increases the individual's suffering

Related to providing care that does not relieve the individual's suffering

Related to conflicts between wanting to disclose poor medical practice and wanting to maintain trust in the physician

Professional Conflicts

Related to insufficient resources for care (e.g., time, staff)

Related to failure to be included in the decision-making process

Related to more emphasis on technical skills and tasks than relationships and caring

Cultural Conflicts

Related to decisions made for women by male family members

Related to cultural conflicts with the American health-care system

 Author's Note

This NANDA-I nursing diagnosis, accepted in 2006, has application in all settings where nurses practice. The literature to support this diagnosis when submitted was focused primarily on moral distress in nursing.

If moral distress occurs in an individual or family, this author suggests a referral to a professional expert in this area; for example, a counselor, therapist, or nurse spiritual advisor. Refer also to *Spiritual Distress*. Nurses should expect to experience moral distress as they struggle to make clinical decisions involving conflicting ethical principles (Zuzelo, 2007).

This author will present *Moral Distress* as a Department of Nursing—Standard of Practice. This standard addresses prevention of moral distress with specific individual nurse, unit, and department interventions. Strategies for addressing moral distress for individual nurses, on units, in the department of nursing, and in the institution will be presented.

This author has developed and included *Risk for Moral Distress*.

Moral Distress represents proactive strategies for individuals, groups, and institutions to prevent moral distress in nurses. This diagnosis has not yet been submitted to NANDA-I.

Most Americans fear how they will die than death itself (*Beckstrand, Callister, & Kirchhoff, 2006). Eighty-six percent of Americans polled reported nurses have very high or high ethical standards, ranking nurses at the top of other professions (Gallup poll, 2009).

Non applicable

Goals

The nurse will relate strategies to address moral distress, as evidenced by the following indicators:

- Identify source(s) of moral distress
- Share their distress with a colleague
- Identify two strategies to enhance decision making with individuals and family
- Identify two strategies to enhance discussion of the situation with the physician

Non applicable

Interventions

Identify Sources of Moral Stress (*AACN, 2004)

- Staffing
- Competency of nurses, physicians
- Nurse–physician communication

- Futile care
- Needless pain and suffering
- End-of-life conflicts
- Deception/incomplete information
- Inadequate symptom management
- Disrespectful interactions
- Violence in the workplace

Avoid Rationalization

"Use the Chain of Command to Share and Discuss Issues That Have Escalated Beyond the Problem-Solving Ability and/or Scope of Those Immediately Involved" (LaSala & Bjarnason, 2010)

Investigate How Clinical Situations That Are Morally Problematic Are Managed in the Institution; If an Ethics Committee Exists, Determine Its Mission and Procedures

Initiate Dialogue With the Individual, If Possible, and Family

- Explore what the perception of the situation is (e.g., How do you think your ___ is doing?)
- Pose questions (e.g., "What options do you have in this situation?") Elicit feelings about the present situation. Does the family know that the individual is terminal? Is the individual improving?
- Access the physician to clarify misinformation. Stay in the room to promote sharing.
- Encourage the individual/family to write down questions for the physician.
- Be present during physician's round to ensure individual's/family's understanding.
- Avoid deception or supporting deception.

Gently Explore Individual/Family End-of-Life Decisions

- Explain the options (e.g., "If you or your loved one dies, what interventions are preferred or desired?")
  - Medications, oxygen
  - Cardio defibrillation (shock)
  - Cardiopulmonary resuscitation
  - Intubation and use of respirator
- Advise the individual/family that they can choose all, some, or none of the above.
- Differentiate between prolonging life versus prolonging dying.
- Document the discussion and decisions according to institute on policy.

If Indicated, Explain "No Code" Status and Explain the Focus of Palliative Care That Replaces Aggressive and Futile Care (e.g., Pain Management, Symptom Management, Less or No Intrusive/Painful Procedures)

Seek To Transfer Individual From Intensive Care Unit, If Possible

Dialogue With Unit Colleagues About the Situation That Causes Moral Distress

Seek support and Information From Nurse Manager

Enlist a Colleague as a Coach or Engage as a Coach for a Coworker

• For advice, seek out colleagues who implement actions when they are distressed.

Start With an Approach to Address an Unsatisfactory Moral Clinical Situation That Has a Low Risk; Evaluate the Risks Before Taking Action; Be Realistic

Engage in Open Communication With Involved Physicians or Nurse Manager; Start the Conversation With Your Concern, for Example, "I Am Not Comfortable With. . . ," "The Family Is Asking/Questioning/Feeling. . . ," "Mr. X Is Asking/Questioning/Feeling. . ."

Dialogue With Other Professionals: Chaplains, Social Workers, or Ethics Committee

Advocate for End-of-Life Decision Dialogues With All Individuals and Their Families, Especially When the Situation Is Not Critical; Direct the Individual to Create Written Documents of Their Decisions, and Advise Family About the Document

Risk for Moral Distress

Definition[22]

The state in which a person is at risk to experience psychological disequilibrium, physical discomforts, anxiety, and/or anguish that result when a person makes a moral decision but does not follow through with the moral behavior

---

[22]This definition has been added by Lynda Juall Carpenito, the author, for clarity and clinical usefulness.

Risk Factors

Refer to *Moral Distress* Related Factors.

Non applicable

 Author's Note

Refer to *Moral Distress*.

Goals

The nurse will relate strategies to prevent moral distress, as evidenced by the following indicators:

* Identify risk situations for moral distress
* Share their distress with a colleague
* Identify two strategies to enhance decision making with individuals and families
* Identify two strategies to enhance communication patterns with physicians
* Engage institutional programs to prevent or decrease moral distress

Non applicable

Interventions

The following interventions are indicated for the institution and department of nursing.

Create a Just Culture That Fosters Moral Courage (ANA, 2010 a, b)

* Commitment to organizational improvement
* Resilience
* Mission, vision, and values that support high-quality individual outcomes and increasing situational awareness
* Identifying at-risk behavior creates incentives for healthy behaviors.
* Address the problem of behaviors that threaten the performance of the health-care team.
* Make choices that align with organizational values.

Explore Moral Work and Action

- Educate yourself about moral distress. Refer to articles on Bibliography.
- Share your stories of moral distress. Elicit stories from coworkers.
- Read stories of moral action. Refer to Gordon's *Life Support: Three Nurses on the Front Lines* and Kritek's *Reflections on Healing: A Central Construct* (see Bibliography).

Investigate How Clinical Situations That Are Morally Problematic Are Managed in the Institution; If an Ethics Committee Exists, Determine Its Mission, Procedures, and Accessibility.

Clarify the Difference of Medical/Surgical Unit Care, ICUs, and Palliative/Hospice Care

Advocate for the Individual/Family With Their Physician Before Conflicts Arise

- Explore the physician's understanding of the situation, prognosis.
- Elicit the individual's and/or family's perception of the situation.
- Explore individual's and family's expectations.
- Explore if the individual's and/or family's expectations are realistic.
- Offer your observations of the individual's/family's understanding of the situation to involved health-care professionals (e.g., manager, nurse colleagues, physicians).
- Develop strategies to transition individuals from acute care to palliative care.

If Indicated, Explain "No Code" Status and Explain the Focus of Palliative Care That Replaces Aggressive and Futile Care (e.g., Pain Management, Symptom Management, Less or No Intrusive/Painful Procedures)

- If their code status has not been determined, ask if you (your ___) die (s) what do you want done or what does your ___ want if he or she dies?
- Enlist the services of palliative or hospice nurses, when indicated.
- Seek to transfer the individual from ICU, if possible.
- If feasible, plan a transition of individual out of the hospital. Explore the "Going Home Initiative" at Baystate Medical Center, Springfield, MA (Lusardi et al., 2011).

Advocate for End-of-Life Decision Dialogues With All Individuals and Their Families, Especially When the Situation Is Not Critical. Direct the Individual to Create Written Documents of Their Decisions and Advise Family of the Document

Integrate Health Promotion and Stress Reduction in Your Lifestyle (e.g., Smoking Cessation, Weight Management, Regular Exercise, Meaningful Leisure Activities)

- Refer to *Altered Health Maintenance.*

SELF-NEGLECT

NANDA-I Definition

A constellation of culturally framed behaviors involving one or more self-care activities in which there is a failure to maintain a socially accepted standard of health and well-being (Gibbons, Lauder, & Ludwick, 2006)

Defining Characteristics*

Inadequate personal hygiene
Inadequate environmental hygiene
Nonadherence to health activities

Related Factors*

Capgras syndrome
Cognitive impairment
   (e.g., dementia)
Depression
Learning disability
Fear of institutionalization
Frontal lobe dysfunction and
   executive processing ability
Functional impairment

Lifestyle choice
Maintaining control
Malingering
Obsessive-compulsive
   disorder
Schizotypal personality
   disorders
Substance abuse
Major life stressor

Author's Note

This diagnosis focuses on three problems: self-care problems, home hygiene, and noncompliance. Presently, three nursing diagnoses would more specifically describe the focus as *Self-Care Deficit*, *Altered Home Management*, and *Ineffective Self-Health Management*. Refer to these diagnoses in the index.

UNILATERAL NEGLECT

NANDA-I Definition

Impairment in sensory and motor response, mental representation, and special attention of the body, and the corresponding environment characterized by inattention to one side and over-attention to the opposite side. Left-side neglect is more severe and persistent than right-side neglect.

Defining Characteristics

Major (Must Be Present, One or More)

Neglect of involved body parts and/or extrapersonal space (hemispatial neglect), and/or denial of the existence of the affected limb or side of body (anosognosia)

Minor (May Be Present)

Difficulty with spatial–perceptual tasks
Hemiplegia (usually of the left side)

Related Factors

Pathophysiologic

Related to brain injury secondary to:
Cerebrovascular accident*   Trauma*
Cerebral aneurysms   Tumors*
Cerebrovascular problems*

Author's Note

Unilateral Neglect represents a disturbance in the reciprocal loop that occurs most often in the right hemisphere of the brain. This diagnosis could also be viewed as a syndrome diagnosis, *Unilateral Neglect Syndrome*. Syndrome diagnoses encompass a cluster of nursing diagnoses related to the situation. The nursing interventions for *Unilateral Neglect Syndrome* would focus on *Self-Care Deficit*, *Anxiety*, and *Risk for Injury*.

NOC

Heedfulness of Affected Side; Neurological Status: Peripheral; Sensory Function: Proprioception; Adaption to Physical Disability; Self Care Status

Goals

The individual will demonstrate an ability to scan the visual field to compensate for loss of function/sensation in affected limbs, as evidenced by the following indicators:

- Identify safety hazards in the environment
- Describe the deficit and the rationale for treatment

NIC

Unilateral Neglect Management, Self-Care Assistance, Body Image Enhancement; Environmental Management: Safety, Exercise Therapy

Interventions

Consult With a Neuropsychologist, Physical Therapist, Occupational Therapist, and a Nurse Rehabilitation Specialist to Create a Multidisciplinary Plan With and for the Individual

- Ensure the individual/family understands unilateral neglect and the nursing and other treatment plans, for example, visual scanning training (VST), limb activation treatment (LAT), prism adaptation (PA).

Assist the Individual to Recognize the Perceptual Deficit

- Initially adapt the environment to the deficit:
  - Position the individual, call light, bedside stand, television, telephone, and personal items on the unaffected side.
  - Position the bed with the unaffected side toward the door.
- Approach and speak to the individual from the unaffected side.
- If you must approach the individual from the affected side, announce your presence as soon as you enter the room to avoid startling the individual.

- Teach to scan from left to right frequently.
- Gradually change the individual's environment as you teach him or her to compensate and to learn to recognize the forgotten field; move furniture and personal items out of the visual field. Speak to the individual from the affected side (after introducing yourself on the unaffected side).
- Provide a simplified, well-lit, uncluttered environment:
  - Provide a moment between activities.
  - Provide concrete cues: "You are on your side facing the wall."
- Provide a full-length mirror to help with vertical orientation and to diminish the distortion of the vertical and horizontal plane, which manifests itself in the individual leaning toward the affected side.
- For an individual in a wheelchair, obtain a lapboard (preferably Plexiglas); position the affected arm on the lapboard with the fingertips at midline. Encourage the individual to look for the arm on the board.
- For an ambulatory individual, obtain an arm sling to prevent the arm from dangling and causing shoulder subluxation.
- When in bed, elevate the affected arm on a pillow to prevent dependent edema.
- Constantly cue to the environment.
- Encourage to wear a watch, favorite ring, or bracelet on affected arm to draw attention to it.

Assist With Adaptations Needed for Self-Care and Other Activities of Daily Living (ADLs)

- Encourage the individual to wear prescribed corrective lenses or hearing aids for bathing, dressing, and toileting.
- Instruct the individual to attend to the affected extremity side first when performing ADLs.
- Instruct the individual always to look for the affected extremity when performing ADLs, to know where it is at all times.
- Teach the individual to dress and groom in front of a mirror.
- Suggest using color-coded markers sewn or placed inside shoes or clothes to help distinguish right from left.
- Encourage the individual to integrate affected extremity during bathing and to feel extremity by rubbing and massaging it.
- Use adaptive equipment as appropriate.
- Refer to *Self-Care Deficit* for additional interventions.
- For feeding:
  - Set up meals with a minimum of dishes, food, and utensils.
  - Instruct the individual to eat in small amounts and place food on unaffected side of mouth.

- Instruct the individual to use the tongue to sweep out "pockets" of food from the affected side after every bite.
- After meals/medications, check oral cavity for pocketed food/medication.
- Provide oral care TID and PRN.
- Initially place food in the individual's visual field; gradually move the food out of the field and teach the individual to scan entire visual field.
- Use adaptive feeding equipment as appropriate.
- Refer to *Self-Care Deficit: Feeding* for additional interventions.
- Refer to *Imbalanced Nutrition: Less Than Body Requirements related to swallowing difficulties* if the individual has difficulty chewing and swallowing food.

Teach Measures to Prevent Injury

- Ensure a clutter-free, well-lit environment.
- Retrain the individual to scan entire environment.
  - Instruct the individual to turn the head past midline to view the scene on the affected side.
  - Perform activities that require turning the head.
  - Remind the individual to scan when ambulating or propelling a wheelchair.

Use Tactile Sensation to Reintroduce Affected Arm/Extremity to the Individual

- Have the individual stroke the involved side with the uninvolved hand and watch the arm or leg while stroking it.
- Rub different-textured materials to stimulate sensations (hot, cold, rough, soft).

Initiate Health Teaching and Referrals

- Ensure referrals to nursing, physical therapy, and occupational therapy post transition.
- Ensure that both the individual and the family understand the cause of unilateral neglect and the purpose of and rationale for all interventions.
- Have the family demonstrate how to facilitate relearning techniques (e.g., cueing, scanning visual field).
- Teach principles of maintaining a safe environment.

NONCOMPLIANCE[23]

Definition

Behavior of person and/or caregiver that fails to coincide with a health-promoting or therapeutic plan agreed on by the person (and/or family and/or community) and health-care professional. In the presence of an agreed-upon, health-promoting, or therapeutic plan, the person's or caregiver's behavior is fully or partially nonadherent and may lead to clinically ineffective or partially ineffective outcomes.

Defining Characteristics

Development-related complication
Exacerbation of symptoms
Failure to meet outcomes
Missing appointments
Nonadherance behavior

Related Factors

Health System
Difficulty in client–provider relationship
Inadequate access to care
Inconvenience of care
Ineffective communication skills of provider
Insufficient follow-up with provider
Insufficient health insurance

Insufficient provider reimbursement
Insufficient teaching skill of provider
Low satisfaction with care
Perceived low credibility of provider
Provider discontinuity

Health-Care Plan
Complex treatment regimen
Financial barriers
High-cost regimen

Intensity of regimen
Lengthy duration of regimen

---

[23]This author has chosen retire this nursing diagnosis and replace it with *Compromised Engagement* and *Risk for Compromised Engagement*. Refer to thePoint® to access these diagnoses.

Individual

Cultural incongruence

Health beliefs incongruent with plan

Insufficient knowledge about regimen

Insufficient skills to perform regimen

Expectation incongruent with
developmental phase

Insufficient motivation

Insufficient social
support

Insufficient motivation

Values incongruent
with plan

Network

Insufficient involvement of members
in plan

Perception that beliefs of significant
other differ from plan

Low social value
attributed to plan

 Author's Note

The nursing diagnosis *Noncompliance* was last revised in 1998. The label *Noncompliance* has never reflected a proactive approach to an individual/family who was not participating in recommended treatments or lifestyle changes. Criticism of the term noncompliant surfaced in the literature a decade ago. Recent health-care literature is full of alternative strategies for health-care professionals to improve health outcomes with individuals/families.

Merriam-Webster defines compliance as the act or process of complying to a desire, demand, proposal, or regimen, or to coercion. Compliance occurs when an individual obeys a directive from a health-care provider.

Gruman (2011) wrote, "Saying 'engagement' when meaning 'compliance' supports the belief that we are the only ones who must change our behavior. . . Doing so misrepresents the magnitude of shifts in attitude, expectations and effort that are required for all health care stakeholders to ensure that we have adequate knowledge and support to make well-informed decisions. . . And it fails to recognize that our behaviors are powerfully shaped by many contingencies, money, culture, time, illness status, and personal preference. . . Being engaged in our health and care does not mean following our clinician's instructions to the letter. . . Rather, it means being able to accurately weigh the benefits and risks of a new medication, of stopping smoking or getting a PSA test in the context of the many other demands and opportunities that influence our pursuit of lives that are free of suffering for ourselves and those we love."

Note: We = consumer/clients/family

IMBALANCED NUTRITION

Imbalanced Nutrition

Impaired Dentition

Impaired Swallowing

Ineffective Infant Feeding Pattern

NANDA-I Definition

Intake of nutrients insufficient to meet metabolic needs

Defining Characteristics

The individual who is not NPO reports or is found to have food intake less than the recommended daily allowance (RDA) with or without weight loss

and/or

Actual or potential metabolic needs in excess of intake with weight loss

Weight 10% to 20% or more below ideal for height and frame

Triceps skinfold, mid-arm circumference, and mid-arm muscle circumference less than 60% standard measurement

Muscle weakness and tenderness

Mental irritability or confusion

Decreased serum albumin

Decreased serum transferrin or iron-binding capacity

Sunken fontanel in infant

Related Factors

Pathophysiologic

Related to increased caloric requirements and difficulty in ingesting sufficient calories secondary to:

Burns (postacute phase)
Cancer
Infection
Trauma
Chemical dependence

Preterm infants
Gastrointestinal (GI) complications/deformities
AIDS

Related to dysphagia secondary to:

Cerebrovascular accident (CVA) Cerebral palsy
Parkinson's disease Cleft lip/palate
Möbius syndrome Amyotrophic lateral sclerosis
Muscular dystrophy Neuromuscular disorders

Related to decreased absorption of nutrients secondary to:

Crohn's disease Necrotizing enterocolitis
Lactose intolerance Cystic fibrosis

Related to decreased desire to eat secondary to altered level of consciousness

Related to self-induced vomiting, physical exercise in excess of caloric intake, or refusal to eat secondary to anorexia nervosa

Related to reluctance to eat for fear of poisoning secondary to paranoid behavior

Related to anorexia and excessive physical agitation secondary to bipolar disorder

Related to anorexia and diarrhea secondary to protozoal infection

Related to vomiting, anorexia, and impaired digestion secondary to pancreatitis

Related to anorexia, impaired protein and fat metabolism, and impaired storage of vitamins secondary to cirrhosis

Related to anorexia, vomiting, and impaired digestion secondary to GI malformation or necrotizing enterocolitis

Related to anorexia secondary to gastroesophageal reflux

Treatment Related

Related to protein and vitamin requirements for wound healing and decreased intake secondary to:

Surgery Medications (chemotherapy)
Surgical reconstruction of mouth Wired jaw
Radiation therapy

Related to inadequate absorption as a medication side effect of (specify):

Colchicine *para*-Aminosalicylic acid
Neomycin Antacid
Pyrimethamine

Related to decreased oral intake, mouth discomfort, nausea, and vomiting secondary to:

Radiation therapy Chemotherapy
Tonsillectomy Oral trauma

Related to inadequate absorption as a medication side effect of (specify):
Example (Gröber & Kisters, 2007):

Colchicine
Neomycin
Pyrimethamine
Antacid
Antiepileptics
Antineoplastic drugs
Antibiotics (Clotrimazole, Rifampicin)

Dexamethasone
Antihypertensives (nifedipine, spironolactone)
Antiretroviral drugs (ritonavir, saquinavir)
Herbal medicines: Kava kava
St. John's wort (hyperforin)

Situational (Personal, Environmental)

Related to decreased desire to eat secondary to:

Anorexia
Social isolation
Depression

Nausea and vomiting
Stress
Allergies

Related to inability to procure food (physical limitation or financial or transportation problems)

Related to inability to chew (damaged or missing teeth, ill-fitting dentures)

Related to diarrhea secondary to (specify)*

Maturational

Infant/Child

Related to inadequate intake secondary to:

Lack of emotional/sensory stimulation
Lack of knowledge of caregiver

Inadequate production of breast milk

Related to malabsorption, dietary restrictions, and anorexia secondary to:

Celiac disease
Lactose intolerance
Necrotizing enterocolitis

Cystic fibrosis
GI malformation
Gastroesophageal reflux

Related to sucking difficulties (infant) and dysphagia secondary to:

Cerebral palsy
Cleft lip and palate

Neurologic impairment

Related to inadequate sucking, fatigue, and dyspnea secondary to:

Congenital heart disease
Viral syndrome syndrome
Hyperbilirubinemia

Prematurity
Respiratory distress

Developmental delay

Author's Note

Because of their 24-hour presence, nurses are usually the primary profes-sionals responsible for improving nutritional status. Although *Imbalanced Nutrition* is not a difficult diagnosis to validate, interventions for it can challenge the nurse. Secondary screening for individual determined to be at increased risk for nutritional deficits are performed by clinical nutrition-ists. This nursing diagnosis will focus on nutritional deficits in individuals in health-care settings. In addition, assessments and interventions will be presented to assist the individual or family to improve nutrition and food security

Many factors influence food habits and nutritional status: personal, family, cultural, financial, functional ability, nutritional knowledge, disease and injury, and treatment regimens. *Imbalanced Nutrition: Less Than Body Requirements* describes people who can ingest food but eat an inadequate or imbalanced quality or quantity. For instance, the diet may have insuf-ficient protein or excessive fat. Quantity may be insufficient because of increased metabolic requirements (e.g., cancer, pregnancy, trauma, or interference with nutrient use [e.g., impaired storage of vitamins in cirrhosis]).

The nursing focus for *Imbalanced Nutrition* is assisting the individual or family to improve nutritional intake. Nurses should not use this diagnosis to describe individuals who are NPO or cannot ingest food. They should use the collaborative problems *RC of Electrolyte Imbalance* or *RC of Nega-tive Nitrogen Balance* to describe those situations.

NOC
Nutritional Status, Teaching: Nutrition, Symptom Control

Goals

The individual will ingest daily nutritional requirements in ac-cordance with activity level and metabolic needs, as evidenced by the following indicators:

- Relate importance of good nutrition
- Identify deficiencies in daily intake
- Relate methods to increase appetite

Interventions

Explain the Need for Adequate Consumption of Carbohydrates, Fats, Protein, Vitamins, Minerals, and Fluids

Consult With a Nutritionist to Establish Appropriate Daily Caloric and Food-Type Requirements for the Individual

Discuss With the Individual Possible Causes of Decreased Appetite

Encourage the Individual to Rest Before Meals

Offer Frequent, Small Meals Instead of a Few Large Ones; Offer Foods Served Cold

With Decreased Appetite, Restrict Liquids With Meals and Avoid Fluids 1 Hour Before and After Meals

Encourage and Help the Individual to Maintain Good Oral Hygiene

Arrange to Have High-Calorie and High-Protein Foods Served at the Times That the Individual Usually Feels Most Like Eating

Take Steps to Promote Appetite

- Determine the individual's food preferences and arrange to have them provided, as appropriate.
- Eliminate any offensive odors and sights from the eating area.
- Control any pain and nausea before meals.
- Encourage the individual's family to bring permitted foods from home, if possible.
- Provide a relaxed atmosphere and some socialization during meals.

Provide for Supplemental Dietary Needs Amplified by Acute Illness

Give the Individual Printed Materials Outlining a Nutritious Diet That Includes the Following

- High intake of complex carbohydrates and fiber
- Decreased intake of sugar, salt, cholesterol, total fat, and saturated fats
- Alcohol use only in moderation
- Proper caloric intake to maintain ideal weight

Pediatric Interventions

- Teach parents the following regarding infant nutrition:
  - Adequate infant feeding schedule and weight gain requirements for growth: 100 to 120 kcal/kg/day for growth
  - Proper preparation of infant formula
  - Proper storage of breast milk and infant formula
  - Proper elevation of infant's head during and immediately after feedings
  - Proper chin/cheek support techniques for orally compromised infants

- The age-related nutritional needs of their children (consult an appropriate textbook on pediatrics or nutrition for specific recommendations).
- If eating "fast foods," teach healthier choices as follows:
  - Encourage portion control; educate children/adolescents that "large," "extra," "double," or "triple" will be high in calories and fat.
  - Recommend smaller portions, since a regular serving is enough for most children, or sharing with a parent or sibling.
  - Look for whole grain foods, fruits, vegetables, and calcium-rich foods.
  - When planning a fast food meal, select an establishment that promotes healthier options at the point of purchase.
- Address strategies to improve nutrition when eating fast foods:
  - Drink skim milk.
  - Avoid French fries or share one order.
  - Choose grilled foods.
  - Eat salads and vegetables.
- Explore healthier fast foods at home (e.g., frozen dinners with three food groups).
- Suggest healthy snacks at home. Offer fresh fruits, vegetables, cheese and crackers, low-fat milk, calcium-fortified juices, and frozen yogurt as snacks.
- Avoid describing foods as bad or good. Explain nutrient density of foods (*Hunter & Cason, 2006).
- Foods that are nutrient dense:
  - Fruits and vegetables that are bright or deeply colored
  - Foods that are fortified
  - Lower fat versions of meats, milk, dairy products, and eggs
- Foods that are less nutrient dense:
  - Be lighter or whiter in color
  - Contain a lot of refined sugar
  - Be refined products (white bread as compared to whole grains)
  - Contain high amounts of fat for the amount of nutrients compared to similar products (fat-free milk vs. ice cream)
  - For example:
    ○ Apple is a better choice than a bag of pretzels with the same number of calories, but apple provides fiber, vitamin C, and potassium.
    ○ An orange is better than orange juice because it has fiber.
- Allow the child to select one type of food he or she does not have to eat.
- Provide small servings (e.g., 1 tablespoon of each food for every year of age).

- Make snacks as nutritiously important as meals (e.g., hard-boiled eggs, raw vegetable sticks, peanut butter/crackers, fruit juices, cheese, and fresh fruit).
- Offer a variety of foods.
- Involve the child in monitoring healthy eating (e.g., create a chart where the child checks off intake of healthy foods daily).
- Replace passive television watching with a group activity (e.g., Frisbee tossing, biking, walking).
- Substitute quick, nutritious fast meals (e.g., frozen dinners).
- Discuss the importance of limiting snacks high in salt, sugar, or fat (e.g., soda, candy, chips) to limit risks for cardiac disorders, obesity, and diabetes mellitus. Advise families to substitute healthy snacks (e.g., fresh fruits, plain popcorn, frozen fruit juice bars, fresh vegetables).
  - More total energy (2,236 vs. 2,049 kcal/day)
  - More total fat (84 vs. 75 g/day)
  - More total carbohydrates (303 vs. 277 g/day
  - More added sugars (122 vs. 94 g/day)
  - More sugar-sweetened carbonated beverages (471 vs. 243 g/day)
  - Less milk (236 vs. 302 g/day)
  - Less fiber (13.2 vs. 14.3 g/day)
  - Fewer fruits and nonstarchy vegetables (103 vs. 148 g/day)

🕴 Maternal Interventions

- Teach the importance of adequate calorie and fluid intake while breastfeeding in relation to breast milk production.
- Explain physiologic changes and nutritional needs during pregnancy.
- Discuss the effects of alcohol, caffeine, and artificial sweeteners on the developing fetus.
- Discuss with pregnant adolescents that their nutritional needs are greater since they are still developing and now are pregnant (Pillitteri, 2014). Emphasize the growing fetus.

〰 Geriatric Interventions

Consider a Consult With Registered Dietician When the Individual (Chima, 2004; Hammond, 2011)

- Has significant unintentional weight loss ≥10 lb in past 1 to 2 months
- Desires education on a more nutritious diet

- Is unable to take oral or other feedings ≥ 5 days prior to admission
- Is on enteral or parenteral feedings
- Is 80+ years and admitted for surgical procedure
- With skin breakdown (decubitus ulcer) consumes foods fortified with vitamin B_{12}, such as fortified cereals, or dietary supplement

Determine the Individual's Understanding of Nutritional Needs With

- Aging
- Medication use
- Illness
- Activity

Assess Whether Any Factors Interfere With Ingesting Foods (Lutz, Mazur, & Litch, 2015; Miller, 2015)

- Anorexia from medications, grief, depression, or illness
- Impaired mental status, leading to inattention to hunger or selecting insufficient kinds/amounts of food
- Voluntary fluid restriction for fear of urinary incontinence
- Small frame or history of undernutrition
- New dentures or poor dentition
- Dislike of cooking and eating alone
- Regularly eats alone
- Has more than two alcoholic drinks daily

Assess Whether Any Factors Interfere With Preparing and/or Procuring Foods (Miller, 2015)

- Inadequate income to purchase food
- Lack of transportation to buy food
- Inadequate facility to cook
- Impaired mobility or manual dexterity (paresis, tremors, weakness, joint pain, or deformity)
- Safety issues (e.g., fires, spoiled foods)

Assess for Food Insecurity

Explain Decline in Sensitivity to Sweet and Salty Tastes, But Not Bitter and Sour (Lutz et al., 2015). **Caution Against Oversalting Foods.**

If Indicated, Consult With Home Health Nurse to Evaluate Home Environment (e.g., Safety Issues, Cooking Facilities, Food Supply, and Cleanliness)

Access Community Agencies as Indicated (e.g., Nutritional Programs, Community Centers, Home-Delivered Grocery Services)

- Teach the importance of adequate calorie and fluid intake while breastfeeding in relation to breast milk production.
- Explain physiologic changes and nutritional needs during pregnancy.
- Discuss the effects of alcohol, caffeine, and artificial sweeteners on the developing fetus.
- Explain the different nutritional requirements for pregnant girls 11 to 18 years of age, pregnant young women 19 to 24 years of age, and women older than 25 years.

Impaired Dentition

NANDA-I Definition

Disruption in tooth development/eruption patterns or structural integrity of individual teeth

Defining Characteristics*

Excessive plaque	Loose teeth
Asymmetric facial expression	Malocclusion or tooth misalignment
Halitosis	Incomplete eruption for age (may be primary or permanent teeth)
Crown or root caries	
Toothache	Premature loss of primary teeth
Tooth enamel discoloration	Tooth fracture(s)
Excessive calculus	Missing teeth or complete absence
	Erosion of enamel

Impaired Swallowing

NANDA-I Definition

Abnormal functioning of the swallowing mechanism associated with deficits in oral, pharyngeal, or esophageal structure or function

Defining Characteristics (Fass, 2014)

Oral Dysfunction
Drooling   Piecemeal swallows
Food spillage   Sialorrhea (hypersalivation)
Dysarthria

Pharyngeal dysfunction
Coughing or choking during food consumption
Dysphonia (defective use of the voice)

Esophageal Dysphagia
Difficulty swallowing several seconds after initiating a swallow
A sensation of food getting stuck in the suprasternal notch or
    behind the sternum

Related Factors

Pathophysiologic

*Related to decreased/absent gag reflex, mastication difficulties, or
decreased sensations secondary to:*
Cerebral palsy*   CVA
Muscular dystrophy   Neoplastic disease affecting brain
Poliomyelitis   Right or left hemispheric brain
Parkinson's disease   damage
Guillain–Barré syndrome   Vocal cord paralysis
Myasthenia gravis   Cranial nerve damage
Amyotrophic lateral scle-   (V, VII, IX, X, XI)
    rosis

Related to constriction of esophagus secondary to:
Vascular ring anomaly
Large aneurysm of the thoracic aorta

Related to tracheoesophageal tumors, edema

Related to irritated oropharyngeal cavity

Related to decreased saliva

Treatment Related

Related to surgical reconstruction of the mouth, throat, jaw, or nose

Related to decreased consciousness secondary to anesthesia

Related to mechanical obstruction secondary to tracheostomy tube

Related to esophagitis secondary to radiotherapy

Situational (Personal, Environmental)

Related to fatigue

Related to limited awareness, distractibility

Maturational

Infants/Children

Related to decreased sensations or difficulty with mastication

Related to poor suck/swallow/breathe coordination

Older Adult

Related to reduction in saliva, taste

 Author's Note

See *Imbalanced Nutrition: Less Than Body Requirements*.

NOC
Aspiration Control, Swallowing Status

Goals

The individual will report improved ability to swallow, as evidenced by the following indicators:

• Describe causative factors when known
• Describe rationale and procedures for treatment

Interventions

Assure individual and/or family have discussed the advantages and risks of dysphagia management (e.g., oral nutrition, intravenous, nasogastric, or percutaneous-endoscopic-gastrostomy tube with a specialist). Document the discussion event and decisions.

Assess for Causative or Contributing Factors

• Refer to Related Factors.
• Consult with a speech therapist for a bedside swallowing assessment and recommended plan of care.
• Alert all staff that individual has impaired swallowing.

- Consult with swallowing specialist for the best position when taking food or fluids (Sura, Madhavan, Carnaby, & Crary , 2012).
- Head posture
  - With food—head extension/chin up—raise chin—better bolus transport
  - Head rotation/head turn—turning head towards the weaker side
- Modify the consistency of solid food and/or liquid for individuals with dysphagia. All individuals on texture-modified diets should be assessed by the dietitian for nutritional support (Sura, 2012; Wright, 2005)

Reduce or Eliminate Causative/Contributing Factors in People With

Mechanical Impairment of Mouth

- Assist individual with moving the bolus of food from the anterior to the posterior part of mouth. Place food in the posterior mouth, where swallowing can be ensured, using
  - Soft, moist food of a consistency that can be manipulated by the tongue against the pharynx, such as gelatin, custard, or mashed potatoes
- Prevent/decrease thick secretions with
  - Frequent mouth care
- Increase fluid intake to eight glasses of liquid (unless contraindicated).
- Check medications for potential side effects of dry mouth/decreased salivation.

Muscle Paralysis or Paresis

- Plan meals when individual is well rested; ensure that reliable suction equipment is on hand during meals. Discontinue feeding if individual is tired.
- If indicated, use modified supraglottic swallow technique (*Emick-Herring & Wood, 1990).
- Note the consistency of food that is problematic. Select consistencies that are easier to swallow, such as
  - Highly viscous foods (e.g., mashed bananas, potatoes, gelatin, gravy)
  - Thick liquids (e.g., milkshakes, slushes, nectars, cream soups)
- If a bolus of food is pocketed in the affected side, teach individual how to use tongue to transfer food or apply external digital pressure to cheek to help remove the trapped bolus (Emick-Herring & Wood, 1990).

Reduce the Possibility of Aspiration

- Before beginning feeding, assess that the individual is adequately alert and responsive, can control the mouth, has cough/gag reflex, and can swallow saliva.
- Have suction equipment available and functioning properly.
- Position individual correctly:
  - Sit individual upright (60° to 90°) in chair, or dangle his or her feet at side of bed, if possible (prop with pillows if necessary).
  - Individual should assume this position 10 to 15 minutes before eating and maintain it for 10 to 15 minutes after finishing eating.
  - Flex individual's head forward on the midline about 45° to keep esophagus patent.

Ineffective Infant Feeding Pattern

NANDA-I Definition

Impaired ability of an infant to suck or coordinate the suck/swallow response, resulting in inadequate oral nutrition for metabolic needs

Defining Characteristics

Inability to initiate or sustain an effective suck*
Inability to coordinate sucking, swallowing, and breathing*
Regurgitation or vomiting after feeding

Related Factors

Pathophysiologic

Related to increased caloric need secondary to:

Body temperature instability
Tachypnea with increased respiratory effort
Infection
Möbius syndrome

Growth needs
Wound healing
Major organ system disease or failure
Cleft lip/palate

Related to muscle weakness/hypotonia secondary to:

Malnutrition

Congenital defects

Prematurity*

Major organ system disease or failure

Hyperbilirubinemia

Acute/chronic illness

Neurologic impairment/delay*

Lethargy

Treatment Related

Related to hypermetabolic state and increased caloric needs secondary to:

Surgery

Painful procedures

Cold stress

Sepsis

Fever

Related to muscle weakness and lethargy secondary to:

Medications

Muscle relaxants (antiseizure medications, past use of paralyzing agents, sedatives, narcotics)

Sleep deprivation

*Related to oral hypersensitivity**

Related to previous prolonged NPO state

Situational (Personal, Environmental)

Related to inconsistent caretakers (feeders)

Related to lack of knowledge or commitment of caretaker (feeder) to special feeding needs or regimen

Related to presence of noxious facial stimuli or absence of oral stimuli

Related to inadequate production of breast milk

 Author's Note

Ineffective Infant Feeding Pattern describes an infant with sucking or swallowing difficulties. This infant experiences inadequate oral nutrition for growth and development, which is exacerbated when caloric need increases, as with infection, illness, or stress. Nursing interventions assist infants and their caregivers with techniques to achieve nutritional intake needed for weight gain. In addition, the goal is for the intake eventually to be exclusively oral.

Infants with sucking or swallowing problems who have not lost weight need nursing interventions to prevent weight loss. *Ineffective Infant Feeding Pattern* is clinically useful for this situation.

NOC

Muscle Function, Nutritional Status, Swallowing Status

Goals

The infant will

- Receive adequate and appropriate calories (carbohydrate, protein, fat) for age with weight gain at a rate consistent with an individualized plan based on age and needs. Infant needs caloric intake of 100 to 120 kcal/kg/day for growth
- Take all feedings orally

The parent will

- Demonstrate increasing skill in infant feeding
- Identify techniques that increase effective feeding

NIC

Nonnutritive Swallowing, Swallowing Therapy, Aspiration, Precautions, Bottle Feeding, Parent Education: Infant

Interventions

- Assess volume, duration, and effort during feeding; respiratory rate and effort; and signs of fatigue.
- Assess past caloric intake, weight gain, trends in intake and output, renal function, and fluid retention.
- Identify physiologic ability to feed (Pillitteri, 2014).
  - Can infant stop breathing when sucking and swallowing?
  - Does infant gasp or choke during feedings?
  - What happens to oxygen level, heart rate, and respiratory rate when sucking/swallowing?
  - Does the infant need rest periods? How long? Are there problems in initiating sucking/swallowing again?
- Assess nipple-feeding skills (Pillitteri, 2014).
  - Does the infant actively suck with a bottle?
  - Does the infant initiate a swallow in coordination with suck?
  - Does the infant coordinate sucking, swallowing, and breathing?
  - Is the feeding completed in a reasonable time?

- Collaborate with clinical dietitian to set calorie, volume, and weight gain goals.
- Collaborate with occupational therapist and speech therapist to identify oral motor skills and planned intervention, if needed.
- Collaborate with parent(s) about effective techniques used with this infant or other children, temperament, and responses to environmental stimuli.

Provide Specific Interventions to Promote Effective Oral Feeding
(Hockenberry & Wilson, 2015)

- Ensure a quiet, calm, and dim environment.
- Eliminate painful procedures prior to feeding.
- Ensure uninterrupted sleep periods.
- Encourage nonnutritive sucking not in response to noxious stimuli.
- Ensure nutritive sucking for an identified period.
- Control adverse environmental stimuli and noxious stimuli to face and mouth.
- Avoid the following actions that can hinder feeding:
  - Twisting or turning the nipple
  - Moving the nipple up, down, around in the mouth
  - Putting the nipple in and out of the mouth
  - Putting pressure on the jaw or moving the infant's jaw up and down
  - Placing the infant in a head-back position
  - Caregiver anxiousness and impatience
- Refer to *Risk for Aspiration* for interventions for feeding an infant with cleft lip and/or palate.

Establish Partnership With Parent(s) in All Stages of Plan

- Create a supportive environment for the parents to have the primary role in providing feeding-related intervention, when they are present. Whenever possible, nurses use the parents' approach when a parent is not present. In addition, when parents are not present, nurses can support the parents' role by imitating their approach to the infant, and communicate the infant's responses to the parents at a later time.
- Negotiate and identify transition plans with parents and incorporate into the overall feeding plan; provide ongoing information about special needs, and assist parents to establish needed resources (equipment, nursing care, other caretakers) when needed.

OBESITY

Obesity
Overweight

Risk for Overweight

NANDA-I Definition

A condition in which an individual accumulates abnormal or excessive fat for age and gender that exceeds overweight

Defining Characteristics

Adult: BMI of >30 kg/m^2

Child <2 years: Term not applicable/not used with infants/children at this age

Child 2 to 18 years: BMI of >30 kg/m^2 or >95th percentile for age and gender

Related Factors

Average daily physical activity is less than recommended for gender and age

Consumption of sugar-sweetened beverages

Disordered eating behaviors

Disordered eating perceptions

Economically disadvantaged

Energy expenditure below energy intake based on standard assessment (e.g., WAVE assessment[24])

Excessive alcohol consumption

Fear regarding lack of food supply

Formula- or mixed-fed infants

Frequent snacking

Genetic disorder

Heritability of interrelated factors (e.g., adipose tissue distribution, energy expenditure, lipoprotein lipase activity, lipid synthesis, lipolysis)

High disinhibition and restraint eating behavior score

---

[24]WAVE assessment = weight, activity, variety in diet, excess.

High frequency of restaurant or fried food
Low dietary calcium intake in children
Maternal diabetes mellitus
Maternal smoking
Overweight in infancy
Parental obesity
Portion sizes larger than recommended
Premature pubarche
Rapid weight gain during childhood
Rapid weight gain during infancy, including the first week, first
   4 months, and first year
Sedentary behavior occurring for > 2 hr/day
Shortened sleep time
Sleep disorder
Solid foods as major food source at <5 months of age

 Author's Note

Given the public health problem of *Overweight* and *Obesity* across the lifespan, the above three diagnoses are excellent additions to NANDA-I Classification.

The interventions for these diagnoses will focus on strategies to motivate and engage individuals/families to proceed to a healthy lifestyle.[25]

Obesity is a complex condition with sociocultural, psychological, and metabolic implications. When the focus is primarily on limiting food intake, as with many weight-loss programs, bariatric surgery, the chance of permanent weight loss is slim. To be successful, a weight-loss program in an individual needs to focus on behavior modification and lifestyle changes, through exercise, decreased intake, and addressing their emotional component of overeating.

If someone is at a healthy weight, but routinely eats foods low in nutrients.

Risk-Prone Health Behavior related to intake of insufficient nutrients and/or inactivity in the present of a healthy weight that does not meet recommended dietary intake. For some people with dysfunctional eating, *Ineffective Coping* related to increased eating in response to stressors would be valid and require a referral after discharge.

WAVE (Weight, Activity, Variety, and Excess) (Barner et al., 2001; Gans et al., 2003). Wave is an abbreviated model for addressing nutrition in an individual and achieving healthy weight. With assessment questions and targeted interventions, it was designed to be utilized in health-care

---

[25] *Imbalanced and Risk for Imbalanced Nutrition: More Than Body Requirement* has been deleted from the NANDA-I Classification.

settings as a brief intervention to activate an individual to evaluate their nutritional intake and activity level. It also can be useful with the family member responsible for food shopping and preparation, to evaluate food groups served, frequency, and serving sizes eaten. Refer to MyPlate under *Imbalanced Nutrition: Less Than Body Requirements.* Refer to references cited for **WAVE** > **Assessment and Recommendations.**

NOC

Nutritional Status: Nutrient Intake, Weight Control, Exercise Participation, Infant Nutritional Status, Weight Body Mass, Adherence Behavior: Healthy Diet, Weight Loss Behavior

Goals

The individual will commit to a weight-loss program, as evidenced by the following indicators:

- Identify the patterns of eating, associated with consumption/energy expenditure imbalance
- Give examples of nutrient dense foods versus those with "empty calories"
- Identify three ways to increase his or her activity
- Commit to increasing foods with high nutrient density and less with "empty calories"
- Commit to making 3 to 5 changes in food/fluid choices, which are healthier

The child (over 8) will verbalize what is healthy eating by the following indicators:

- Describe "MyPlate"
- Describe what "empty calories" mean
- Name "empty calories" beverages and healthier substitutions
- Name foods high in nutrients
- Name food high in sugar and "empty calories" and healthier substitutions

The pregnant woman will verbalize healthy eating and recommended weight gain during pregnancy by the following indicators:

- Describe vitamin, mineral, protein, fat needs during pregnancy
- Give examples of nutrient dense foods versus those with "empty calories"
- Identify three ways to increase his or her activity
- Relate the weight gain specific to her weight prior to pregnancy
- Explain why "dieting" is problematic

NIC

Self-Efficacy Enhancement, Self-Responsibility Enhancement, Nutritional Counseling, Weight Management, Teaching: Nutrition (age appropriate), Behavioral Modification, Exercise Promotion, Coping Enhancement

Interventions

Refer to Appendix C: Strategies to Promote Engagement of Individual/Families for Healthier Outcomes for specific techniques to improve activation and engagement.

Initiate Discussion: "How Can You Be Healthier?"

- Focus on the person's response (e.g., stop smoking, exercise more, eat healthier, and cut down on drinking).
- Refer to index for interventions for the targeted lifestyle change.

Before a Person Can Change, They Must (*Martin, Haskard, Zolnierek, & DiMatteo, 2010)

- Know what change is necessary (information and why)
- Desire the change (motivation)
- Have the tools to achieve and maintain the change (strategy)
- Trust the health-care professional, who has a sympathetic presence (Pelzang, 2010)

If Appropriate, Gently and Expertly Discuss the Hazards of Obesity But Respect a Person's Right to Choose, the Right of Self-Determination

- How do you think being overweight affects you?
- Focus on what the person tells you (e.g., my sugar is high, my knees hurt). Do not overload him or her with advice or information

To Help to Activate Engagement in an Individual

- Ask them one of the questions below. Pick the best question that applies to this person. Use language they understand (e.g., blood veins or that carry blood).
  - Do your legs swell during the day and go back to normal during the night?
    - Explain fat tissue compresses tubes in your legs and prevent fluids from circulating well. Eventually the swelling will be permanent, 24 hours a day, causing difficulty walking and wearing shoes.
  - Do you have high blood pressure or is it getting a little higher each year?

- ○ Explain that blood vessels are damaged when excess weight puts pressure on them and they stretch, become thinner and lose their strength. Your heart now has to pump harder, causing high blood pressure. Over time the heart enlarges and cannot pump well. This is heart failure.
- Is your cholesterol level increasing each year?
  - ○ Explain that the stretching of your blood vessels damages the inside of the blood tubes. Cholesterol sticks to the damaged tubes and slows the blood flow to your kidneys, eyes, brain, and legs. This can cause strokes, renal failure, vision problems, and blood clots in your legs.
- So you may not feel that anything is wrong, but high blood pressure can permanently damage your heart, brain, eyes, and kidneys before you feel anything. Even losing 10 lb can reduce your blood pressure.
- Is your blood glucose test getting a little higher each year? Is there diabetes in your family?
  - ○ Explain the more fatty tissue you have, the more resistant your cells become to insulin.
  - ○ Insulin carries glucose from blood to the cells. When you are overweight, the cells are damaged and will not absorb the insulin. So your blood glucose goes up. High blood glucose damage blood vessels in the eyes, kidneys, and heart.
- Does your back, knees, or other joints hurt?
  - ○ Explain that extra weight puts pressure on your joints and bones. This pressure wears away the cartilage, the cushion at the ends of your bones. This causes the bone to rub against another bone causing pain.
- Do you think people who are overweight have problem healing from injuries or surgery?
  - ○ Explain that fat tissue has less blood supply, which is needed for healing. The incision has more pressure against, when you are overweight, which can cause the wound to open up. If antibiotics are needed for infection, the medicine does not work well because of poor circulation to the wound.
  - ○ If the person does not identify any negative effects of excess weight that they feel, explain the effects of excess weight are insidious and often not felt by the person until the effects threaten their health or cause pain (e.g., joint).

Eating Healthier

Review Usual Daily Intake to Identify Patterns That Contribute to Excess Weight

- Usual breakfast, usual lunch, usual dinner
- Snacks, nighttime eating
- Skipping meals

Promote Activation to Engage the Individual in Healthier Behavior. Focus on What the Person Wants to Change. Limit to Three Changes

Address What Excesses or Deficiencies Exist, Using the Information He or She Gave, For Example

- I ate fried chicken wings last night for dinner.
- Anything else? No.
- How could you change what you ate to improve nutrients and decrease fat?
- Listen. If no response
  - Suggest one or two piece(s) of fried chicken instead of 12 wings.
  - One piece of fried chicken with no batter has 158 calories/ thigh or 131 calories/breast.
  - One medium fried chicken wing with no batter has 102 calories.
  - Ten (10) wings have 1,020 calories.
- What could you eat in addition to the fried chicken that is a vegetable (e.g., salad)?

Avoid Describing Foods as Bad or Good. Explain Nutrient Density of Foods (*Hunter & Cason, 2006)

- Foods that are nutrient dense (low in calories):
  - Fruits and vegetables that are bright or deeply colored
  - Foods that are fortified
  - Lower fat versions of meats, milk, dairy products, and eggs
- Foods that are less nutrient dense (high in calories, low or no nutrients)
  - Are lighter or whiter in color
  - Contain a lot of refined sugar
  - Contain refined products (white bread as compared to whole grains)
  - Contain high amounts of fat for the amount of nutrients compared to similar products (fat-free milk versus ice cream)

- For example:
  - ○ An apple is a better choice than a bag of pretzels with the same number of calories, but the apple provides fiber, vitamin C, and potassium.
  - ○ An orange is better than orange juice because it has fiber.
  - ○ Water is better than any sugar drink even 100% fruit juice.
- Keep a list of positive outcomes and health benefits (e.g., sleep better, lower blood pressure)

Initiate Health Teaching and Referrals, as Indicated

- Refer to support groups (e.g., Weight Watchers, Overeaters Anonymous, TOPS).
- Suggest that the individual plan to walk or exercise with someone.

Overweight

Definition

A condition in which an individual accumulates abnormal or excessive fat for age and gender

Defining Characteristics

Adult: BMI of >25 kg/m^2
Child <2 years: Weight-for-length >95th percentile
Child 2 to 18 years: BMI of >85th but <95th percentile, or 25 kg/m^2 (whichever is smaller)

Related Factors

Physiological

Genetic disorder
Heritability of interrelated factors (e.g., adipose tissue distribution, energy expenditure, lipoprotein lipase activity, lipid synthesis, lipolysis)

Treatment-Related

Prolonged steroid therapy
Diminished sense of taste and/or smell (will diminish satiety)

Situational (Personal, Environment)

Economically disadvantaged
Fear regarding lack of food supply
Intake in excess of metabolic requirements
Reported undesirable eating patterns
   Frequent snacking
   High disinhibition and restrained eating behavior score
   High frequency of restaurant or fried food
   Portion sizes larger than recommended
   Consumption of sugar-sweetened beverages
   Disordered eating behaviors (e.g., binge eating, extreme
     weight control)
   Disordered eating perceptions
Energy expenditure below energy intake based on standard assessment (e.g., WAVE assessment[24])
   Sedentary activity patterns
   Sedentary behavior occurring for >2 hr/day
   Average daily physical activity is less than recommended for
     gender and age
Sleep disorder, shortened sleep time
Excessive alcohol consumption
Low dietary calcium intake in children
Obesity in childhood
Parental obesity

Pregnancy
Maternal diabetes mellitus
Maternal smoking

Maturational

Neonates/Infants
Formula- or mixed-fed infants
Premature pubarche
Rapid weight gain during childhood
Rapid weight gain during infancy, including the first week, first
  4 months, and first year
Solid foods as major food source at <5 months of age

NOC
Nutritional Status: Nutrient Intake, Weight Control, Exercise Participation, Infant Nutritional Status, Weight Body Mass, Adherence Behavior: Healthy Diet, Weight Loss Behavior

Goals

The individual will commit to a weight-loss program, as evidenced by the following indicators:

- Identify the patterns of eating associated with consumption/energy expenditure imbalance
- Give examples of nutrient dense foods versus those with empty calories
- Identify three ways to increase his or her activity
- Commit to increasing foods with high nutrient density and less with empty calories
- Commit to making 3 to 5 changes in food/fluid choices, which are healthier

The child (over 8) will verbalize what is healthy eating by the following indicators:

- Describe the "MyPlate"
- Describe what "empty calories" mean
- Name empty calories beverages and healthier substitutions
- Name foods high in nutrients
- Name food high in sugar and empty calories, and healthier substitutions

The pregnant woman will verbalize healthy eating and recommended weight gain during pregnancy by the following indicators:

- Describe vitamin, mineral, protein, and fat needs during pregnancy
- Give examples of nutrient dense foods versus those with empty calories
- Identify three ways to increase his or her activity
- Relate the weight gain specific to her weight prior to pregnancy
- Explain why "dieting" is problematic

NIC
Self-Efficacy Enhancement, Self-Responsibility Enhancement, Nutritional Counseling, Weight Management, Teaching: Nutrition (age appropriate), Behavioral Modification, Exercise Promotion, Coping Enhancement

Interventions

Refer to *Risk for Overweight* for interventions for overweight individuals.

Risk for Overweight

Definition

Vulnerable to abnormal or excessive fat accumulation for age and gender, which may compromise health

Risk Factors

Adult: BMI approaching >25 kg/m^2
Average daily physical activity is less than recommended for gender and age
Child <2 years: Weight-for-length approaching 95th percentile
Child 2 to 18 years: BMI approaching 85th percentile, or 25 kg/m^2 (whichever is smaller)
Children who are crossing BMI percentiles upward
Children with high BMI percentiles
Consumption of sugar-sweetened beverages
Disordered eating behaviors (e.g., binge eating, extreme weight control)
Disordered eating perceptions
Eating in response to external cues (e.g., time of day, social situations)
Eating in response to internal cues other than hunger (e.g., anxiety)
Economically disadvantaged
Energy expenditure below energy intake based on standard assessment (e.g., WAVE assessment[25])
Excessive alcohol consumption
Fear regarding lack of food supply
Formula- or mixed-fed infants
Frequent snacking
Genetic disorder
Heritability of interrelated factors (e.g., adipose tissue distribution, energy expenditure, lipoprotein lipase activity, lipid synthesis, lipolysis)
High disinhibition and restrained eating behavior score
High frequency of restaurant or fried food
Higher baseline weight at beginning of each pregnancy
Low dietary calcium intake in children
Maternal diabetes mellitus
Maternal smoking

Obesity in childhood
Parental obesity
Portion sizes larger than recommended
Premature pubarche
Rapid weight gain during childhood
Rapid weight gain during infancy, including the first week, first 4 months, and first year
Sedentary behavior occurring for >2 hr/day
Shortened sleep time
Sleep disorder
Solid foods as major food source at <5 months of age

Situational (Personal, Environmental)

Related to risk of gaining more than 25 to 30 lb when pregnant

Related to lack of basic nutrition knowledge

Maturational

Adult/Older Adult
Related to decreased activity patterns, decreased metabolic needs

NOC
Nutritional Status, Weight Control

Goals

The person will describe why he or she is at risk for weight gain, as evidenced by the following indicators:

- Describe reasons for increased intake with taste or olfactory deficits
- Discuss the nutritional needs during pregnancy
- Discuss the effects of exercise on weight control

NIC
Self-Efficacy Enhancement, Self-Responsibility Enhancement, Nutritional Counseling, Weight Management, Teaching: Nutrition (age appropriate), Behavioral Modification, Exercise Promotion, Coping Enhancement

Interventions

Initiate Discussion: "How Can You Be Healthier?"

- Focus on the person's response (e.g., stop smoking, exercise more, eat healthier, and cut down on drinking).
- Refer to index for interventions for the targeted lifestyle change.

Before a Person Can Change, They Must (*Martin et al., 2010)

- Know what change is necessary (information and why)
- Desire the change (motivation)
- Have the tools to achieve and maintain the change (strategy)
- Trust the health-care professional, who has a sympathetic presence (Pelzang, 2010)

If Appropriate, Gently and Expertly Teach the Hazards of Obesity But Respect a Person's Right to Choose, the Right of Self-Determination

- How do you think being overweight affects you?

If the Person Does Not Identify Any Negative Effects of Excess Weight That They Feel

- Ask them one of the questions below; pick the best question that applies to this person, use language they understand (blood vessels or blood tubes) as:
  - Do your legs swell during the day and go back to normal during the night?
    - Explain fat tissue compresses tubes in your legs and prevent fluids from circulating well. Eventually the swelling will be permanent, 24 hours a day, causing difficulty walking and wearing shoes.
  - Do you have high blood pressure or is it getting a little higher each year?
    - Explain that blood vessels are damaged when excess weight puts pressure on them and they stretch, become thinner and lose their strength. Your heart now has to pump harder, causing high blood pressure. Over time, the heart enlarges and cannot pump well. This is heart failure.
  - Is your cholesterol level increasing each year?
    - Explain that the stretching of your blood vessels damages the inside of the blood tubes. Cholesterol sticks to the damaged tubes and slows the blood flow to your kidneys, eyes, brain, and legs. This can cause strokes, renal failure, vision problems, and blood clots in your legs.

- ○ So you may not feel that anything is wrong, but high blood pressure can permanently damage your heart, brain, eyes, and kidneys before you feel anything. Even losing 10 lb can reduce your blood pressure.
- Is your blood glucose test getting a little higher each year? Is there diabetes in your family?
  - ○ Explain the more fatty tissue you have, the more resistant your cells become to insulin.
  - ○ Insulin carries glucose from blood to the cells. When you are overweight, the cells are damaged and will not absorb the insulin. So your blood glucose goes up. High blood glucose damages blood vessels in the eyes, kidneys, and heart.
- Does your back, knees, or other joints hurt?
  - ○ Explain that extra weight puts pressure on your joints and bones. This pressure wears away the cartilage, the cushion at the ends of your bones. This causes the bone to rub against another bone causing pain.
- Do you think people who are overweight have problem healing from injuries or surgery?
  - ○ Explain that fat tissue has less blood supply, which is needed for healing. The incision has more pressure against, when you are overweight, which can cause the wound to open up. If antibiotics are needed for infection, the medicine does not work well because of poor circulation to the wound.
- Advise them to focus on a goal of losing 5 lb. Emphasize how heavy 5 lb of sugar is and that every 5 lb lost is less work for their heart and less strain on their joints. A reduction in calories and increase in activity can cause a weight loss of about 2 lb a week
- Refer interested individual to the National Institute of Diabetes and Digestive and Kidney Diseases (NIDDK) website article, "Do You Know Some of the Health Risks of Being Overweight?"

Eating Healthier

Refer to Eating Healthier under *Obesity* nursing diagnosis.

🦵 Maternal Interventions

Discuss the Total Weight Gain Appropriate For the Individual
(Institute of Medicine, 2009)

- 25 to 35 lb if you were a healthy weight before pregnancy, with a BMI of 18.5 to 24.9.

- 28 to 40 lb if you were underweight before pregnancy with a BMI of less than 18.5.
- 15 to 25 lb if you were overweight before pregnancy with a BMI of 25 to 29.9.
- 11 to 20 lb if you were obese before pregnancy with a BMI of over 30.

Explain Healthy Weight Gain for Each Trimester (Institute of Medicine, 2009)

- 1 to 4.5 lb during the first trimester
- Approximately, 1 to 2 lb/week in the second trimester
- Approximately, 1 to 2 lb/week in the third trimester

Explain the Problems That Can Occur With Too Much Weight Gain During Pregnancy (Institute of Medicine, 2009)

- Gestational diabetes
- Leg pain
- Varicose veins
- High blood pressure
- Backaches
- Increased fatigue
- Increased risk of cesarean delivery

Stress the Importance of Not Dieting and Skipping Meals But Instead Consume Recommended Portions and Avoid High-Fat/ Carbohydrate Foods

- Refer to *Imbalanced Nutrition* for dietary recommendation for pregnant woman (e.g., "MyPlate," vitamins, calcium)

Initiate Discussion: "How Can You Be Healthier?"

- Focus on response (e.g., stop smoking, exercise more, eat healthier, and stop drinking alcohol).
- Refer to index for interventions for the targeted lifestyle change.

Discuss Nutritional Intake and Weight Gain During Pregnancy

Discuss the Total Weight Gain Appropriate For the Client (Institute of Medicine, 2009)

- 25 to 35 lb if you were a healthy weight before pregnancy, with a BMI of 18.5 to 24.9.
- 28 to 40 lb if you were underweight before pregnancy with a BMI of less than 18.5.
- 15 to 25 lb if you were overweight before pregnancy with a BMI of 25 to 29.9.
- 11 to 20 lb if you were obese before pregnancy with a BMI of over 30.

⚛ Pediatric Interventions

Try to Engage the Child and Family to Realize the Importance of Good Nutrition and Exercise

Discuss With Family the Hazards of Being Overweight as a Child

- Childhood obesity leads to adult obesity.
- Excess weight elevates blood pressure, heart rate, and cardiac output in children (see Key Concepts, Pediatric Considerations for other health dangers).
- As weight increases, activity decreases.

Address the Barriers to Parents Taking Action to Help Their Child Eat Better and Exercise More (under Pediatric Interventions)

- A belief that children will outgrow their excess weight
- Overweight parents feel they do not set a good example.
- A lack of knowledge about how to help their children control their weight
- A fear that they will cause an eating disorder in their children

Provide a Color Copy of "MyPlate"

- Refer to *Imbalance Nutrition* for interventions for healthy eating in children and adolescents.

Use Creative Methods With Younger Children to Teach Good Nutrition

- Create a felt board with each day of the week on it. Using pictures of food groups, vegetables, grains, milk, meat, cheese, yogurt, and fruits, have the child stick them to the board for that day.
- Read books that emphasize good food with more energy, strong muscles and bones, etc.

If Eating "Fast Foods" Points Out Healthier Choices

- Encourage portion control; educate children/adolescents that "large," "extra," "double," or "triple" will be high in calories and fat.
- Recommend smaller portions, since a regular serving is enough for most children, or sharing with a parent or sibling.
- Look for whole grain foods, fruits, vegetables, and calcium-rich foods.
- When planning a fast food meal, select an establishment that promotes healthier options at the point of purchase.

- Address strategies to improve nutrition when eating fast foods:
  - Drink skim milk.
  - Avoid French fries or share one order.
  - Choose grilled foods.
  - Eat salads and vegetables.
- Explore healthier fast foods at home (e.g., frozen dinners with three food groups).

Suggest Healthy Snacks at Home

- Offer fresh fruits, vegetables, cheese and crackers, low-fat milk, calcium-fortified juices, and frozen yogurt as snacks.

Initiate Health Teaching and Referrals, as Indicated

- Community programs (YM/WCA, adolescent support groups).
- Access additional information at www.uptodate.com/contents/fast-food-for-children-and-adolescents.

IMPAIRED PARENTING

NANDA-I Definition

Inability of the primary caregiver to create, maintain, or regain an environment that promotes the optimum growth and development of the child

Defining Characteristics

The home environment must be assessed for safety before discharge: location of bathroom, access to water, cooking facilities, and environmental barriers (e.g., stairs, narrow doorways).
Inappropriate and/or nonnurturing parenting behaviors
Lack of behavior indicating parental attachment
Inconsistent behavior management
Inconsistent care
Frequent verbalization of dissatisfaction or disappointment with infant/child
Verbalization of frustration with role

Verbalization of perceived or actual inadequacy
Diminished or inappropriate visual, tactile, or auditory stimulation of infant
Evidence of abuse or neglect of child
Growth and development challenges in infant/child

Related Factors

Individuals or families who may be at risk for developing or experiencing parenting difficulties

Parent(s)
Financial resources
Single
Addicted to drugs
Adolescent
Terminally ill

Abusive
Acutely disabled
Psychiatric disorder
Accident victim
Alcoholic

Child
Of unwanted pregnancy
With undesired characteristics
Terminally ill
With hyperactive characteristics

Mentally handicapped
Of undesired gender
Physically handicapped

Situational (Personal/Environmental)

Related to interruption of bonding process secondary to:
Illness (child/parent)
Relocation/change in cultural
environment

Incarceration

Related to separation from nuclear family

Related to lack of knowledge

Related to inconsistent caregivers or techniques

Related to relationship problems (specify):
Marital discord
Stepparents
Divorce

Live-in partner
Separation
Relocation

Related to little external support and/or socially isolated family

Related to lack of available role model

Related to ineffective adaptation to stressors associated with:
Illness
Economic problems
New baby

Substance abuse
Elder care

Maturational

Adolescent Parent

Related to the conflict of meeting own needs over child's

Related to history of ineffective relationships with own parents

Related to parental history of abusive relationship with parents

Related to unrealistic expectations of child by parent

Related to unrealistic expectations of self by parent

Related to unrealistic expectations of parent by child

Related to unmet psychosocial needs of child by parent

 Author's Note

The family environment should provide the basic needs for a child's physical growth and development: stimulation of the child's emotional, social, and cognitive potential; consistent, stable reinforcement to learn impulse control; it is the role of parents to provide such an environment. Most parenting difficulties stem from lack of knowledge or inability to manage stressors constructively. The ability to parent effectively is at high risk when the child or parent has a condition that increases stress on the family unit (e.g., illness, financial problems) (*Gage, Everett, & Bullock, 2006).

Impaired Parenting describes a parent experiencing difficulty creating or continuing a nurturing environment for a child. *Parental Role Conflict* describes a parent or parents whose previously effective functioning is challenged by external factors. In certain situations, such as illness, divorce, or remarriage, role confusion and conflict are expected; thus, *Risk for Impaired Parenting* would be useful. At present, *Risk for Impaired Parenting* is not an approved NANDA-I nursing diagnosis.

NOC

Parenting Performance; Specify age (e.g., adolescent, toddler); Child Development; Abuse Cessation; Abuse Recovery

Goals

The parent/primary caregiver demonstrates two effective skills to increase parenting effectiveness, as evidenced by the following indicators:

- Will acknowledge an issue with parenting skills
- Will identify resources available for assistance with improvement of parenting skills that are culturally considerate

NIC

Anticipatory Guidance; Counseling; Developmental Enhancement; Family Support; Family Therapy; Parenting Promotion; Family Integrity: Promotion

Interventions

Encourage Parents to Express Frustrations Regarding Role Responsibilities, Parenting, or Both

- Convey empathy.
- Reserve judgment.
- Convey/offer educational information based on assessment.
- Help foster realistic expectations.
- Encourage discussion of feelings regarding unmet expectations.
- Discuss individualized, achievable, and culturally considerate strategies (e.g., discussing with partner, child; setting personal goals).

Educate Parents About Normal Growth and Development and Age-Related Expected Behaviors

- Refer to *Delayed Growth and Development*.

Explore With Parents the Child's Problem Behavior

- Frequency, duration, context (when, where triggers)
- Consequences (parental attention, discipline, inconsistencies in response)
- Behavior desired by parents

Discuss Guidelines for Promoting Acceptable Behavior in Children (Hockenberry & Wilson, 2015)

- Convey to the child that he or she is loved.
- Positive reinforcement is an effective and recommended discipline technique for all ages.
- Redirecting is effective for infants to school-age, whereas verbal instruction/explanation is most effective for school-age and adolescents.
- Set realistic expectations for behavior based on child's level of understanding and developmental stage.
- When reprimanding child, focus on the bad behavior or action, not insinuating that the child is bad.
- Watch for potential scenarios where child might be likely to misbehave such as the child being overtired or overexcited. Change conditions when able to or have strategies in place to minimize bad behavior.

- Help child develop self-control techniques.
- Demonstrate and discuss acceptable and expected social behaviors.
- Minimize bad behavior by ignoring minor transgressions which will eventually stop the act or behavior (Ball, Bindler, & Cowen, 2015).
- Make promises only when they can be kept (Ball et al., 2015).

Explain the Discipline Technique of "Time-Out" (Ball et al., 2015)

- "Time-out," refers to a discipline technique that places child in a designated, isolated area. This area does not include toys or games and serves a consequence of undesirable behavior. Typically the length of time recommended is 1 min/year of age.
- Time-out provides a cooling-off period for both child and parent.
- Explain to the child what to expect from the time-out as well as why they have found themselves in it.
- Start the timer only when the child is quiet, and reset timer for acting out that occurs while in time-out.
- Make sure the individual minimize any distractions while child is in time-out (e.g., turn off television or make sure television cannot be seen or heard).

Acknowledge Cultural Impacts on Parent/Caregiver's Disciplinary Methods (Ball et al., 2015)

- Expected behaviors emerge from the family's preexisting cultural values and beliefs.
- The child learns cultural values and expected roles and behaviors as they grow.
- Immigrant families may face challenges as they work toward not only raising their child in their inherent culture but also adapting to the culture of which they have immigrated to.
- Different cultures place varying levels of importance on different aspects of childrearing (e.g., grandparents as active caregivers, families with large numbers of children, responsibilities expected of the child).

Acknowledge and Encourage Parent/Caregiver's Strengths in Their Parenting Role (Ball et al., 2015)

- Focus on family competence.
- Validate family member's emotions.
- Help family member recognize that they can bring prior positive life experiences to their current situation in coping with a child's health-care concern.

Provide General Parenting Guidelines (Hockenberry & Wilson, 2015)

- Be consistent with disciplinary techniques in terms of type of punishment for type of infraction.
- Be adaptable and flexible when it comes to child's behavior and setting.
- As child gets older, provide privacy to administer punishment to avoid public shaming.
- Avoid repeated lecturing or bringing up of infraction once punishment for a specific incident is completed and addressed.
- Show unity among parents/caregivers when it comes to discipline and expected behavior.
- Follow through with punishments and the initial details set forth. Avoid becoming distracted.
- Praise children for acceptable or desired behavior.
- Serve as a role model in acting in a way that you wish your child to act.
- Address misbehavior upon its discovery.
- Set and explain clear and expected rules for behavior with consideration to child's age and level of understanding.

Initiate Appropriate Referrals as Indicated

POST-TRAUMA SYNDROME

Post-Trauma Syndrome

Risk for Post-Trauma Syndrome

Rape-Trauma Syndrome (Sexual Assault Trauma Syndrome)

NANDA-I Definition

Sustained maladaptive response to a traumatic, overwhelming event

A response to a horrific, overwhelming event "characterized by intrusive thoughts, nightmares and flashbacks of past traumatic events, avoidance of reminders of trauma, hypervigilance, and sleep disturbance, all of which lead to considerable social, occupational, and interpersonal dysfunction" (Ciechanowski, 2014)

Defining Characteristics

Stressor criterion
"Has been exposed to a catastrophic event involving actual or threatened death or injury, or a threat to the physical integrity of himself or herself or others (such as sexual violence).[26] Indirect exposure includes learning about the violent or accidental death or perpetration of sexual violence to a loved one" (Friedman, 2016).

Intrusive recollection criterion
Persistent re-experience of the traumatic event through recurrent intrusive recollections of the event, dreams about the event, flashbacks

Avoidance criterion
Avoidance of the stimuli associated with the event, talking about it, avoiding activities, people or places that arouse memories, feeling numb, constricted affect, detachment, alienation[1]

Negative cognitions and mood criterion
Alterations in mood, chronic depression

Alterations in arousal or reactivity criterion
Persistent symptoms of increased arousal, hypervigilance, difficulty sleeping, difficulty concentration

Duration criterion
Symptoms must persist for at least one month before posttraumatic stress disorder (PTSD) may be diagnosed.

Functional significance criterion
Must experience significant social, occupational, or other distress as a result of these symptoms.

NANDA-I Defining Characteristics

Flashbacks, intrusive dreams, intrusive thoughts
Repetitive nightmares
Guilt*
Shames, anxiety*, or panic attacks*
Hopelessness

Dissociative amnesia
Aggression, alienation
Alteration in concentration
Alteration in mood
Compulsive behaviors
Reports of feeling numb*, alienation*

---

[26]DSM-5 Seven Criteria for PTSD Diagnosis (American Psychiatric Association, 2014; Friedman, 2016).

Fear* of repetition, death, or loss of bodily control
Anger, rage, horror
Hypervigilance, avoidance behaviors
Exaggerated startle response
Avoidance behaviors, reports feeling numb
Confusion
Reduced interest in significant activities
Substance abuse*
Thrill-seeking activities
Avoidance behaviors, enuresis (in children)*
Irritability*

Related Factors

Situational (Personal, Environmental)

Related to traumatic events of natural origin, including:
Floods
Earthquakes
Volcanic eruptions
Storms
Avalanches
Epidemics*
Disasters*

Related to traumatic events of human origin, such as:
Concentration camp confinement
Serious accidents (e.g., industrial, motor vehicle)*
Assault
Torture*
Rape
Bombing
Large fires
Witnessing violent death*
Terrorist attacks
War*
Witnessing mutilation*
Being held prisoner of war*
Criminal victimization*
Airplane crashes
Abuse (e.g., physical, psychological)*

Related to industrial disasters(nuclear, chemical, or other life-threatening accidents)*

Related to serious threat or injury to loved ones and/or self

Related to tragic occurrence involving multiple deaths

Related to events outside the range of unusual human experience

Related to sudden destruction of one's home and/ or community

 Author's Note

Post-Trauma Syndrome represents a group of emotional responses to a traumatic event of either natural origin (e.g., floods, volcanic eruptions, earthquakes) or human origin (e.g., war, torture). The emotional responses (e.g., hypervigilance, avoidance, flashbacks, fear, anger) can interfere with interpersonal relationships and daily-life responsibilities. This assessment will provide data to formulate nursing diagnoses. It is through these nursing diagnoses that direct nursing interventions not *Post-Trauma Syndrome*, which is too broad.

From an historical perspective, the significant change ushered in by the PTSD concept was the stipulation that the etiological agent was outside the individual (i.e., a traumatic event) rather than an inherent individual's weakness (i.e., a traumatic neurosis). The key to understanding the scientific basis and clinical expression of PTSD is the concept of "trauma" (Friedman, 2016).

NANDA-I retired the diagnosis *Rape-Trauma Syndrome* in 2011 because no revisions have been submitted. The author has revised this diagnosis since 1975 and therefore it will be retained in this work. This diagnosis should be renamed *Sexual Assault Syndrome*. This label change will more clearly describe the event as a violent attack and may decrease the biases surrounding rape (e.g., was in a dangerous neighborhood, went on a date with him).

Based on the most recent definition of syndrome nursing diagnoses as a cluster of associated nursing diagnoses, this diagnosis does not represent a syndrome and would be more accurately labeled *Rape-Trauma Response*. The inclusion of causative or contributing factors with this category is unnecessary, because the etiology is always rape. Thus, the nurse omits the second part of the diagnostic statement; however, he or she can add the individual's report of the rape to the statement. For example, *Rape-Trauma Response as evidenced by the report of a sexual assault and sodomy on June 22 and multiple facial bruises* (refer to ER record for description).

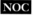

NOC
Abuse Recovery, Coping, Fear Control

Goals

In the short term, the individual will do the following:

- Acknowledge the traumatic event and begin to work with the trauma
- Make connections with support persons/resources
- Engage in activities that reduce stress and improve coping

As evidenced by the following indicators:

- Talk about the experience and express feelings such as fear, anger, and guilt
- Identify sources of support

- Identify three coping strategies that may improve their quality of life (e.g., exercise, hobby, nature walks, thought-stopping)

In the long term, the individual will assimilate the experience into a meaningful whole and go on to pursue his or her life, as evidenced by goal setting and the following indicators:

- Report a lessening of re-experiencing the trauma or numbing symptoms
- Report feelings of support and comfort from individuals and/or support groups (Halter, 2014; Varcarolis, 2011)
- Report engaging in regular activities (daily, weekly) that enhance coping
- Report cognitive coping strategies that have their improved sense of control

NIC

Counseling, Anxiety Reduction, Emotional Support, Family Support, Support System Enhancement, Coping Enhancement, Active Listening, Presence, Grief Work, Facilitation, Referral

Interventions

Screen individuals of all ages for abuse; someone may be holding on to this secret for a lifetime.

Determine If the Person Has Experienced a Traumatic Event

- During the interview, secure a quiet room where there will be no interruptions but easy access to other staff in case of management problems.
- Be aware that talking about a traumatic experience may cause significant discomfort to the person.
- If the individual becomes too anxious, discontinue the assessment and help the individual regain control of the distress or provide other appropriate interventions.

Document the Person's Responses

Evaluate the Severity of the Responses and Effects on Current Functioning

- Assess for any suicidal or homicidal thoughts (Varcarolis, 2011).
- Refer to *Risk for Suicide*. Consult with law enforcement if needed.

- If alcohol/drug abuse is present, determine whether at risk for withdrawal (e.g., alcohol, opioids). Consult physician, NP, or PA for prevention.

Assist Individual to Decrease Extremes of Re-experiencing or Numbing Symptoms

- Provide a safe, therapeutic environment where the individual can regain control.
- Reassure the individual that others who have experienced such traumatic events often experienced these feelings/symptoms.
- Stay with the individual and offer support during an episode of high anxiety (see *Anxiety* for additional information).
- Assist individual to control impulsive acting-out behavior by setting limits, promoting ventilation, and redirecting excess energy into physical exercise or activity (e.g., walking, jogging). (See *Risk for Self-Harm* and *Risk for Violence* for additional information.)
- Provide techniques to reduce anxiety (e.g., progressive relaxation, deep breathing).

Assist Individual to Identify and Make Connections With Support People and Resources

- Help individual to identify his or her strength and resources.
- Explore available support systems.
- Assist individual to make connections with support and resources according to his or her needs.
- Assist individual to resume old activities and explore some new ones, such as exercise, nature walks, and hobbies.

Assist Family/Significant Others

- Assist them to understand what is happening to the individual.
- Be specific about the various responses the individual can display.
- Encourage expression of their feelings.
- Provide counseling sessions or link them with appropriate community resources, as necessary.

Provide Nursing Care Appropriate to Each Individual's Traumatic Experience and Needs

Provide or Arrange Follow-Up Treatment in Which the Individual Can Continue to Work Through the Trauma and to Integrate the Experience into a New Self-Concept

Risk for Post-Trauma Syndrome

NANDA-I Definition

Vulnerable for sustained maladaptive response to a traumatic, overwhelming event, which may compromise health

Risk Factors

Refer to Related Factors in *Post-Trauma Syndrome*.

Goals

The individual will continue to function appropriately after the traumatic event and relate he or she will seek professional help, as evidenced by the following indicators:

- Identify signs or symptoms that necessitate professional consultation
- Express feelings regarding traumatic event

Interventions

Refer to *Post-Trauma Syndrome*.

Rape-Trauma Syndrome[27] (Sexual Assault Trauma Syndrome)

Definition

Sustained maladaptive response to a forced, violent sexual penetration against the victim's will and consent (NANDA-I)

---

[27]This diagnosis has been retired by NANDA-I because it has not been revised and updated. The author has revised and updated this diagnosis and thus will retain it for its clinical usefulness.

State in which an individual experiences a forced, violent sexual assault (vaginal or anal penetration) against his or her will and without his or her consent. The trauma syndrome that develops from this attack or attempted attack includes an acute phase of disorganization of the victim and family's lifestyle and a long-term process of reorganization of lifestyle (Burgess, 1995).[28]

Defining Characteristics

Reports or evidence of sexual assault
If the victim is a child, parents may experience similar responses.

Acute Phase

Somatic Responses

Physical Trauma (Bruises, Soreness)
Gastrointestinal irritability (nausea, vomiting, anorexia, diarrhea)
Genitourinary discomfort (pain, pruritus, vaginal discharge)
Skeletal muscle tension (spasms, pain, headaches, sleep
  disturbances)

Psychological Responses

Overt
Crying, sobbing
Feelings of revenge
Change in relationships*

Hyperalertness*
Volatility, anger
Confusion, incoherence,
  disorientation*

Ambiguous Reaction
Confusion*, incoherence,
  disorientation*
Masked facies
Calm, numbness

Shock*, numbness, confusion*,
  or disbelieving
Distractibility and difficulty
  making decisions

Emotional Reaction
Self-blame
Fear*—of being alone or that the rapist will return (a child
  victim fears punishment, repercussions, abandonment,
  rejection)
Denial, shock, humiliation, and embarrassment*

---

[28]The author has added to the NANDA-I definition to enhance usefulness and
  clarity.

Desire for revenge; anger*
Guilt, shame
Fatigue

Sexual Responses

Mistrust of men (if victim is a woman)
Change in sexual behavior, sexual dysfunction*

Long-Term Phase (Varcarolis, Carlson, & Shoemaker, 2006)

Any response of the acute phase may continue if resolution does not occur. In addition, the following reactions can occur 2 or more weeks after the assault.

Psychological Responses

Change in relationship(s) associated with nonsupportive parent, partner, relative, friend (e.g., blames victim for event, "taking too long to get over it")
Intrusive thoughts (anger toward assailant, flashbacks of the traumatic event, dreams, insomnia)
Increased motor activity (moving, taking trips, staying some other place)
Increased emotional lability (intense anxiety, mood swings, crying spells, depression)
Fears and phobias (of indoors, or outdoors, where the rape occurred, of being alone, of crowds, of sexual encounters (with partner or potential partners)

◷ Author's Note

Department of Justice's National Crime Victimization Survey (NCVS)—there is an average of 293,066 victims (age 12 or older) of rape and sexual assault each year (U.S. Department of Justice, 2014).

The word rape has a history of being viewed as a crime of passion not a crime of violence. Sexual assault is defined as any sexual activity involving a person who does not or cannot (due to alcohol, drugs, or some sort of incapacitation) consent. The phrase sexual assault denotes unprovoked violence, which defines the perpetrator as the criminal and the victim as a "victim of a crime." Rape/Sexual Assault can be defined differently by states. The author has interacted with numerous girls and women who have shared their sexual assault; some for the first time in their lives. Two themes are woven into their stories: (1) guilt that they contributed to the assault and (2) profound disappointment with their mother's response.

Many mothers blamed their daughter for the event and sometimes refuse to believe their daughter if a relative or paramour is involved; or they suggest their daughter provoked the event. Perhaps that was the only reaction a mother could have at the time, because she could not face the truth. I discussed forgiveness with these women. Forgiveness never means you accept what happened, only that you are going to release the pain from yourself. It is a gift you give yourself.

Girls and women shared stories that the rape would not have happened if they had not:

Worn that short skirt
Drank too much
Walked home in the dark
Had engaged in kissing and hugging
Had not went somewhere alone with him

The author shares with each girl or woman this scenario: Instead of being sexually assaulted, imagine that you were hit over the head with a shovel. Would it have mattered what you were wearing, doing, or saying at the time? Sexual assault is not sex, it is a violent act like hitting someone with a shovel. The author suggests when thoughts of self-blame surface, these women think of the shovel.

NOC
Abuse Protection, Abuse Recovery, Coping

Goals

The individual, parents, spouse, or significant other will return to precrisis level of functioning, and the child will express feelings concerning the assault and the treatment based on the following indicators:

Short-Term Goals
* Share feelings
* Describe rationale and treatment procedures
* Sexual Assault Response Team (SART)

Interventions

Ask the Person: How Can I Help You?

* If sexual assault is suspected, access the institution's protocol (e.g., Sexual Assault Nursing Examiners [SANE], Sexual Assault Response Team [SART], Women against Rape [WAR]).

Assist the Individual in Identifying Major Concerns (Psychological, Medical, and Legal) and Perception of Help Needed

- Assess vulnerable older adults for abuse.
- Researchers analyzed data from 5,777 adults aged 60 years or older in a randomly selected national sample. One-year prevalence was 4.6% for emotional abuse, 1.6% for physical abuse, 0.6% for sexual abuse, 5.1% for potential neglect, and 5.2% for current financial abuse by a family member. Slightly under 7% reported sexual mistreatment before age 60 (Acierno et al., 2010).

Explain What the Person Will Experience

- The interview
- Examination, evidence collection
- Prevention of sexually transmitted diseases, pregnancy
- Police investigation

Fulfill Medical–Legal Responsibilities by Documentation (Ledray, 2001)

- Follow institution's protocol.

Explain the Risks of Sexually Transmitted Infections (Centers for Disease Control and Prevention, 2008; Ledray, 2001)

- Sexually transmitted diseases (specimens, blood tests): Gonorrhea, Human immunodeficiency virus (HIV), Trichomoniasis, Syphilis, Hepatitis B, A, C, Chlamydia.
- Consult with protocol or physician/nurse practitioner/physician assistant for prophylaxis for Chlamydia, HIV, Trichomoniasis, and Gonorrhea.
- Vaccinate individuals if needed for tetanus and Hepatitis A, B.
- Determine if the woman is at risk for pregnancy and, if at risk, explain emergency contraceptive pills (ECP).

Eliminate or Reduce Somatic Symptomatology

Genitourinary Discomfort
Pain
- Assess for quality and duration.
- Monitor intake and output.
- Inspect urine and external genitalia for bleeding.
- Listen attentively to the victim's description of pain.
- Give pain medication per physician's order (see *Impaired Comfort*).

Discharge
- Assess amount, color, and odor of discharge.
- Allow the victim time to wash and change garments after initial examination has been completed.

Itching
- Encourage bathing in cool water.
- Avoid use of detergent soaps.
- Avoid touching the area causing discomfort.

Skeletal Muscle Tension
Headaches
- Avoid any sudden change of the victim's position.
- Approach the victim calmly.
- Slightly elevate the bed (unless contraindicated).
- Discuss pain-reducing measures that have been effective in the past.

Fatigue
- Assess present sleeping patterns if altered (see *Disturbed Sleep Pattern*).
- Discuss precipitating factors for sleep disturbance; try to eliminate them, if possible.
- Provide frequent rest periods throughout the day.
- Avoid interruptions during sleep.
- Avoid stress-producing situations.

Generalized Bruising and Edema
- Avoid constrictive garments.
- Handle affected body parts gently.
- Elevate affected body part, if edema is present.
- Apply a cool, moist compress to the edematous area for the first 24 hours, then a warm compress after 24 hours.
- Encourage the victim to verbalize discomfort.
- Record any bruises, lacerations, edema, or abrasions.

Proceed With Health Teaching to Victim and Family

- Before the victim leaves the hospital, provide a card with information about follow-up appointments and names and telephone numbers of local crisis and counseling centers.
- Plan a home visit or telephone call.
- Arrange for legal or pastoral counseling, if appropriate.
- Recommend and make referrals to a psychotherapist, mental health clinic, citizen action, or community group advocacy-related service.

POWERLESSNESS

Powerlessness

Risk for Powerlessness

NANDA-I Definition

The lived experience of lack of control over a situation, including a perception that one's actions do not significantly affect an outcome

Defining Characteristics

Overt (anger, apathy) or covert expressions of dissatisfaction over inability to control a situation (e.g., work, illness, prognosis, care, recovery rate) that negatively affects outlook, goals, and lifestyle

Inability to access valued resources (food, shelter, income, education, employment)

Belief that one has little or no control over the cause or the solutions of one's problems

Lack of Information-Seeking Behaviors

Excessive dependence on others

Acting-out behavior

Violent behavior

Inability to effectively problem solve

Passivity

Apathy

Anger

Feelings of alienation

Low self-efficacy

Resignation

Anxiety

Depression

Sense of vulnerability

Feelings of helplessness

Related Factors

Pathophysiologic

Any disease process, acute or chronic, can cause or contribute to powerlessness. Some common sources are the following:

Related to inability to communicate secondary to:
Stroke
Alzheimer's or Parkinson's disease (dysarthria)
Intubation, mechanical ventilation, or tracheostomy

Related to inability to perform activities of daily living secondary to such conditions as:

Stroke

Cervical trauma

Myocardial infarction

Pain

Related to inability to perform role responsibilities secondary to surgery, trauma, or arthritis

Related to progressive debilitating disease secondary to such diseases as multiple sclerosis, terminal cancer, or AIDS

Related to substance abuse

Related to cognitive distortions secondary to mental health disorders

Situational (Personal, Environmental)

Related to change from curative status to palliative status

Related to feeling of loss of control and lifestyle restrictions secondary to (specify)

Related to overeating patterns

Related to personal characteristics that highly value control (e.g., internal locus of control)

Related to effects of hospital or institutional limitations

Related to elevated fear of disapproval

Related to consistent negative feedback

Related to long-term abusive relationships

Related to oppressive patriarchal values with women

Related to the presence of an abusive relationships with a history of mental illness (Orzeck, Rokach, & Chin, 2010)

Maturational

Older Adult

Related to multiple losses secondary to aging (e.g., retirement, sensory deficits, motor deficits, money, significant others)

 Author's Note

Powerlessness is a feeling that all people experience to varying degrees in various situations. Stephenson (* 1979) described two types of powerlessness: (1) *Situational powerlessness* occurs in a specific event and is probably short-lived and (2) *trait powerlessness* is more pervasive, affecting general outlook, goals, lifestyle, and relationships.

Hopelessness differs from powerlessness in that a hopeless individual sees no solution to problems or no way to achieve what is desired, even if he or she feels in control. A powerless individual may see an alternative yet is unable to do anything about it because of perception of lack of control and resources. Prolonged powerlessness may lead to hopelessness.

NOC
Depression Control, Health Beliefs, Health Beliefs: Perceived Control, Participation: Health Care Decisions

Goals

The individual will verbalize ability to control or influence situations and outcomes, as evidenced by the following indicators:

- Identify the factors that the individual can control
- Make decisions regarding his or her care, treatment, and future when possible

NIC
Mood Management, Teaching: Individual, Decision-Making Support, Self-Responsibility Facilitation, Health System Guidance, Spiritual Support

Interventions

Assess for Causative and Contributing Factors

- Lack of knowledge
- Previous inadequate coping patterns (e.g., depression; for discussion, see *Ineffective Coping* related to depression)
- Insufficient decision-making opportunities

Eliminate or Reduce Contributing Factors, If Possible

Lack of Knowledge
- Increase effective communication between individual and health-care provider.
- Explain all procedures, rules, and options to the individual; avoid medical jargon. Help the individual anticipate situations that will occur during treatments (provides reality-oriented cognitive images that bolster a sense of control and coping strategies).

- Allow time to answer questions; ask the individual to write questions down so that he or she does not forget them.
- Provide a specific time (10 to 15 minutes) per shift that the individual knows can be used to ask questions or discuss subjects as desired.
- Anticipate questions/interest and offer information. Help the individual to anticipate events and outcomes.
- While being realistic, point out positive changes in the individual's condition, such as serum enzymes decreasing after myocardial infarction or surgical incision healing well.
- Provide opportunities for the individual and family to identify with a primary nurse to establish continuity in provision of care and implementation of the care plan.
- If contributing factors are pain or anxiety, provide information about how to use behavioral control techniques (e.g., relaxation, imagery, deep breathing).

Provide Opportunities for the Individual to Control Decisions and to Identify Personal Goals of Care

- Allow the individual to manipulate surroundings, such as deciding what is to be kept where (shoes under bed, picture on window).
- If the individual desires, and as hospital policy permits, encourage the individual to bring personal effects from home (e.g., pillows, pictures).
- Do not offer options if there are none (e.g., a deep intramuscular [IM] Z-track injection must be rotated). Offer options that are personally relevant.
- Record the individual's specific choices in care plan to ensure that others on staff acknowledge preferences ("dislikes orange juice," "takes showers," "plan dressing change at 7:30 AM before shower").
- Keep promises.
- Provide opportunities for the individual and family to participate in care.
- Be alert for signs of paternalism/maternalism in health-care providers (e.g., making decisions for).
- Plan a care conference to allow staff to discuss methods of individualizing care; encourage each nurse to share at least one action that he or she discovered a particular individual likes.
- Shift emphasis from what one cannot do to what one can do.
- Set goals that are short term, behavioral, practical, and realistic (walk 5 more feet every day; then in 1 week, individual can walk to the television room).

Allow the Individual to Experience Outcomes That Result From His or Her Own Actions

Actively Involve an Individual With External Locus of Control to Encourage Participation

- Have the individual keep a record (e.g., food intake for 1 week; weight loss chart; exercise program; type and frequency of medications taken).
- Use telephone or e-mail contact to monitor the individual, if feasible.
- Provide explicit written directions (e.g., meal plans; exercise regimen—type, frequency, duration; speech practice lessons for aphasia).

Assist the Individual in Deriving Power From Other Sources

- Support use of other power sources (e.g., prayer, stress reduction techniques). Provide privacy and support for other measures the individual or family may request (e.g., meditation, imagery, special rituals).
- Suggest self-help groups focusing on empowerment.
- Offer referral to faith-based community resources (e.g., religious leaders, faith community nurse, house of worship).

Initiate Health Teaching and Referrals as Indicated (Social Worker, Psychiatric Nurse/Physician, Visiting Nurse, Religious Leader, Self-Help Groups)

Evaluate the Situation With the Individual

- When feelings of powerlessness have subsided, review with the individual what worked best to diminish or alleviate the intensity of the experience.

Pediatric Interventions

- Provide opportunities for the child to make decisions (e.g., set time for bath, hold still for injection).
- Engage the child in play therapy before and after a traumatic situation (refer to *Delayed Growth and Development* for specific interventions for age-related development needs).

Risk for Powerlessness

NANDA-I Definition

Vulnerable for the lived experience of lack of control over a situation, including a perception that one's actions do not significantly affect an outcome, which can compromise health

Risk Factors

Refer to Related Factors in *Powerlessness*.

Goals

The individual will continue to make decisions regarding his or her life, health care, and future, as evidenced by the following indicators:

- Engage in discussions of options
- Raise questions regarding choices

Interventions

Refer to *Powerlessness*.

INEFFECTIVE PROTECTION

Ineffective Protection

Risk for Corneal Injury

Risk for Dry Eye

Impaired Oral Mucous Membrane

Risk for Impaired Oral Mucous Membrane

Impaired Tissue Integrity

Impaired Skin Integrity

Risk for Impaired Skin Integrity

Pressure Ulcer

Risk for Pressure Ulcer

NANDA-I Definition

Decrease in the ability to guard self from internal or external threats, such as illness or injury

Defining Characteristics*

Deficient immunity

Impaired healing

Altered clotting

Maladaptive stress response

Neurosensory alterations

Pressure ulcers

Chilling

Insomnia

Perspiring

Fatigue

Dyspnea

Anorexia

Cough

Weakness

Itching

Immobility

Restlessness

Disorientation

 Author's Note

This broad diagnosis describes an individual with compromised ability to defend against microorganisms, bleeding, or both because of immuno-suppression, myelosuppression, abnormal clotting factors, or all these. Use of this diagnosis entails several potential problems.

The nurse is cautioned against substituting *Ineffective Protection* for an immune system compromise, acquired immunodeficiency syndrome (AIDS), disseminated intravascular coagulation, diabetes mellitus, or other disorders. Rather, the nurse should focus on diagnoses describing the individual's functional abilities that are or may be compromised by altered protection, such as *Fatigue*, *Risk for Infection*, and *Risk for Social Isolation*. The nurse also should address the physiologic complications of altered protection that require nursing and medical interventions for management, identifying appropriate collaborative problems as *RC of Sickle Cell Crisis* and *RC of Opportunistic Infections*.

NANDA-I approved two new nursing diagnoses—*Pressure Ulcer* and *Risk for Pressure Ulcers*. These new diagnoses make *Impaired Skin Integrity* and *Risk for Impaired Skin Integrity* unnecessary and inconsistent with the appropriate clinical language—*Pressure Ulcer*.

Risk Factors

Pathophysiologic

Autoimmune diseases (rheumatoid arthritis, diabetes mellitus, thyroid disease, gout, osteoporosis, etc.)*
Collagen vascular disease
History of allergy*
Structural eyelid problems
Neurologic lesions with sensory or motor reflex loss (lagophthalmos, lack of spontaneous blink reflex due to decreased consciousness, and other medical conditions)*
Ocular surface damage*
Vitamin A deficiency*
Deficient tear-producing glands
Tear gland damage from inflammation
Difficulty blinking due to eyelid problems (e.g., ectropion [turning out]; entropion [turning in])

Treatment Related

Pharmaceutical agents such as angiotensin-converting enzyme inhibitors, antihistamines, diuretics, steroids, antidepressants, tranquilizers, analgesics, sedatives, neuromuscular blockage agents*
Surgical operations*
Anti-inflammatory agents (e.g., ibuprofen, naproxen, birth control pills, decongestants)
After laser eye surgery
Tear gland damage from radiation
After cosmetic eyelid surgery
Oral contraceptives
Mechanical ventilation therapy*

Personal (Situational, Environmental)

Long hours looking at computer screen
Smoking
Heavy drinking
Contact lenses*

Environmental factors (air-conditioning, excessive wind, sunlight exposure, air pollution, low humidity),* hot, dry, windy climate
Place of living*
Female gender*
Lifestyle (e.g., smoking, caffeine use, prolonged reading)*
Air travel

Maturational

Aging
Postmenopause

Risk for Corneal Injury

Definition

Vulnerable to infection or inflammatory lesion in the corneal tissue that can affect superficial or deep layers, which may compromise health.

Risk Factors

- Blinking <5 times/min
- Exposure of the eyeball
- Glasgow Coma Scale score <7
- Intubation
- Mechanical ventilation
- Periorbital edema
- Pharmaceutical agent
- Prolonged hospitalization
- Tracheostomy
- Use of supplemental oxygen

NOC
Knowledge: Illness Care, Infection Control, Symptom Control, Hydration

Goals

The individual will exhibit minimal or no signs or symptoms of complications of dry eye, as evidenced by the following indicators:

- Pink conjunctiva
- No increase in drainage or purulent drainage
- Clear cornea

NIC
Eye Care Infection Protection; Medication Administration: Eye, Comfort Level, Hydration, Anxiety Reduction (family)

Interventions

Identify High-Risk Individuals

- Unconscious
- Sedated for >48 hours
- Paralyzed
- Ventilatory support

Monitor for Keratitis

- Red and watery eyes
- Pain in the eye (if can report)
- White to gray area on cornea (late sign)

Report Any Changes in the Eye Appearance or Report of Eye Pain or Blurring (If Able) Immediately

Provide Eye Care as Prescribed

- Eye drops, lubricants, antibiotics
- Patches, gauze, eye shields, polyethylene covers

If No Eye Care Protocol Has Been Prescribed, Consult With Physician/Nurse Practitioner Immediately

Prevent Infection

- Wear gloves with all eye care.
- Instruct family not to touch or wipe the eye area of an individual.
- Gently pull lower lid and instill drops or a line of ointment in pocket of the lid.
- Avoid any contamination of eye care products. Never touch dropper or tube tip to eyelid. If this occurs, discard the medicine.
- Offer to demonstrate to a new nurse or student nurse.

Evaluate Hydration Status Frequently

Prior to Seeing Individual, Explain to Individual and/or Significant Others the Reason for the Eye Care Treatments (e.g., Use of Shields, Polyethylene Covers [Plastic Wrap]).

Initiate Health Teaching as Indicated

- Advise to see primary care provider or an eye specialist if there are signs and symptoms of dry eyes, infection, and eye pain.

Risk for Dry Eye

NANDA-I Definition

Vulnerable for eye discomfort or damage to the cornea and conjunctiva due to reduced quantity or quality of tears to moisten the eye, which may compromise health

Risk Factors

Pathophysiologic

Autoimmune diseases (rheumatoid arthritis, diabetes mellitus, thyroid disease, gout, osteoporosis, etc.)*
History of allergy*
Neurologic lesions with sensory or motor reflex loss (lagophthalmos, lack of spontaneous blink reflex due to decreased consciousness, and other medical conditions)*
Ocular surface damage*
Vitamin A deficiency*

Treatment Related

Pharmaceutical agents such as angiotensin-converting enzyme inhibitors, antihistamines, diuretics, steroids, antidepressants, tranquilizers, analgesics, sedatives, neuromuscular blockage agents*
Surgical operations*
Mechanical ventilation therapy*

Personal (Situational, Environmental)

Contact lenses*
Environmental factors (air-conditioning, excessive wind, sunlight exposure, air pollution, low humidity),* hot, dry, windy climate
Place of living*
Female gender*
Lifestyle (e.g., smoking, caffeine use, prolonged reading)*

Maturational

Aging
Postmenopause

Author's Note

This new NANDA-I nursing diagnosis represents a common problem experienced by most persons acutely or chronically. For some individuals, the problem is annoying, for others it causes a significant chronic discomfort, and for a few individuals dry eye is a serious risk factor that can cause corneal abrasions. Therefore, this diagnosis can be used to prevent or reduce dry eyes.

For those individuals who are at risk for corneal abrasion, such as those with chronic dry eyes or those so debilitated that the natural lubrication system in the eye is compromised (e.g., comatose), *Risk for Corneal Abrasion* would be more clinically useful. NANDA-I accepted *Risk for Corneal Injury* in 2014.

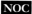 **NOC**

Environmental, Health Promotion Behavior, Symptom Control

Goals

The individual will report reduction of dry eye symptoms, as evidenced by the following indicators:

- Describe causes of dry eye
- Identify strategies to prevent dry eyes

 NIC

Comfort Level, Hydration, Environmental Management, Nutritional Counseling

Interventions

Explain Factors That Contribute to Dry Eyes

- Refer to Risk Factors.

Teach to Use Over-the-Counter Artificial Tears or Ocular Lubricants as Needed

- To use before reading or other activities that increase eye movements
- To use preservative-free eye drops if they are used more than four times a day
- To avoid using drops that "get the red out," which are not effective in lubricating eyes

Increase Environmental Humidity, Especially in the Winter and Dry Climates

- Avoid hot rooms, high winds

Wear Wraparound Sunglasses or Other Type With Foam or Other Seals; When Swimming, Wear Goggles

Avoid Eye Irritants
- Hair sprays
- Tobacco smoke
- Air blowing in eyes (e.g., hair dryer, fans)

For Contact Lens Wearers
- If eye drops are used, be aware if lens must be removed before instillation of drops and not replaced for 15 minutes.
- Rewetting drops may be effective if eye dryness is mild.
- Wear lens for few hours daily if needed.

Advise of Nutritional and Hydration Effects on Eye Dryness
- Avoid dehydration. Advise to monitor hydration by keeping urine color pale.
- Advise that coffee and tea are diuretics and of the need to increase water intake, unless contraindicated.
- Discuss the relationship of nutritional intake of omega-3 fatty acids, such as cold-water fish, sardines, tuna, salmon, cod, herring, flax seed oil, soybean oil, canola oil, fish oil supplements, and vitamin A (e.g., carrots, broccoli supplements).

When Reading or Using a Computer for Long Periods (Mayo Clinic, 2010):
- Take eye breaks, close eyes for a few minutes.
- Blink repeatedly for a few seconds.

Advise to See Primary Care Provider or an Eye Specialist If There Are Prolonged Signs and Symptoms of Dry Eyes

Impaired Oral Mucous Membrane

NANDA-I Definition

Disruption of the lips and/or soft tissue of the oral cavity

Defining Characteristics

Disrupted oral mucous membranes
Color changes—erythema, pallor, white patches, lesions, and
  ulcers
Moisture changes—increased or decreased saliva
Cleanliness changes—debris, malodor, discoloration of the teeth
Mucosal integrity changes—difficulty swallowing, decreased
  taste, difficulty weaning
Perception changes—difficulty swallowing, decreased taste, dif-
  ficulty wearing dentures, burning, pain, and change in voice
  quality

Related Factors

Pathophysiologic

Related to inflammation/drying effects secondary to:

Allergy	Immunodeficiency
Autoimmune disease	Immunosuppression
Autosomal disorder	Infection
Behavior disorder (e.g., attention	Syndrome (e.g., Sjögren's)
deficit, oppositional defiant)	Trauma

Related to inflammation secondary to oral cancer

Related to periodontal disease

Treatment Related

Related to drying effects of:
NPO more than 24 hours
Radiation to head or neck
Prolonged use of steroids or other immunosuppressive agents
  and other medications, including opioids, antidepressants,
  phenothiazines, antihypertensives, antihistamines, diuretics,
  and sedatives
Use of antineoplastic drugs
Oxygen therapy
Mouth breathing
Blood and marrow stem cell transplant

Related to mechanical irritation secondary to:
Endotracheal tube
NG tube

Situational (Personal, Environmental)

Related to chemical irritants secondary to:*

Acidic foods	Alcohol
Drugs	Tobacco
Noxious agents	High sugar intake

Related to mechanical trauma secondary to:

Broken or jagged teeth	Braces
Ill-fitting dentures	

*Related to malnutrition**

Related to inadequate oral hygiene

Related to lack of knowledge of oral hygiene

 Author's Note

See *Impaired Tissue Integrity.*

Oral health directly influences many activities of daily living (eating, fluid intake, and breathing) and interpersonal relations (appearance, self-concept, communication). Many oral diseases or infarctions begin quietly and are painless until significant involvement has taken place. Unfortunately, mouth care is often not a priority in health-care facilities. Even those who can provide their own oral hygiene but need assistance with setup and supplies are not encouraged.

 NOC

Oral Tissue Integrity

Goals

The individuals will be free of oral mucosa irritation or exhibit signs of healing with decreased inflammation, as evidenced by the following indicators:

- Describe factors that cause oral injury
- Demonstrate knowledge of optimal oral hygiene

NIC

Oral Health Restoration, Chemotherapeutic Management, Oral Health Maintenance, Oral Health Promotion

Interventions

Assess for Causative or Contributing Factors

- Assess with a valid and reliable tool as a first step to preventing and treating oral mucositis (Eilers, Harris, Henry, & Johnson, 2014).
- Evaluate person's ability to perform oral hygiene. Allow person to perform as much oral care as possible. For high-risk individuals, inspect the oral cavity for lesions (e.g., white patches, broken teeth, and signs of infection).
- Advise staff/student to report any complaints of mouth sores, white patches, broken, sharp teeth, and problems with swallowing.

Teach Preventive Oral Hygiene to Individuals at Risk for Development of Mucositis

- Instruct to
  - Perform the regimen including brushing, flossing, rinsing, and moisturizing after meals and before sleep.
  - For people with their own teeth, brush following the procedure outlined above. Use sodium bicarbonate (1 tsp:8 oz water), water, or normal saline solution (may be contraindicated in people with sodium restrictions).
  - Avoid mouthwashes with alcohol content, lemon/glycerin swabs, or prolonged use of hydrogen peroxide.
  - Apply lubricant to lips every 2 hours and PRN (e.g., lanolin, A&D ointment).
  - Inspect mouth daily for lesions and inflammation and report alterations.
  - Avoid foods that are spicy, salty, hot, rough, or acidic.
  - Report following symptoms: temperature greater than 101° F, new lesions or sores in mouth, bleeding from gums, difficulty swallowing or inability to take in fluids, and pain in the mouth.
  - Keep mouth clean and moist.
- Initiating oral care protocols have decreased both ventilator-associated pneumonia (Feider, Mitchell, & Bridges, 2010) and non–ventilator-acquired pneumonia (Quinn et al., 2014).

Consult With Prescriber for Possible Need for Prophylactic Antifungal or Antibacterial Agent for Immunocompromised Individuals at Risk for Mucositis (National Comprehensive Cancer Network, 2008)

- Instruct individual to see a dentist 2 to 3 weeks before therapy begins for diagnosis and treatment of infections and to ensure adequate time for healing.

- Consult with dentist for a regimen of daily fluoride treatments and oral hygiene.
- Instruct individual to see a dentist during treatment as needed and 2 months after treatment.
- Refer any suspicious oral lesions to health-care provider for culture to identify organism.
- Administer antibiotics, antifungals, or antivirals as prescribed.
- Monitor temperature every 4 hours, and report abnormal readings to health-care provider.
- Replace toothbrush after treatment of suspected or documented oral infection.

Perform Oral Hygiene on Individuals Who Are Intubated and/or Mechanically Ventilated

- Position head of bed higher than 30° unless medically contraindicated.
- Brush teeth, tongue, and gums as described above twice a day, with brush not foam brush.
- Swab oral cavity every 2 to 4 hours and as needed with normal saline or mouth rinse solution.
- Use a bulb syringe to rinse mouth; aspirate rinse with suction or use an aspirating toothbrush.
- Use oral chlorhexidine gluconate rinses or gels as per protocols or orders.
- Apply mouth moisturizer to mouth and lips.
- Remove excess oral secretions by using the suction.
- Further studies are needed to determine what mouth care solutions are the most effective.

Promote Healing and Reduce Progression of Mucositis

- Inspect oral cavity three times daily with tongue blade and light; if mucositis is severe, inspect mouth every 4 hours.
- Ensure that oral hygiene regimen is done every 1 to 2 hours while awake and every 4 hours during the night.
- Use normal saline solution as a mouthwash.
- Floss teeth only once in 24 hours.
- Omit flossing if bleeding is excessive.

Evaluate for the Presence or Risks for Decreased Salivation

- Dehydration and anemia
- Radiation treatment to head and neck
- Vitamin deficiencies
- Removal of salivary glands
- Allergies

- Side effects of drugs (e.g., antihistamines, anticholinergics, phenothiazine, narcotics, chemotherapy, laxatives, and other antineoplastic medications)

Reduce Oral Pain and Maintain Adequate Food and Fluid Intake

- Assess individual's ability to chew and swallow. Refer to speech therapy for a comprehensive evaluation if indicated.
- Administer mild analgesic every 3 to 4 hours as ordered.
- Instruct to
  - Avoid commercial mouthwashes, citrus fruit juices, spicy foods, extremes in food temperature (hot, cold), crusty or rough foods, alcohol, and mouthwashes with alcohol.
  - Eat bland, cool foods (e.g., sherbets).
  - Drink cool liquids every 2 hours and PRN.
- Consult with dietitian for specific interventions.
- Consult with prescriber for an oral pain-relief solution.
  - Lidocaine viscous 2% oral: Swish and expectorate every 2 hours and before meals. (If throat is sore, the solution can be swallowed; if swallowed, Lidocaine produces local anesthesia and may affect the gag reflex.) The dose of the viscous Lidocaine is not to exceed 25 mL/day (National Comprehensive Cancer Network, 2008).
  - Gelclair is a concentrated gel that provides a protective barrier and requires frequent applications because of limited duration. Prophylaxis is not recommended.
  - Topical morphine provides a reduction in pain severity and duration of pain. If the morphine is in an alcohol-based formula, it may cause burning.
- If not contraindicated, use salt or baking soda rinses.
- Use regular toothbrushes not foam brushes.

Initiate Health Teaching and Referrals, as Indicated

- Teach the factors that contribute to stomatitis and its progression.
- Have the individual/family describe or demonstrate home care regimen.
- Have individual describe or demonstrate home care regimen.

⟨⟨ Pediatric Interventions

Teach Parents to

- Provide their child with fluoride supplements if not present in concentrations higher than 0.7 parts per million in drinking water.
- Avoid taking tetracycline drugs during pregnancy or giving them to children younger than 8 years.

- Refrain from putting an infant to bed with a bottle of juice or milk.
- Provide child with safe objects for chewing during teething.
- Replace toothbrushes frequently (every 3 months).
- Schedule dental checkups every 6 months after 2 years of age.
- Supervise and assist preschool child with brushing and flossing in front of mirror.
- Talk to child when brushing.
- "Ask child to 'tweet like a bird' to brush front teeth and 'roar like a lion' to brush back teeth" (Perry et al., 2014).
- Incorporate brushing and flossing teeth into bedtime rituals.

R: *Plaque, microbial flora found in the mouth, is the primary cause of dental cavities and periodontal disease. Daily removal of plaque through brushing and flossing can help prevent dental decay and disease.*

Maternal Interventions

- Stress the importance of good oral hygiene and dental examinations.
- Remind to advise dentist of pregnancy.
- Explain that gum hypertrophy and tenderness are normal during pregnancy.

Risk for Impaired Oral Mucous Membrane

Definition

Vulnerable to injury to the lips, soft tissues, buccal cavity, and/or oropharynx, which may compromise health

Risk Factors

Pathophysiologic

Related to inflammation/drying effects secondary to:
Examples:
Allergy   Immunosuppression
Autoimmune disease   Infection
Autosomal disorder   Syndrome (e.g., Sjögren's)

Behavior disorder (e.g., attention deficit, oppositional defiant)
Immunodeficiency

Trauma

Treatment Related

Related to drying effects of:
NPO more than 24 hours
Radiation to head or neck*
Prolonged use of steroids or other immunosuppressive agents (e.g., chemotherapy and other medications including opioids, antidepressants, phenothiazines, antihypertensives, antihistamines, diuretics, and sedatives)
Use of antineoplastic drugs
Oxygen therapy
Mouth breathing
Blood and marrow stem cell transplant

Related to mechanical irritation secondary to:
Endotracheal tube
NG tube

Situational (Personal, Environmental)

Related to chemical irritants* secondary to:
Acidic foods
Drugs
Noxious agents

Alcohol*
Tobacco*
High sugar intake

Related to mechanical trauma secondary to*:
Broken or jagged teeth
Ill-fitting dentures

Braces

Related to malnutrition*

Related to inadequate oral hygiene

Related to lack of knowledge of oral hygiene*

Related to barriers to dental care secondary to* (e.g., economically disadvantaged*, alteration in cognitive functioning*)

Related to barriers to oral self-care* (e.g., stressors*)

Maturational

Decrease in hormone level in women*
Children/adolescents
Low motivation
Lack of mouth care supplies (e.g., toothbrush, toothpaste, floss)
Inadequate knowledge

Author's Note

Risk for Impaired Oral Mucous Membrane is a newly accepted NANDA-I nursing diagnosis. The assessments and interventions for this diagnosis are standard in all health-care facilities. However, if an individual is at high risk for *Impaired Oral Mucous Membrane*, the diagnosis should appear on the individual's problem list with the high-risk factors cited in the diagnostic statement, as *Risk for Impaired Oral Mucous Membrane related to malnourished state and the effects of chemotherapy.*

Goals/Interventions

Refer to *Impaired Oral Mucous Membrane.*

Impaired Tissue Integrity

NANDA-I Definition

Damage to mucous membranes, corneal integumentary, or subcutaneous tissues

Defining Characteristics

Damaged tissue or destroyed tissue (e.g., cornea, mucous membranes, integumentary, subcutaneous)

Related Factors

Pathophysiologic

Related to inflammation of dermal–epidermal junctions secondary to:

Autoimmune Alterations	Bacterial
Lupus erythematosus	Impetigo
Scleroderma	Folliculitis
Metabolic and Endocrine Alterations	Cellulitis
Diabetes mellitus	Viral
Jaundice	Herpes zoster (shingles)
Hepatitis	Herpes simplex
Cancer	Gingivitis
Cirrhosis	Fungal

Thyroid dysfunction
sis)
Renal failure

Ringworm (dermatophyto-

Athlete's foot
Vaginitis

Related to decreased blood and nutrients to tissues secondary to:

Diabetes mellitus
Peripheral vascular alterations
Anemia
Venous stasis
Cardiopulmonary disorders

Arteriosclerosis
Obesity
Malnutrition
Emaciation
Edema*

Treatment Related

Related to decreased blood and nutrients to tissues secondary to:
Therapeutic extremes in body
temperature
NPO status

Surgery

Related to imposed immobility secondary to sedation

Related to mechanical trauma
Therapeutic fixation devices
    Wired jaw
    Casts
    Traction
Orthopedic devices/braces

Related to effects of radiation on epithelial and basal cells*

Related to effects of mechanical factors or pressure secondary to:*
Inflatable or foam donuts
Tourniquets
Footboards
Restraints
Dressings, tape, solutions
External urinary catheters

Nasogastric (NG) tubes
Shear
Friction
Endotracheal tubes
Oral prostheses/braces
Contact lenses

Related to the effects of medicines (specify) (e.g., steroids, antibiotics)

Situational (Personal, Environmental)

Related to chemical irritants secondary to:*
Excretions
Secretions

Noxious agents/substances

Related to environmental irritants secondary to:
Radiation/sunburn
Humidity
Bites (insect, animal)
Poisonous plants

Temperature extremes*
Parasites
Inhalants

*Related to the effects of pressure of impaired physical mobility**
secondary to:

Pain	Motivation
Fatigue	Cognitive, sensory, or motor deficits

Related to inadequate personal habits (hygiene/dental/dietary/sleep)

Related to thin body frame

Maturational

Related to dry, thin skin and decreased dermal vascularity secondary to aging

 Author's Note

With the newly accepted *Risk for Pressure Ulcer*, *Risk for Corneal Injury*, *Risk for Urinary Tract Injury*, and the addition of *Pressure Ulcer* by this author, *Impaired Tissue Integrity* and *Risk for Impaired Tissue Integrity* are too broad nursing diagnosis for clinical usefulness.

Impaired Tissue Integrity is the broad diagnosis under which fall the more specific diagnoses *Impaired Skin Integrity* and *Impaired Oral Mucous Membranes*. Because tissue is composed of epithelium, connective tissue, muscle, and nervous tissue, *Impaired Tissue Integrity* correctly describes some pressure ulcers that are deeper than the dermis. *Impaired Skin Integrity* should be used to describe disruptions of epidermal and dermal tissue only.

When a pressure ulcer is stage IV, necrotic, or infected, it may be more appropriate to label the diagnosis a collaborative problem, such as *Risk for Complications of Stage IV Pressure Ulcer*. This would represent a situation in which a nurse manages with physician- and nurse-prescribed interventions. When a stage II or III pressure ulcer needs a dressing that requires a physician's order in an acute care setting, the nurse should continue to label the situation a nursing diagnosis, *Pressure Ulcer*, because it would be appropriate and legal for a nurse to treat the ulcer independently in other settings (e.g., in the community).

If an individual is immobile and multiple systems are threatened (respiratory, circulatory, musculoskeletal, as well as integumentary), the nurse can use *Disuse Syndrome* to describe the entire situation. If an individual is at risk for damage to corneal tissue, the nurse can use a diagnosis such as *Risk for Corneal Integrity* related to corneal drying and lower lacrimal production secondary to unconscious state.

Impaired Skin Integrity

NANDA-I Definition

Altered epidermis and/or dermis

Defining Characteristics*

Destruction of skin layers
Disruption of skin surface
Invasion of body structures

Related Factors

See *Impaired Tissue Integrity*.

 Author's Note

Refer to Author's Notes under *Impaired Tissue Integrity*.

Risk for Impaired Skin Integrity

NANDA-I Definition

Vulnerable for alteration in epidermis and/or dermis, which may compromise health

Risk Factors

Refer to related factors under *Impaired Skin Integrity*.

Tissue Integrity: Skin and Mucous Membrane

Author's Note

Refer to Author's Notes under *Impaired Tissue Integrity*.

Pressure Ulcers[30]

Definition

A pressure ulcer is a localized injury to the skin and/or underlying tissue, usually over a bony prominence, as a result of pressure, or pressure in combination with shear (e.g., sacrum, calcaneus, ischium) (National Pressure Ulcer Advisory Panel, European Pressure Ulcer Advisory Panel, 2014)

Defining Characteristics
(National Pressure Ulcer Advisory Panel, European Pressure Ulcer Advisory Panel, 2014)

Category/Stage I: Nonblanchable Erythema

Intact skin with nonblanchable redness of a localized area usually over a bony prominence. The area may be painful, firm, soft, warmer, or cooler as compared to adjacent tissue.

Category/Stage II: Partial Thickness

Partial thickness loss of dermis, presenting as a shallow open ulcer with a red pink wound bed, without slough. May also present as an intact or open/ruptured serum-filled or serosanguinous-filled blister. Presents as a shiny or dry shallow ulcer without slough or bruising. Bruising indicates deep tissue injury.

Category/Stage III: Full Thickness Skin Loss

Full thickness tissue loss. Subcutaneous fat may be visible but bone, tendon, or muscle is *not* exposed. Slough may be present but does not obscure the depth of tissue loss. May include undermining and tunneling. Bone/tendon is not visible or directly palpable.
The depth of a category/stage III pressure ulcer varies by anatomical location.

---

[30]This nursing diagnosis has been added by Lynda Juall Carpenito for its clarity and clinical usefulness.

Category/Stage IV: Full Thickness Tissue Loss

Full thickness tissue loss with exposed bone, tendon, or muscle.
Slough or eschar may be present. Often includes undermining and tunneling. The depth of a category/stage IV pressure
ulcer varies by anatomical location. Category/Stage IV ulcers
can extend into muscle and/or supporting structures (e.g.,
fascia, tendon, or joint capsule), making osteomyelitis or oste-
itis likely to occur. Exposed bone/muscle is visible or directly
palpable

Additional Categories/Stages for the United States

Unstageable/Unclassified: Full Thickness Skin or Tissue Loss—
Depth Unknown

Full thickness tissue loss in which actual depth of the ulcer is
completely obscured by slough (yellow, tan, gray, green, or
brown) and/or eschar (tan, brown, or black) in the wound bed.
Until enough slough and/or eschar are removed to expose the
base of the wound, the true depth cannot be determined; but it
will be either a category/stage III or IV.

Suspected Deep Tissue Injury—Depth Unknown

Purple or maroon localized area of discolored intact skin or
blood-filled blister due to damage of underlying soft tissue
from pressure and/or shear. The area may be preceded by
tissue that is painful, firm, mushy, boggy, warmer, or cooler as
compared to adjacent tissue. Deep tissue injury may be difficult to detect in individuals with dark skin tones. Evolution
may include a thin blister over a dark wound bed. The wound
may further evolve and become covered by thin eschar. Evolution may be rapid exposing additional layers of tissue even
with optimal treatment.

Author's Note

The staging of pressure ulcers denotes the interventions needed. As indicated above, Stages I and II pressure ulcers are primarily managed by
nursing-prescribed interventions, thus they are appropriate to be classified as a nursing diagnosis, *Pressure Ulcer*.

Categories/Stages III and IV, unstageable/unclassified, suspected deep
tissue injuries require complex medical and nursing treatments. However, in many institutions in the United States and other countries, wound
care nurse specialist coordinate to care of most pressure ulcers, thus
the nursing diagnosis of *Pressure Ulcer* may be utilized regardless of the
stage. Stage IV pressure ulcers should also have an additional collaborative

problems as Risk for Sepsis. In addition, appropriate nursing diagnoses as *Risk for Infection*, *Impaired Physical Mobility*, *Imbalanced Nutrition*, and *Risk for Health Management* could also be indicated.

Related Factors

Pathophysiologic

Related to decreased blood and nutrients to tissues secondary to:

Peripheral vascular alterations	Arteriosclerosis
Obesity	Dehydration
Anemia	Malnutrition
Venous stasis	Edema
Cardiopulmonary disorders	Emaciation

Treatment Related

Related to decreased blood and nutrients to tissues secondary to:

Therapeutic extremes in body	Obesity
temperature	NPO status
Surgery	

Related to imposed immobility secondary to sedation

Related to mechanical trauma

Therapeutic fixation devices	Traction
Wired jaw	Orthopedic devices/braces
Casts	

Related to effects of radiation on epithelial and basal cells

Related to effects of mechanical irritants or pressure secondary to:

Inflatable or foam donuts	Dressings, tape, solutions	Friction
Tourniquets	External urinary catheters	Endotracheal tubes
Footboards	NG tubes	Oral prostheses/ braces
Restraints	Shear	Contact lenses

Situational (Personal, Environmental)

Related to chemical irritants secondary to:

Excretions	Noxious agents/substances
Secretions	

Related to environmental irritants secondary to:

Radiation/sunburn	Temperature extremes
Humidity	Parasites

Bites (insect, animal)   Inhalants
Poisonous plants

Related to the effects of pressure of impaired physical mobility
secondary to:

Pain   Motivation
Fatigue   Cognitive, sensory, or motor deficits

Related to dry, thin skin, and decreased dermal vascularity secondary
to aging

 Carp's Cues

- Pressure ulcers are among the most common conditions encountered in acutely hospitalized individuals (0% to 46%), those in critical care (13.1% to 45.5%), or those requiring long-term institutional care (4.1% to 32.2%). An estimated 2.5 million pressure ulcers are treated each year in acute care facilities in the United States alone (National Pressure Ulcer Advisory Panel, European Pressure Ulcer Advisory Panel).
- According to the Agency for Healthcare Research & Quality (AHRQ, 2011), pressure ulcers cost the US health-care system an estimated $9.1 to $11.6 billion annually.
- Studies have shown that the development of a pressure ulcer independently increases the length of a patient's hospital stay by 4 to 10 days. These prolonged hospital stays are also associated with an increased incidence of nosocomial infections and other complications.
- In the 4th quarter of 2011, on average, nursing homes had 6.9% of their long-stay high-risk residents with pressure ulcers and (Berlowitz, 2014; Ling & Mandl, 2013):
  - The 10% of nursing homes who performed the best had 2% or less prevalence of pressure ulcers among their high-risk residents.
  - The 10% of nursing homes who performed the poorest had 12% or more prevalence of pressure ulcers among their high-risk residents.
  - 6.9% of facilities reported no pressure ulcers.
- Among short-stay nursing home residents, the following risk factors for pressure ulcers were identified at admission (Ling & Mandl, 2013).
  - 89.2% had an impairment in bed mobility.
  - 34.5% had bowel incontinence (occasional or more).
  - 42.4% had diabetes or peripheral vascular disease.
  - 9.8% had a low body mass index.

Goals

The individual will demonstrate, as evidenced by the following indicators:

- Progressive healing of pressure ulcer
- Participate in risk reduction (specify)

The individual/family will accurately

- Demonstrate pressure ulcer care
- Identify signs of improvement and/or deterioration
- Explain rationale for interventions

 NIC

Teaching Interventions, Surveillance, Nutritional Management, Pressure Prevention, Positioning, Incontinence, Pressure Ulcer Care

Interventions

Ensure Assessment and Documentation of Skin and Tissue Condition at Intervals Depending on Individual's Risk (National Pressure Ulcer Advisory Panel, 2014)

- Blanching response
- Localized heat
- Edema
- Induration (hardness)
- Localized pain

Ask the Individual If They Have Any Areas of Discomfort or Pain That Could be Attributed to Pressure Damage

- Observe the skin for pressure damage caused by medical devices (for example, catheters and cervical collars).

For Individuals With Darkly Pigmented Skin, Consider (*Bennett, 1995; Clark, 2010, p. 17) **the Following**

- The color of intact dark pigmented skin may remain unchanged (does not blanch) when pressure is applied over a bony prominence.
- Local areas of intact skin that are subject to pressure may feel either warm or cool when touched. This assessment should be performed without gloves to make it easier to distinguish differences in temperature after any body fluids are cleansed before making this direct contact.

- Areas of skin subjected to pressure may be purplish/bluish/violet in color. This can be compared with the erythema seen in people with lighter skin tones.
- Complains of, or indicate, current or recent pain or discomfort at body sites where pressure has been applied.
- Ensure a nutritional assessment is completed by a registered dietician/nutritionist using the MNA, if possible.
- Report to prescribing provider when food and/or fluid intake is decreased.

Advise Family/Friends the Importance of Nutrition-Dense Foods/Beverages Versus Calorie-Dense Foods/Beverages

- Calorie-dense foods, also called energy-dense foods, contain high levels of calories per serving in fat and carbohydrates. Many processed foods are considered calorie-dense, such as cakes, cookies, snacks, donuts, and candies.
- Nutrient-dense foods contain high levels of nutrients, such as protein, carbohydrates, fats, vitamins, and minerals, but with less calories. Some nutrient-dense foods are fresh fruits, vegetables, berries, melons, dark-green vegetables, sweet potatoes, tomatoes, and whole grains, including quinoa, barley, bulger, and oats. Lean beef and pork are high in protein and contain high levels of zinc, iron, and B-vitamins.
- Refer to *Imbalance Nutrition* for interventions related to promoting optimal intake of required nutrients.

Follow the Wound Care Procedure as Prescribed by a Wound Specialist or Prescribing Professional (Physician, Nurse Practitioner, Physician Assistant)

- Wound bed preparation (tissue management, infection/inflammation control, moisture barrier, epithelial edge advancement) (National Pressure Ulcer Advisory Panel, 2014)
- Prevention, assessment, treatment of infection:
  - Suspect an infection when:
    - Lack of signs of healing for 2 weeks
    - Friable (easily bleeds) granulation tissue
    - Malodor
    - Increased pain in ulcer
    - Increased heat in area around ulcer
    - Increased drainage
    - Unsatisfactory change in character of drainage (e.g., bloody, purulent)
    - Increase in necrotic tissue in the wound bed
    - Pocketing or bridging in the wound bed

- Suspect biofilm in pressure ulcer when:
  - Ulcer is present more than 4 weeks
  - Lacks signs of any healing in the previous 2 weeks
  - Has clinical signs and symptoms of inflammation
  - It does not respond to antimicrobial therapy
- Wound dressings: should keep wound moist, contain exudate, protect peri-ulcer skin, comply with the size and location, presence of tunneling
- When the dressing does not address the characteristics of the ulcer or the ulcer has deteriorated, consult with specialist.

Consult with Wound Care Nursing Specialist to Consider

- Pressure-dispersing devices, microclimate manipulations, and fabrics (e.g., silk-like texture designed to reduce shear/friction as appropriate (National Pressure Ulcer Advisory Panel, 2014).
- Applying polyurethane foam dressing to bony prominences (e.g., heel, elbows, sacrum). Avoid dressing that cannot easily be removed (National Pressure Ulcer Advisory Panel, 2014).

Encourage Highest Degree of Mobility to Avoid Prolonged Periods of Pressure: Exercise and Mobility Increase Blood Flow to All Areas

- Principles of pressure ulcer prevention include reducing or rotating pressure on soft tissue. If pressure on soft tissue exceeds intracapillary pressure (approximately 32 mm Hg), capillary occlusion and resulting hypoxia can cause tissue damage. The greater the duration of immobility, the greater the likelihood of the development of small vessel thrombosis and subsequent tissue necrosis (National Pressure Ulcer Advisory Panel, 2014).
- Do not position person on reddened and/or tender areas.
- Avoid all inflatable donuts or rings.
- Reduce immobility; refer to *Impaired Physical Mobility*.

Assess Dependent Skin Areas With Every Position Turn

- Use finger or transparent disk to assess whether skin is blanchable or nonblanchable.

Do Not Rub or Massage Reddened Areas

- Assess skin temperature, edema, and change in tissue consistency as compared to surrounding tissue.
- Increase frequency of the turning schedule if any nonblanchable erythema is noted. Consult with prescribing professional for the utilization of pressure-dispersing devices and microclimate manipulation devices in addition to repositioning.
- Place the individual in normal or neutral position with body weight evenly distributed. Use 30° laterally inclined position when possible.

- Keep the bed as flat as possible to reduce shearing forces; limit semi-Fowler's position to only 30 minutes at a time.
- Alternate or reduce the pressure on the skin with an appropriate support surface.
- Suspend heels off bed surface.
- Use enough personnel to lift the individual up in bed or a chair rather than pull or slide skin surfaces.
- To reduce shearing forces, support the feet with a footboard to prevent sliding.

Promote Optimal Circulation When the Person Is Sitting

- Limit sitting time for those at high risk for ulcer development.
- Instruct to lift self using chair arms every 10 minutes, if possible, or assist in rising up off the chair at least every hour, depending on risk factors present.
- Do not elevate the legs unless calves are supported to reduce the pressure over the ischial tuberosities.
- Pad the chair with pressure-relieving cushion.
- Inspect areas at risk of developing ulcers with each position change.

Protect Skin Near Feeding Tubes or Endotracheal Tubes With a Protective Barrier

- Change skin barrier when loose or leaking.
- Instruct to report discomforts.

Initiate Health Teaching and Referrals as Needed

- Teach the individual/family appropriate measures to prevent pressure, shear, friction, and maceration and to not use inflatable donuts or rings (*Bergstrom et al., 1994; National Pressure Ulcer Advisory Panel, 2014; *Wound Ostomy Continence Nursing [WOCN], 2003).
- If indicated, observe family member perform wound care.
- Ensure a home health evaluation is scheduled for the day the individual returns to home.

Risk for Pressure Ulcer

NANDA-I Definition

Vulnerable to localized injury to the skin and/or underlying tissue usually over a bony prominence as a result of pressure, or pressure in combination with shear (National Pressure Ulcer Advisory Panel, 2014).

Risk Factors

Pathophysiologic

Adult: Braden Scale score of <18
Alteration in cognitive functioning
Alteration in sensation
American Society of Anesthesiologists (ASA) Physical Status
    classification score ≥2
Anemia
Cardiovascular disease
Child: Braden Q Scale of ≤16
Decrease in serum albumin level
Electrolyte imbalances, elevated urea, elevated creatinine above
    1 mg/dL, lymphopenia, elevated C-reactive protein*)
Decrease in tissue oxygenation
Decrease in tissue perfusion* (e.g., hypertension, hypotension,
    cerebrovascular accident (CVA), diabetes mellitus, renal
    disease, peripheral vascular disease)
Dehydration
Diabetes mellitus*
Edema
Elevated skin temperature by 1° C to 2° C
History of CVA
History of pressure ulcer
History of trauma
Hyperthermia
Impaired circulation
Low score on Risk Assessment Pressure Sore (RAPS) scale
Lymphopenia
New York Heart Association (NYHA) Functional Classification
    ≥2
Hip fracture
Nonblanchable erythema (Author's Note: This is not a risk fac-
    tor but instead represents stage I pressure ulcer.)

Treatment Related

Pharmaceutical agents (e.g., general anesthesia, vasopressors,
    antidepressant, norepinephrine)
Extended period of immobility on hard surface (e.g., surgical
    procedure ≥ 2 hours)
Shearing forces
Surface friction
Use of linen with insufficient moisture wicking property

Situational (Personal, Environmental)

Extremes of weight
Inadequate nutrition
Incontinence
Insufficient caregiver
Knowledge of pressure ulcer prevention
Physical immobilization
Pressure over bony prominence
Reduced triceps skin fold thickness

Scaly skin
Dry skin
Self-care deficit
Skin moisture
Smoking
Female gender
Decreased cognition[30]
Dibilitated[30]

Maturational

Extremes of age

 Author's Note

Refer to *Pressure Ulcer.*

Focus Assessment Criteria

Braden Scale For Predicting Pressure Sore Risk
Sensory Perception: ability to respond meaningfully to
    pressure-related discomfort
Moisture: degree to which skin is exposed to moisture
Activity: degree of physical activity
Mobility: ability to change and control body position
Nutrition: usual food intake pattern
Friction & Shear

NOC
Tissue Integrity: Skin and Mucous Membrane

Goals

The individual will demonstrate skin integrity free of pressure ulcers (if able), as evidenced by the following indicators:

- Describe etiology and prevention measures
- Participate in risk reduction

---

[30]Added by author source: National Pressure Ulcer Advisory Panel (2014).

- Consume recommended daily dietary intakeNIC
- Pressure Management, Skin Surveillance, Positioning, Teaching Interventions, Surveillance, Nutritional Management, Pressure Prevention, Positioning, Incontinence

NIC

Pressure Management, Skin Surveillance, Positioning, Teaching Interventions, Surveillance, Nutritional Management, Pressure Prevention, Positioning, Incontinence

Interventions

Use a Formal Risk Assessment Scale to Identify Individual Risk Factors in Addition to Activity and Mobility Deficits

- Refer to Focus Assessment Criteria.

Perform Regular Skin Assessments as Frequently as Indicated

- Skin inspection should include assessment for localized heat, edema, or induration (hardness), especially in individuals with darkly pigmented skin.
- Inspect areas at risk of developing ulcers with each position change.
  - Ears
  - Elbows
  - Occiput
  - Trochanter[31]
  - Heels
  - Ischia
  - Sacrum
  - Scapula
  - Scrotum

Assess Dependent Skin Areas With Every Position Turn

- Use finger or transparent disk to assess whether skin is blanchable or nonblanchable.
- Assess skin temperature, edema, and change in tissue consistency as compared to surrounding tissue.
- Observe the skin for pressure damage caused by medical devices (for example, catheters and cervical collars).
- Ask individuals to identify any areas of discomfort or pain that could be attributed to pressure damage.
- Document all skin assessments, noting details of any pain possibly related to pressure damage.

---

[31]Areas with little soft tissue over a bony prominence are at greatest risk.

- Ask the individual, if they have any areas of discomfort or pain that could be attributed to pressure damage.

For Individuals With Dark Pigmented Skin, Consider (*Bennett, 1995; Clark, 2010, p. 17) **the Following**

- The color of intact dark pigmented skin may remain unchanged (does not blanch) when pressure is applied over a bony prominence.
- Local areas of intact skin that are subject to pressure may feel either warm or cool when touched. This assessment should be performed without gloves to make it easier to distinguish differences in temperature after any body fluids are cleansed before making this direct contact.
- Areas of skin subjected to pressure may be purplish/bluish/violet in color. This can be compared with the erythema seen in people with lighter skin tones.
- Complains of, or indicate, current or recent pain or discomfort at body sites where pressure has been applied.
- Increase frequency of the turning schedule if any nonblanchable erythema is noted. Consult with prescribing professional for the utilization of pressure-dispersing devices and microclimate manipulation devices in addition to repositioning.
- Repositioning should be undertaken using the 30°-tilted side-lying position (alternately, right side, back, left side) or the prone position if the individual can tolerate this and her or his medical condition allows. Avoid postures that increase pressure, such as the 90° side-lying position, or the semirecumbent position.
- Ensure that the heels are free of the surface of the bed. Position knee in slight flexion. Use a pillow under the calves so that heels are elevated (i.e., "floating").
- Use transfer aids to reduce friction and shear. Lift—don't drag—the individual while repositioning.
- Avoid positioning the individual directly onto medical devices, such as tubes or drainage systems.
- Avoid positioning the individual on bony prominences with existing nonblanchable erythema.
- If sitting in bed is necessary, avoid head-of-bed elevation or a slouched position that places pressure and shear on the sacrum and coccyx.

Repositioning the Seated Individual

- Position the individual so as to maintain his or her full range of activities.
- Select a posture that is acceptable for the individual, and minimizes the pressures and shear exerted on the skin and soft

tissues. Place the feet of the individual on a footstool or footrest when the feet do not reach the floor.
- Limit the time an individual spends seated in a chair without pressure relief.

Use of Support Surfaces to Prevent Pressure Ulcers

- Use a pressure-redistributing seat cushion for individuals sitting in a chair whose mobility is reduced.
- Limit the time an individual spends seated in a chair without pressure relief.
- Use alternating-pressure active support overlays or mattress as indicated.

Attempt to Modify Contributing Factors to Lessen the Possibility of a Pressure Ulcer Developing

Incontinence of Urine or Feces

- Determine the etiology of the incontinence.
- Maintain sufficient fluid intake for adequate hydration (approximately 2,500 mL daily, unless contraindicated); check oral mucous membranes for moisture and check urine specific gravity.
- Establish a schedule for emptying the bladder (begin with every 2 hours).
- If the individual is confused, determine what his or her incontinence pattern is and intervene before incontinence occurs.
- Explain problem to the individual; secure his or her cooperation for the plan.
- When incontinent, wash the perineum with a liquid soap.
- Apply a protective barrier to the perineal region (incontinence film barrier spray or wipes).
- Check the individual frequently for incontinence when indicated.
- For additional interventions, refer to *Impaired Urinary Elimination*.

Skin Care

- Whenever possible, do not turn the individual onto a body surface that is still reddened from a previous episode of pressure loading.
- Do not use massage for pressure ulcer prevention or do not vigorously rub skin that is at risk for pressure ulceration.
- Use skin emollients to hydrate dry skin in order to reduce risk of skin damage. Protect the skin from exposure to excessive moisture with a barrier product.

- Avoid use of synthetic sheepskin pads; cutout, ring, or donut-type devices; and water-filled gloves.
- Monitor serum prealbumin levels.
  - Less than 5 mg/dL predicts a poor prognosis.
  - Less than 11 mg/dL predicts high risk and requires aggressive nutritional supplementation.
  - Less than 15 mg/dL predicts an increased risk of malnutrition (Dudek, 2014).

Nutrition

- Ensure a nutritional assessment is completed by a registered dietician/nutritionist using the mini nutritional assessment (MNA), if possible.
- Report to prescribing provider when food and/or fluid intake is decreased.
- Advise family/friends the importance of nutrition-dense foods/beverages versus calorie-dense foods/beverages.
- Calorie-dense foods, also called energy-dense foods, contain high levels of calories per serving in fat and carbohydrates. Many processed foods are considered calorie-dense, such as cakes, cookies, snacks, donuts, and candies.
- Nutrient-dense foods contain high levels of nutrients, such as protein, carbohydrates, fats, vitamins, and minerals, but with fewer calories. Some nutrient-dense foods are fresh fruits, vegetables, berries, melons, dark-green vegetables, sweet potatoes, tomatoes, and whole grains, including quinoa, barley, bulgur, and oats. Lean beef and pork are high in protein and contain high levels of zinc, iron, and B-vitamins.
- Refer to *Imbalance Nutrition* for interventions related to promoting optimal intake of required nutrients.

Initiate Health Teaching as Indicated

- Instruct the individual/family in specific techniques to use at home to prevent pressure ulcers.
- Teach how to use their finger to assess whether skin is blanchable or nonblanchable and when to notify primary care provider.
- Stress the importance of prevention and early identification of nonblanchable redness.
- Consider the use of long-term pressure-relieving devices for permanent disabilities.
- Initiate a referral to a home health nurse for an in-home assessment.

INEFFECTIVE RELATIONSHIP

Ineffective Relationship

Risk for Ineffective Relationship

NANDA-I Definition

A pattern of mutual partnership that is insufficient to provide for each other's needs

Defining Characteristics*

No demonstration of mutual respect between partners
No demonstration of mutual support in daily activities between partners
No demonstration of understanding of partner's insufficient (physical, social, psychological) functioning
No demonstration of well-balanced autonomy between partners
No demonstration of well-balanced collaboration between partners
No identification of partner as a key person
Inability to communicate in a satisfying manner between partners
Report of dissatisfaction with complementary relation between partners
Report of dissatisfaction with fulfilling emotional needs by one's partner
Report of dissatisfaction with fulfilling physical needs by one's partner
Report of dissatisfaction with the sharing of ideas between partners
Report of dissatisfaction with the sharing of information between partners
Does not meet development goals appropriate for family life-cycle stage

Related Factors*

Cognitive changes in one partner
Developmental crises
History of domestic violence
Poor communication skills
Stressful life events
Substance abuse
Unrealistic expectations

Author's Note

This NANDA-I diagnosis represents problems or situations that can disrupt partner relationships. The list of related factors presents substantial different foci for interventions. For example, the interventions for relationship problems associated with substance abuse versus domestic violence and incarceration versus stressful life events are very different.

This book contains assessment and interventions for all of the related factors listed above, for example:

- Related to domestic violence, refer to *Dysfunctional Family Processes*
- Related to substance abuse, refer to *Disturbed Self-Concept*, *Ineffective Denial*, and/or *Dysfunctional Family Processes*
- Related to unrealistic expectations, refer to *Compromised Family Processes*
- Related to poor communication skills and stressful life events, refer to *Compromised Family Processes* and *Readiness for Enhanced Relationships*
- Related to cognitive changes, refer to *Chronic Confusion* and *Altered Thought Processes*

Thus, when *Ineffective or Risk for (Partner) Relationship* is validated, the nurse can find goals and interventions in sections listed above or can use one of the above diagnoses instead, if found to be more descriptive.

Risk for Ineffective Relationship[32]

NANDA-I Definition

Vulnerable for a pattern of mutual partnership that is insufficient to provide for each other's needs

Risk Factors

Cognitive changes in one's partner
Developmental crises
Domestic violence
Incarceration of one's partner

Poor communication skills
Stressful life events
Substance abuse
Unrealistic expectations

---

[32]This diagnosis may be more clinically useful as *Risk for Ineffective Partner Relationships* because it is defined for partners.

RELOCATION STRESS [SYNDROME]

Relocation Stress [Syndrome]
Risk for Relocation Stress [Syndrome]

NANDA-I Definition

Physiologic and/or psychological disturbance following transfer from one environment to another

Note: Other terms found in the literature that describe relocation stress include admission stress, postrelocation crisis, relocation crisis, relocation shock, relocation trauma, transfer stress, transfer trauma, translocation syndrome, and transplantation shock.

Defining Characteristics[33]

Major (80% to 100%)

Responds to transfer or relocation with:

Loneliness	Apprehension
Depression	Anxiety
Anger	Increased confusion (older adult population)

Minor (50% to 79%)

Change in former eating habits	Decrease in leisure activities
Change in former sleep patterns	Gastrointestinal disturbances
Increased verbalization of needs	Need for excessive reassurance
Demonstration of dependency	Restlessness
Demonstration of insecurity	Withdrawal
Demonstration of lack of trust	Allergic symptoms
Hypervigilance	Unfavorable comparison of posttransfer to pretransfer staff
Weight change	

[33]*Sources*: Harkulich, J. & Bruggler, C. (1988). *Nursing Diagnosis–translocation syndrome: Expert validation study*. Partial funding granted by the Peg Schlitz Fund, Delta Ix Chapter, Sigma Theta Tau International; Barnhouse, A. (1987). *Development of the nursing diagnosis of translocation syndrome with critical care patients* (Unpublished Master's Thesis). Kent State University, Kent, OH.

Sad affect
Decrease in self-care activities

Verbalization of being concerned/upset about transfer
Verbalization of insecurity in new living situation

Related Factors

Pathophysiologic

Related to compromised ability to adapt to a unit transfer (e.g., ICU, relocation, living condition changes secondary to):

Decreased physical health status*
Physical difficulties

Decreased psychosocial health status
Increased/perceived stress before relocation

Situational (Personal, Environmental)

Related to little or no preparation for the impending move

Related to insufficient finances, foreclosures

Related to high degree of changes associated with:
Admission to a care facility

Related to:
Loss of social and familial ties
Abandonment

Maturational

School-Aged Children and Adolescents
Related to losses associated with moving secondary to:
Fear of rejection, loss of peer group, or school-related problems
Decreased security in new adolescent peer group and school

Older Adult
Related to the need to be closer to family members for assistance

Related to admission to a care facility

 Author's Note

NANDA-I has accepted *Relocation Stress* as a syndrome diagnosis. It does not fit the criterion for a syndrome diagnosis, which is a cluster of actual or risk nursing diagnoses as defining characteristics. The defining characteristics associated with *Relocation Stress* are observable or reportable cues consistent with *Relocation Stress*, not *Relocation Stress Syndrome*. The author recommends deleting "Syndrome" from the label.

Relocation represents a disruption for all parties involved. It can accompany a transfer from one unit to another or from one facility to another. It can involve a voluntary or forced permanent move to a long-term–care facility or new home. Since 2009, 4.4 million housing units have been foreclosed in the United States. In 2013, the rate trended down 18%.

In December 2015, 9.3 million properties, or 19% of all homes, were reported to be "deeply underwater," meaning borrowers owed at least 25% more on their mortgage than the homes was worth (Christie, 2014). This explosion of foreclosures in the United States and abroad has severely compromised individuals and families. The relocation disturbs all age groups involved. When physiologic and psychological disturbances compromise functioning, the nursing diagnosis *Relocation Stress Syndrome* is appropriate.

The optimal nursing approach to relocation stress is to initiate preventive measures, using *Risk for Relocation Stress* as the diagnosis.

NOC

Anxiety Self-Control, Coping, Loneliness, Psychosocial Adjustment: Life Change, Quality of Life

Goals

The individual/family will report adjustment to the new environment with minimal disturbances, as evidenced by the following indicators:

- Share in decision-making activities regarding the new environment
- Express concerns regarding the move to a new environment
- Verbalize one positive aspect of the relocation
- Establish new bonds in the new environment
- Become involved in activities in the new environment

NIC

Anxiety Reduction, Coping Enhancement, Counseling, Family Involvement Promotion, Support System Enhancement, Anticipatory Guidance, Family Integrity Promotion, Transfer, Relocation Stress Reduction

Interventions

Encourage Each Family Member to Share Feelings About the Move

- Provide privacy for each individual.
- Encourage family members to share feelings with one another.
- Discuss the possible and different effects of the move on each family member.
- Inform parents regarding potential changes in children's conduct with relocation, such as regression, withdrawal, acting out, and changes with eating (breast/bottle-feeding).
- Instruct parents to obtain all pertinent documents regarding children's medical/dental history (e.g., immunizations, communicable diseases, dental work).
- Allow for some ritual(s) when leaving the old environment. Encourage reminiscing, which will bring closure for many family members.

Teach Parents Techniques to Assist Their Children With the Move

- Remain positive about the move before, during, and after accepting that the child may not be optimistic.
- Explore various options with children on how to communicate with friends/families in previous environment. Children's relationships with friends in the previous community are important, especially for "peer reassurance" after relocation.
- Keep regular routines in the new environment; establish them as soon as possible.
- Acknowledge the difficulty of peer losses with the adolescent.
- Join the organizations to which the child previously belonged (e.g., Scouts, sports).
- Assist children to focus on similarities between old and new environments (e.g., clubs, Scouts, church groups).
- Plan a trip to school during a class and lunch period to reduce fear of unknown.
- Allow children some choices regarding room arrangements, decorating, and the like.
- Ask teacher or counselor at the new school to introduce the adolescent to a student who recently relocated to that school.
- Allow children to mourn their losses as a result of the move.

Assess the Following Areas When Counseling a Relocated Adolescent

- Perceptions about the move
- Concurrent stressors
- Usual and present coping skills
- Support (family, peers, and community)

Initiate Health Teaching and Referrals, as Indicated

- Alert the family to the possible need for counseling before, during, or after the move.
- Furnish a written directory of relevant community organizations, such as area churches, children's groups, Parents Without Partners, senior citizens' groups, and Welcome Wagon or other local new-neighbor groups.
- Instruct the family about appropriate community services.
- Consult the school nurse regarding school programs for new students.

 Geriatric Interventions

Promote Integration After Transfer Into a Long-Term–Care Nursing Facility

- Allow as many choices as possible.
- Encourage person to bring familiar objects from home.
- Encourage person to interact with other individuals in new facility.
- Assist person to maintain previous interpersonal relationships.

Risk for Relocation Stress [Syndrome]

NANDA-I Definition

Vulnerable for physiologic and/or psychological disturbance following transfer from one environment to another, which may compromise health

Risk Factors

Refer to *Relocation Stress Syndrome* Related Factors.

Anxiety Self-Control, Coping, Loneliness, Psychosocial Adjustment: Life Change, Quality of Life, Fear Control

Goals

The individual/family members will report adjustment to the new environment with minimal disturbances, as evidenced by the following indicators:

* Share in decision-making activities regarding the new environment
* Express concerns regarding the move to a new environment
* Verbalize one positive aspect of the relocation
* Establish new bonds in the new environment
* Become involved in activities in the new environment

NIC

Anxiety Reduction, Coping Enhancement, Counseling, Family Involvement Promotion, Support System Enhancement, Anticipatory Guidance, Family Integrity Promotion, Transfer, Relocation Stress Reduction

Interventions

Determine the Reason for the Move (Whittenhal, 2008l)

* Voluntary move—usually related to a parent's/caregiver's. Usually positive; however the new job may be a less desirable. These moves are typically the least stressful of the three for adolescents.
* Forced move—can be the result of eviction, fleeing, and migratory work or going back to live with extended family. These situations are almost always negative with numerous stressors on the family unit.
* Legal move—is enforced and bound by law. Examples are relocation under witness protection, a foster child or steward of the state, and most frequently child custody with divorce.
* Refer individual to the publication at the Northern Illinois University website, "Helping an Adolescent Student Cope with Moving."

Advise Parents/Caregiver to Access School Personnel Before School Starts

* If desired, share with teacher whether this is a planned move, forced, or legal.
* Is there a program for welcoming new students?
* Ask if an appropriate student be assigned to buddy with the new student.

- Ask about clubs, organizations, and others that may be of interest to the new student.
- Suggest each student introduces himself or herself in addition to the new student.

Encourage Each Family Member to Share Feelings About the Move

- Provide privacy for each person.
- Encourage family members to share feelings with one another.
- Discuss the possible and different effects of the move on each family member.
- Inform parents regarding potential changes in children's conduct with relocation, such as regression, withdrawal, acting out, and changes with eating (breast/bottle-feeding).
- Instruct parents to obtain all pertinent documents regarding children's medical/dental history (e.g., immunizations, communicable diseases, dental work).
- Allow for some ritual(s) when leaving the old environment. Encourage reminiscing, which will bring closure for many family members.

Teach Parents Techniques to Assist Their Children With the Move

- Remain positive about the move before, during, and after accepting that the child may not be optimistic.
- Explore various options with children on how to communicate with friends/families in previous environment. Children's relationships with friends in the previous community are important, especially for "peer reassurance" after relocation.
- Keep regular routines in the new environment; establish them as soon as possible.
- Acknowledge the difficulty of peer losses with the adolescent.
- Join the organizations to which the child previously belonged (e.g., Scouts, sports).
- Assist children to focus on similarities between old and new environments (e.g., clubs, Scouts, church groups).
- Plan a trip to school during a class and lunch period to reduce fear of unknown.
- Allow children some choices regarding room arrangements, decorating, and the like.
- Ask teacher or counselor at the new school to introduce the adolescent to a student who recently relocated to that school.
- Allow children to mourn their losses as a result of the move.

Advise Parents/Caregivers to Routinely Discuss Their School Experience

- Avoid asking "How is school?"

- Ask instead:
  - Who did you eat lunch with? What did you do at recess?
  - What do you like about this new school?
  - What do you not like?

Assess the Following Areas When Counseling a Relocated Adolescent

- Perceptions about the move
- Concurrent stressors
- Usual and present coping skills
- Support (family, peers, and community)

Initiate Health Teaching and Referrals, as Indicated

- Alert the family to the possible need for counseling before, during, or after the move.
- Furnish a written directory of relevant community organizations, such as area churches, children's groups, parents without partners, senior citizens' groups, and Welcome Wagon or other local new-neighbor groups.
- Instruct the family about appropriate community services.
- Consult the school nurse regarding school programs for new students.

Promote Integration After Admission/Transfer Into a Long-Term–Care Nursing Facility

- Allow as many choices as possible regarding physical surroundings and daily routines.
- Encourage the individual or family to bring familiar objects from the individual's home.
- Orient to the physical layout of the environment.
- Introduce relocated individuals to new staff and fellow residents.
- Encourage interaction with other people in the new facility.
- Assist the individual in maintaining previous interpersonal relationships.
- Clearly state smoking rules and orient the individual to areas where smoking is permitted.
- Promote the development or maintenance of a relationship with a confidante.
- Re-establish normal routines, while initially increasing staffing and lighting, when a large number of long-term–care residents are involved in a secondary relocation.
- Assist nursing home residents to meet people from their previous geographic area.
- Arrange frequent contacts by a volunteer or staff member with each newly admitted resident. Also, match a successfully relocated resident with the new resident to begin the networking process.

RISK FOR COMPROMISED RESILIENCE

NANDA-I Definition

Vulnerable for decreased ability to sustain a pattern of positive responses to an adverse situation or crisis, which may compromise health

Risk Factors*

Chronicity of existing crises

Multiple coexisting adverse situations

Presence of additional new crisis (e.g., unplanned pregnancy, death of spouse, loss of job, illness, loss of housing, death of family member)

 Author's Note

This NANDA-I diagnosis is not a response but an etiology of a coping problem. Resilience is a strength that can be taught to and nurtured in children. Resilient individuals and families can cope in adverse situations and crises. They problem solve and adapt their functioning to the situation. For example, when a mother of a family of five had to undergo chemotherapy, the family formulated a plan together to divide the responsibilities previously managed by the mother.

When an individual or family is experiencing chronic, multiple adverse situations or a new crisis, refer to *Risk for Ineffective Coping*. In situations involving the loss of family member, significant other, or friend, refer to *Grieving* for Goals and Interventions.

IMPAIRED INDIVIDUAL RESILIENCE

NANDA-I Definition

Decreased ability to sustain a pattern of positive responses to an adverse situation or crisis

Defining Characteristics*

Decreased interest in academic activities

Decreased interest in vocational activities

Depression, guilt, shame

Isolation

Low self-esteem

Lower perceived health status

Renewed elevation of distress

Social isolation

Using maladaptive coping skills (e.g., drug use, violence)

Related Factors*

Demographics that increase chance of maladjustment

Drug use

Inconsistent parenting

Low intelligence

Low maternal education

Large family size

Minority status

Parental mental illness

Poor impulse control

Poverty, violence

Psychological disorders

Vulnerability factors that encompass indices that exacerbate the negative effects of the risk condition

 Author's Note

This NANDA-I diagnosis does not represent a nursing diagnosis. The defining characteristics are not defining resilience but in fact a variety of coping problems or mental disorders. Most of the related factors are prejudicial, pejorative, and cannot be changed by interventions. One related factor listed—poor impulse control—is a sign/symptom of hyperactivity disorders and some mental disorders. Resilience is a strength that can be taught to and nurtured in children. Resilient individuals and families can cope in adverse situations and crises. They problem solve and adapt their functioning to the situation. For example, when a mother of a family of five had to undergo chemotherapy, the family formulated a plan together to divide the responsibilities previously managed by the mother. When an individual or family has inadequate resilience, they are at risk for ineffective coping. Refer to *Ineffective Coping, Compromised or Disabled Family Coping* for Goals and Interventions.

RISK FOR INEFFECTIVE RESPIRATORY FUNCTION[34]

Risk for Ineffective Respiratory Function

Dysfunctional Ventilatory Weaning Response

Risk for Dysfunctional Ventilatory Weaning Response

Ineffective Airway Clearance

Ineffective Breathing Pattern

Impaired Gas Exchange

Impaired Spontaneous Ventilation

Definition

At risk for experiencing a threat to the passage of air through the respiratory tract and/or to the exchange of gases (O_2–CO_2) between the lungs and the vascular system

Risk Factors

Presence of risk factors that can change respiratory function (see Related Factors)

Related Factors

Pathophysiologic

Related to excessive or thick secretions secondary to:

Infection	Cardiac or pulmonary disease
Inflammation	Smoking
Allergy	Exposure to noxious chemical

Related to immobility, stasis of secretions, and ineffective cough secondary to:

Diseases of the nervous system (e.g., Guillain–Barré syndrome, multiple sclerosis, myasthenia gravis)

---

[34]This diagnosis is not currently on the NANDA list but has been included for clarity or usefulness.

Central nervous system (CNS) depression/head trauma
Cerebrovascular accident (stroke)
Quadriplegia

Treatment Related

Related to immobility secondary to:
Sedating or paralytic effects of medications, drugs, or chemicals
 (specify)
Anesthesia, general or spinal

Related to suppressed cough reflex secondary to (specify)

Related to effects of tracheostomy (altered secretions)

Situational (Personal, Environmental)

Related to immobility secondary to:

Surgery or trauma	Perception/cognitive impairment
Fatigue	Fear
Pain	Anxiety

Related to extremely high or low humidity
For infants, related to placement on stomach for sleep
Exposure to cold, laughing, crying, allergens, smoke

 Author's Note

Nurses' many responsibilities associated with problems of respiratory function include identifying and reducing or eliminating risk (contributing) factors, anticipating potential complications, monitoring respiratory status, and managing acute respiratory dysfunction.

The author has added *Risk for Ineffective Respiratory Function* to describe a state that may affect the entire respiratory system, not just isolated areas, such as airway clearance or gas exchange. Allergy and immobility are examples of factors that affect the entire system; thus, it is incorrect to say *Impaired Gas Exchange* related to immobility, because immobility also affects airway clearance and breathing patterns. The nurse can use the diagnoses *Ineffective Airway Clearance* and *Ineffective Breathing Patterns* when nurses can definitely alleviate the contributing factors influencing respiratory function (e.g., ineffective cough, stress).

The nurse is cautioned not to use this diagnosis to describe acute respiratory disorders, which are the primary responsibility of medicine and nursing together (i.e., collaborative problems). Such problems can be labeled *RC of Acute Hypoxia* or *RC of Pulmonary Edema*. When an individual's immobility is prolonged and threatens multiple systems—for example, integumentary, musculoskeletal, vascular, as well as respiratory—the nurse should use *Disuse Syndrome* to describe the entire situation.

NOC

Aspiration Control, Respiratory Status

Goals

The individual will have a respiratory rate within normal limits compared with baseline, as evidenced by the following indicators:

- Express willingness to be actively involved in managing respiratory symptoms and maximizing respiratory function
- Relate appropriate interventions to maximize respiratory status (varies depending on health status)
- Have satisfactory pulmonary function, as measured by PFTs

NIC

Airway Management, Cough Enhancement, Respiratory Monitoring, Positioning

Interventions

Determine Causative Factors

- Refer to Related Factors.

Eliminate or Reduce Causative Factors, If Possible

- Encourage ambulation as soon as consistent with the medical plan of care.
- If the individual cannot walk, establish a regimen for being out of bed in a chair several times a day (e.g., 1 hour after meals and 1 hour before bedtime).
- Increase activity gradually. Explain that respiratory function will improve and dyspnea will decrease with practice.
- For neuromuscular impairment:
  - Vary the position of the bed, thereby gradually changing the horizontal and vertical position of the thorax, unless contraindicated.
  - Assist the individual to reposition, turning frequently from side to side (hourly if possible).
  - In the hospital, especially if the individual is on a ventilator, use beds with continuous lateral rotation (when available) (Swadener-Culpepper, 2010).
  - Encourage deep breathing and controlled coughing exercises five times every hour.

- Teach the individual to use a blow bottle or incentive spirometer every hour while awake. (With severe neuromuscular impairment, the individual may have to be wakened during the night as well.)
- For individuals with quadriplegia, teach individual and caregivers the "quad cough." (Caregiver places a hand on the individual's diaphragm and thrusts upward and inward.)
- For a child, use colored water in a blow bottle; have him or her blow up balloons.
- Ensure optimal hydration status and nutritional intake.
- For the individual with a decreased level of consciousness:
  - Position the individual from side to side with a set schedule (e.g., left side on even hours, right side on odd hours); do not leave the individual lying flat on his or her back.
  - Position the individual on the right side after feedings (nasogastric tube feeding, gastrostomy) to prevent regurgitation and aspiration.
- Keep the head of the bed elevated at 30° unless contraindicated (Institute for Healthcare Improvement, 2008).
- See also *Risk for Aspiration*.

Prevent the Complications of Immobility

- See *Disuse Syndrome*.

Dysfunctional Ventilatory Weaning Response

NANDA-I Definition

Inability to adjust to lowered levels of mechanical ventilator support that interrupts and prolongs the weaning process

Defining Characteristics

Dysfunctional ventilatory weaning response (DVWR) is a progressive state, and experienced nurses have identified three levels (*Logan & Jenny, 1990): mild, moderate, and severe. The defining characteristics occur in response to weaning.

Mild

Restlessness

Slight increase of respiratory rate from baseline

Expressed feelings of increased oxygen need, breathing discomfort, fatigue, and warmth

Queries about possible machine dysfunction

Increased concentration on breathing

Moderate

Slight increase from baseline blood pressure (<20 mm Hg)*

Slight increase from baseline in heart rate (<20 beats/minute)*

Increase from baseline in respiratory rate (<5 breaths/minute)

Hypervigilance to activities

Inability to respond to coaching

Inability to cooperate

Apprehension

Diaphoresis

Wide-eyed look

Decreased air entry heard on auscultation

Color changes: pale, slight cyanosis

Slight respiratory accessory muscle use

Severe

Agitation*

Deterioration in arterial blood gases from current baseline

Increase from baseline blood pressure (≥20 mm Hg)

Increase from baseline heart rate (≥ 20 beats/min)

Shallow breaths

Cyanosis

Gasping breaths

Paradoxical abdominal breathing

Adventitious breath sounds

Full respiratory accessory muscle use

Profuse diaphoresis

Asynchronized breathing with the ventilator

Decreased level of consciousness

Paradoxical abdominal breathing

Related Factors

Pathophysiologic

Related to muscle weakness and fatigue secondary to:

Unstable hemodynamic status

Decreased level of consciousness

Chronic neuromuscular disability

Metabolic/acid–base

Abnormality

Severe disease process

Chronic respiratory disease

Multisystem disease

Fluid/electrolyte imbalance

Anemia

Infection

Chronic nutritional deficit

Debilitated condition

Pain

*Related to ineffective airway clearance**

Treatment Related

Related to obstructed airway

Related to muscle weakness and fatigue secondary to:
Excess sedation, analgesia
Uncontrolled pain

*Related to inadequate nutrition (deficit in calories, excess carbohydrates, inadequate fats, and protein intake)**

Related to prolonged ventilator dependence (more than 1 week)

Related to previously unsuccessful ventilator weaning attempt(s)

Related to too-rapid pacing of the weaning process

Situational (Personal, Environmental)

*Related to insufficient knowledge of the weaning process**

Related to excessive energy demands (self-care activities, diagnostic and treatment procedures, visitors)

*Related to inadequate social support**

Related to insecure environment (noisy, upsetting events, busy room)

Related to fatigue secondary to interrupted sleep patterns

Related to inadequate self-efficacy

Related to moderate to high anxiety related to breathing efforts

Related to fear of separation from ventilator

*Related to feelings of powerlessness**

*Related to feelings of hopelessness**

 Author's Note

Dysfunctional Ventilatory Weaning Response is a specific diagnosis within the category of *Risk for Ineffective Respiratory Function*. *Ineffective Airway Clearance*, *Ineffective Breathing Patterns*, and *Impaired Gas Exchange* can also be encountered during weaning, either as indicators of lack of weaning readiness or as factors related to the onset of DVWR. DVWR is a separate individual state. Its distinctive etiologies and treatments arise from the process of separating the individual from the mechanical ventilator.

The process of weaning is an art and a science. Because weaning is a collaborative process, the nurse's ability to gain the individual's trust and willingness to work is an important determinant of the weaning outcomes, especially with long-term individuals. This trust is fostered by the knowledge and self-confidence nurses display and by their ability to deal with individuals' specific concerns (*Jenny & Logan, 1991).

NOC

Anxiety Control, Respiratory Status, Vital Signs Status, Knowledge: Weaning, Energy Conservation

Goals

The individual will achieve progressive weaning goals, as evidenced by the following indicators:

- Have spontaneous breathing for 24 hours without ventilatory support
- Demonstrate a positive attitude toward the next weaning trial
  - Collaborate willingly with the weaning plan
  - Communicate comfort status during the weaning process
  - Attempt to control the breathing pattern
  - Try to control emotional responses
- Be tired from the work of weaning, but not exhausted

NIC

Anxiety Reduction, Preparatory Sensory Information, Respiratory Monitoring, Ventilation Assistance, Presence, Endurance

Interventions

If Applicable, Assess Causative Factors for Previous Unsuccessful Weaning Attempts

- Refer to Related Factors.

Follow the Institution's Multidiscipline Weaning Protocol (If Available)

- Document the specifics of the plan with a timetable.
- Establish predetermined criteria for terminating the weaning process.
- Outline each discipline's responsibilities.

Box I.I OBJECTIVE CRITERIA FOR WEANING (Epstien, 2015)

Required

The cause of the respiratory failure has improved.

$PaO_2/FiO_2 \geq 150$ or $SpO_2 \geq 90\%$ on $FiO_2 \leq 40\%$ and positive end-expiratory pressure (PEEP) ≤ 5 cmH_2O, pH >7.25

Some individuals require higher levels of PEEP to avoid atelectasis during mechanical ventilation.

Hemodynamic stability (no or low dose vasopressor medications)

Able to initiate an inspiratory effort

Additional criteria (optional criteria)

Hemoglobin ≥ 10 to 10 mg/dL

Core temperature $\leq 38°$ C to 38.5° C

Mental status awake and alert, or easily arousable.

- Review goals and progress at each shift. Document response.
- Collaborate if revisions are needed.

Determine Readiness for Weaning (*Morton, Fontaine, Hudak, & Gallo, 2005)

- Refer to Box I.1

Refer to Unit Protocols for Specific Weaning Procedures

Explain the Individual's Role in the Weaning Process

- Negotiate progressive weaning goals.
- Create a visual display of goals that uses symbols to indicate progression (e.g., bar or line graph to indicate increasing time off ventilator).
- Explain that these goals will be reexamined daily.
- From initial intubation, promote the understanding that mechanical ventilation is temporary.

Strengthen Feelings of Self-Esteem, Self-Efficacy, and Control

- Reinforce self-esteem, confidence, and control through normalizing strategies such as grooming, dressing, mobilizing, and conversing socially about things of interest to the individual.
- Permit as much control as possible by informing of the situation and his or her progress, permitting shared decision making about details of care, following the individual's preferences as far as possible, and improving comfort status.

- Increase confidence by praising successful activities, encouraging a positive outlook, and reviewing positive progress to date. Explain that people usually succeed in weaning; reassure the individual that you will be with him or her every step of the way.
- Maintain the individual's confidence by adopting a weaning pace that ensures success and minimizes setbacks.[35]
- Note concerns that hinder comfort and confidence (family members, topics of conversation, room events, previous weaning failures); discuss them openly and reduce them, if possible.

Reduce Negative Effects of Anxiety and Fatigue

- Monitor status frequently to avoid undue fatigue and anxiety. Use a systematic, comprehensive tool. A pulse oximeter is a noninvasive and unobtrusive way to monitor oxygen saturation levels.
- Provide regular periods of rest before fatigue advances.
- During a rest period, dim lights, post "do not disturb" signs, and play instrumental music with 60 to 80 beats/min. Allow the individual to select type of music (*Chan, 1998).
- Encourage calmness and breath control by reassuring the individual that he or she can and will succeed.
- Consider use of alternative relaxation therapies such as music, hypnosis, and biofeedback.
- If the individual is becoming agitated, coach him or her to regain breathing control. Monitor oxygen saturation and vital signs. Use ventilator support at night if necessary to increase sleep time, and try to avoid unnecessary awakening.
- If the weaning trial is discontinued, address the individual's perceptions of weaning failure. Reassure the individual that the trial was a good exercise and a useful form of training. Remind the individual that the work is good for the respiratory muscles and will improve future performance.

Risk for Dysfunctional Ventilatory Weaning Response

NANDA-I Definition

Vulnerable to compromised ability to adjust to lowered levels of mechanical ventilator support during the weaning process, related

---

[35]May require a primary professional's order

to physical and/or psychological unreadiness to wean, which may compromise health

Risk Factors

Pathophysiologic

Related to airway obstruction

Related to muscle weakness and fatigue secondary to:

Impaired respiratory functioning	Severe disease
Metabolic abnormalities	Unstable hemodynamic status
Dysrhythmia	
Fluid and/or electrolyte	Acid–base abnormalities
Decreased level of consciousness	Mental confusion
Fever	Infection
Anemia	Multisystem disease

Treatment Related

Related to ineffective airway clearance

Related to excess sedation, analgesia

Related to uncontrolled pain

Related to fatigue

Related to inadequate nutrition (deficit in calories, excess carbohydrates, inadequate fat, and protein intake)

Related to prolonged ventilator dependence (more than 1 week)

Related to previous unsuccessful ventilator weaning attempt(s)

Related to too-rapid pacing of the weaning process

Situational (Personal, Environmental)

Related to muscle weakness and fatigue secondary to:

Chronic nutritional deficit	Ineffective sleep patterns
Obesity	

Related to knowledge deficit related to the weaning process

Related to inadequate self-efficacy related to weaning

Related to moderate to high anxiety related to breathing efforts

Related to fear of separation from ventilator

Related to feelings of powerlessness

Related to depressed mood

Related to feelings of hopelessness

Related to uncontrolled energy demands (self-care activities, diagnostic and treatment procedures, visitors)

Related to inadequate social support

Related to insecure environment (noisy, upsetting events, busy room)

 Author's Note

This diagnosis is not a NANDA-I approved nursing diagnosis. The author has included this diagnosis for its clinical usefulness when individuals are in the process of weaning from a ventilator. If the process of weaning is problematic, use *Dysfunctional Weaning Response*.

See *Dysfunctional Ventilatory Weaning Response*.

NOC

Refer to *Dysfunctional Ventilatory Weaning Response*.

Goals

The individual will

- Demonstrate a willingness to start weaning
- Demonstrate a positive attitude about ability to succeed
  - Maintain emotional control
  - Collaborate with planning of the weaning

NIC

Cough Enhancement, Airway Suctioning, Positioning, Energy Management

Interventions

Refer to *Dysfunctional Ventilatory Weaning Response*.

Ineffective Airway Clearance

NANDA-I Definition

State in which an individual experiences inability to clear secretions or obstructions from the respiratory tract to maintain a clear airway

Defining Characteristics

Ineffective or absent cough
Inability to remove airway
  secretions

Abnormal breath sounds
Abnormal respiratory
  rate, rhythm, and depth

Related Factors

See *Risk for Ineffective Respiratory Function*.

Aspiration Control, Respiratory Status

Goals

The individual will not experience aspiration, as evidenced by the following indicators:

- Demonstrate effective coughing
- Demonstrate increased air exchange

NIC
Refer to *Dysfunctional Ventilatory Weaning Response*.

Interventions

The nursing interventions for the diagnosis *Ineffective Airway Clearance* represent interventions for any individual with this nursing diagnosis, regardless of the related factors.

Assess for Causative or Contributing Factors

• Refer to Related Factors.

Assess and Evaluate

• Sputum (color, volume, odor)
• Respiratory status before and after coughing exercises (breath sounds, rate, rhythm)

Supervise or Provide Oral Care Every 4 Hours as Indicated

If on Ventilator, Every 2 Hours or 12 Times in 24 Hours

• Brushed teeth at 8 AM and 8 PM with chlorhexidine
• Cleansed the mouth with tooth sponges 10 times per day
• Refer to *Risk for Oral Mucous Membrane* for additional interventions.

Reduce or Eliminate Barriers to Airway Clearance

Inactivity
• Encourage ambulation as soon as consistent with the medical plan of care.
• If the individual cannot walk, establish a regimen for being out of bed in a chair several times a day (e.g., 1 hour after meals and 1 hour before bedtime).
• Increase activity gradually. Explain that respiratory function will improve and dyspnea will decrease with practice.
• Assist with positioning upright; monitor for *Risk for Aspiration* (see *High Risk for Aspiration*).

R: *Lying flat causes the abdominal organs to shift toward the chest, thereby crowding the lungs and making it more difficult to breathe.*
Ineffective Cough
• Instruct on the proper method of controlled coughing.
• Breathe deeply and slowly while sitting up as high as possible.
• Use diaphragmatic breathing.
• Hold the breath for 3 to 5 seconds, then slowly exhale as much of this breath as possible through the mouth (lower rib cage and abdomen should sink down).
• Take a second breath; hold, slowly exhale, and cough forcefully from the chest (not from the back of the mouth or throat), using two short, forceful coughs.
• Increase fluid intake if not contraindicated.

Identify Individuals Who Are Unsuccessful in Attempts to Clear Secretions and Who May Require Suctioning (Nance-Floyd, 2011)

- Evidence:
  - Increased work of breathing
  - Changes in respiratory rate
  - Decreased oxygen saturation
  - Copious secretions, wheezing
- Proceed to suction (Sharma, Sarin, & Bala, 2014)
  - Place the person in supine position with head slightly extended.
  - Place the person on pulse oximeter to assess oxygenation.
  - Hyperoxygenate for 30 to 60 seconds before suctioning.
  - Make sure not to apply suction while inserting the suction catheter.
  - Apply continuous suction by covering the suction control hole.
  - Remove catheter in rotating movement.
  - The single episode of suctioning from removing of ventilator to reattachment of ventilator should not exceed 10 to 15 seconds.
  - Monitor O_2 saturation level of patient between each episode of suctioning.
  - Check the suction levels as follows:
    - 30 (100.00) 60 to 80 mm Hg for infants
    - 80 to 100 mm Hg for those under 10 to 12 years
    - 100 to 120 mm Hg for older children
  - Use suction pressure of up to 120 mm Hg for open-system suctioning and up to 160 mm Hg for closed-system suctioning with adults.
- Do not use normal saline solution (NSS) or normal saline bullets routinely to loosen tracheal secretions because this practice (Nance-Floyd, 2011)
  - May reach only limited areas
  - May flush particles into the lower respiratory tract
  - May lead to decreased postsuctioning oxygen saturation
  - Increases bacterial colonization
  - Damages bronchial surfactant
- See also *Risk for Aspiration*.
- Consult with physical therapy and respiratory therapy as indicated.

R: *Interventions that can enhance pulmonary function include exercise conditioning to improve lung compliance, relaxation and breathing training, chest percussion, postural drainage, and psychosocial rehabilitation.*

Prevent the Complications of Immobility

- See *Disuse Syndrome*.

Pediatric Interventions

- Instruct parents on the need for the child to cough, even if it is painful.
- Allow an adult and older child to listen to the lungs and describe if clear or if rales are present.
- Consult with a respiratory therapist for assistance, if needed.

Ineffective Breathing Pattern

NANDA-I Definition

Inspiration and/or expiration that does not provide adequate ventilation

Defining Characteristics*

Tachypnea, hyperpnea[36]
Panic and anxiety[36]
Complaints of headache, dyspnea, numbness and tingling, light-headedness, chest pain,[36] palpitations, and, occasionally, syncope,[36] bradycardia
Decreased expiratory pressure
Decreased inspiratory pressure
Alterations in depth of breathing
Orthopnea
Dysrhythmic respirations
Altered chest excursion

Assumption of three-point position
Decreased minute ventilation
Dyspnea
Increased anterior-posterior diameter
Prolonged expiration phase
Use of accessory muscles to breathe
Splinted/guarded respirations
Nasal flaring
Pursed-lip breathing

Related Factors

- See *Risk for Ineffective Respiratory Function*.

---

[36]Signs/symptoms of hyperventilation (Grossman & Porth, 2014)

Author's Note

This diagnosis has limited clinical utility except to describe situations that nurses definitively treat, such as hyperventilation. For individuals with chronic pulmonary disease with *Ineffective Breathing Patterns*, refer to *Activity Intolerance*. Individuals with periodic apnea and hypoventilation have a collaborative problem that can be labeled *Risk for Complications of Hypoxemia* to indicate that they are to be monitored for various respiratory dysfunctions. If the person is more vulnerable to a specific respiratory complication, the nurse can write the collaborative problem as *Risk for Complications of Pneumonia* or *Risk for Complications of Pulmonary Embolism*. Hyperventilation is a manifestation of anxiety or fear. The nurse can use *Anxiety* or *Fear related to (specify event) as manifested by hyperventilation* as a more descriptive diagnosis.

NOC

Respiratory Status, Vital Signs Status, Anxiety Control

Goals

The individual will achieve improved respiratory function, as evidenced by the following indicators:

- Demonstrate respiratory rate within normal limits, compared with baseline (8 to 24 breaths/min)
- Express relief of or improvement in feelings of shortness of breath
- Relate causative factors
- Demonstrate rebreathing techniques

NIC

Respiratory Monitoring, Progressive Muscle Relaxation, Teaching, Anxiety Reduction

Interventions

Assess History of Hyperventilating, Symptoms, and Causative Factors

- Previous episodes—when, where, circumstances
- Organic and physiologic
- Emotional (e.g., panic/anxiety disorder)
- Faulty breathing habits

Consider Other Medical Conditions That Can Present With Hyperventilation as (Schwartzstein & Richards, 2014)

- Metabolic disorders (ketoacidosis, less frequently hypoglycemia or hypocalcemia)
- Acute coronary syndrome
  - Arrhythmia
  - Heart failure
  - Pulmonary embolism
  - Pneumothorax
  - Asthma exacerbation
  - Chronic obstructive pulmonary disease exacerbation
  - Seizure disorder
  - Hyperthyroidism

Explain the Signs and Symptoms the Person May Be Experiencing (Schwartzstein & Richards, 2014)

- Feeling anxious, nervous, or tense
- Sense of impending doom
- Frequent sighing or yawning
- Feeling that he or she cannot get enough air (air hunger) or need to sit up to breathe
- A pounding and racing heartbeat
- Problems with balance, light-headedness, or vertigo
- Numbness or tingling in the hands, feet, or around the mouth
- Chest tightness, fullness, pressure, tenderness, or pain
- Carpopedal spasm (tetany)
- Headache
- Gas, bloating, or burping
- Twitching
- Sweating
- Vision changes, such as blurred vision or tunnel vision
- Problems with concentration or memory
- Loss of consciousness (fainting)

During an Acute Episode, Instruct the Person to Breathe With You, As You Do (WebMD, 2012). Do Not Leave Alone.

- Breathe through pursed lips, as if you are whistling, or pinch one nostril and breathe through your nose. It is harder to hyperventilate when you breathe through your nose or pursed lips, because you cannot move as much air.
- Slow your breathing to 1 breath every 5 seconds, or slow enough that symptoms gradually go away.
- Try belly-breathing, which fills your lungs fully, slows your breathing rate, and helps you relax.
- Place one hand on your belly just below the ribs. Place the other hand on your chest. You can do this while standing, but it

may be more comfortable while you are lying on the floor with your knees bent.

- Take a deep breath through your nose. As you inhale, let your belly push your hand out. Keep your chest still.
- As you exhale through pursed lips, feel your hand go down. Use the hand on your belly to help you push all the air out. Take your time exhaling.
- Repeat these steps 3 to 10 times. Take your time with each breath.

Instruct to Always Try Measures to Control Their Breathing or Belly Breathe First

- If these techniques do not work and there are no other health problems as heart or lung problems, such as coronary artery disease, asthma, chronic obstructive pulmonary disease (COPD, emphysema), or a history of deep vein thrombosis, stroke, or pulmonary embolism, try breathing in and out of a paper bag (WebMD, 2012).
- Take 6 to 12 easy, natural breaths, with a small paper bag held over your mouth and nose. Then remove the bag from your nose and mouth and take easy, natural breaths (WebMD, 2012).
- Next, try belly-breathing (diaphragmatic breathing).
- Alternate these techniques until your hyperventilation stops.
- Call 911 for emergency care (do not drive yourself to the hospital).

Remove or Control Causative Factors

- If hyperventilation continues for longer than 30 minutes, instruct to seek.
- If fear or panic has precipitated the episode:
  - Remove the cause of the fear, if possible.
  - Reassure that measures are being taken to ensure safety.
  - Distract the individual from thinking about the anxious state by having him or her maintain eye contact with you (or perhaps with someone else he or she trusts); say, "Now look at me and breathe slowly with me, like this."
  - Reassure the individual that he or she can control breathing; tell him or her that you will help.

Initiate Health Teaching and Referrals as Needed

- Explain a high altitude (above 6,000 feet [1,829 m]) rapid breathing faster than normal.
- Refer to pulmonary rehabilitation for breathing retraining.
- Refer to mental health if panic or anxiety disorder is suspected.

Impaired Gas Exchange

NANDA-I Definition

Excess or deficit in oxygenation and/or carbon dioxide elimination at the alveolar-capillary membrane

Defining Characteristics*

Abnormal arterial blood gases
Abnormal arterial pH
Abnormal breathing (e.g., rate, rhythm, depth)
Abnormal skin color (e.g., pale, dusky)
Confusion
Cyanosis (in neonates only)
Decreased carbon dioxide
Diaphoresis

Dyspnea
Headache upon awakening
Hypercapnia
Hypoxemia
Hypoxia
Irritability
Nasal flaring
Somnolence
Tachycardia
Visual disturbances

Related Factors

See Related Factors for *Risk for Ineffective Respiratory Function.*

 Author's Note

This diagnosis does not represent a situation for which nurses prescribe definitive treatment. Nurses do not treat *Impaired Gas Exchange*, but nurses can treat the functional health patterns that decreased oxygenation can affect, such as activity, sleep, nutrition, and sexual function. Thus, *Activity Intolerance related to insufficient oxygenation for activities of daily living* better describes the nursing focus. If an individual is at risk for or has experienced respiratory dysfunction, the nurse can describe the situation as *Risk for Complications of Hypoxemia* or be even more specific with *Risk for Complications of Pulmonary Embolism.* Refer to Section II Collaborative Problems.

Impaired Spontaneous Ventilation

NANDA-I Definition

Decreased energy reserves resulting in an inability to maintain independent breathing that is adequate to support life

Defining Characteristics*

Major

Dyspnea
Increased metabolic rate

Minor

Increased restlessness
Increased heart rate
Reports apprehension
Decreased PO_2
Increased use of accessory muscles

Increased PCO_2
Decreased tidal volume
Decreased cooperation
Decreased SaO_2

 Author's Note

This diagnosis represents respiratory insufficiency with corresponding metabolic changes that are incompatible with life. This situation requires rapid nursing and medical management, specifically resuscitation and mechanical ventilation. *Inability to Sustain Spontaneous Ventilation* is not appropriate as a nursing diagnosis; it is hypoxemia, a collaborative problem. *Hypoxemia* is insufficient plasma oxygen saturation from alveolar hypoventilation, pulmonary shunting, or ventilation-perfusion inequality. As a collaborative problem, physicians prescribe the definitive treatments; however, both nursing- and medical-prescribed interventions are required for management. The nursing accountability is to monitor status continuously and to manage changes in status with the appropriate interventions using protocols. For interventions, refer to *Risk for Complications of Hypoxemia* in Section 3 in Carpenito, L. J. (2016). *Nursing Diagnosis: Application to Clinical Practice* [15th ed.]. Philadelphia: Wolters Kluwer.

INEFFECTIVE ROLE PERFORMANCE

NANDA-I Definition

Patterns of behavior and self-expression that do not match environmental context, norms, and expectations

Defining Characteristics*

Altered role perceptions, anxiety
Inadequate adaptation to change
Role ambivalence

Role conflict, confusion, denial, dissatisfaction
Uncertainty
Role strain

Related Factors

Knowledge

Unrealistic role expectations
Inadequate role preparation (e.g., role transition, skill, rehearsal, validation)

Lack of education
Lack of role model

Physiologic

Body image alteration
Low self-esteem

Neurologic defects

Social

Conflict
Inadequate support system
Inappropriate linkage with the health-care system
Job schedule demands
Young age
Cognitive deficits
Depression, mental illness
Pain

Developmental level
Domestic violence
Inadequate role socialization
Lack of resources
Lack of rewards
Low socioeconomic status
Stress

Author's Note

The nursing diagnosis *Ineffective Role Performance* has a defining characteristic of "conflict related to role perception or performance." All people have multiple roles. Some are prescribed, such as gender and age; some are acquired, such as parent and occupation; and some are transitional, such as elected office or team member.

Various factors affect an individual's role, including developmental stage, societal norms, cultural beliefs, values, life events, illness, and disabilities. When an individual has difficulty with role performance, it may be more useful to describe the effect of the difficulty on functioning, rather than to describe the problem as *Ineffective Role Performance*. For example, an individual who has experienced a cerebrovascular accident (CVA) may undergo a change from being the primary breadwinner to becoming unemployed. In this situation, the nursing diagnosis *Interrupted Family Processes* and/or *Fear* related to loss of role as financial provider secondary to effects of CVA would be appropriate. In another example, if a woman could not continue her household responsibilities because of illness and other family members assumed these responsibilities, the situations that may arise would better be described as *Risk for Disturbed Self-Concept* related to recent loss of role responsibility secondary to illness and *Risk for Impaired Home Maintenance Management* related to lack of knowledge of family members.

A conflict in a family regarding others meeting role obligations or expectations can represent related factors for the diagnosis of *Ineffective Family Processes* related to conflict regarding expectations of members meeting role obligations.

Until clinical research defines this diagnosis and the associated nursing interventions, use *Ineffective Role Performance* as a related factor for another nursing diagnosis (e.g., *Anxiety*, *Grieving*, *Stress Overload*, or *Disturbed Self-Concept*).

SELF-CARE DEFICIT SYNDROME

Self-Care Deficit Syndrome[37]

Feeding Self-Care Deficit

Bathing Self-Care Deficit

---

[37]These diagnoses are not currently on the NANDA-I list but have been included by the author, for clarity or usefulness.

Dressing Self-Care Deficit

Instrumental Self-Care Deficit[37]

Toileting Self-Care Deficit

Definition[38]

A state in which an individual experiences an impaired motor function or cognitive function, causing a decreased ability in performing each of the five self-care activities

Defining Characteristics

Major (One Deficit Must Be Present in Each Activity)

Feeding Self-Care Deficit
Inability (or unwilling) to[38]:

Bring food from a receptacle to the mouth

Complete a meal

Place food onto utensils

Handle utensils

Ingest food in a socially acceptable manner

Open containers

Pick up cup or glass

Prepare food for ingestion

Use assistive device

Self-Bathing Deficits (Including Washing Entire Body, Combing Hair, Brushing Teeth, Attending to Skin and Nail Care, and Applying Makeup)[38]
Inability (or unwilling) to[38]:

Access bathroom

Get bath supplies

Wash body

Dry body

Obtain a water source

Regulate bath water

Self-Dressing Deficits (Including Donning Regular or Special Clothing, Not Nightclothes)[38]
Inability or unwillingness to[38]:

Choose clothing or put clothing on lower body

Put clothing on upper body

Put on/remove socks

Use assistive devices

Use zippers

---

[38]This characteristic has been included by the author for clarity or usefulness.

Put on necessary items of clothing
Maintain appearance at a satisfactory level
Pick up clothing
Put on shoes/remove shoes

Fasten, unfasten clothing
Obtain clothing

Self-Toileting Deficits
Unable or unwillingness to[38]:
Get to toilet or commode
Carry out proper hygiene
Manipulate clothing for toileting

Rise from toilet or commode
Sit on toilet or commode
Flush toilet or empty commode

Instrumental Self-Care Deficits[38]
Difficulty using telephone
Difficulty accessing transportation
Difficulty laundering, ironing
Difficulty managing money

Difficulty preparing meals
Difficulty with medication administration
Difficulty shopping

Related Factors

Pathophysiologic

Related to lack of coordination secondary to (specify)

Related to spasticity or flaccidity secondary to (specify)

Related to muscular weakness secondary to (specify)

Related to partial or total paralysis secondary to (specify)

Related to atrophy secondary to (specify)

Related to muscle contractures secondary to (specify)

Related to visual disorders secondary to (specify)

Related to nonfunctioning or missing limb(s)

Related to regression to an earlier level of development

Related to excessive ritualistic behaviors

Related to somatoform deficits (specify)

Treatment Related

Related to external devices (specify: casts, splints, braces, intravenous [IV] equipment)

Related to postoperative fatigue and pain

Situational (Personal, Environmental)

Related to cognitive deficits

Related to fatigue

Related to pain

Related to decreased motivation

Related to confusion

Related to disabling anxiety

Maturational

Older Adult
Related to decreased visual and motor ability, muscle weakness

 Author's Note

Self-care encompasses the activities needed to meet daily needs, commonly known as activities of daily living (ADLs), which are learned over time and become lifelong habits. Self-care activities involve not only what is to be done (hygiene, bathing, dressing, toileting, feeding), but also how much, when, where, with whom, and how (Miller, 2015).

In every individual, the threat or reality of a self-care deficit evokes panic. Many people report that they fear loss of independence more than death. A self-care deficit affects the core of self-concept and self-determination. For this reason, the nursing focus for self-care deficit should not be on providing the care measure, but on identifying adaptive techniques to allow the individual the maximum degree of participation and independence possible.

The diagnosis *Total Self-Care Deficit* once was used to describe an individual's inability to complete feeding, bathing, toileting, dressing, and grooming (*Gordon, 1982). The intent of specifying "Total" was to describe an individual with deficits in several ADLs. Unfortunately, sometimes its use invites, according to Magnan (1989, personal communication), "preconceived judgments about the state of an individual and the nursing interventions required." The individual may be viewed as in a vegetative state, requiring only minimal custodial care. *Total Self-Care Deficit* has been eliminated because its language does not denote potential for growth or rehabilitation.

Currently not on the NANDA-I list, the diagnosis *Self-Care Deficit Syndrome* has been added here to describe an individual with compromised ability in all five self-care activities. For this individual, the nurse assesses functioning in each area and identifies the level of participation of which the individual is capable. The goal is to maintain current functioning, to increase participation and independence, or both. The syndrome distinction clusters all five self-care deficits together to enable grouping of interventions when indicated, while also permitting specialized interventions for a specific deficit.

The danger of applying a *Self-Care Deficit* diagnosis lies in the possibility of prematurely labeling an individual as unable to participate at any level, eliminating a rehabilitation focus. It is important that the nurse classifies the individual's functional level to promote independence. Use this scale with the nursing diagnosis (e.g., *Toileting Self-Care Deficit* 2 = minimal help). Continuous reevaluation is also necessary to identify changes in the individual's ability to participate in self care.

NOC

See Bathing, Feeding, Dressing, Toileting, and/or Instrumental Self-Care Deficit

Goals

The individual will participate in feeding, dressing, toileting, and bathing activities, as evidenced by the following indicators (specify what the individual can perform with assistance and unassisted):

* Identify preferences in self-care activities (e.g., time, products, location)
* Demonstrate optimal hygiene after assistance with care

NIC

See Feeding, Bathing, Dressing, Toileting, and/or Instrumental Self-Care Deficit

Interventions

Assess for Causative or Contributing Factors

* Refer to Related Factors.

Promote Optimal Participation

* Consult with a physical therapist to assess present level of participation and for a plan.
    * Determine areas for potentially increased participation in each self-care activity.
    * Explore the individual's goals and determine what the individual perceives as his or her own needs.
    * Compare what the nurse believes are the individual's needs and goals, and then work to establish mutually acceptable goals.

- Allow the individual ample time to complete activities without help. Promote independence, but assist when the individual cannot perform an activity.

Promote Self-Esteem and Self-Determination

- Determine preferences for
  - Schedule
  - Products
  - Methods
  - Clothing selection
  - Hair styling
- During self-care activities, provide choices and request preferences.
- Do not focus on disability.
- Offer praise for independent accomplishments.

Evaluate the Individual's Ability to Participate in Each Self-Care Activity (Feeding, Dressing, Bathing, Toileting)

- Reassess ability frequently and revise code as appropriate.

Refer to Interventions Under Each Diagnosis—Feeding, Bathing, Dressing, Toileting, and Instrumental Self-Care Deficit—as Indicated

Feeding Self-Care Deficit

NANDA-I Definition

Impaired ability to perform or complete self-feeding activities

Defining Characteristics*

Inability (or unwilling) to[39]:

Bring food from a receptacle to the mouth

Complete a meal

Get food onto utensils

Handle utensils

Ingest food in a socially acceptable manner

Open containers

Pick up cup or glass

Prepare food for ingestion

Use assistive device

---

[39]These characteristics have been added by the author for clarity and usefulness.

Related Factors

Refer to *Self-Care Deficit Syndrome.*

 Author's Note

This diagnosis is appropriate for an individual who has difficulty with the activities of self-feeding. Individuals who have difficulty chewing and ingesting sufficient calories need an additional diagnosis of *Imbalanced Nutrition.*

NOC

Nutritional Status, Self-Care: Eating, Swallowing Status

Goals

The individual will demonstrate increased ability to feed self or report that he or she needs assistance, as evidenced by the following indicators:

* Demonstrate ability to make use of adaptive devices, if indicated
* Demonstrate increased interest and desire to eat
* Describe rationale and procedure for treatment
* Describe causative factors for feeding deficit

NIC

Feeding, Self-Care Assistance: Feeding, Swallowing Therapy, Teaching, Aspiration Precautions

Interventions

Assess Causative Factors

* Refer to Related Factors.

Use the Following Scale to Rate the Individual's Ability to Perform. Add the Number to the Individual's Nursing Diagnosis as Feeding Self-Care Deficit (3)

* 0 = Is completely independent
* 1 = Requires use of assistive device
* 2 = Needs minimal help
* 3 = Needs assistance and/or some supervision
* 4 = Needs total supervision
* 5 = Needs total assistance or unable to assist

Provide Opportunities to Relearn or Adapt to Activity

Common Nursing Interventions for Feeding

- Ascertain what foods the individual likes or dislikes.
- Provide meals in the same setting with pleasant surroundings that are not too distracting.
- Maintain correct food temperatures (hot foods hot, cold foods cold).
- Provide pain relief because pain can affect appetite and ability to feed self.
- Provide good oral hygiene before and after meals.
- Encourage the individual to wear dentures and eyeglasses.
- Assist the individual to the most normal eating position suited to his or her physical disability (best is sitting in a chair at a table).
- Provide social contact during eating.

Specific Interventions for People With Sensory/Perceptual Deficits

- Encourage the individual to wear prescribed corrective lenses.
- Describe the location of utensils and food on the tray or table.
- Describe food items to stimulate appetite.
- For perceptual deficits, choose different colored dishes to help distinguish items (e.g., red tray, white plates).
- Ascertain usual eating patterns and provide food items according to preference (or arrange food items in clock-like pattern); record on the care plan the arrangement used (e.g., meat, 6 o'clock; potatoes, 9 o'clock; vegetables, 12 o'clock).
- Encourage eating of "finger foods" (e.g., bread, bacon, fruit, hot dogs) to promote independence.
- Avoid placing food to the blind side of the individual with field cut until visually accommodated to surroundings; then encourage him or her to scan the entire visual field.

Specific Interventions for People With Missing Limbs

- Provide an eating environment that is not embarrassing to the individual; allow sufficient time for eating.
- Provide only the supervision and assistance necessary for relearning or adaptation.
- To enhance independence, provide necessary adaptive devices:
  - Plate guard to avoid pushing food off the plate
  - Suction device under the plate or bowl for stabilization
  - Padded handles on utensils for a more secure grip
  - Wrist or hand splints with clamp to hold eating utensils
  - Special drinking cup
  - Rocker knife for cutting

- Assist with setup if needed: opening containers, napkins, condiment packages; cutting meat; and buttering bread.
- Arrange food, so individual has enough space to perform the task of eating.

Specific Interventions for People With Cognitive Deficits
- Provide an isolated, quiet atmosphere until the individual can attend to eating and is not easily distracted from the task.
- Supervise the feeding program until there is no danger of choking or aspiration.
- Orient the individual to location and purpose of feeding equipment.
- Avoid external distractions and unnecessary conversation.
- Place the individual in the most normal eating position he or she can physically assume.
- Encourage the individual to attend to the task, but be alert for fatigue, frustration, or agitation.
- Provide one food at a time in usual sequence of eating until the individual can eat the entire meal in normal sequence.
- Encourage the individual to be tidy, to eat in small amounts, and to put food in the unaffected side of the mouth if paresis or paralysis is present.
- Check for food in cheeks.
- Refer to *Impaired Swallowing* for additional interventions.

Initiate Health Teaching and Referrals, as Indicated

- Ensure that both individual and family understand the reason and purpose of all interventions.
- Proceed with teaching as needed.
  - Maintain safe eating methods.
  - Prevent aspiration.
  - Use appropriate eating utensils (avoid sharp instruments).
  - Test the temperature of hot liquids and wear protective clothing (e.g., paper bib).
  - Teach the use of adaptive devices.

Bathing Self-Care Deficit

NANDA-I Definition

Impaired ability to perform or complete bathing activities for self

Defining Characteristics*

Self-bathing deficits (including washing the entire body, combing hair, brushing teeth, attending to skin and nail care, and applying makeup)[40]

Inability (or unwilling) to[40]:

Access bathroom

Get bath supplies

Wash and/or dry body

Obtain a water source

Regulate bath water

Related Factors

Refer to *Self-Care Deficit Syndrome*.

 Author's Note

Refer to *Self-Care Deficit Syndrome*.

NOC

Self-Care: Activities of Daily Living, Self-Care: Bathing

Goals

The individual will perform bathing activities at expected optimal level or report satisfaction with accomplishments despite limitations, as evidenced by the following indicators:

• Relate a feeling of comfort and satisfaction with body cleanliness
• Demonstrate the ability to use adaptive devices
• Describe causative factors of the bathing deficit

NIC

Self-Care Assistance: Bathing Teaching: Individual

Interventions

Assess Causative Factors

• Refer to Related Factors.

---

[40]These characteristics have been added by the author for clarity and usefulness.

Use the Following Scale to Rate the Individual's Ability to Perform. Add the Number to the Individual's Nursing Diagnosis as *Bathing Self-Care Deficit* (3)

- 0 = Is completely independent
- 1 = Requires use of assistive device
- 2 = Needs minimal help
- 3 = Needs assistance and/or some supervision
- 4 = Needs total supervision
- 5 = Needs total assistance or unable to assist

Provide Opportunities to Relearn or Adapt to Activity

General Nursing Interventions for Inability to Bathe

- Bathing time and routine should be consistent to encourage optimal independence.
- Encourage the individual to wear prescribed corrective lenses or hearing aid.
- Keep the bathroom temperature warm; ascertain the individual's preferred water temperature.
- Provide for privacy during bathing routine.
- Elicit from the individual his or her usual bathing routine.
- Keep the environment simple and uncluttered.
- Observe skin condition during bathing.
- Provide all bathing equipment within easy reach.
- Provide for safety in the bathroom (nonslip mats, grab bars).
- When the individual is physically able, encourage the use of either a tub or shower stall, depending on which he or she uses at home. (The individual should practice in the hospital in preparation for going home).
- Provide for adaptive equipment as needed:
  - Chair or stool in bathtub or shower
  - Long-handled sponge to reach back or lower extremities
  - Grab bars on bathroom walls where needed to assist in mobility
  - Bath board for transferring to tub chair or stool
  - Safety treads or nonskid mat on floor of bathroom, tub, and shower
  - Washing mitts with pocket for soap
  - Adapted toothbrushes
  - Shaver holders
  - Handheld shower spray
- Provide for relief of pain that may affect the individual's ability to bathe self.[41]

---

[41]May require a primary care professional's order.

Specific Bathing Interventions for People With Visual Deficits

- Place bathing equipment in a location most suitable to the individual.
- Avoid placing bathing equipment to the blind side if the individual has a field cut and is not visually accommodated to surroundings.
- Keep the call bell within reach if the individual is to bathe alone.
- Give the individual with visual impairment the same degree of privacy and dignity as any other individual.
- Announce yourself before entering or leaving the bathing area.
- Observe the individual's ability to perform mouth care, hair combing, and shaving.

Specific Bathing Interventions for People With Cognitive Deficits

- Determine the best method to bathe individual (e.g., towel bath, shower, tub bath).
- Provide a consistent time for bathing as part of a structured program to help decrease confusion.
- Keep instructions simple and avoid distractions; orient the individual to the purpose of bathing equipment and put toothpaste on the toothbrush.
- Preserve dignity.
- Provide verbal warning prior to doing anything (e.g., touching, spraying with water).
- Apply firm pressure to the skin when bathing; it is less likely to be misinterpreted than a gentle touch.
- Use a warm shower or bath to help a confused or agitated individual to relax.

Initiate Health Teaching and Referrals, as Indicated

- Teach the use of adaptive devices.
- Ascertain bathing facilities at home and assist in determining if there is any need for adaptations; refer to occupational therapy or social service for help in obtaining needed home equipment.
- Teach the individual to use the tub or shower stall, depending on what is used at home.

Dressing Self-Care Deficit

NANDA-I Definition

Impaired ability to perform or complete dressing activities for self

Defining Characteristics

Self-dressing deficits (including donning regular or special clothing, not nightclothes)[42]

Inability (or unwillingness) to[42]:

Choose clothing
Put clothing on lower or upper body
Maintain appearance at a satisfactory level
Pick up clothing
Put on/remove shoes

Put on/remove socks
Use assistive devices
Use zippers
Fasten, unfasten clothing
Obtain clothing

Related Factors

Refer to *Self-Care Deficit Syndrome*.

 Author's Note

Refer to *Self-Care Deficit Syndrome*.

NOC

Self-Care: Activities of Daily Living, Self-Care: Dressing

Goals

The individual will demonstrate increased ability to dress self or report the need to have someone else assist him or her to perform the task, as evidenced by the following indicators:

- Demonstrate ability to use adaptive devices to facilitate independence in dressing
- Demonstrate increased interest in wearing street clothes
- Describe causative factors for dressing deficits
- Relate rationale and procedures for treatments

NIC

Self-Care Assistance: Dressing/Grooming, Teaching: Individual, Dressing

---

[42]These characteristics have been added by the author for clarity and usefulness.

Interventions

Assess for Causative Factors

- Refer to Related Factors.

Use the Following Scale to Rate the Individual's Ability to Perform Add the Number to the Individual's Nursing Diagnosis as *Dressing Self-Care Deficit* (3)

- 0 = Is completely independent
- 1 = Requires use of assistive device
- 2 = Needs minimal help
- 3 = Needs assistance and/or some supervision
- 4 = Needs total supervision
- 5 = Needs total assistance or unable to assist

General Nursing Interventions for Self-Dressing

- Obtain clothing that is larger-sized and easier to put on, including clothing with elastic waistbands, wide sleeves and pant legs, dresses that open down the back for women in wheelchairs, and Velcro fasteners or larger buttons.
- Encourage the individual to wear prescribed corrective lenses or hearing aid.
- Promote independence in dressing through continual and unaided practice.
- Provide dressing aids as necessary (some commonly used aids include dressing stick, Swedish reacher, zipper pull, buttonhook, long-handled shoehorn, and shoe fasteners adapted with elastic laces).

Specific Dressing Interventions for People With Visual Deficits

- Allow the individual to select the most convenient location for clothing and adapt the environment to accomplish the task best (e.g., remove unnecessary barriers).
- Announce yourself before entering or leaving the dressing area.
- If the individual has a field cut, avoid placing clothing to the blind side until he or she is visually accommodated to the surroundings; then encourage him or her to turn the head to scan the entire visual field.

Specific Dressing Interventions for People With Cognitive Deficits (Miller, 2015)

- Keep verbal communication simple.
  - Ask yes/no questions.
  - Use one-step requests (e.g., "put your sock on").

- Praise after each step.
- Call the individual by name.
- Use the same word for the same thing (e.g., "shirt").
- Dress the bottom half, and then the top half.
- Prepare an uncluttered environment.
  - Lay clothes face down.
  - Place clothes in the order that they will be used.
  - Allow the individual a choice from only two pieces.
  - Place matching clothes together on hangers.
  - Remove dirty clothes from the dressing area.
- Provide nonverbal cues.
  - Hand one clothing item at a time in correct order.
  - Place shoes beside the correct foot.
  - Point or touch the body part to be used.
  - If the individual cannot complete all the steps, always allow him or her to finish the dressing step, if possible—zipper pants, buckle belt.
  - Decrease assistance gradually.

Initiate Health Teaching and Referrals, as Indicated

- Access a home health nurse for an in-home evaluation.

Instrumental Self-Care Deficit[43]

Definition

Impaired ability to perform certain activities or access certain services essential for managing a household

Defining Characteristics

Observed or reported difficulty with one or more of the following:

Using a telephone	Shopping (food, clothes)
Accessing transportation	Managing money
Laundering and ironing	Administering medication
Preparing meals	

---

[43]This diagnosis is not currently on the NANDA-I list but has been included by the author for clarity or usefulness.

Related Factors

Refer to *Self-Care Deficit Syndrome*.

 Author's Note

Instrumental Self-Care Deficit is not currently on the NANDA-I list but has been added here for clarity and usefulness. This diagnosis describes problems with performing certain activities or accessing certain services, including housekeeping, preparing and procuring food, shopping, laundering, ability to self-medicate safely, ability to manage money, and access to transportation (Miller, 2015). Instrumental ADLs require more complex tasks than ADLs.

 NOC

Self-Care: Instrumental Activities of Daily Living (IADL)

Goals

The individual or family will report satisfaction with household management, as evidenced by the following indicators:

* Demonstrate use of adaptive devices (e.g., telephone, cooking aids)
* Describe a method to ensure adherence to medication schedule
* Report ability to make calls and answer the telephone
* Report regular laundering by self or others
* Report daily intake of at least two nutritious meals
* Identify transportation options to stores, physician, house of worship, and social activities
* Demonstrate management of simple money transactions
* Identify people who will assist with money matters

 NIC

Teaching: Individual, Referral, Family Involvement Promotion

Interventions

Assess for Causative and Contributing Factors

* Refer to Related Factors.

Use the Following Scale to Rate the Individual's Ability to Perform. Add the Number to the Individual's Nursing Diagnosis as *Instrumental Self-Care Deficit* (0)

- 0 = Is completely independent
- 1 = Requires use of assistive device
- 2 = Needs minimal help
- 3 = Needs assistance and/or some supervision
- 4 = Needs total supervision
- 5 = Needs total assistance or unable to assist

Ensure an Occupational Therapist is Consulted and an In-Home Assessment Planned

Evaluate the Individual's Ability to Select, Procure, and Prepare Nutritious Food Daily

- Prepare a permanent shopping list with cues for essential foods and products.
- Teach the individual to review the list before shopping, check items needed, and, in the store, check off items selected. (Use a pencil that can be erased to reuse list.)
- Teach the individual how to shop for single-person meals (refer to *Imbalanced Nutrition* for specific techniques).
- If possible, teach the individual to use a microwave to reduce the risk of heat-related injuries or accidents.

Offer Hints to Improve Adherence to Medication Schedule

- Have someone place medications in a commercial pill holder divided into 7 days.
- Take out the exact amount of pills for the day. Divide them in small cups, each labeled with time of day.
- If needed, draw a picture of the pills and the quantity on each cup.
- Teach the individual to transfer the pills from cup to small plastic bag when planning to be away from home.
- Tell the individual whom to call for instructions if he or she misses a dose.

Initiate Health Teaching and Referrals, as Indicated

- Ensure a home assessment is scheduled (e.g., nursing, social services, occupational therapy, physical therapy).
- Determine available sources of transportation (neighbors, relatives, community centers)
  - Refer the individual to church groups or social service agency.
  - Refer the individual to community agencies for assistance (e.g., Department of Social Services, area agency on aging, senior neighbors, public health nursing, Meals on Wheels).

Toileting Self-Care Deficit

NANDA-I Definition

Impaired ability to perform or complete toileting activities for self

Defining Characteristics[*]

Unable (or unwilling) to[44]:
Get to toilet or commode
Carry out proper hygiene
Manipulate clothing for toileting

Rise from toilet or commode
Sit on toilet or commode
Flush toilet or empty
commode

Related Factors

Refer to *Self-Care Deficit Syndrome*.

 Author's Note

Refer to *Self-Care Deficit Syndrome*.

NOC
Self-Care: Activities of Daily Living, Self-Care: Hygiene, Self-Care: Toileting

Goals

The individual will demonstrate increased ability to toilet self or report the need to have someone assist him or her to perform the task, as evidenced by the following indicators (specify when assistance is needed):

• Demonstrate the ability to use adaptive devices to facilitate toileting
• Describe causative factors for toileting deficit
• Relate the rationale and procedures for treatment

---

[44]These characteristics have been added by the author for clarity and usefulness.

NIC

Self-Care Assistance: Toileting, Self-Care Assistance: Hygiene, Teaching Individual, Mutual Goal Setting

Interventions

Assess Causative Factors

• Refer to Related Factors.

Use the Following Scale to Rate the Individual's Ability to Perform. Add the Number to the Individual's Nursing Diagnosis as *Toileting Self-Care Deficit* (3)

• 0 = Is completely independent
• 1 = Requires use of assistive device
• 2 = Needs minimal help
• 3 = Needs assistance and/or some supervision
• 4 = Needs total supervision
• 5 = Needs total assistance or unable to assist

Common Nursing Interventions for Toileting Difficulties

• Obtain bladder and bowel history from the individual or family (see *Impaired Bowel Elimination* or *Impaired Urinary Elimination*).
• Ascertain the individual knows how to use the communication system to request assistance.
• Avoid development of "bowel fixation" by less frequent discussion and inquiries about bowel movements.
• Be alert to the possibility of falls when toileting the individual (be prepared to ease him or her to the floor without injuring either of you).
• Allow sufficient time for the task of toileting to avoid fatigue. (Lack of sufficient time to toilet may cause incontinence or constipation.)

Specific Toileting Interventions for People With Visual Deficits

• Keep the call bell easily accessible so the individual can quickly obtain help to toilet; answer the call bell promptly to decrease anxiety.
• If the bedpan or urinal is necessary for toileting, be sure it is within the individual's reach.
• Avoid placing toileting equipment to the side of an individual with field cut. (When he or she is visually accommodated to surroundings, you may suggest he or she search the entire visual field for equipment.)
• Announce yourself before entering or leaving the toileting area.

- Observe the individual's ability to obtain equipment or get to the toilet unassisted.

Specific Toileting Interventions for People With Cognitive Deficits

- Offer toileting reminders every 2 hours, after meals, and before bedtime.
- When the individual can indicate the need to toilet, begin toileting at 2-hour intervals, after meals, and before bedtime.
- Answer the call bell immediately to avoid frustration and incontinence.
- Encourage wearing ordinary clothes. (Many confused people are continent while wearing regular clothing.)
- Avoid the use of bedpans and urinals; if physically possible, provide a normal atmosphere of elimination in bathroom. (The toilet used should remain constant to promote familiarity.)
- Give verbal cues as to what is expected of the individual and positive reinforcement for success.
- Refer to *Impaired Urinary Elimination* for additional information on incontinence.

Initiate Health Teaching and Referrals, as Indicated

- Assess the understanding and knowledge of the individual and family of foregoing interventions and rationales.

DISTURBED SELF-CONCEPT

Disturbed Self-Concept

Disturbed Body Image

Disturbed Personal Identity

Risk for Disturbed Personal Identity

Disturbed Self-Esteem

Chronic Low Self-Esteem

Risk for Chronic Low Self-Esteem

Situational Low Self-Esteem

Risk for Situational Low Self-Esteem

Definition[45]

A negative state of change about the way a person feels, thinks, or views himself or herself. It may include a change in body image, self-esteem, or personal identity (Boyd, 2012)

Defining Characteristics

This diagnosis reflects a broad diagnostic category that can be used initially until more specific assessment data can support a more specific nursing diagnosis, such as *Disturbed Body Image* or *Disturbed Self-Esteem*.

Some examples of signs and symptoms (observed or reported) are:

Verbal or nonverbal negative response to actual or perceived change in structure, function, or both (e.g., shame, embarrassment, guilt, revulsion)

Expression of shame or guilt

Rationalization or rejection of positive feedback and exaggeration of negative feedback about self

Hypersensitivity to slight criticism

Episodic occurrence of negative self-appraisal in response to life events in an individual with a previously positive self-evaluation

Verbalization of negative feelings about self (helplessness, uselessness)

Related Factors

A disturbed self-concept can occur as a response to a variety of health problems, situations, and conflicts. Some common sources follow.

Pathophysiologic

Related to change in appearance, lifestyle, role, response of others secondary to:

Chronic disease   Pain
Severe trauma   Loss of body functions
Loss of body parts

---

[45]This definition has been added by the author for clarity and usefulness.

Situational (Personal, Environmental)

Related to feelings of abandonment or failure secondary to:
Divorce, separation from, or death of a significant other
Loss of job or ability to work

Related to immobility or loss of function

Related to unsatisfactory relationships (parental, spousal)

Related to sexual preferences (homosexual, lesbian, bisexual, abstinent)

Related to teenage pregnancy

Related to gender differences in parental child-rearing

Related to experiences of parental violence

Related to change in usual patterns of responsibilities

Maturational

Middle-Aged
Loss of role and responsibilities

Older Adult
Loss of role and responsibilities

 Author's Note

Self-concept reflects self-view, encompassing body image, esteem, role performance, and personal identity. Self-concept develops over a lifetime and is difficult to change. It is influenced by interactions with the environment and others and by the individual's perceptions of how others view him or her.

Disturbed Self-Concept represents a broad diagnostic category under which fall more specific nursing diagnoses. Initially, the nurse may not have sufficient clinical data to validate a more specific diagnosis, such as Chronic Low Self-Esteem or Disturbed Body Image; thus, he or she can use Disturbed Self-Concept until data can support a more specific diagnosis.

Self-esteem is one of the four components of self-concept. Disturbed Self-Esteem is the general diagnostic category. Chronic Low Self-Esteem and Situational Low Self-Esteem represent specific types of Disturbed Self-Esteem and thus involve more specific interventions. Initially, the nurse may not have sufficient clinical data to validate a more specific diagnosis, such as Chronic Low Self-Esteem or Situational Low Self-Esteem; thus, Disturbed Self-Esteem may be appropriate to use. Refer to the major Defining Characteristics under these categories for validation.

Situational Low Self-Esteem is an episodic event; repeated occurrence, continuous negative self-appraisals over time, or both can lead to *Chronic Low Self-Esteem* (Willard, 1990, personal communication).

NOC

Quality of Life, Depression Level, Depression, Self-Control, Self-Esteem, Coping

Goals

The individual will demonstrate healthy adaptation and coping skills, as evidenced by the following indicators:

- Appraise self and situations realistically without distortions
- Verbalize and demonstrate increased positive feelings

NIC

Hope Instillation, Mood Management, Values Clarification, Counseling, Referral, Support Group, Coping Enhancement

Interventions

Contact the Individual Frequently and Treat Him or Her With Warm, Positive Regard

Encourage the Individual to Express Feelings and Thoughts About the Following:

- Condition
- Progress
- Prognosis
- Effects on lifestyle
- Support system
- Treatment

Provide Reliable Information and Clarify Any Misconceptions

Document the Person's Own Words, Not an Interpretation of the Words

Help Individual to Identify Positive Attributes and Possible New Opportunities

Assist With Hygiene and Grooming, as Needed

Encourage Visitors

Help Individual Identify Strategies to Increase Independence and to Maintain Role Responsibilities

- Prioritizing activities
- Using mobility aids and assistive devices, as needed

Promote the Most Involvement in Self-Care as Possible

- Prioritizing activities
- Using mobility aids and assistive devices, as needed

Discuss With Individual's Family the Importance of Communicating the Individual's Value and Importance to Them

Initiate Health Teaching, as Indicated

- Teach individual what community resources are available, if needed (e.g., mental health centers, self-help groups such as Reach for Recovery, Make Today Count).
- Refer to specific health teaching issues under *Disturbed Body Image*, *Disturbed Self-Esteem* (*Chronic* and *Situational*).

⚜ Pediatric Interventions

- Allow the child to bring his or her own experiences into the situation (e.g., "Some children say that an injection feels like an insect sting; some say they don't feel anything. After we do this, you can tell me how it feels"; *Johnson, 1995).
- Avoid using "good" or "bad" to describe behavior. Be specific and descriptive (e.g., "You really helped me by holding still. Thank you for helping"; *Johnson, 1995).
- Connect previous experiences with the present one (e.g., "The X-ray camera will look different from the last time. You will have to hold real still again. The table will move, too"; *Johnson, 1995).
- Convey optimism with positive self-talk (e.g., "I am so busy today. I wonder if I will get all my work done? I bet I can." or "When you come back from surgery you will need to stay in bed. What would you like to do when you come back?").
- Help the child plan playtime with choices. Encourage crafts that produce an end product.
- Encourage interactions with peers and supportive adults.
- Encourage child to decorate room with crafts and personal items.

Disturbed Body Image

NANDA-I Definition

Confusion in mental picture of one's physical self

Defining Characteristics

Major (Must Be Present)

Verbal or nonverbal negative response to actual or perceived
    change in structure and/or function (e.g., shame, embarrass-
    ment, guilt, revulsion)

Minor (May Be Present)

Not looking at body part*
Not touching body part*
Intentional hiding or overexposing body part*
Change in social involvement*
Negative feelings about body; feelings of helplessness, hopeless-
    ness, powerlessness, vulnerability
Preoccupation with change or loss
Refusal to verify actual change
Depersonalization of part or loss
Self-destructive behaviors (e.g., mutilation, suicide attempts,
    overeating/undereating)

Related Factors

Pathophysiologic

Related to changes in appearance secondary to:

Chronic disease	Illness*
Loss of body part or body function	Aging
Severe trauma	

Related to unrealistic perceptions of appearance secondary to:

Psychosis	Bulimia
Anorexia nervosa	

Treatment Related

Related to changes in appearance secondary to:

Hospitalization	Radiation
Surgery*	Treatment regimen*
Chemotherapy	

Situational (Personal, Environmental)

Related to physical trauma secondary to:*

Sexual abuse	Rape (perpetrator known or unknown)
Accidents	Assault

Related to effects of (specify) on appearance:
Obesity

Related to cognitive/perceptual factors*

Related to morbid fear of obesity (Varcarolis, 2011)

Maturational

Related to developmental changes*
Immobility
Pregnancy

 Author's Note

An amputation results in several limitations in performing professional, leisure, and social activities. It reduces mobility, pain, and physical integrity, which disturbs the integrity of the human body and lowers the quality of life (QoL). Psychological issues range from depression, anxiety and to suicide in severe cases (*Atherton & Robertson, 2006; Holzer et al., 2014). The loss of a body part also affects the perception of someone's own body and its appearance (Holzer et al., 2014).

NOC

Body Image, Child Development: (specify age), Grief Resolution, Psychosocial Adjustment: Life Change, Self-Esteem

Goals

The person will implement new coping patterns and verbalize and demonstrate acceptance of appearance (grooming, dress, posture, eating patterns, presentation of self), as evidenced by the following indicators:

- Demonstrate a willingness and ability to resume self-care/role responsibilities
- Initiate new or reestablish contacts with existing support systems

NIC

Self-Esteem Enhancement, Counseling, Presence, Active Listening, Body Image Enhancement, Grief Work Facilitation, Support Group, Referral

Interventions

Establish a Trusting Nurse–Individual Relationship

- Encourage person to express feelings, especially about the way he or she feels, thinks, or views self.
- Encourage to ask questions about health problem, treatment, progress, and prognosis.
- Provide reliable information and reinforce information already given.
- Clarify any misconceptions about self, care, or caregivers.
- Provide privacy and a safe environment.

Promote Social Interaction

- Encourage movement.
- Prepare significant others for physical and emotional changes.
- Support family as they adapt.
- Encourage visits from peers and significant others.
- Encourage contact (letters, telephone) with peers and family.
- Encourage involvement in unit activities.
- Provide opportunity to share with people going through similar experiences.

Provide Specific Interventions in Selected Situations

Loss of Body Part or Function

- Assess the meaning of the loss for the individual and significant others, as related to visibility of loss, function of loss, and emotional investment.
- Explore and clarify misconceptions and myths regarding loss or ability to function with loss.
- Expect the individual to respond to the loss with denial, shock, anger, and depression.
- Be aware of the effect of the responses of others to the loss; encourage sharing of feelings between significant others.
- Validate feelings by allowing the individual to express his or her feelings and to grieve.
- Use role-playing to assist with sharing; if the individual says, "I know my husband will not want to touch me with this colostomy," take the husband's role and discuss her colostomy, then switch roles so she can act out her feelings about her husband's response.
- Explore strengths and resources with person.

- Assist with the resolution of a surgically created alteration of body image:
  - Replace the lost body part with prosthesis as soon as possible.
  - Encourage viewing of site.
  - Encourage touching of site.
  - Encourage activities that encompass new body image (e.g., shopping for new clothes).
- Begin to incorporate person in care of operative site.
- Gradually allow individual to assume full self-care responsibility, if feasible.

Changes Associated With Chemotherapy (*Camp-Sorrell, 2007)
- Discuss the possibility of hair loss, absence of menses, temporary or permanent sterility, decreased estrogen levels, vaginal dryness, and mucositis.
- Encourage individual to share concerns, fears, and perception of the effects of these changes on life.
- Explain where hair loss may occur (head, eyelashes, eyebrows; axillary, pubic, and leg hair).
- Explain that hair will grow back after treatment but may change in color and texture.
- Encourage individual to select and wear a wig before hair loss. Suggest consulting a beautician for tips on how to vary the look (e.g., combs, clips).
- Encourage the wearing of scarves or turbans when wig is not on.
- Teach individual to minimize the amount of hair loss by
  - Cutting hair short
  - Avoiding excessive shampooing
  - Using a conditioner twice weekly
  - Patting hair dry gently
  - Avoiding electric curlers, dryers, and curling irons
  - Avoiding pulling hair with bands, clips, or bobby pins
  - Avoiding hair spray and hair dye
  - Using wide-tooth comb, avoiding vigorous brushing
- Refer individual to American Cancer Society for information about new or used wigs. Inform the individual that the wig is a tax-deductible item.
- Discuss the difficulty that others (spouse, friends, coworkers) may have with visible changes.
- Encourage individual to initiate calls and contacts with others who may be having difficulty.
- Encourage individual to ask for assistance of friends and relatives. Ask person if the situation were reversed, what he or she would want to do to help a friend.
- Allow significant others opportunities to share their feelings and fears.

- Assist significant others to identify positive aspects of the individual and ways this can be shared.
- Provide information about support groups for couples.

Anorexia Nervosa, Bulimia Nervosa
- Differentiate between body image distortion and body image dissatisfaction.
- Provide factual feedback on low weight and determents to health. Do not argue or challenge their distorted perceptions (Varcarolis, 2011).
- Know that the person's distorted image is their reality (Varcarolis, 2011).
- Assist to identify their positive traits (Varcarolis, 2011).
- Refer individuals for psychiatric counseling.

Psychoses
- Refer to *Confusion* for specific information and interventions.

Sexual Abuse
- Refer to *Disabled Family Coping* for specific information and interventions.

Sexual Assault
- Refer to *Rape-Trauma Syndrome* for specific information and interventions.

Assault
- Refer to *Post-Trauma Response* for specific information and interventions.

Initiate Health Teaching, as Indicated

- Teach what community resources are available, if needed (e.g., mental health centers, self-help groups such as Reach for Recovery, Make Today Count).
- Teach wellness strategies.

Pediatric Interventions

For Hospitalized Child
- Prepare child for hospitalization, if possible, with an explanation and a visit to the hospital to meet personnel and examine the environment.
- Provide familiarities/routines of home as much as possible (e.g., favorite toy or blanket, story at bedtime).
- Provide nurturance (e.g., hug).

- Provide child with opportunities to share fears, concerns, and anger:
  - Provide play therapy.
  - Correct misconceptions (e.g., that the child is being punished; that parents are angry).
  - Encourage family to stay with or visit child, despite the child's crying when they leave; teach them to provide accurate information about when they will return to reduce fears of abandonment.
  - Allow parents to help with care.
  - Ask child to draw a picture of self, and then ask for a verbal description.
- Assist child to understand experiences:
  - Provide an explanation ahead of time, if possible.
  - Explain sensations and discomforts of condition, treatments, and medications.
  - Encourage crying.

Discuss With Parents How Body Image Develops and What Interactions Contribute to Their Child's Self-Perception

- Teach the names and functions of body parts.
- Acknowledge changes (e.g., height).
- Allow some choices for what to wear.

For Adolescents
- Discuss with parents the adolescent's need to "fit in":
  - Do not dismiss concerns too quickly.
  - Be flexible and compromise when possible (e.g., clothes are temporary, tattoos are not).
  - Negotiate a time period to think about options and alternatives (e.g., 4 to 5 weeks).
  - Provide with reasons for denying a request. Elicit adolescent's reasons. Compromise if possible (e.g., parents want curfew at 11:00; adolescent wants 12:00; compromise at 11:30).
  - Provide opportunities to discuss concerns when parents are not present.
  - Prepare for impending developmental changes.

🧍 Maternal Interventions

- Encourage the woman to share her concerns.
- Attend to each concern, if possible, or refer her to others for assistance.
- Discuss the challenges and changes that pregnancy and motherhood bring.
- Encourage her to share expectations: her own and those of her significant others.

- Assist her to identify sources for love and affection.
- Provide anticipatory guidance to both parents-to-be concerning:
  - Fatigue and irritability
  - Appetite swings
  - Gastric disturbances (nausea, constipation)
  - Back and leg aches
  - Changes in sexual desire and activity (e.g., sexual positions as pregnancy advances)
  - Mood swings
  - Fear (for self, for unborn baby, of loss of attractiveness, of inadequacy as a parent)
- Encourage sharing of concerns between spouses.

Disturbed Personal Identity

NANDA-I Definition

Inability to maintain an integrated and complete perception of self

Defining Characteristics
(Varcarolis, 2011)

Appears unaware of or uninterested in others or their activities
Unable to identify parts of the body or body sensations (e.g., enuresis)
Excessively imitates other's activities or words
Fails to distinguish parent/caregiver as a whole person
Becomes distressed with bodily contact with others
Spends long periods of time in self-stimulating behaviors (self-touching, sucking, rocking)
Needs ritualistic behaviors and sameness to control anxiety
Cannot tolerate being separated from parent/caregiver

Related Factors
(Varcarolis, 2011)

Pathophysiologic

Related to biochemical imbalance

Related to impaired neurologic development or dysfunction

Maturational

Related to failure to develop attachment behaviors, resulting in fixation at autistic phase of development

Related to interrupted or uncompleted separation/individualization process, resulting in extreme separation anxiety

 Author's Note

Disturbed Personal Identity is a very complex diagnosis and should not be used to label autism. It may be more clinically useful in nursing to use *Anxiety* and/or *Impaired Social Interactions* for the nursing focus.

Risk for Disturbed Personal Identity

NANDA-I Definition

Vulnerable for the inability to maintain an integrated and complete perception of self, which may compromise health

Risk Factors*

Chronic low self-esteem
Psychiatric disorders (e.g., psychoses, depression, dissociative disorder)
Cult indoctrination
Situational crises
Situational low self-esteem
Cultural discontinuity
Social role change
Discrimination
Stages of development
Dysfunctional family processes
Stages of growth
Ingestion/inhalation of toxic chemicals
Use of psychoactive pharmaceutical agents
Manic states
Multiple personality disorder
Organic brain syndromes
Perceived prejudice

 Author's Note

Refer to *Disturbed Personal Identity*.

Disturbed Self-Esteem[46]

Definition

State in which a person experiences or is at risk of experiencing negative self-evaluation about self or capabilities

Defining Characteristics
Leuner, Coler, & Norris, 1994; *Norris & Kunes-Connell, 1987)

Major (Must Be Present, One or More)

Observed or Reported

Self-negating verbalization
Expressions of shame or guilt
Evaluates self as unable to deal with events
Rationalizes away or rejects positive feedback and exaggerates negative feedback about self

Lack of or poor problem-solving ability
Hesitant to try new things or situations
Rationalizes personal failures
Hypersensitivity to slight criticism

Minor (May Be Present)

Lack of assertion
Overly conforming
Indecisiveness
Passive

Seeks approval or reassurance excessively
Lack of culturally appropriate body presentation (posture, eye contact, movements)
Denial of problems obvious to others
Projection of blame or responsibility for problems

Related Factors

Disturbed Self-Esteem can be either episodic or chronic. Failure to resolve a problem or multiple sequential stresses can result in chronic low self-esteem (CLSE). Those factors that occur over time and are associated with CLSE are indicated by CLSE in parentheses.

---

[46]This diagnosis is not presently on the NANDA-I list but has been added for clarity and usefulness.

Pathophysiologic

Related to change in appearance secondary to:

Loss of body parts
Loss of body functions

Disfigurement (trauma, surgery, birth defects)

Related to biochemical/neurophysiologic imbalance

Situational (Personal, Environmental)

Related to unmet dependency needs

Related to feelings of abandonment secondary to:

Death of significant other
Separation from significant other

Child abduction/murder

Related to feelings of failure secondary to:

Loss of job or ability to work
Increase/decrease in weight
Unemployment
Financial problems
Premenstrual syndrome

Relationship problems
Marital discord
Separation
Stepparents
In-laws

Related to assault (personal, or relating to the event of another's assault—e.g., same age, same community)

Related to failure in school

Related to history of ineffective relationship with parents (CLSE)

Related to history of abusive relationships (CLSE)

Related to unrealistic expectations of child by parent (CLSE)

Related to unrealistic expectations of self (CLSE)

Related to unrealistic expectations of parent by child (CLSE)

Related to parental rejection (CLSE)

Related to inconsistent punishment (CLSE)

Related to feelings of helplessness and/or failure secondary to institutionalization:

Mental health facility
Orphanage

Jail
Halfway house

Related to history of numerous failures (CLSE)

Maturational

Infant/Toddler/Preschool
Related to lack of stimulation or closeness (CLSE)

Related to separation from parents/significant others (CLSE)

Related to continual negative evaluation by parents

Related to inability to trust significant other (CLSE)

School-Aged
Related to failure to achieve grade-level objectives

Related to loss of peer group

Related to repeated negative feedback

Related to loss of independence and autonomy secondary to (specify)

Related to disruption of peer relationships

Related to scholastic problems

Related to loss of significant others

Middle-Aged
Related to changes associated with aging

Older Adult
Related to losses (people, function, financial, retirement)

 Author's Note

See *Disturbed Self-Concept*.

NOC
Refer to *Chronic Low Self-Esteem.*

Goals

The individual will express a positive outlook for the future and resume previous level of functioning, as evidenced by the following indicators:

- Identify source of threat to self-esteem and work through that issue
- Identify positive aspects of self
- Analyze own behavior and its consequences
- Identify one positive aspect of change

NIC
Refer to *Chronic Low Self-Esteem.*

Interventions

Establish a Trusting Nurse–Individual Relationship

- Encourage individual to express feelings, especially about the way he or she thinks or views self.
- Encourage individual to ask questions about health problem, treatment, progress, prognosis.
- Provide reliable information and reinforce information already given.
- Clarify any misconceptions the individual has about self, care, or caregivers. Avoid criticism.

Promote Social Interaction

- Assist individual to accept help from others.
- Avoid overprotection while still limiting the demands made on the individual.
- Encourage movement.

Explore Strengths, Resources, and Expectations With Individual

- Explore realistic alternatives.

Refer to Community Resources as Indicated (e.g., Counseling, Assertiveness Courses)

Chronic Low Self-Esteem

NANDA-I Definition

Long-standing negative self-evaluating/feelings about self or self-capabilities

Defining Characteristics
(Leuner et al., 1994; *Norris & Kunes-Connell, 1987)

Major (80% to 100%)

Long-Standing or Chronic

Self-negating verbalization
Reports feelings of shame/ guilt*

Rationalizes away/rejects positive feedback and exaggerates negative feedback about self*

Evaluates self as unable to deal with events*

Hesitant to try new things/ situations*

Exaggerating negative feedback about self*

Minor (50% to 79%)

Frequent lack of success in work or other life events*

Overly conforming, dependent on others' opinions*

Lack of culturally appropriate body presentation (eye contact, posture, movements)

Nonassertive/passive*

Indecisive

Excessively seeks reassurance*

Related Factors

See *Disturbed Self-Esteem*.

 Author's Note

See *Disturbed Self-Concept*.

NOC

Depression Level, Depression Self-Control, Anxiety Level, Quality of Life, Self-Esteem

Goals

The individual will identify positive aspects of self and a realistic appraisal of limitations, as evidenced by the following indicators (Halter, 2014; Varcarolis, 2011):

- Identify two strengths
- Identify two unrealistic expectations and modify more realistic life goals
- Verbalize acceptance of limitations
- Cease self-abusive descriptions of self (e.g., I am stupid)

NIC

Hope Instillation, Anxiety Reduction, Self-Esteem Enhancement, Coping Enhancement, Socialization Enhancement, Referral

Interventions

Assist the Person to Reduce Present Anxiety Level

- Be supportive, nonjudgmental.
- Accept silence, but let him or her know you are there.
- Orient as necessary.
- Clarify distortions; do not use confrontation.
- Be aware of your own anxiety and avoid communicating it to the person.
- Refer to *Anxiety* for further interventions.

Enhance the Person's Sense of Self

- Be attentive.
- Respect personal space.
- Validate your interpretation of what he or she is saying or experiencing ("Is this what you mean?").
- Help him or her to verbalize what he or she is expressing nonverbally.
- Assist individual to reframe and redefine negative expressions (e.g., not "failure," but "setback").
- Use communication that helps to maintain his or her individuality ("I" instead of "we").
- Pay attention to person, especially new behavior.
- Encourage good physical habits (healthy food and eating patterns, exercise, proper sleep).
- Provide encouragement as he or she attempts a task or skill.
- Provide realistic positive feedback on accomplishments.
- Teach person to validate consensually with others.
- Teach and encourage esteem-building exercises (self-affirmations, imagery, mirror work, use of humor, meditation/prayer, relaxation).

Promote Use of Coping Resources

- Identify the individual's areas of personal strength:
  - Sports, hobbies, crafts
  - Health, self-care
  - Work, training, education
  - Imagination, creativity
  - Writing skills, math
  - Interpersonal relationships
- Share your observations with the individual.
- Provide opportunities for individual to engage in the activities.

Assist to Identify Cognitive Distortions That Increase Negative Self-Appraisal (Varcarolis, 2011)

- Overgeneralization: Teach to focus on each event as separate.
- Self-Blame: Teach to evaluate if she/he is really responsible and why.
- Mind-Reading: Advise to clarify verbally what he or she thinks is happening.
- Discounting positive responses of others: Teach to respond with only "thank you."

Set Limits on Problematic Behavior Such as Aggression, Poor Hygiene, Ruminations, and Suicidal Preoccupation

- Refer to *Risk for Suicide* and/or *Risk for Violence* if these are assessed as problems.

Initiate Health Teaching and Referrals as Indicated

- Refer for vocational counseling.
- Involve the individual in volunteer organizations.
- Encourage participation in activities with others of same age.
- Arrange for continuation of education (e.g., literacy class, vocational training, art/music classes).

Risk for Chronic Low Self-Esteem

NANDA-I Definition

Vulnerable for long-standing negative self-evaluating/feelings about self or self-capabilities, which may compromise health

Risk Factors*

Ineffective adaptation to loss
Lack of affection
Lack of membership in group
Perceived discrepancy between self and cultural norms
Perceived discrepancy between self and spiritual norms
Perceived lack of belonging
Perceived lack of respect from others
Psychiatric disorder
Repeated failures
Repeated negative reinforcement
Traumatic event
Traumatic situation

NOC

Depression Level, Depression Self-Control, Anxiety Level, Quality of Life, Self-Esteem

Goals

The individual will identify positive aspects of self and a realistic appraisal of limitations, as evidenced by the following indicators (Varcarolis, 2011):

- Identify two strengths
- Identify two unrealistic expectations and modify more realistic life goals
- Verbalize acceptance of limitations
- Cease self-abusive descriptions of self (e.g., I am stupid, etc.)

NIC

Hope Instillation, Anxiety Reduction, Self-Esteem Enhancement, Coping Enhancement, Socialization Enhancement, Referral

Interventions

Refer to *Chronic Low Self-Esteem*.

Situational Low Self-Esteem

NANDA-I Definition

Development of a negative perception of self-worth in response to a current situation

Defining Characteristics
(Leuner et al., 1994; *Norris & Kunes-Connell, 1987)

Major (80% to 100%)

Episodic occurrence of negative self-appraisal in response to life events in a person with a previously positive self-evaluation
Verbally reports current situational challenge to self-worth*
Verbalization of negative feelings about self (helplessness, uselessness)*

Minor (50% to 79%)

Self-negating verbalizations*
Expressions of shame/guilt

Evaluates self as unable to handle
   situations/events*
Difficulty making decisions

Related Factors

See *Disturbed Self-Esteem.*

 Author's Note

See *Disturbed Self-Concept.*

NOC
Decision-Making, Grief Resolution, Psychosocial Adjustment: Life Change, Self-Esteem

Goals

The individual will express a positive outlook for the future and
resume previous level of functioning, as evidenced by the following indicators:

* Identify source of threat to self-esteem and work through that
  issue
* Identify positive aspects of self
* Analyze his or her own behavior and its consequences
* Identify one positive aspect of change

NIC
Active Listening, Presence, Counseling, Cognitive Restructuring, Family Support,
Support Group, Coping Enhancement

Interventions

Assist the Individual to Identify and to Express Feelings

* Be empathic, nonjudgmental.
* Listen; do not discourage expressions of anger, crying, and so
  forth.
* Ask what was happening when he or she began feeling this way.
* Clarify relationships between life events.

Assist the Individual to Identify Positive Self-Evaluations

- How has he or she handled other crises?
- How does he or she manage anxiety—through exercise, withdrawal, drinking/drugs, talking?
- Reinforce adaptive coping mechanisms.
- Examine and reinforce positive abilities and traits (e.g., hobbies, skills, school, relationships, appearance, loyalty, industriousness).
- Help individual accept both positive and negative feelings.
- Do not confront defenses.
- Communicate confidence in the individual's ability.
- Involve individual in mutual goal setting.
- Have individual write positive true statements about self (for his or her eyes only); have individual read the list daily as a part of normal routine.
- Reinforce use of esteem-building exercises (self-affirmations, imagery, meditation/prayer, relaxation, use of humor).

Assist to Identify Cognitive Distortions That Increase Negative Self-Appraisal (Varcarolis, 2011)

- Overgeneralization
- Teach to focus on each event as separate.
- Self-blame
- Teach to evaluate if he or she is really responsible and why.
- Mind-reading
- Advise to clarify verbally what he or she thinks is happening.
- Discount positive responses of others.
- Teach to respond with only "thank you."

Assist to Learn New Coping Skills

- Practice positive self-talk (Martin, 2013; *Murray, 2000).
- Avoid jumping to negative conclusions (Martin, 2013).
- Write a brief description of the change and its consequence (e.g., My work evaluation was poor, evaluation was terrible).
- Review each negative comment. Is it true? If yes, how can you improve this?
  - If not true, tell yourself why it is not true. Is it partially true?
  - Are there any other ways that I could look at this situation? (Martin, 2013)
- Challenge to imagine positive futures and outcomes.
- Encourage a trial of new behavior.
- Reinforce the belief that the individual does have control over the situation.
- Obtain a commitment to action.
- Stop destructive self-talk as soon as it starts.

Assist the Individual to Manage Specific Problems

- Rape—Refer to Rape-Trauma Syndrome.
- Loss—Refer to *Grieving*.
- Hospitalization—Refer to *Powerlessness* and *Parental Role Conflict*.
- Ill family member—Refer to *Interrupted Family Processes*.
- Change or loss of body part—Refer to *Disturbed Body Image*.
- Depression—Refer to *Ineffective Coping* and *Hopelessness*.
- Domestic violence—Refer to *Disabled Family Coping*.

Pediatric Interventions

- Provide opportunities for child to be successful and needed.
- Personalize the child's environment with pictures, possessions, and crafts he or she made.
- Provide structured and unstructured playtime.
- Ensure continuation of academic experiences in the hospital and home. Provide uninterrupted time for schoolwork.

Geriatric Interventions

- Acknowledge the individual by name.
- Use a tone of voice that you use for your peer group.
- Avoid words associated with infants (e.g., "diapers").
- Ask about family pictures, personal items, and past experiences.
- Avoid attributing disabilities to "old age."
- Knock on door of bedrooms and bathrooms.
- Allow enough time to accomplish tasks at own pace.

Risk for Situational Low Self-Esteem

NANDA-I Definition

Vulnerable for developing a negative perception of self-worth in response to a current situation, which may compromise health

Risk Factors

See *Situational Low Self-Esteem*.

Author's Note

See *Situational Low Self-Esteem*.

Goals

The individual will continue to express a positive outlook for the future to identify positive aspects of self, as evidenced by the following indicators:

- Identify threats to self-esteem
- Identify one positive aspect of change

Interventions

See *Situational Low Self-Esteem*.

RISK FOR SELF-HARM[47]

Risk for Self-Harm

Self-Mutilation

Risk for Self-Mutilation

Risk for Suicide

Definition

State in which a client is at risk for inflicting direct harm on himself or herself. This may include one or more of the following: self-abuse, self-mutilation, and suicide.

Defining Characteristics

Major (Must Be Present, One or More)

Expresses desire or intent to harm self
Expresses desire to die or commit suicide
History of attempts to harm self

---

[47]This diagnosis is not currently on the NANDA-I list but has been added for clarity or usefulness.

Minor (May Be Present)

Reported or Observed

Depression	Emotional pain
Helplessness	Agitation
Substance abuse	Poor self-concept
Hostility	Lack of support system
Hopelessness	Poor impulse control
Hallucinations/delusions	

Related Factors

Risk for Self-Harm can occur as a response to a variety of health problems, situations, and conflicts. Some sources are listed next.

Pathophysiologic

Related to feelings of helplessness, loneliness, or hopelessness secondary to:

Disabilities	Chemical dependency
Terminal illness	Substance abuse
Chronic illness	New diagnosis of positive human
Chronic pain	immunodeficiency virus (HIV)
	status
Psychiatric disorder	Mental impairment (organic or
	traumatic)
Schizophrenia	Adolescent adjustment disorder
Personality disorder	Posttrauma syndrome
Bipolar disorder	Somatoform disorders

Treatment Related

Related to unsatisfactory outcome of treatment (medical, surgical, psychological)

Related to prolonged dependence on:

Dialysis	Insulin injections
Chemotherapy/radiation	Ventilator

Situational (Personal, Environmental)

Related to:

Incarceration	Parental/marital conflict
Depression	Substance abuse in family
Ineffective coping skills	Child abuse

Real or perceived loss secondary to:

Finances/job	Status/prestige
Death of significant others	Someone leaving home

Separation/divorce   Natural disaster
Threat of abandonment

*Related to wish for revenge on real or perceived injury
(body or self-esteem)*

Maturational

Related to indifference to pain secondary to autism

Adolescent
Related to feelings of abandonment

Related to peer pressure

Related to unrealistic expectations of child by parents

Related to depression

Related to relocation

Related to significant loss

Older Adult
Related to multiple losses secondary to:
Retirement   Significant loss
Social isolation   Illness

 Author's Note

In 2013, the most recent year for which data is available, 494,169 people visited a hospital for injuries due to self-harm behavior, suggesting that approximately 12 people harm themselves (not necessarily intending to take their lives) for every reported death by suicide.

Risk for Self-Harm represents a broad diagnosis that can encompass self-abuse, self-mutilation, and/or risk for suicide. Although initially they may appear the same, the distinction lies in the intent. Self-mutilation and self-abuse are pathologic attempts to relieve stress temporarily, whereas suicide is an attempt to die to relieve stress permanently (Carscadden, 1992, personal communication).

Risk for Self-Harm also can be a useful early diagnosis when insufficient data are present to differentiate one from the other. In some clinical situations, the person may have delirium or dementia. This person is at risk of harming themselves (e.g., pulling out a Foley catheter or IV). *Risk for Self-Harm* would be clinically useful.

Risk for Suicide has been in this author's work for more than 20 years. *Risk for Suicide* was added to the NANDA list in 2006. Previously, *Risk for Violence to Self* was included under *Risk for Violence*. The term violence is defined as a swift and intense force or a rough or injurious physical force. As the reader knows, suicide can be either violent or nonviolent (e.g., overdose of barbiturates). Using the term violence in this diagnostic context, unfortunately, can lead to nondetection of an individual at risk for suicide because of the perception that the individual is not capable of violence.

Risk for Suicide clearly denotes an individual at high risk for suicide and in need of protection. Treatment of this diagnosis involves validating the risk, contracting with the individual, and providing protection. Treatment of the individual's underlying depression and hopelessness should be addressed with other applicable nursing diagnoses (e.g., *Ineffective Coping*, *Hopelessness*).

NOC

Aggression Self-Control, Impulse Self-Control

Goals

The individual will choose alternatives that are not harmful, as evidenced by the following indicators:

- Acknowledge self-harm thoughts
- Admit to use of self-harm behavior if it occurs
- Be able to identify personal triggers
- Learn to identify and tolerate uncomfortable feelings

NIC

Presence, Anger Control, Environmental Management: Violence Prevention, Behavior Modification, Security Enhancement, Therapy Group, Coping Enhancement, Impulse Control Training, Crisis Intervention

Interventions

Establish a Trusting Nurse–Individual Relationship

- Demonstrate acceptance of the individual as a worthwhile person through nonjudgmental statements and behavior.
- Ask questions in a caring, concerned manner.
- Encourage expression of thoughts and feelings.
- Actively listen or provide support by just being there if the individual is silent.
- Be aware of the individual's supersensitivity.
- Label the behavior, not the individual.
- Be honest in your interactions.
- Assist the individual in recognizing hope and alternatives.

- Provide reasons for necessary procedures or interventions.
- Maintain the individual's dignity throughout your therapeutic relationship.

Help Reframe Old Thinking/Feeling Patterns (*Carscadden, 1993)

- Assist to identify thought–feeling–behavior concept.
- Help to assess payoffs and drawbacks to self-harm.
- Rename words that have a negative connotation (e.g., "setback," not "failure").
- Assist in exploring viable alternatives.

Facilitate the Development of New Behavior

- Validate good coping skills already in existence.
- Encourage journaling: keeping a diary of triggers, thoughts, feelings, and alternatives that work or do not work.
- Assist the individual to develop body awareness as a method of ascertaining triggers and determining levels of impending self-harm.

Endorse an Environment That Demotes Self-Harm

- Follow policies/procedures to prevent and/or intervene in self-harm attempts.

Promote the Use of Alternatives

- Stress that there are always alternatives.
- Stress that self-harm is a choice, not something uncontrollable. Tell me about a time you resisted the urge to hurt yourself?
- Relieve pent-up tension and purposeless hyperactivity with physical activity (e.g., brisk walk, dance therapy, aerobics).
- Provide acceptable physical outlets (e.g., yelling, pounding pillow, tearing up newspapers, using clay or Play-Doh, taking a brisk walk).
- Provide for less physical alternatives (e.g., relaxation tapes, soft music, warm bath, diversional activities).

Reduce Excessive Stimuli

- Provide a quiet, serene atmosphere.
- Establish firm, consistent limits while giving the individual as much control/choice as possible within those boundaries.
- Intervene at the earliest stages to assist the individual in regaining control, prevent escalation, and allow treatment in the least restrictive manner.
- Keep communication simple. Agitated people cannot process complicated communication.

- Provide an area where the individual can retreat to decrease stimuli (e.g., time-out room, quiet room; individuals on hallucinogens need a darkened, quiet room with a nonintrusive observer).
- Remove potentially dangerous objects from the environment (if the individual is in crisis stage).

Determine Present Level of Impending Self-Harm, If Indicated
Beginning Stage (Thought Stage)

- Remind that this is an "old tape" and to replace it with new thinking and belief patterns.
- Provide nonintrusive, calming alternatives.

Climbing Stage (Feeling Stage)

- Remind to consider alternatives.
- Give as much control to the person as possible to support his or her accountability.
- Are you in control? How can I help? Would you like me to assist?
- Provide more intense interventions at this stage.

Crisis Stage (Behavior Stage)

- Give positive feedback if the individual chooses an alternative and does not harm himself or herself.
- Ask to put down any object of harm if he or she possesses one.
- Continue to emphasize there are always alternatives.
- As soon as possible give responsibility back to him or her. "Are you in control now?" "Are you feeling safe?"
- Attend to practical issues in a nonpunitive, nonjudgmental manner.

Postcrisis Stage

- Give positive reinforcements if the person did not harm himself or herself.
- Assist in problem solving on how to divert himself or herself before the crisis stage.
- Assess the degree of injury/harm if the person did not choose the alternative.
- Pay as little attention as possible to the act of self-harm and focus on prior stages (e.g., "Can you remember what triggered you?" "What kinds of things were going through your mind?" "What do you think you might have done instead?").
- Return the person to normal activities/routine as soon as possible.

Initiate Support Systems to Community, When/Where Indicated

Teach Family
- How to assist with appropriate interventions.
- How to deal with self-harm behavior/results.

Supply Phone Number of 24-Hour Emergency Hotlines
Provide Referral to
- Individual therapist
- Family counseling
- Peer support group
- Leisure/vocational counseling
- Halfway houses

Self-Mutilation

NANDA-I Definition

Deliberate self-injurious behavior causing tissue damage with the intent of causing nonfatal injury to attain relief of tension

Defining Characteristics*

Expresses desire or intent to harm self[48]
Past history of attempts to harm self, including:

Cuts on body	Self-inflicted burns
Scratches on body	Severing
Picking at wounds	Inhalation of harmful substances
Abrading	Insertion of object into body orifice
Constricting a body part	Hitting
Biting	Ingestion of harmful substances

Related Factors

See *Risk for Self-Harm.*

---

[48]This has been added by the author for clarity and usefulness.

Author's Note

See *Risk for Self-Harm*.

Goals

See *Risk for Self-Harm*.

Interventions

See *Risk for Self-Harm*.

Risk for Self-Mutilation

NANDA-I Definition

At risk for deliberate self-injurious behavior causing tissue damage with the intent of causing nonfatal injury to attain relief of tension

Related Factors
(Varcarolis, 2011)

Pathophysiologic

Related to biochemical/neurophysiologic imbalance secondary to:
Bipolar disorder   Autism
Psychotic states   Mentally impaired

Personal

Related to:
History of self-injury   Eating disorders
Desperate need for   Inability to verbally express
   attention   tensions
History of physical,   Impulsive behavior
   emotional, or sexual   Feelings of depression, rejection,
   abuse   self-hatred, separation anxiety,
Ineffective coping skills   guilt, and/or depersonalization

Maturational

Children/Adolescents

Related to emotional disturbed or battered children

 Author's Note

Individuals, who self-injure, have been mentally harmed previously in life and who because of this is vulnerable in relationships with other people (Tofthagen, Talsethand, & Fagerström, 2014).

 NOC

Impulse Self-Control, Self-Mutilation Restraint

Goals

The individual will identify persons to contact if thoughts of self-harm occur, as evidenced by the following indicators:

Long Term (Varcarolis, 2011)

- Demonstrate a decrease in frequency and intensity of self-inflicted injury by (date)
- Participate in therapeutic regimen
- Demonstrate two new coping skills that work for the individual when tension mounts and impulse is present instead of acting-out behaviors by (date)

Short Term

- Respond to external limits
- Express feelings related to stress and tension instead of acting-out behaviors by (date)
- Discuss alternative ways the individual can meet demands of current situation by (date)

NIC

Active Listening, Coping Enhancement, Impulse Control Training, Behavior Management: Self-Harm, Hope Instillation, Contracting, Surveillance: Safety

Interventions
(Varcarolis, 2011)

Convey Confidence That the Person Can Change Their Behavior With a Caring Attitude

- Initiate agency procedure to identify and remove all sources of potential harm (e.g., person search, belongings search). Limit personal belongings.
- Try to learn about the person (e.g., interests, goals).
- Assess history of self-mutilation (Varcarolis, 2011):
  - Types of mutilating behaviors (e.g., cutting, burning, self-hitting, strangulation, hair pulling, aggravation of chronic wounds, and/or insertion of objects into the body)
  - Frequency of behaviors
  - Triggers preceding events (e.g., being alone, rejection, conversations with a physician or nurse, evenings, and/or private circumstances). Some individuals may be unclear of triggers.

Explore for Feeling Before the Act of Mutilation and What They Mean (e.g., Gain Control Over Others, Attention, Method to Feel Alive, Expression of Guilt, or Self-Hate)

If a Self-Injury Occurs

- Respond to self-mutilation episode without emotion; maintained the belief that the person can improve.
- Collaborate on alternative behaviors to self-mutilation.
- Avoid certain activities that trigger behavior.
- Discuss their feelings before self-mutilation.
- Clearly establish limits on behavior.

Be Vigilant for Signs of Worsening and Increased Risk for Suicide

- Refer to *Risk for Suicide*.

Initiate Referrals as Needed

- Connect with community resources (therapist, support groups).

Risk for Suicide

NANDA-I Definition

At risk for self-inflicted, life-threatening injury

Risk Factors

Suicidal behavior (ideation, talk, plan, available means) (Varcarolis, 2011)
Persons at high risk for suicide
Poor support system*
Family history of suicide*
Hopelessness/helplessness*
Poor support system
History of prior suicidal attempts*
Alcohol and substance abuse*
Legal or disciplinary problems*
Grief/bereavement (loss of person, job, home)
Suicidal cues (Varcarolis, 2011)
Overt ("No one will miss me," "I am better off dead," "I have nothing to live for")
Covert (making out a will, giving valuables away, writing forlorn love notes, acquiring life insurance)

 Author's Note

In 2013, the highest suicide rate (19.1) was among people 45 to 64 years old. The second highest rate (18.6) occurred in those 85 years and older. Younger groups have had consistently lower suicide rates than middle-aged and older adults. In 2013, adolescents and young adults aged 15 to 24 had a suicide rate of 10.9. Of those who died by suicide in 2013, 77.9% were male and 22.1% were female. After cancer and heart disease, suicide accounts for more years of life lost than any other cause of death (American Foundation for Suicide Prevention, 2015).

NOC
Impulse Self-Control, Suicide Self-Restraint

Goals

The individual will identify persons to contact if suicidal thoughts occur, and he or she will not commit suicide, as evidenced by the following indicators:

Long Term (Varcarolis, 2011)

- State the desire to live
- Name two people he or she can call if thoughts of suicide recur before discharge

- Name at least one acceptable alternative to his or her situation
- Identify at least one realistic goal for the future

Short Term

- Remain safe while in the hospital
- Stay with a friend or family if person has a potential for suicide (if in the community)
- Keep an appointment for the next day with a crisis counselor (if in the community)
- Join family in crisis family counseling
- Have links to self-help groups in the community

NIC

Active Listening, Coping Enhancement, Suicide Prevention, Impulse Control Training, Behavior Management: Self-Harm, Hope Instillation, Contracting, Surveillance: Safety

Interventions

Assist the Individual in Reducing His or Her Present Risk for Self-Destruction

- Assess level of present risk.
- Refer to Table I.5.
  - High
  - Moderate
  - Low
- Assess level of long-term risk.
  - Lifestyle
  - Lethality of plan
  - Usual coping mechanisms
  - Support available

Provide a Safe Environment Based on Level of Risk; Notify All Staff That the Individual Is at Risk for Self-Harm; Use Both Written and Oral Communication to Convey Risk

- Initiate suicide precaution for immediate management for the high-risk individual.
- When the person is being constantly observed, he or she is not to be allowed out of sight, even though privacy is lost.
- Arm's length is the most appropriate space for a high-risk individual.
- Initiate suicide observation for risk persons.
- Provide 15-minute visual check of mood, behaviors, and verbatim statements (Varcarolis, 2011).
- Initiate suicide observation for risk persons.

Table I.5 ASSESSING THE DEGREE OF SUICIDAL RISK (Halter, 2014; Hockenberry & Wilson, 2015; Varcarolis, 2011)

Behavior or Symptom	Intensity of Risk		
	Low	Moderate	High
Anxiety	Mild, moderate	High or panic state	Severe or a sudden change to a happy or peaceful state
Depression	Mild	Moderate	Hopeless, withdrawn, and self-deprecating, isolation
Isolation/withdrawal	Some feelings of isolation, no withdrawal	Some feelings of hopelessness, and withdrawal	Depressed
Daily functioning	Effective	Moody	Depressed
	Good grades in school[a]	Some friends	Poor grades[a]
	Close friends	Prior suicidal thoughts	Few or no close friends
	No prior suicide attempt		Prior suicide attempts
	Stable job		Erratic or poor work history
Lifestyle	Stable	Moderately stable	Unstable
Alcohol/drug use	Infrequently to excess	Frequently to excess	Continual abuse
Previous suicide attempts	None or of low lethality (few pills)	One or more (pills, superficial wrist slash)	One or more (entire bottle of pills, gun, hanging)

562

Associated events	None or an argument	Disciplinary action[a] Failing grades[a] Work problems Family illness	Relationship breakup Death of a loved one Loss of job Pregnancy[a]
Purpose of act	None or not clear	Relief of shame or guilt To punish others To get attention	Wants to die Escape to join deceased Debilitating disease
Family's reaction and structure	Supportive Intact family Good coping and mental health No history of suicide	Mixed reaction Divorced/separated Usually copes and understands	Angry and unsupportive Disorganized Rigid/abusive Prior history of suicide in family
Suicide plan (method, location, time); Lethality of suicide attempts	No plan	Frequent thoughts, occasional ideas about a plan Wrist slashing Overdose of nonprescription drugs except aspirin and acetaminophen	Specific plan Firearms Hanging Jumping Carbon monoxide Overdose of antidepressants, barbiturates, aspirin, acetaminophen

[a]Applies only to children and adolescents.

563

- Provide 15-minute visual check of mood, behaviors, and verbatim statements.
- Restrict glass, nail files, scissors, nail polish remover, mirrors, needles, razors, soda cans, plastic bags, lighters, electric equipment, belts, hangers, knives, tweezers, alcohol, and guns.
- Provide meals in a closely supervised area, usually on the unit or in individual's room:
  - Ensure adequate food and fluid intake.
  - Use paper/plastic plates and utensils.
  - Check to be sure all items are returned on the tray.
- When administering oral medications, check to ensure that all medications are swallowed.
- Designate a staff member to provide checks on the individual as designated by the institution's policy. Provide relief for the staff member.
- Restrict the individual to the unit unless specifically ordered by physician. When the individual is off unit, provide a staff member to accompany him or her.
- Instruct visitors on restricted items (e.g., ensure they do not give the individual food in a plastic bag).
- The individual may use restricted items in the presence of staff, depending on level of risk.
- For acutely suicidal individuals, provide a hospital gown to deter the individual from leaving the facility. As risk decreases, the individual may be allowed own clothing.
- Conduct room searches periodically according to institution policy.
- Use seclusion and restraint if necessary (refer to *Risk for Violence* for discussion).
- Notify the police if the individual leaves the facility and is at risk for suicide.
- Keep accurate and thorough records of the individual's behaviors and all nursing assessments and interventions.

Emphasize the Following

- The crisis is temporary.
- Unbearable pain can be survived.
- Help is available.
- You are not alone (Varcarolis, 2011).

Observe for a Sudden Change in Emotions From Sad, Depressed to Elated, Happy, or Peaceful

Assist the Individual to Identify and Contact Support System

- Inform family and significant others.
- Enlist support.

- Do not provide false reassurance that behavior will not recur.
- Encourage an increase in social activity.
- Refer the individual to read "If You Are Thinking About Suicide... Read This First," found at www.metanoia.org/suicide.

Initiate Health Teaching and Referrals, When Indicated

- Provide teaching that prepares the individual to deal with life stresses (relaxation, problem-solving skills, how to express feelings constructively).
- Refer for peer or group therapy.
- Refer for family therapy, especially when a child or adolescent is involved.
- Teach the family limit-setting techniques.
- Teach the family constructive expression of feelings.
- Instruct significant others in how to recognize an increase in risk: change in behavior, verbal or nonverbal communication, withdrawal, or signs of depression.
- Supply the phone number of 24-hour emergency hotline.
- Refer to vocational training if appropriate.
- Refer to halfway house or other agencies, as appropriate.
- Refer for ongoing psychiatric follow-up.
- Refer to senior citizen centers or other agencies to increase leisure activities.
- Initiate referral for family intervention after a completed suicide.

Pediatric Interventions

- Take all suicide threats seriously. Listen carefully.
- Determine whether the child understands the finality of death (e.g., "What does it mean to die?").
- "Have you ever seen a dead animal on the road? Can it get up and run?"
- Engage parents, friends, school personnel, and the individual in behavior contracts to "keep safe."
- Explore feelings and reason for suicidal feelings.
- Consult with a psychiatric expert regarding the most appropriate environment for treatment.
- Participate in programs in school to teach about the symptoms of depression and signs of suicidal behavior.
- With adolescents, explore (Hockenberry and Wilson, 2015):
  - Family problems
  - Mental status
  - Strength of support systems
  - Disruption of friendship or romantic relationship

- Seriousness of the attempt
- Presence of performance failure (e.g., examination, course)
- Recent or upcoming change (change of school, relocation)
- Sexual orientation
- Convey empathy regarding problems and/or losses.
- Be alert for symptoms of a masked depression (e.g., boredom, restlessness, irritability, difficulty concentrating, somatic preoccupation, excessive dependence on or isolation from others, especially adults).

INEFFECTIVE SEXUALITY PATTERN

Ineffective Sexuality Pattern

Sexual Dysfunction

NANDA-I Definition

Expressions of concern regarding own sexuality

Defining Characteristics

Actual concerns regarding sexual behaviors, sexual health, sexual functioning, or sexual identity

Expression of concern about impact a medical diagnosis or treatment for a medical condition may have on sexual functioning or sexual desirability.

Related Factors

Ineffective sexual patterns can occur as a response to various health problems, situations, and conflicts. Some common sources are listed next.

Pathophysiologic

Related to biochemical effects on energy and libido secondary to:

Endocrine
Diabetes mellitus
Hyperthyroidism
Addison's disease

Decreased hormone production
Myxedema
Acromegaly

Genitourinary
Chronic renal failure

Neuromuscular and Skeletal
Arthritis
Amyotrophic
   lateral sclerosis

Multiple sclerosis
Disturbances of nerve supply to
   brain, spinal cord, sensory nerves,
   or autonomic nerves

Cardiorespiratory
Peripheral vascular disorders
Cancer
Myocardial infarction

Congestive heart failure
Chronic respiratory disorders

Related to fears associated with (sexually transmitted diseases [STDs]) *
(specify):

Human immunodefi-
   ciency virus (HIV)/
   Acquired immuno-
   deficiency syndrome
   (AIDS)
Human papilloma virus
Herpes

Gonorrhea
Chlamydia
Syphilis

Related to effects of alcohol on performance

Related to decreased vaginal lubrication secondary to (specify)

Related to fear of premature ejaculation

Related to pain during intercourse

Treatment Related

Related to effects of:
Medications
Radiation therapy

Related to altered self-concept from change in appearance (trauma, radical surgery)

Related to knowledge/skill deficit about alternative responses to health-related transitions, altered body function or structure, illness, or medical treatment *

Situational (Personal, Environmental)

Related to fear of pregnancy *

*Related to lack of significant other**

*Related to conflicts with sexual orientation preferences**

Related to conflicts with variant preferences

Related to partner problem (specify):
Unwilling   Conflicts
Not available   Abusive
Uninformed   Separated, divorced

*Related to lack of privacy**

*Related to ineffective role model**

Related to stressors secondary to:
Job problems   Financial worries
Value conflicts   Relationship conflicts

Related to misinformation or lack of knowledge

Related to fatigue

Related to fear of rejection secondary to obesity

Related to pain

Related to fear of sexual failure

Related to fear of pregnancy

Related to depression

Related to anxiety

Related to guilt

Related to history of unsatisfactory sexual experiences

Maturational

Adolescent

*Related to ineffective/absent role models**

Related to negative sexual teaching

Related to absence of sexual teaching

Adult

Related to adjustment to parenthood

Related to effects of menopause on libido and vaginal tissue atrophy

Related to values conflict

Related to effects of pregnancy on energy levels and body image

Related to effects of aging on energy levels and body image

Author's Note

The diagnoses *Ineffective Sexuality Pattern* and *Sexual Dysfunction* are difficult to differentiate. *Ineffective Sexuality Pattern* represents a broad diagnosis, of which sexual dysfunction can be one part. *Sexual Dysfunction* may be used most appropriately by a nurse with advanced preparation in sex therapy. Until *Sexual Dysfunction* is well differentiated from *Ineffective Sexuality Pattern*, most nurses should not use it.

NOC

Body Image, Self-Esteem, Role Performance, Sexual Identity

Goals

The individual will resume previous sexual activity or engage in alternative satisfying sexual activity, as evidenced by the following indicators:

- Identify effects of stressors, loss, or change on sexual functioning
- Modify behavior to reduce stressors
- Identify limitations on sexual activity caused by a health problem
- Identify appropriate modifications in sexual practices in response to these limitations
- Report satisfying sexual activity

NIC

Behavioral Management, Sexual Counseling, Emotional Support, Active Listening, Teaching: Sexuality

Interventions

Assess for Causative or Contributing Factors

- See Related Factors.

Explore the Individual's Patterns of Sexual Functioning Using the PLISSITT model (*Annon, 1976)

- Encourage him or her to share concerns; assume that individuals of all ages have had some sexual experience, and convey a willingness to discuss feelings and concerns.
  - Permission: Convey to the individual and significant other a willingness to discuss sexual thoughts and feelings (e.g., "Some people with your diagnosis have concerns about how it will affect sexual functioning. Is this a concern for you or your partner?").

- Limited information: Provide the individual and significant other with information on the effects certain situations (e.g., pregnancy), conditions (e.g., cancer), and treatments (e.g., medications) can have on sexuality and sexual function.
- Specific suggestions: Provide specific instructions that can facilitate positive sexual functioning (e.g., changes in coital positions).
- Intensive therapy: Refer people who need more help to an appropriate health-care professional (e.g., sex therapist, surgeon).

Discuss the Relationship Between Sexual Functioning and Life Stressors

- Clarify the relation between stressors and problem in sexual functioning.
- Explore options available for reducing the effects of the stressor on sexual functioning (e.g., increase sleep, increase exercise, modify diet, explore stress reduction methods).

Reaffirm the Need for Frank Discussion Between Sexual Partners

- Explain how the individual and the partner can use role-playing to discuss concerns about sex.
- Reaffirm the need for closeness and expressions of caring through touching, massage, and other means.
- Suggest that sexual activity need not always culminate in vaginal intercourse, but that the partner can reach orgasm through noncoital manual or oral stimulation.

Address Factors for Individuals With Acute or Chronic Illness

- Eliminate or reduce causative or contributing factors, if possible, and teach the importance of adhering to medical regimen designed to reduce or control disease symptoms.
- Provide limited information and specific suggestions.
- Provide appropriate information to individual and partner concerning actual limitations on sexual functioning caused by the illness (limited information).
- Teach possible modifications in sexual practices to assist in dealing with limitations caused by illness.

Provide Referrals as Indicated

- Enterostomal therapist
- Physician
- Nurse specialist
- Sex therapist

Older Adults Interventions

- Use the PLISSIT model to assess sexual concerns and issues with older adults.
- The PLISSIT model and the questions suggested may be used with older adults in a variety of clinical settings. Despite the findings that sexuality continues throughout all phases of life, little material, scientific or otherwise, exists in the literature to guide nurses toward assessing the sexuality of older adults (Kazer, 2012b).

Prove Factual Information of Treatment-Related Negative Effects on Sexual Desire/Function

- Discuss normal age-related physiologic changes.
  - Women experience decreased breast tone, thinning and loss of elasticity of the vaginal wall, decreased vaginal lubrication, and shortening of vaginal length from loss of circulating estrogen (Miller, 2015).
  - Men experience decreased production of spermatozoa, decreased ejaculatory force, and smaller, less firm testicles. Direct stimulation may be required to achieve an erection; however, the erection may be maintained for a longer time (Miller, 2015).

Facilitate Communication With Older Adults Regarding Sexual Health as Desired, Including the Following

- Encourage family meetings with open discussion of issues if indicated.
- Teach about safe sex practices.
- Discuss use of condoms to prevent transmission of sexually transmitted infections (STIs) and HIV (Kazer, 2012a).
- Ensure privacy and safety among long-term care and community-dwelling residents.
- Ensure privacy, dignity, and respect surrounding their sexuality.
- Provide communication and education regarding sexual health as desired.
- Teach to pursue sexual health free of pathologic and problematic sexual behaviors.

Ensure the Residential Community Facility Has a Program for

- Provision of education on the ongoing sexual needs of older adults and appropriate interventions to manage these needs with dignity and respect
- Inclusion of sexual health questions in routine history and physical assessment

- Frequent reassessment of individuals for changes in sexual health
- Provision of needed privacy for individuals to maintain intimacy and sexual health (e.g., in long-term care)

⁂ Pediatric Interventions

Adolescents

- To reduce the tension, have the conversation in the car or while cooking to reduce the need for eye contact and reduce the early termination of the dialogue.
- Do not abstain from educating your own children (Ginsburg, 2015).
- Choose right time and right place (Ginsburg, 2015).
- Avoid sexuality conversations that are all *don'ts* (Ginsburg, 2015).
- Find out what your child is thinking when talking about their relationships or sexual experiences (Ginsburg, 2015).
- Talking about sex is difficult. When necessary, identify and encourage them to ask for help from other trusted adults; it does not always have to be you.
- Emphasize no means no to female and male adolescents.

Sexual Dysfunction

NANDA-I Definition

The state in which an individual experiences a change in sexual function during the sexual response phases of desire, excitation, and/or orgasm, which is viewed as unsatisfying, unrewarding, or inadequate

Defining Characteristics*

Alterations in achieving sexual satisfaction and/or perceived sex role
Actual or perceived limitations imposed by disease and/or therapy
Change in interest in others and/or in self
Inability to achieve desired satisfaction
Perceived alteration in sexual excitement

Perceived deficiency of sexual desire
Seeking confirmation of desirability
Verbalization of problem

Related Factors

See *Ineffective Sexuality Pattern*.

 Author's Note

See *Ineffective Sexuality Pattern*.

RISK FOR SHOCK

See also *Risk for Complications of Hypovolemia* in Section 3, Collaborative Problems.

NANDA-I Definition

At risk for inadequate blood flow to the body's tissues, which may lead to life-threatening cellular dysfunction

Risk Factors*

Hypertension	Infection
Hypovolemia	Sepsis
Hypoxemia	Systemic inflammatory response syndrome
Hypoxia	

 Author's Note

This NANDA-I diagnosis represents several collaborative problems. To decide which of the following collaborative problems is appropriate for an individual, determine what you are monitoring for. Which of the following describes the focus of nursing for this individual?

- *Risk for Complications of Hypertension*
- *Risk for Complications of Hypovolemia*
- *Risk for Complications of Sepsis*
- *Risk for Complications of Decreased Cardiac Output*
- *Risk for Complications of Hypoxemia*
- *Risk for Complications of Allergic Reaction*

Refer to http://thePoint.lww.com/CarpenitoHB14e for related Goals and Interventions.

DISTURBED SLEEP PATTERN

Disturbed Sleep Pattern

Insomnia

Sleep Deprivation

NANDA-I Definition

Time-limited interruptions of sleep amount and quality due to external factors

Defining Characteristics

Major (Must Be Present)

Adults
Difficulty falling or remaining asleep

Minor (May Be Present)

Adults
Fatigue on awakening or during the day   Agitation
Dozing during the day   Mood alterations

Children
Reluctance to retire   Frequent awakening during the night
Persists in sleeping with   parents

Related Factors

Many factors can contribute to disturbed sleep patterns. Some common factors follow.

Pathophysiologic

Related to frequent awakenings secondary to:

Impaired oxygen transport
  Angina
  Respiratory disorders
  Peripheral arteriosclerosis
  Circulatory disorders
Impaired elimination; bowel or bladder
Diarrhea
Retention

Constipation
Dysuria
Incontinence
Frequency
Impaired metabolism
Hyperthyroidism
Hepatic disorders
Gastric ulcers

Treatment Related

Related to Interruptions (e.g., for therapeutic monitoring, laboratory tests)*

Related to physical restraints*

Related to difficulty assuming usual position secondary to (specify)

Related to excessive daytime sleeping or hyperactivity secondary to (specify medication):

Tranquilizers
Sedatives
Amphetamines
Monoamine oxidase inhibitors
Hypnotics

Barbiturates
Antidepressants
Corticosteroids
Antihypertensives

Situational (Personal, Environmental)

Related to lack of sleep privacy/control*

Related to lighting, noise, noxious odors*

Related to sleep partner (e.g., snoring)*

Related to unfamiliar sleep furnishings*

Related to ambient temperature, humidity*

Related to caregiving responsibilities*

Related to change in daylight/darkness exposure*

Related to excessive hyperactivity secondary to:
Bipolar disorder   Panic anxiety
Attention-deficit disorder   Illicit drug use

Related to excessive daytime sleeping

Related to depression

Related to inadequate daytime activity

Related to pain

Related to anxiety response

Related to discomfort secondary to pregnancy

Related to lifestyle disruptions
Occupational   Sexual
Emotional   Financial
Social

Related to environmental changes (specify)
Hospitalization (noise, disturbing roommate, fear)
Travel

Related to fears

Related to circadian rhythm changes

Maturational

Children
Related to fear of dark

Related to fear

Related to enuresis

Related to inconsistent parenteral responses

Related to inconsistent sleep rituals

Adult Women
Related to hormonal changes (e.g., perimenopausal)

 Author's Note

Sleep disturbances can have many causes or contributing factors. Some examples are asthma, tobacco use, stress, marital problems, and traveling. *Disturbed Sleep Pattern* describes a situation that is probably transient due to a change in the individual or environment (e.g., acute pain, travel, hospitalization). *Risk for Disturbed Sleep Pattern* can be used when an individual is at risk due to travel or shift work. *Insomnia* describes an individual with a persistent problem falling asleep or staying asleep because of chronic pain and multiple chronic stressors. It may be clinically useful to view sleep problems as a sign or symptom of another nursing diagnosis such as *Stress Overload, Pain, Ineffective Coping, Dysfunctional Family Coping,* or *Risk-Prone Health Behavior.*

NOC

Rest, Sleep, Well-Being, Parenting Performance

Goals

The individual will report an optimal balance of rest and activity, as evidenced by the following indicators:

* Describe factors that prevent or inhibit sleep
* Identify techniques to induce sleep

NIC

Energy Management, Sleep Enhancement, Relaxation Therapy, Exercise Promotion, Environmental Management, Parent Education: Childrearing Family

Interventions

Although many believe that a person needs 8 hours of sleep each night, no scientific evidence supports this. Individual sleep requirements vary greatly. Generally, a person who can relax and rest easily requires less sleep to feel refreshed. With aging, less time is spent in the sleep cycle stages 3 and 4, which are the most restorative stages of sleep. The results are difficulty falling asleep and staying asleep (Cole & Richards, 2007). The following suggests general interventions for promoting sleep and specific interventions for selected clinical situations.

Identify Causative Contributing Factors

* Refer to Related Factors.
* Explain that sleep cycles include REM, NREM, and wakefulness, and explain sleep requirements.
* Encourage or provide evening care:
  * Bathroom or bedpan
  * Personal hygiene (mouth care, bath, shower, partial bath)
  * Clean linen and bedclothes (freshly made bed, sufficient blankets)

- Cluster procedures to minimize the times you need to wake the individual at night. If possible, plan for at least four periods of 90-minute uninterrupted sleep.
- If the individual is being awoken for monitoring, use SBAR with prescribing professional.

SBAR

Situation: Mr. Nelo has only slept _ hours the last 24 hours.

Background: He is not sleeping because . . ..

Assessment: He is complaining of more pain, wants a sleeping pill.

Recommendation: It would be useful to. . . (e.g., stop vital signs 10 PM to 6 AM) unless needed, change the times for medication administration.

Provide Treatments Before 10 PM and After 6 AM When Possible

- Discuss with physician/NP/PA the use of a "Sleep Protocol." This will allow the nursing staff the authority not to wake a person for blood draws or vital signs if appropriate (Bartick, Thai, Schmidt, Altaye, & Solet, 2010):
  - Implementation of the sleep hygiene protocol permitted acutely injured or ill patients in our intensive care unit to fall asleep more quickly and to experience fewer sleep disruptions (Faraklas et al., 2013).
  - Close the door to the room or pull the curtains.
  - Designate "quiet time" between 10 PM and 6 AM.
  - Lullabies were played over public address system.
  - Overhead hallway lights went off on a timer at 10 PM.
  - Mute phones close to individual rooms, avoid intercom use except in emergencies.
  - Vital signs were taken at 10 PM, and started again at 6 AM unless otherwise indicated.
  - Medications are ordered bid, tid, qid, not "q" certain hours when possible.
  - No administering a diuretic after 4 PM.
  - Avoid blood transfusions during "quiet time" due to frequent monitoring.

Advise Ancillary Staff/Student to Report the Amount of Time Spent Sleeping (Including Naps and Nighttime Sleep)

Initiate Health Teaching as Indicated

- If poor sleep is contributing to daytime fatigue and pain, try the following tips to improve sleep at home (Arthritis Foundation, 2012):
  - Maintain a regular daily schedule of activities, including a regular sleep schedule.

- Exercise, but not late in the evening.
- Set aside an hour before bedtime for relaxation.
- Eat a light snack before bedtime. You should not go to bed hungry, nor should you feel too full.
- Make your bedroom as quiet and as comfortable as possible. Maintain a comfortable room temperature. Invest in a comfortable mattress and/or try a body-length pillow to provide more support.
- Use your bedroom only for sleeping and for being physically close to your partner.
- Arise at the same time every day, even on weekends and holidays.

Reduce or Eliminate Environmental Distractions and Sleep Interruptions

Noise
- Close the door to the room.
- Pull the curtains.
- Unplug the telephone.
- Use "white noise" (e.g., fan, quiet music, tape of rain, waves).
- Eliminate 24-hour lighting.
- Provide night lights.
- Decrease the amount and kind of incoming stimuli (e.g., staff conversations).
- Cover blinking lights with tape.
- Reduce the volume of alarms and televisions.
- Place the individual with a compatible roommate, if possible.

Interruptions
- Organize procedures to minimize disturbances during sleep period (e.g., when the individual awakens for medication, also administer treatments and obtain vital signs).
- Avoid unnecessary procedures during sleep period.
- Limit visitors during optimal rest periods (e.g., after meals).
- If voiding during the night is disruptive, have the individual limit nighttime fluids and void before retiring.

Increase Daytime Activities, as Indicated

- Establish with the individual a schedule for a daytime program of activity (walking, physical therapy).
- Discourage naps longer than 90 minutes.
- Encourage naps in the morning.
- Limit the amount and length of daytime sleeping if excessive (i.e., more than 1 hour).

- Encourage others to communicate with the individual and stimulate wakefulness.

Promote a Sleep Ritual or Routine

- Maintain a consistent daily schedule for waking, sleeping, and resting (weekdays, weekends).
- Arise at the usual time even after not sleeping well; avoid staying in bed when awake.
- Use the bed only for activities associated with sleeping; avoid TV watching.
- If the individual is awakened and cannot return to sleep, tell him or her to get out of bed and read in another room for 30 minutes.
- Take a warm bath.
- Consume a desired bedtime snack (avoid highly seasoned and high-roughage foods) and warm milk.
- Use herbs that promote sleep (e.g., lavender, ginseng, chamomile, valerian, rose hips, lemon balm, passion flower; Miller, 2015). Consult with the primary care provider prior to use.
- Avoid alcohol, caffeine, and tobacco at least 4 hours before retiring.
- Go to bed with reading material.
- Get a back rub or massage.
- Listen to soft music or a recorded story.
- Practice relaxation/breathing exercises.
- Ensure that the individual has at least four or five periods of at least 90 minutes each of uninterrupted sleep every 24 hours.
- Document the amount of the individual's uninterrupted sleep each shift.

Provide Health Teaching and Referrals, as Indicated

- Teach an at-home sleep routine (Miller, 2015). See above for specifics.
- Teach the importance of regular exercise (walking, running, aerobic dance) for at least 30 minutes three times a week (if not contraindicated). Avoid exercise in the evening.
- Explain risks of hypnotic medications with long-term use.
- Refer an individual with a chronic sleep problem to a sleep disorders center.
- For peri- and postmenopausal women, explain the following:
  - Sedative and hypnotic drugs begin to lose their effectiveness after 1 week of use, requiring increasing dosages and leading to the risk of dependence.
  - Warm milk contains L-tryptophan, which is a sleep inducer.
  - Caffeine and nicotine are CNS stimulants that lengthen sleep latency and increase nighttime wakening (Miller, 2015).

- Alcohol induces drowsiness but suppresses REM sleep and increases the number of awakenings (Miller, 2015).
- Early-morning naps produce more REM sleep than do afternoon naps. Naps longer than 90 minutes decrease the stimulus for longer sleep cycles in which REM sleep is obtained.

☶ Pediatric Interventions

Explain the Sleep Differences of Infants and Toddlers (*Murray, Zentner, & Yakimo, 2009)

15 months	Shorter morning nap, needs afternoon nap
17 to 24 months	Has trouble falling asleep
	Has a favorite sleep toy, pillow, or blanket
18 months	Tries to climb out of bed
19 months	May awake with nightmares
20 months	Sleeps better, shorter afternoon naps
21 months	Wants to delay bedtime, needs afternoon nap, sleeps less time
24 months	
2 to 3 years	Can change to bed from crib, needs closely spaced side rails

- Explain night to the child (stars and moon).
- Discuss how some people (nurses, factory workers) work at night.
- Explain that when night comes for them, day is coming for other people elsewhere in the world.
- If a nightmare occurs, encourage the child to talk about it, if possible. Reassure the child that it is a dream, even though it seems very real. Share with the child that you have dreams too.

Stress the Importance of Establishing a Sleep Routine (*Murray et al., 2009)

- Set a definite time and bedtime routine. Begin 30 minutes before bedtime. Try to prevent the child from becoming overtired and agitated.
- Establish a bedtime ritual with bath, reading a story, and soft music.
- Ensure that the child has his or her favorite bedtime object/toy, pillow, blanket, etc.
- Quietly talk and hold the child.
- Avoid TV and videos.
- If the child cries, go back in for a few minutes and reassure for less than a minute. Do not pick up the child. If crying continues, return in 5 minutes and repeat the procedure.
- "If extended crying continues, lengthen the time to return to the child to 10 minutes" (*Murray et al., 2009). Eventually the child will fatigue and fall asleep.

- "The child should remain in his or her bed rather than co-sleep for part or all of the night with parents" (*Murray et al., 2009). Occasional exceptions can be made for family crises, trauma, and illness.
- Provide a night light or a flashlight to give the child control over the dark.
- Reassure the child that you will be nearby all night.

Maternal Interventions

- Discuss reasons for sleeping difficulties during pregnancy (e.g., leg cramps, backache, fetal movements).
- Teach the individual how to position pillows in side-lying position (one between legs, one under abdomen, one under top arm, one under head).
- Refer to Interventions for *Sleep Promotion Strategies.*

Geriatric Interventions

Explain the Age-Related Effects on Sleep

Explain That Medications (Prescribed, Over the Counter) Should Be Avoided Because of Their Risk for Dependence and the Risks of Drowsiness

- If the individual needs sleeping pills occasionally, advise him or her to consult primary care provider for a type with a short half-life.

Insomnia

NANDA-I Definition

A disruption in amount and quality of sleep that impairs functioning

Defining Characteristics*

Observed changes in effect
Increased absenteeism (e.g., school, work)
Reports:
    Changes in mood
    Decreased health status
    Dissatisfaction with sleep (current)

Increased accidents
Lack of energy
Waking up too early
Observed lack of energy
Decreased quality of life
Difficulty concentrating
Difficulty falling or staying asleep
Nonrestorative sleep
Sleep disturbances that produce next-day consequences

Related Factors

Refer to *Disturbed Sleep Pattern*.

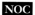 **NOC**

Refer to *Disturbed Sleep Pattern*.

Goals

Refer to *Disturbed Sleep Pattern*.

 NIC

Refer to *Disturbed Sleep Pattern*.

Interventions

- Have the individual keep a sleep–awake diary for 1 month to include bedtime, arising time, difficulty getting sleep, number of awakenings (reason), and naps.
- Evaluate if there is a physiologic condition or medication that is interfering with sleep. Refer to Related Factors under Pathophysiologic and Treatment Related under *Disturbed Sleep Pattern*. Refer to the primary care provider for management.
- Evaluate if a psychological state is interfering with sleep. Refer to Situational Related Factors. Refer to mental health professions.
- Determine if the lifestyle or life events are interfering with sleep. Refer to other nursing diagnoses if appropriate: *Grieving, Stress Overload, Ineffective Coping,* or *Risk-Prone Health Behavior*.

Refer to *Disturbed Sleep Pattern* for Interventions to Establish a Sleep Ritual or Routine

Sleep Deprivation

NANDA-I Definition

Prolonged periods without sleep (sustained natural, periodic suspension of relative unconsciousness)

Defining Characteristics

Refer to *Disturbed Sleep Pattern*.

Related Factors

Refer to *Disturbed Sleep Pattern*.

 Author's Note

This diagnostic label represents a situation in which the individual's sleep is insufficient. It is difficult to differentiate this diagnosis from the others. Refer to *Disturbed Sleep Pattern* for interventions.

Goals /Interventions

Refer to *Disturbed Sleep Pattern*.

SOCIAL ISOLATION

NANDA-I Definition

Aloneness experienced by the individual and perceived as imposed by others and as a negative or threatening state

Defining Characteristics

Absence of support system
Desires to be alone
Cultural incongruence
Developmental delay
Developmentally inappropriate
   interests
Disabling condition
Aloneness imposed by others and/
   or rejection*
Inability to meet expectations of
   others*
Insecurity in public*
Withdrawn
History of rejection
Feeling different than others

Illness
Meaningless actions
Member of a subculture
Purposelessness
Repetitive actions
Values incongruent with
   cultural norms
Hostility*
Withdrawn*
Sad affect*
Flat affect
Poor eye contact
Preoccupied with own
   thoughts

Related Factors

Alteration in mental status
Alteration in physical appearance
Alteration in wellness
Developmentally inappropriate interests
Factors impacting satisfying personal relationships (e.g., developmental delay)
Inability to engage in satisfying personal relationships
Insufficient personal resources (e.g. poor achievement, poor insight—affect unavailable and poorly controlled)
Social behavior incongruent with norms
Values incongruent with cultural norms

 Author's Note

In 1994, NANDA added a new diagnosis: *Risk for Loneliness*. It more accurately adheres to the NANDA definition of "response to." In addition, an individual can experience loneliness even with many people around. In reviewing the defining characteristics and related factors listed above, some are repeated in both categories. This author recommends deleting *Social Isolation* from clinical use and using *Loneliness* or *Risk for Loneliness* instead. An individual with difficulty communicating one to one or in group may avoid social interactions or experience negative responses from others. *Impaired Social Interactions* can be used to describe this person.

CHRONIC SORROW

Definition

Cyclical, recurring, and potentially progressive pattern of pervasive sadness experienced (by parent, caregiver, individual with chronic illness or disability) in response to continual loss throughout the trajectory of an illness or disability (NANDA-I)

A state in which an individual experiences, or is at risk to experience, permanent pervasive psychic pain and sadness, variable in intensity, in response to a loved one forever changed by an event or condition and the ongoing loss of normalcy (*Teel, 1991)

Defining Characteristics

Lifelong episodic sadness to loss of a loved one or loss of
 normalcy in a loved one who has been changed by an event,
 disorder, or disability
Variable intensity
Expresses feelings that interfere with ability to reach highest
 level of personal and/or social well-being*
Negative feelings of variable intensity, periodic, recurrent*
Anger
Loneliness
Sadness
Frustration
Guilt
Self-blame
Fear
Overwhelmed
Emptiness
Helplessness
Confusion
Disappointment

Related Factors

Situational (Personal, Environmental)

Related to the chronic loss of normalcy secondary to a child's or adult child's condition, for example:

Asperger's syndrome   Mental retardation
Autism   Spina bifida

Severe scoliosis	Sickle cell disease
Chronic psychiatric condition	Type I diabetes mellitus
Down syndrome	Human immunodeficiency virus

Related to lifetime losses associated with infertility

Related to ongoing losses associated with a degenerative condition (e.g., multiple sclerosis, Alzheimer's disease)

Related to loss of loved one

Related to losses associated with caring for a child with fatal illness

 Author's Note

Olchansky identified *Chronic Sorrow* in 1962. Chronic sorrow differs from grieving, which is time-limited and results in adaptation to the loss. Chronic sorrow varies in intensity but persists as long as the individual with the disability or chronic condition lives (*Burke, Hainsworth, Eakes, & Lindgren, 1992). Chronic sorrow can also accompany the loss of a child with heightened sorrow as time passes and events of birthdays, graduations, marriage are notable missing. Chronic sorrow can also occur in an individual, who suffers from a chronic disease that regularly impairs his or her ability to live a "normal life" (e.g., paraplegic, AIDS, sickle cell disease). "Chronic sorrow does not mean that the families don't love or feel pride in their children. These feelings, and many other feelings, exist alongside the sadness. It is as if many threads are woven side-by-side, bright and dark, in the fabric of the parents/caregivers' lives" (Rhode Island Department of Health, 2011, p. 22).

NOC

Depression Level, Coping, Mood Equilibrium Acceptance: Health Status

Goals

The individual will be assisted in anticipating events that can trigger heightened sadness, as evidenced by the following indicators:

- Express sadness
- Discuss the loss(es) periodically

NIC

Anticipatory Guidance, Coping Enhancement, Referral, Active Listening, Presence, Resiliency Promotion

Interventions

Explain Chronic Sorrow

- Normal response
- Focus on loss of normalcy
- Not time-limited
- Episodic
- Persists throughout life

Encourage to Share Feelings Since the Change (e.g., Birth of Child, Accident)

Promote Hopefulness (Hockenberry & Wilson, 2015)

- Advise of age-related health promotion needs.
- Provide anticipatory guidance for maturational stages (e.g., puberty).
- Discuss possible age-related self-care responsibilities.

Explore Activities That the Child and/or the Parent Enjoys Doing

Acquire a Consult with Play Therapist

Convey an Interest of Each Individual and Family

- Provide siblings opportunities to share their feelings.

Explore Activities That Can Improve Coping on a Day-to-Day Basis as (Gordon, 2009)

- Accessing resources to learn more about condition (e.g., library, internet)
- Regular stress-reducing activities, for example, exercising (yoga at home, walking, reading, crafts)
- Keeping a journal
- Help planning how to have "a night out"
- Stressing the importance of maintaining support systems and friendships

Prepare for Subsequent Crises Over the Life Span

- Gently encourage the individual to share lost dreams or hopes.
- Assist the individual to identify developmental milestones that will exacerbate the loss of normalcy (e.g., school play, sports, prom, dating).
- Clarify that feelings will fluctuate (intense, diminished) over the years, but the sorrow will not disappear.
- Advise individual that these crises may feel like the first response to the "news."

Encourage Participation in Support Groups With Others Experiencing Chronic Sorrow

- Share the difficulties of the following (*Monsen, 1999):
  - Living worried
  - Treating the child like other children
  - Staying in the struggle

Acknowledge That Parent(s) Is the Child's Expert Caregiver (Melnyk et al., 2001)

- Prepare the family for transition to another health-care provider (e.g., child to adult providers).

Link the Family With Appropriate Services (e.g., Home Health, Respite Counselor)

- Differentiate between chronic sorrow and depression. If depression is suspected, parent(s) should be referred to a psychiatrist/psychiatric nurse practitioner for proper assessment and diagnosis (Gordan, 2009).

Refer to *Caregiver Role Strain* for Additional Interventions

SPIRITUAL DISTRESS

Spiritual Distress

Risk for Spiritual Distress

Impaired Religiosity

Risk for Impaired Religiosity

NANDA-I Definition

Impaired ability to experience and integrate meaning and purpose in life through connectedness with self, others, art, music, literature, nature, and/or a power greater than oneself

Defining Characteristics

Questions meaning of life, death, and suffering
Reports no sense of meaning and purpose in life

Lacks enthusiasm for life, feelings of joy, inner peace, or love

Demonstrates discouragement or despair

Feels a sense of emptiness

Experiences alienation from spiritual or religious community

Expresses need to reconcile with self, others, God, or creator

Presents with sudden interest in spiritual matters (reading spiritual or religious books, watching spiritual or religious programs on television)

Displays sudden changes in spiritual practices (rejection, neglect, doubt, fanatical devotion)

Verbalizes that family, loved ones, peers, or health-care providers opposed spiritual beliefs or practices

Questions credibility of religion or spiritual belief system

Requests assistance for a disturbance in spiritual beliefs or religious practice

Related Factors

Pathophysiologic

Related to challenge in spiritual health or separation from spiritual ties secondary to:

Hospitalization

Pain

Terminal illness

Loss of body part or function

Trauma

Debilitating disease

Miscarriage, stillbirth

Treatment Related

Related to conflict between (specify prescribed regimen) and beliefs:

Abortion

Isolation

Surgery

Blood transfusion

Medications

Dietary restrictions

Medical procedures

Dialysis

Situational (Personal, Environmental)

Related to death* or illness of significant other

Related to embarrassment of expressions of spirituality or religion, such as prayers, meditation, or other rituals

Related to barriers to practicing spiritual rituals:

Restrictions of intensive care

Lack of privacy

Unavailability of special foods/diet or ritual objects

Confinement to bed or room

Related to spiritual or religious beliefs opposed by family, peers, health-care providers

Related to divorce, separation from loved one, or other perceived loss

 Author's Note

Wellness represents a response to an individual's potential for personal growth, involving use of all of an individual's resources (social, psychological, cultural, environmental, spiritual, and physiologic). Nurses profess to care for the whole individual, but several studies report that they commonly avoid addressing the spiritual dimension of individuals, families, and communities (*Kendrick & Robinson, 2000; Puchalski & Ferrell, 2010; Swift, Calcutawalla, & Elliott, 2007).

To promote positive spirituality with individuals and families, the nurse must possess spiritual self-knowledge. For the nurse, self-evaluation must precede assessment of spiritual concerns, and assessment of spiritual health should be confined to the context of nursing. The nurse can assist people with spiritual concerns or distress by providing resources for spiritual help, by listening nonjudgmentally, and by providing opportunities to meet spiritual needs (*O'Brien, 2010; *Wright, 2004).

Spirituality and religiousness are two different concepts. Burkhart and Solari-Twadell (*2001) define spirituality as the "ability to experience and integrate meaning and self; others, art, music, literature, nature, or a power greater than oneself." Religiousness is "the ability to exercise participation in the beliefs of a particular denomination of faith community and related rituals" (*Burkhart & Solari-Twadell, 2001). Although the spiritual dimension of human wholeness is always present, it may or may not exist within the context of religious traditions or practices.

Impaired Religiousness was approved by NANDA in 2004. This diagnosis can be used for *Spiritual Distress* when an individual has a barrier to practicing his or her religious rituals that the nurse can assist by decreasing or removing. *Impaired Religiosity* would be appropriate.

NOC

Hope, Spiritual Well-Being

Goals

The individual will find meaning and purpose in life, even during illness, as evidenced by the following indicators:

- Expresses his or her feelings related to beliefs and spirituality
- Describes his or her spiritual belief system as it relates to illness
- Finds meaning and comfort in religious or spiritual practice

NIC
Spiritual Growth Facilitation, Hope Instillation, Active Listening, Presence, Emotional Support, Spiritual Support

Interventions

Create an Environment of Trust (Puchalski & Ferrell, 2010)

- Be open to listening to the patient's story, not just the medical facts.
- Listen for the content, emotion and manner, and spiritual meanings.
- Give "permission" to discuss spiritual matters with the nurse by bringing up the subject of spiritual welfare, if necessary.
- Be fully present.

Conflict Between Religious or Spiritual Beliefs and Prescribed Health Regimen

Assess for Causative and Contributing Factors

- Lack of information about or understanding of spiritual restrictions
- Lack of information about or understanding of health regimen
- Informed, true conflict
-

Eliminate or Reduce Causative and Contributing Factors, If Possible

Feeling Threatened and Vulnerable Because of Symptoms or Possible Death
- Inform individuals and families about the importance of finding meaning in illness.
- Suggest using prayer, imagery, and meditation to reduce anxiety and provide hope and a sense of control.

Failure of Spiritual Beliefs to Provide Explanation or Comfort During Crisis of Illness/Suffering/Impending Death
- Use questions about past beliefs and spiritual experiences to assist the individual in putting this life event into wider perspective.
- Offer to contact the usual or a new spiritual leader.
- Offer to pray/meditate/read with the individual if you are comfortable with this, or arrange for another member of the healthcare team if more appropriate.
- Provide uninterrupted quiet time for prayer/reading/meditation on spiritual concerns.

- Parental conflict concerning treatment of their child
- Lack of time for deliberation before emergency treatment or surgery
- Practice as an advocate for the individual and family

Doubting Quality of Own Faith to Deal With Current Illness/ Suffering/Death

- Be available and willing to listen when individual expresses self-doubt, guilt, or other negative feelings.
- Silence, touch, or both may be useful in communicating the nurse's presence and support during times of doubt or despair.
- Offer to contact usual or new spiritual leader.

Anger Toward God/Supreme Deity or Spiritual Beliefs for Allowing or Causing Illness/Suffering/Death

- Express that anger toward God/Supreme Deity is a common reaction to illness/suffering/death.
- Help to recognize and discuss feelings of anger.
- Allow to problem solve to find ways to express and relieve anger.
- Offer to contact the usual spiritual leader or offer to contact another spiritual support person (e.g., pastoral care, hospital chaplain) if the individual cannot share feelings with the usual spiritual lead.

Lack of Information About Spiritual Restrictions

- Have the spiritual leader discuss restrictions and exemptions as they apply to those who are seriously ill or hospitalized.
- Provide reading materials on religious and spiritual restrictions and exemptions.
- Encourage the individual to seek information from and discuss restrictions with spiritual leader and/or others in the spiritual group.
- Chart the results of these discussions.

Informed, True Conflict

- Encourage the individual and physician/nurse practitioner to consider alternative methods of therapy.[49] Support the individual making an informed decision—even if the decision conflicts with nurse's own values.

---

[49]Definitions designated as NANDA-I and characteristics and factors identified with a blue asterisk are from *Nursing Diagnoses: Definitions and Classification 2012–2014*. Copyright © 2012, 2009, 2007, 2003, 2001, 1998, 1996, 1994 by NANDA International. Used by arrangement with Blackwell Publishing Limited, a company of John Wiley & Sons, Inc.

Parental Conflict Over Treatment of the Child

- If parents refuse treatment of the child, follow the interventions under informed conflict above.
- If parents still refuse treatment, the physician or hospital administrator may obtain a court order appointing a temporary guardian to consent to treatment.
- Call the spiritual leader to support the parents (and possibly the child).
- Encourage expression of negative feelings.

Listening Skills (Puchalski & Ferrell, 2010)
- Create an environment of trust.
- Be open to listening to the individual's story, not just the medical facts.
- Listen for the content, emotion and manner, and spiritual meanings.
- Be fully present.
- Communicate acceptance of various spiritual beliefs and practices.
- Convey nonjudgmental attitude.
- Acknowledge importance of spiritual needs.
- Express willingness of health-care team to help in meeting spiritual needs.
  - Maintain diet with religious restrictions when not detrimental to health.
  - Encourage spiritual rituals not detrimental to health.
  - Provide opportunity for individual to pray with others or be read to by members of own religious group or a member of the health-care team who feels comfortable with these activities.

Pediatric Interventions

- Encourage children to maintain bedtime or before-meal prayer rituals.
- If compatible with the child's religious beliefs:
  - Share religious picture books and other religious articles.
  - Consult with the family for appropriate books or objects (e.g., medals, statues).
  - Explore the child's feelings regarding illness as punishment for wrongdoing (Hockenberry & Wilson, 2015).
- Discuss if being sick has changed his or her beliefs (e.g., prayer requests).
- Support an adolescent who may be struggling for understanding of spiritual teachings.

Risk for Spiritual Distress

NANDA-I Definition

Vulnerable for an impaired ability to experience and integrate meaning and purpose in life through connectedness with self, others, art, music, literature, nature, and/or a power greater than oneself, which may compromise health.

Risk Factors

Refer to *Spiritual Distress*.

 Author's Note

Refer to *Spiritual Distress*.

Refer to *Spiritual Distress*.

Goals

The individual will find meaning and purpose in life, including during illness, as evidenced by the following indicators:

- Practice spiritual rituals
- Express comfort with beliefs

Refer to *Spiritual Distress*.

Interventions

Refer to *Spiritual Distress*.

Impaired Religiosity

NANDA-I Definition

Impaired ability to exercise reliance on beliefs and/or participate in rituals of a particular faith tradition

Defining Characteristics

Individuals experience distress because of difficulty with adhering to prescribed religious rituals such as:
Religious ceremonies
Dietary regulations
Certain clothing
Prayer
Request to worship
Holiday observances
Separation from faith community*
Emotional distress regarding religious beliefs, religious social network, or both
Need to reconnect with previous belief patterns and customs
Questioning of religious belief patterns and customs*

Related Factors

Pathophysiologic

*Related to sickness/illness**

Related to suffering

*Related to pain**

Situational (Personal, Environmental)

Related to personal crisis secondary to activity*

*Related to fear of death**

Related to embarrassment at practicing spiritual rituals

Related to barriers to practicing spiritual rituals

Intensive care restrictions
Confinement to bed or the room
Lack of privacy

Lack of availability of
special foods/diets
Hospitalization

Related to crisis within the faith community, which causes distress in the believer

 Author's Note

Refer to *Spiritual Distress*.

 NOC
Spiritual Well-Being

Goals

The individual will express satisfaction with ability to practice or exercise beliefs and practices, as evidenced by the following indicators:

- Continue spiritual practices not detrimental to health
- Express decreasing feelings of guilt and anxiety

 NIC
Spiritual Support

Interventions

Explore Whether the Individual Desires to Engage in an Allowable Religious or Spiritual Practice or Ritual; If So, Provide Opportunities to Do So

Express Your Understanding and Acceptance of the Importance of the Individual's Religious or Spiritual Beliefs and Practices

Assess for Causative and Contributing Factors

- Hospital or nursing home environment
- Limitations related to disease process or treatment regimen (e.g., cannot kneel to pray because of traction; prescribed diet differs from usual religious diet)
- Fear of imposing on or antagonizing medical and nursing staff with requests for spiritual rituals

- Embarrassment over spiritual beliefs or customs (especially common in adolescents)
- Separation from articles, texts, or environment of spiritual significance
- Lack of transportation to spiritual place or service
- Spiritual leader unavailable because of emergency or lack of time

Eliminate or Reduce Causative and Contributing Factors, If Possible

Limitations Imposed by the Hospital or Nursing Home Environment
- Provide privacy and quiet as needed for daily prayer, visit by spiritual leader, and spiritual reading and contemplation.
  - Pull the curtains or close the door.
  - Turn off the television and radio.
  - Ask the desk to hold calls, if possible.
  - Note the spiritual interventions on Kardex and include in the care plan.
- Contact the spiritual leader to clarify practices and perform religious rites or services, if desired.
  - Communicate with the spiritual leader concerning the individual's condition.
  - Address Roman Catholic, Orthodox, and Episcopal priests as "Father," other Christian ministers as "Pastor," and Jewish rabbis as "Rabbi."
- Prevent interruption during the visit, if possible.
- Offer to provide a table or stand covered with a clean white cloth.
- Inform the individual about religious services and materials available within the institution.

Fear of Imposing or Embarrassment
- Communicate acceptance of various spiritual beliefs and practices.
- Convey a nonjudgmental, respectful attitude.
- Acknowledge the importance of spiritual needs.
- Express the willingness of the health-care team to help the individual meet spiritual needs.
- Provide privacy and ensure confidentiality.

Limitations Related to Disease Process or Treatment Regimen
- Encourage spiritual rituals not detrimental to health.
  - Assist individuals with physical limitations in prayer and spiritual observances (e.g., help to hold rosary; help to kneeling position, if appropriate).
  - Assist in habits of personal cleanliness.
  - Avoid shaving if beard is of spiritual significance.

- Allow the individual to wear religious clothing or jewelry whenever possible.
- Make special arrangements for burial of respected limbs or body organs.
- Allow the family or spiritual leader to perform ritual care of the body.
- Make arrangements as needed for other important spiritual rituals (e.g., circumcisions).
- Determine if there are dietary restrictions. Maintain diet with spiritual restrictions when not detrimental to health.
  - Consult with a dietitian.
  - Allow fasting for short periods, if possible.
  - Change the therapeutic diet as necessary.
  - Have family or friends bring in special food, if possible.
  - Have members of the spiritual group supply meals to the individual at home.
  - Be as flexible as possible in serving methods, times of meals, and so forth.

Risk for Impaired Religiosity

NANDA-I Definition

Vulnerable for an impaired ability to exercise reliance on religious beliefs and/or participate in rituals of a particular faith tradition, which may compromise health

Related Factors

Refer to *Impaired Religiosity*.

Spiritual Well-Being

Goals

The individual will express continued satisfaction with religious activities, as evidenced by the following indicators:

- Continue to practice religious rituals
- Described increased comfort after assessment

Spiritual Support

Interventions

Refer to *Impaired Religiosity* for interventions.

STRESS OVERLOAD

NANDA-I Definition

Excessive amounts and types of demands that require action

Defining Characteristics

Reports excessive situational stress (e.g., rates stress level as 7 or above on a 10-point scale)*

Reports negative impact from stress (e.g., physical symptoms, psychological distress, feeling of being sick or of going to get sick)*

Physiologic
Headaches
Sleep difficulties
Fatigue

Indigestion
Restlessness

Emotional
Crying
Edginess
Nervousness
Overwhelmed
Feeling of pressure*

Increased anger*
Increased impatience*
Easily upset
Feeling sick
Feeling of tension*

Cognitive
Memory loss
Forgetfulness
Problems with decision making*

Constant worry
Loss of humor
Trouble thinking clearly

Behavioral
Isolation
Lack of intimacy
Excessive smoking
Difficulty functioning*

Intolerance
Compulsive eating
Resentment

Related Factors

The related factors of *Stress Overload* represent the multiple coexisting stressors that can be pathophysiologic, maturational, treatment related, situational, environmental, personal, or all of these. An individual may be able to reduce or eliminate some factors, while other factors that are chronic may require new strategies to manage these stressors.

Pathophysiologic

Related to coping with:
Acute illness (myocardial infarction, fractured hip)
Chronic illness* (arthritis, depression, chronic obstructive pulmonary disorder)
Terminal illness*
New diagnosis (cancer, genital herpes, HIV, multiple sclerosis, diabetes mellitus)
Disfiguring condition

Situational (Personal, Environmental)

Related to actual or anticipated loss of a significant other secondary to:

Death, dying	Divorce
Moving	Military duty

Related to coping with:

Dying	Assault
War	

Related to actual or perceived change in socioeconomic status secondary to:

Unemployment	Illness
New job	Foreclosure
Promotion	Destruction of personal property

Related to coping with:

Family violence*	Relationship problems
New family member	Declining functional status of
older relative	
Substance abuse	

Maturational

Related to coping with:

Retirement	Loss of residence
Financial changes	Functional losses

Author's Note

This diagnosis represents an individual in an overwhelming situation influenced by multiple varied stressors. If stress overload is not reduced, the individual will deteriorate and may be in danger of injury and illness.

 Carp's Cues

- Health People 2020 has the following goals, which can influence stress and stress management (US Department of Health and Human Service, 2015):
  - Improve health-related quality of life and well-being for all individuals
  - Improve mental health through prevention and by ensuring access to appropriate, quality mental health services
  - Reduce illness, disability, and death related to tobacco use and secondhand smoke exposure
  - Reduce substance abuse to protect the health, safety, and quality of life for all, especially children
  - Improve health, fitness, and quality of life through daily physical activity
  - Improve the health and well-being of women, infants, children, and families

Goals

The individual will verbalize intent to change two behaviors to decrease or manage stressors, as evidenced by the following indicators:

- Identify stressors that can be controlled and those that cannot
- Identify one successful behavior change to increase stress management
- Identify one behavior to reduce or eliminate that will increase successful stress management

 NIC

Anxiety Reduction, Behavioral Modification, Exercise Promotion

Interventions

> **CLINICAL ALERT** At a site Peaceful Parent Institute (2015), the effects of chronic stress overload is described:
>
> The person who grew up in a relatively relaxed and emotionally safe environment will generally be able to identify that their stress levels are too high and will be less tolerant of living with such discomfort on an ongoing basis, hence likely to be more proactive about meeting their self-care needs.
>
> However, when someone grows up in an emotionally stifling, demanding, or chaotic environment, their body becomes accustomed to the regular high peaks of stress and anxiety and rushes of adrenalin. Eventually the child's physiological resting state, even when there is not an apparent threat, remains in a state of heightened stress and low (or high) level anxiety.
>
> The result is always living on the edge to one extent or another, but because this was normal as a child, it is difficult for the person, as an adult, to recognize that they need and deserve to generally live in a more relaxed state.

Assist to Recognize His or Her Thoughts, Feelings, Actions, and Physiologic Responses Refer to Focus Assessment

R: *Self-awareness can help the individual reframe and reinterpret their experiences (Edelman, Kudzma, & Mandle, 2014).*

Teach How to Break the Stress Cycle and How to Decrease Heart Rate, Respirations, and Strong Feelings of Anger (Edelman et al., 2014)

- Purposefully distract yourself by thinking of something pleasant.
- Engage in a diversional activity.
- Teach to use mini-relaxation techniques (Edelman et al., 2014).
  - Inhale through nose for 4 seconds, exhale through mouth for 4 seconds.
  - Repeat this controlled breathing and think about something that makes you smile (e.g., a child, your pet).

- Refer to resources to learn relaxation techniques such as audio-tapes, printed material, and yoga.

R: *Faced with overwhelming multiple stressors, the person can be assisted to differentiate which stressors can be modified or eliminated (Edelman & Mandle, 2010).*

Ask to List One or Two Changes They Would Like to Make in the Next Week

- Diet (eat one vegetable a day)
- Exercise (walk one to two blocks each day)

R: *In a person who is already overwhelmed, small changes in lifestyle may have a higher chance for success and will increase confidence (*Bodenheimer, MacGregor, & Shariffi, 2005).*

If Sleep Disturbances Are Present, Refer to *Insomnia*

If Spiritual Needs Are Identified as Deficient, Refer to *Spiritual Distress*

- Ask what activity brings the individual feelings of peace, joy, and happiness. Ask them to incorporate one of these activities each week.

R: *Overwhelmed individuals usually deny themselves such activities. Leisure can break the stress cycle (Edelman & Mandle, 2014).*

- Ask the individual what is important, and if change is needed in their life.

R: *Values clarification assists the overwhelmed individual to identify what is meaningful and valued and if it is present in their actual living habits (Edelman & Mandle, 2014).*

Assist to Set Realistic Goals to Achieve a More Balanced Health-Promoting Lifestyle

- What is most important?
- What aspects of your life would you like to change most?
- What is the first step?
- When?

R: *Setting realistic goals will increase confidence and success (*Bodenheimer et al., 2005).*

Initiate Health Teaching and Referrals, as Necessary

- If the individual is engaged in substance or alcohol abuse, refer for drug and alcohol abuse.
- If the individual has severe depression or anxiety, refer for professional counseling.
- If family functioning is compromised, refer for family counseling.

RISK FOR SUDDEN INFANT DEATH SYNDROME

NANDA-I Definition

Vulnerable to unpredicted death of infant

Risk Factors

There is no single risk factor. Several risk factors combined may be contributory (refer to Related Factors).

Related Factors
(*McMillan et al., 1999)

Pathophysiologic

Related to increased vulnerability secondary to:

Cyanosis	Tachypnea
Hypothermia	Low birth weight*
Fever	Small for gestational age*
Poor feeding	Prematurity*
Irritability	Low Apgar score (less than 7)
Respiratory distress	History of diarrhea, vomiting, or
Tachycardia	listlessness 2 weeks before death

Related to increased vulnerability secondary to prenatal maternal:

Anemia*	Poor weight gain
Urinary tract infection	Sexually transmitted infections

Situational (Personal, Environmental)

Related to increased vulnerability secondary to maternal:

Cigarette smoking*
Drug use during pregnancy
Lack of breastfeeding* (20)*
Inadequate prenatal care*
Low educational levels*

Single mother*
Multiparity with first
Young age (younger than

Young age during pregnancy*

Related to increased vulnerability secondary to:

Crowded living conditions*
Sleeping on stomach*
Poor family financial status

Cold environment
Low socioeconomic status

Related to increased vulnerability secondary to:

Male gender*
Native Americans*
Multiple births

African descent*
Previous sudden infant death
    syndrome (SIDS) death
    in family

NOC

Knowledge: Maternal–Child Health, Risk Control: Tobacco Use, Risk Control, Knowledge: Infant Safety

Goals

The caregiver will reduce or eliminate risk factors that are modifiable, as evidenced by the following indicators:

- Position the infant on the back or lying on the side
- Eliminate smoking in the home, near the infant, and during pregnancy
- Participate in prenatal and newborn medical care
- Improve maternal health (e.g., treat anemia, promote optimal nutrition)
- Enroll in drug and alcohol programs, if indicated

NIC

Teaching: Infant Safety, Risk Identification

Interventions

Explain SIDS to Caregivers and that SIDS Has Similar Risk Factors to Other Sleep-Related Infant Deaths, Including Those Attributed to Suffocation, Asphyxia, and Entrapment (Corwin, 2015)

Reduce or Eliminate Risk Factors That Can Be Modified
(Corwin, 2015)

- Maternal factors:
  - Young maternal age <20
  - Maternal smoking during pregnancy
  - Late or no prenatal care
- Infant and environmental factors:
  - Preterm birth and/or low birth weight
  - Prone sleeping position
  - Sleeping on a soft surface and/or with bedding accessories such as loose blankets and pillows
  - Bed-sharing (e.g., sleeping in parents' bed)
  - Overheating
- Position infant on his or her back.
- Use a pacifier.
- Avoid overheating the infant during sleep (e.g., excessive clothing, bedding, hot room).
- Reduce risks for suffocation:
  - Avoid loose or soft bedding (e.g., mattresses).
  - Avoid pillows, sleep positioners.
  - Avoid sleeping with the infant (Anderson, 2000).
- Do not expose the infant to any tobacco smoke.
- Avoid using car seats to sleep outside the car. Car seats, strollers, or swings should not be routinely used for sleep because the slumped position can inhibit breathing.

Initiate Health Teaching and Referrals, as Indicated

- Discuss strategies to stop smoking (refer to index—*smoking*).
- Provide emergency numbers, as indicated.
- Refer to social agencies, as indicated.

DELAYED SURGICAL RECOVERY

Delayed Surgical Recovery

Risk for Delayed Surgical Recovery

NANDA-I Definition

Extension of the number of postoperative days required to initiate and perform activities that maintain, life, health, and well-being

Defining Characteristics

Postpones resumption of work/employment activities*
Requires help to complete self-care*
Loss of appetite with or without nausea*
Fatigue*
Perceives that more time is needed to recover*
Evidence of interrupted healing of surgical area (e.g., red, indurated, draining, immobilized)*
Difficulty moving about*
Venous obstruction/pooling

 Author's Note

This diagnosis represents an individual who has not achieved recovery from a surgical procedure within the expected time. Based on the defining characteristics from NANDA-I, some confusion exists regarding the difference between defining characteristics (signs and symptoms) and related factors. A possible use of this diagnosis is as a risk diagnosis. Persons who are at high risk for *Delayed Surgical Recovery*, for example, the the obese, those with diabetes mellitus, or cancer, could be identified. Interventions to prevent this state could be implemented. The diagnosis has not been developed sufficiently for clinical use. This author recommends using other nursing diagnoses, such as *Self-Care Deficit, Acute Pain,* or *Imbalanced Nutrition.*

Risk for Delayed Surgical Recovery

Definition

Vulnerable to an extension of the number of postoperative days required to initiate and perform activities that maintain life, health, and well-being, which may compromise health

Risk Factors

American Society of Anesthesiologist (ASA) Physical Status classification score ≥3
Diabetes mellitus
Edema at surgical site
Extensive surgical procedure
Extremes of age
History of delayed wound healing
Perioperative surgical site infection
Persistent nausea
Persistent vomiting
Pharmaceutical agent
Postoperative emotional response
Prolonged surgical procedure

Impaired mobility
Malnutrition
Obesity
Pain

Psychological disorder in
   postoperative period
Surgical site
   contamination
Trauma at surgical site

 Author's Note

A new NANDA-I nursing diagnosis, *Risk for Delayed Surgical Recovery*, is a clinically useful nursing diagnosis to designate individuals who are at risk for delayed transition to home. Factors that increase an individual's risk for infection are usually associated with delayed transition. Nursing care needs to be more aggressive in reducing factors that contribute to infection as uncontrolled diabetes mellitus and tobacco use. In addition, strict environmental control to prevent transfer of infection to the compromised individual is imperative.

Goals

 NOC
Refer to Delayed Surgical Recovery

Interventions

NIC
Refer to Delayed Surgical Recovery

Assess for the following risk factors. Total the number of Risk Factors from (1 to 10) in (). The higher the score, the greater their risk. For example, an individual, who smokes, has diabetes mellitus and is obese has a total score of 15. The diagnosis can be written as *High Risk for Delayed Surgical Healing* (15) or add the risk factors, for example, as *High Risk for Delayed Surgical Healing* related to obesity, diabetes mellitus, and tobacco use.

- Infection colonization of microorganisms (1)
  - Preoperative nares colonization with *Staphylococcus aureus* noted in 30% of most healthy populations, especially methicillin-resistant *Staph aureus* (MRSA), predisposes individuals to have higher risk of surgical site infection (Price et al., 2008).
- Preexisting remote body site infection (1)

- Preoperative contaminated or dirty wound (e.g., post trauma) (1)
- Glucocorticoid steroids (2)
- Tobacco use (3)
- Malnutrition (4)
- Obesity (5)
- Perioperative hyperglycemia (6)
- Diabetes mellitus (7)
- Altered immune response (8)
- Chronic alcohol use/acute alcohol intoxication (9)

Monitor the Surgical Site for Bleeding, Dehiscence, Hematoma, Inadequate Incisional Closure

Monitor for Signs of Paralytic Ileus

- Absent bowel sounds
- Nausea, vomiting
- Abdominal distention

Explain the Effects of Nicotine (Cigarettes, Cigars, Smokeless) on Circulation

- If the individual quit before the surgery, stress the importance of continued smoking cessation to reduce the risk of infection. Refer to Getting Started to Quit Smoking on thePoint at http://thePoint.lww.com/Carpenito6e and print guideline for individual.

Refer to Specific Nursing Diagnoses to Reduce the Risk Factors If Amenable to Nursing Care as

- *Imbalanced Nutrition*
- *Obesity*
- *Risk Prone Behaviors* (e.g., alcohol, tobacco use)
- *Ineffective Health Management* related to (specify) as evident by uncontrolled glucose levels
- *Nonengagement* related to (specify) as evident by inadequate management of disease (specify)

Initiate Health Teaching and Referrals as Needed

- Explain wound healing and precautions needed.
- Emphasize the importance of good hydration and nutrition.

- Demonstrate wound care; observe a relative or the individual doing wound care.
- Arrange for home nursing consultation.

INEFFECTIVE TISSUE PERFUSION[50]

Ineffective Tissue Perfusion

Risk for Decreased Cardiac Tissue Perfusion

Risk for Ineffective Cerebral Tissue Perfusion

Risk for Ineffective Gastrointestinal Tissue Perfusion

Ineffective Peripheral Tissue Perfusion

Risk for Ineffective Peripheral Tissue Perfusion

Risk for Peripheral Neurovascular Dysfunction

Risk for Ineffective Renal Perfusion

Definition

Decrease in oxygen, resulting in failure to nourish tissues at capillary level

 Author's Note

The use of any *Ineffective Tissue Perfusion* diagnosis other than *Peripheral* merely provides new labels for medical diagnoses, labels that do not describe the nursing focus or accountability.

When using these diagnoses, nurses cannot be accountable for prescribing the interventions for outcome achievement. Instead of using *Ineffective Tissue Perfusion*, the nurse should focus on the nursing diagnoses and collaborative problems that are present or at risk for because of altered renal, cardiac, cerebral, pulmonary, or gastrointestinal (GI) tissue perfusion. Refer to Section 3 for specific collaborative problems, for example *Risk for Complications of Increased Intracranial Pressure*, *Risk for*

---

[50]This diagnosis is presently not on the NANDA-I list but has been added by this author for clarity and usefulness.

Complications of GI Bleeding, Risk for Decreased Cardiac Output, Risk for Renal Insufficiency, Risk for Hypoxemia.

Ineffective Peripheral Tissue Perfusion can be a clinically useful nursing diagnosis if used to describe chronic arterial or venous insufficiency. (In contrast, acute embolism and thrombophlebitis represent collaborative problems as *Risk for Complications of Pulmonary Embolism* or *RC of Deep Vein Thrombosis.* A nurse focusing on preventing deep vein thrombosis in a postoperative client would write the diagnosis *Risk for Ineffective Peripheral Tissue Perfusion related to postoperative immobility and dehydration.*

Risk for Decreased Cardiac Tissue Perfusion

NANDA-I Definition

Vulnerable to a decrease in cardiac (coronary) circulation, which may compromise health

Risk Factors*

Pharmaceutical agent* (medication side effect of combination pills)[51]
Cardiovascular surgery* (treatment)
Cardiac tamponade* (clinical emergency)
Coronary artery spasm* (clinical emergency)
Diabetes mellitus* (medical diagnosis with multiple complications with associated modifiable risk lifestyles)
Drug abuse* (clinical situations with multiple complications)
Elevated C-reactive protein* (positive laboratory test)
Family history of coronary artery disease* (factor with associated modifiable risk lifestyles)
Hyperlipidemia* (medical diagnosis with associated modifiable risk lifestyles)
Hypertension* (medical diagnosis with multiple complications with associated modifiable risk lifestyles)
Hypoxemia* (complication)

---

[51]Text in parentheses has been added by author to indicate that nursing diagnosis is not the clinical terminology to communicate clinical emergencies or to direct medical treatment for complications.

Hypovolemia* (complication)
Hypoxia* (complication)
Substance abuse (medical diagnosis)
Insufficient knowledge of modifiable risk factors (e.g., smoking,
    sedentary lifestyle, obesity)[2]
(These related factors are more appropriate to the nursing
    diagnoses of *Risk-Prone Health Behavior* and/or *Ineffective Self-
    Health Management*.)

 Author's Note

This NANDA-I nursing diagnosis represents a collection of risk factors or
that have different clinical implications. Some include a collection of physiologic complications that relate to the situation and can be labeled as *Risk
for Complications of Cardiac Surgery*, *Risk for Complications of Acute Coronary Syndrome*, and *Risk for Complications of Diabetes Mellitus*. Some are
single complications such as *Risk for Complications of Hypovolemia* and *Risk
for Complications of Hypoxia*. Refer to Section II, Collaborative Problems.

   For example, *Risk for Complications of Cocaine Abuse* would describe
monitoring and management of complications such as cardiac/vascular
shock, seizures, coma, respiratory insufficiency, stroke, and hyperpyrexia.
These complications are different from *Risk for Complications of Alcohol
Abuse* which describes the monitoring and management of complications
of delirium tremors, seizures, autonomic hyperactivity, hypovolemia,
hypoglycemia, alcohol hallucinosis, and cardio/vascular shock.

   Some complications are medical emergencies, such as cardiac tamponade, coronary artery spasm, or occlusion, all of which have protocols
for medical interventions.

   If a diagnosis is needed for this clinical situation, use *Risk for Complications of Medication Therapy Adverse Effects*, specifically *Risk for Complications of Oral Combination Contraception Therapy*.

Risk for Ineffective Cerebral Tissue Perfusion

NANDA-I Definition

Vulnerable to for a decrease in cerebral tissue circulation that may
compromise health

Risk Factors*

Abnormal partial thromboplastin time
Akinetic left ventricular segment
Arterial dissection
Atrial myxoma
Carotid stenosis
Coagulopathies (e.g., sickle cell anemia)
Disseminated intravascular coagulation
Head trauma
Hypertension
Left atrial appendage thrombosis
Mitral stenosis
Recent myocardial infarction
Substance abuse
Treatment-related side effects (cardiopulmonary bypass, pharmaceutical agents)

Abnormal prothrombin time
Aortic atherosclerosis
Atrial fibrillation
Brain tumor
Cerebral aneurysm
Dilated cardiomyopathy
Embolism
Hypercholesterolemia
Endocarditis
Mechanical prosthetic valve
Neoplasm of the brain
Sick sinus syndrome
Thrombolytic therapy

 Author's Note

This NANDA-I nursing diagnosis represents a collection of risk factors that have very different clinical implications. Some are physiologic complications that are related to a medical diagnosis or treatment and can be labeled as *Risk for Complications of Head Trauma*, *Risk for Complications of Brain Tumor*, or *Risk for Complications of Thrombolytic Therapy*. These clinical situations have both nursing diagnoses and collaborative problems that require interventions.

For example, *Risk for Complications of Cranial Surgery* would have the following collaborative problems:

- *Risk for Complications of Increased Intracranial Pressure*
- *Risk for Complications of Hemorrhage and Hypovolemia/Shock*
- *Risk for Complications of Thromboembolism*
- *Risk for Complications of Cranial Nerve Dysfunction*
- *Risk for Complications of Cardiac Dysrhythmias*
- *Risk for Complications of Seizures*
- *Risk for Complications of Sensory/Motor Alterations*

Nursing diagnoses associated with this clinical situation:

- *Anxiety* to impending surgery and fear of outcomes
- *Acute Pain* related to compression/displacement of brain tissue and increased intracranial pressure

- *Risk for Ineffective Heath Management* related to insufficient knowledge of wound care signs and symptoms of complications, restrictions, and follow-up care

Goals /Interventions

Refer to Section 3 for specific collaborative problems under *Risk for Complications of Neurologic Dysfunction.*

Risk for Ineffective Gastrointestinal Tissue Perfusion

NANDA-I Definition

Vulnerable to a decrease in gastrointestinal circulation, which may compromise health

Risk Factors*

Abdominal aortic aneurysm
Abdominal compartment syndrome
Abnormal partial thromboplastin time
Abnormal prothrombin time
Acute gastrointestinal hemorrhage
Age >60 years
Anemia
Coagulopathy (e.g., sickle cell anemia)
Diabetes mellitus
Disseminated intravascular coagulation
Female gender
Gastrointestinal condition
Ulcer, ischemic colitis, ischemic pancreatitis

Cerebrovascular accident; decrease in left ventricular performance
Impaired liver function (e.g., cirrhosis, hepatitis)
Poor left ventricular performance
Hemodynamic instability
Myocardial infarction
Renal disease (e.g. polycystic kidney, renal artery stenosis, failure)
Trauma
Smoking
Treatment regimen
Vascular diseases

Author's Note

This diagnosis is too general for clinical use because it represents a variety of physiologic complications related to GI perfusion. These complications are collaborative problems and should be separated to more specific complications for example as:

* *Risk for Complications of GI Bleeding*
* *Risk for Complications of Paralytic Ileus*
* *Risk for Complications of Hypovolemia/Shock*

Goals /Interventions

Refer to Section 3 for goals and interventions/rationale for *Risk for Complications of GI Bleeding* or *Paralytic Ileus* or *Hypovolemia/Shock*.

Ineffective Peripheral Tissue Perfusion

NANDA-I Definition

Decrease in blood circulation to the periphery that may compromise health

Defining Characteristics

Presence of one of the following types (see Key Concepts for definitions):

Claudication (arterial)*
Rest pain (arterial)
Skin color changes*
Reactive hyperemia (arterial)
Skin temperature changes
Warmer (venous)
Capillary refill longer than 3 seconds (arterial)*
Edema* (venous)
Change in motor function (arterial)
Hard, thick nails
Aching pain (arterial or venous)

Diminished or absent arterial pulses* (arterial)
Pallor (arterial)
Cyanosis (venous)
Cooler (arterial)
Decreased blood pressure (arterial)
Change in sensory function (arterial)
Trophic tissue changes (arterial)
Loss of hair
Nonhealing wound

Related Factors

Pathophysiologic

Related to compromised blood flow secondary to:
Vascular disorders

Arteriosclerosis	Leriche's syndrome	Venous hypertension
Raynaud's disease/syndrome	Aneurysm	Varicosities
Arterial thrombosis	Buerger's disease	Deep vein thrombosis
Sickle cell crisis	Collagen vascular disease	Cirrhosis
Rheumatoid arthritis	Alcoholism	

Diabetes mellitus
Hypotension
Blood dyscrasias
Renal failure
Cancer/tumor

Treatment Related

Related to immobilization

Related to presence of invasive lines

Related to pressure sites/constriction (elastic compression bandages, stockings, restraints)

Related to blood vessel trauma or compression

Situational (Personal, Environmental)

Related to pressure of enlarging uterus on pelvic vessels

Related to pressure of enlarged abdomen on pelvic vessels

Related to vasoconstricting effects of tobacco

Related to decreased circulating volume secondary to dehydration

Related to dependent venous pooling

Related to hypothermia

Related to pressure of muscle mass secondary to weight lifting

 Author's Note

See *Ineffective Peripheral Tissue Perfusion.*

Sensory Functions; Cutaneous, Tissue Integrity, Tissue perfusion: Peripheral

Goals

The individual will report a decrease in pain, as evidenced by the following indicators:

- Define peripheral vascular problem in own words
- Identify factors that improve peripheral circulation
- Identify necessary lifestyle changes
- Identify medical regimen, diet, medications, and activities that promote vasodilation
- Identify factors that inhibit peripheral circulation
- State when to contact physician or health-care professional

Peripheral Sensation Management, Circulatory Care: Venous Insufficiency, Circulatory Care: Arterial Insufficiency, Positioning, Exercise Promotion

Interventions

Assess Causative and Contributing Factors

- Underlying disease
- Inhibited arterial blood flow
- Inhibited venous blood flow
- Fluid volume excess or deficit
- Hypothermia or vasoconstriction
- Activities related to symptom/sign onset

Promote Factors That Improve Arterial Blood Flow

- Keep extremity in a dependent position.
- Keep extremity warm (do not use heating pad or hot water bottle).

Reduce Risk for Trauma

- Change positions at least every hour.
- Avoid leg crossing.
- Reduce external pressure points (inspect shoes daily for rough lining).
- Avoid sheepskin heel protectors (they increase heel pressure and pressure across dorsum of foot).
- Encourage range-of-motion exercises.
- Discuss smoking cessation (see *Ineffective Health Maintenance related to tobacco use*).

Promote Factors That Improve Venous Blood Flow

- Elevate extremity above the level of the heart (may be contraindicated if severe cardiac or respiratory disease is present).
- Avoid standing or sitting with legs dependent for long periods.
- Consider the use of elastic compression stockings.

Teach to

- Avoid pillows behind the knees or Gatch bed, which is elevated at the knees.
- Avoid leg crossing.
- Change positions, move extremities, or wiggle fingers and toes every hour.
- Avoid garters and tight elastic stockings above the knees.
- Measure baseline circumference of calves and thighs if the individual is at risk for deep venous thrombosis, or if it is suspected.

Plan a Daily Walking Program

- Refer to *Sedentary Lifestyle* for specific interventions.

Initiate Health Teaching, as Indicated

- Teach individual to:
  - Avoid long car or plane rides (get up and walk around at least every hour).
  - Keep dry skin lubricated (cracked skin eliminates the physical barrier to infection).
  - Wear warm clothing during cold weather.
  - Wear cotton or woolen socks.
  - Use gloves or mittens if hands are exposed to cold (including home freezers).
  - Avoid dehydration in warm weather.
  - Give special attention to feet and toes:
    - Wash feet and dry well daily.
    - Do not soak feet.
    - Avoid harsh soaps or chemicals (including iodine) on feet.
    - Keep nails trimmed and filed smooth.
    - Inspect feet and legs daily for injuries and pressure points.
    - Wear clean socks.
    - Wear shoes that offer support and fit comfortably.
    - Inspect the inside of shoes daily for rough lining.

Explain the Relation of Certain Risk Factors to the Development of Atherosclerosis

- Smoking
- Vasoconstriction

- Elevated blood pressure
- Decreased oxygenation of the blood
- Increased lipidemia
- Increased platelet aggregation
- Hypertension/hyperlipidemia
- Sedentary lifestyle
- Excess weight (greater than 10% of ideal)
- Refer to community resources for lifestyle changes.

Risk for Ineffective Peripheral Tissue Perfusion

NANDA-I Definition

Vulnerable to a decrease in blood circulation to the periphery, which may compromise health

Risk Factors*

Age >60 years
Deficient knowledge of aggravating factors (e.g., smoking, sedentary lifestyle, trauma, obesity, salt intake, immobility)
Deficient knowledge of disease process (e.g., diabetes mellitus, hyperlipidemia)
Diabetes mellitus
Endovascular procedures
Hypertension
Sedentary lifestyle
Smoking

Goals

Refer to *Ineffective Peripheral Tissue Perfusion*.

Interventions

Refer to *Ineffective Peripheral Tissue Perfusion*.

Risk for Peripheral Neurovascular Dysfunction

Definition

At risk for disruption in the circulation, sensation, or motion of an extremity

Risk Factors

Pathophysiologic

Related to increased volume of (specify extremity) secondary to:
Bleeding (e.g., trauma*, fractures*)   Arterial obstruction
Venous obstruction*/pooling   Coagulation disorder

Related to increased capillary filtration secondary to:
Allergic response (e.g., insect bites)   Nephrotic syndrome
Trauma   Venomous bites (e.g.,
Severe burns (thermal, electrical)   snake)
Frostbite   Hypothermia

Related to restrictive envelope secondary to circumferential burns

Treatment Related

Related to increased capillary filtration secondary to:
Total knee replacement
Total hip replacement

Related to restrictive envelope secondary to:
Tourniquet   Air splints
Ace wraps   Circumferential dressings
Brace   Cast
Restraints   Premature or tight closure
Antishock trousers   of fascial defects
Excessive traction

 Author's Note

This diagnosis represents a situation that nurses can prevent complications by identifying who is at risk and implementing measures to reduce

or eliminate causative or contributing factors. *Risk for Peripheral Neuro-vascular Dysfunction* can change to compartment syndrome. *Risk for Complications of Compartment Syndrome* is inadequate tissue perfusion in a muscle, usually an arm or leg, caused by edema, which obstructs venous and arterial flow and compresses nerves. The nursing focus for compartment syndrome is diagnosing early signs and symptoms and notifying the physician. The medical interventions required to abate the problem are surgical, such as evacuation of hematoma, repair of damaged vessels, or fasciotomy. Refer to *Risk for Complications of Compartment Syndrome* in Section 3 for specific interventions for either diagnosis. Students should consult with their faculty for direction to use either *Risk for Peripheral Vascular Dysfunction* or *Risk for Complications of Compartment Syndrome*.

Goals

Refer to *Risk for Complications of Compartment Syndrome* in Section 3.

Interventions

Refer to *Risk for Complications of Compartment Syndrome* in Section 3.

Risk for Ineffective Renal Perfusion

NANDA-I Definition

At risk for a decrease in blood circulation to the kidney that may compromise health

Risk Factors*

Abdominal compartment syndrome	Malignancy
Advance age	Malignant hypertension
Bilateral cortical necrosis	Metabolic acidosis
Burns	Multitrauma
Cardiac surgery	Polynephritis
Cardiopulmonary bypass	Renal artery stenosis
Diabetes mellitus	Renal disease (polycystic kidney)

Exposure to toxins
Female glomerulonephritis
Hyperlipidemia
Hypertension
Hypovolemia
Hypoxemia
Hypoxia
Infection (e.g., sepsis, localized infection)

Smoking
Systemic inflammatory response syndrome
Treatment-related side effects (e.g., pharmaceutical agents, surgery)
Vascular embolism vasculitis

 Author's Note

This NANDA-I diagnosis represents a potential complication which is a collaborative problem, *Risk for Complications of Renal Insufficiency*.

If the situation is a medical diagnosis of acute kidney failure or chronic renal disease, using *Risk for Complications of Acute Kidney Failure* would include the following collaborative problems[52]:

* *Risk for Complications of Fluid Overload*
* *Risk for Complications of Metabolic Acidosis*
* *Risk for Complications of Acute Albuminemia*
* *Risk for Complications of Hypertension*
* *Risk for Complications of Pulmonary Edema*
* *Risk for Complications of Dysrhythmias*
* *Risk for Complications of Gastrointestinal Bleeding*

Nursing diagnoses associated with this clinical situation:

* *Risk for Infection* related to invasive procedures
* *Imbalanced Nutrition: Less Than Body Requirements* related to anorexia, nausea, vomiting, loss of taste, loss of smell, stomatitis, and dietary restrictions
* *Risk for Impaired Tissue Integrity* related to retention of metabolic wastes, increased capillary fragility, and platelet dysfunction

---

[52]For a more specific care plan with nursing interventions/rationales and outcomes for clinical situations, such as medical diagnoses (e.g., chronic renal disease, acute kidney failure), surgical procedures (e.g., nephrectomy), treatments/procedures (e.g., hemodialysis, peritoneal dialysis), and 70 other clinical situations, refer to Carpenito-Moyet, L. J. (2017). *Nursing Care Plans; Transitional Patient & Family Centered Care* (7th ed.). Philadelphia, PA: Wolters Kluwer.

Goals /Interventions

Refer to Section 3 for goals and interventions for *Risk for Complications of Renal Insufficiency*.
Refer to Section 2 for goals and interventions for specific related nursing diagnoses.

IMPAIRED URINARY ELIMINATION

Impaired Urinary Elimination

Maturational Enuresis

Functional Urinary Incontinence

Reflex Urinary Incontinence

Stress Urinary Incontinence

Continuous Urinary Incontinence

Urge Urinary Incontinence

Risk for Urge Urinary Incontinence

Overflow Urinary Incontinence

NANDA-I Definition

Dysfunction in urinary elimination

Defining Characteristics

Major (Must Be Present, One or More)

Reports or experiences a urinary elimination problem, such as:

Urgency*	Nocturia*
Dribbling	Incontinence*
Frequency*	Dysuria*
Bladder distention	Enuresis
Hesitancy*	Retention*
Large residual urine volumes	

Related Factors
(Burakgazi et al., 2011)

Pathophysiologic

Related to incompetent bladder outlet secondary to:
Congenital urinary tract anomalies

Related to decreased bladder capacity or irritation to bladder secondary to:

Infection*	Carcinoma
Glucosuria	Urethritis
Trauma	

Related to diminished bladder cues or impaired ability to recognize bladder cues secondary to:

Cord injury/tumor/infection	Tabes dorsalis
Diabetic neuropathy	Demyelinating diseases
Brain injury/tumor/infection	Parkinsonism
Alcoholic neuropathy	Multiple sclerosis
Cerebrovascular accident	Alpha adrenergic agents

*Related to sensory motor impairment**

*Related to multiple causality**

*Related to anatomic obstruction**

Treatment Related

Related to effects of surgery on bladder sphincter secondary to:
Postprostatectomy
Extensive pelvic dissection

Related to diagnostic instrumentation

Related to decreased muscle tone secondary to:
General or spinal anesthesia
Drug therapy (iatrogenic)

Antihistamines	Tranquilizers
Immunosuppressant therapy	Sedatives
Epinephrine	Muscle relaxants
Diuretics	After use of indwelling catheters
Anticholinergics	

Situational (Personal, Environmental)

Related to weak pelvic floor muscles secondary to:

Obesity	Aging
Childbirth	Recent substantial weight loss

Related to inability to communicate needs

Related to bladder outlet obstruction secondary to:
Fecal impaction
Chronic constipation

Related to decreased bladder muscle tone secondary to:
Dehydration

Related to decreased attention to bladder cues secondary to:

Depression	Intentional suppression
Delirium	(self-induced deconditioning)
	Confusion

Related to environmental barriers to bathroom secondary to:

Distant toilets	Bed too high
Poor lighting	Side rails
Unfamiliar surroundings	

Related to inability to access bathroom on time secondary to:
Caffeine/alcohol use
Impaired mobility

Maturational

Child
Related to small bladder capacity

Related to lack of motivation

 Author's Note

In the United States, 17 million people are found to have urinary incontinence, creating a financial burden of over $76 million dollars to both individuals as well as the health-care system (Testa, 2015).

   Impaired Urinary Elimination is too broad a diagnosis for effective clinical use; however, it is clinically useful until additional data can be collected. With more data the nurse can use a more specific diagnosis, such as *Stress Urinary Incontinence*, whenever possible. When the etiologic or contributing factors for incontinence have not been identified, the nurse could write a temporary diagnosis of *Impaired Urinary Elimination* related to unknown etiology, as evidenced by incontinence.

   The nurse performs a focus assessment to determine whether the incontinence is transient, in response to an acute condition (e.g., infection, medication side effects), or established in response to various chronic neural or genitourinary conditions (Miller, 2015). In addition, the nurse should differentiate the type of incontinence: functional, reflex, stress, or urge.

Goals

The person will be continent (specify during day, night, 24 hours), as evidenced by the following indicators:

- Be able to identify the cause of incontinence
- Provide rationale for treatments

Interventions

Determine If There Is Acute Cause of Problem

- Infection (e.g., urinary tract, sexually transmitted disease, gonorrhea)
- Renal disease
- Renal calculi
- Medication effects
- Anesthesia effects

Refer to an Urologist If Acute Cause Is Determined

Assess to Determine Type If Incontinence Is the Problem

- History of continence
- Onset and duration (day, night, just certain times)
- Factors that increase incidence:
  - Coughing
  - Laughing
  - Standing
  - Turning in bed
  - Delay in getting to bathroom
  - When excited
  - Leaving bathroom
  - Running
- Perception of need to void: present, absent, diminished
- Ability to delay urination after urge
- Relief after voiding:
  - Complete
  - Continued desire to void after bladder is emptied

Refer to Specific Type of Incontinence Using Data From Assessment

Maturational Enuresis[53]

Definition

State in which a child experiences involuntary voiding during sleep that is not pathophysiologic in origin

Defining Characteristics

Reports or demonstrates episodes of involuntary voiding during sleep

Related Factors

Situational (Personal, Environmental)

Related to stressors (school, siblings)

Related to inattention to bladder cues

Related to unfamiliar surroundings

Maturational

Child

Related to small bladder capacity

Related to lack of motivation

Related to attention-seeking behavior

 Author's Note

Enuresis can result from physiologic or maturational factors. Certain etiologies, such as strictures, urinary tract infection, constipation, nocturnal epilepsy, and diabetes, should be ruled out when enuresis is present. These situations do not represent nursing diagnoses.

When enuresis results from small bladder capacity, failure to perceive cues because of deep sleep, inattention to bladder cues, or is associated

---

[53]This diagnosis is not presently on the NANDA-I list but has been included for clarity and usefulness.

with a maturational issue (e.g., new sibling, school pressures), the nursing diagnosis *Maturational Enuresis* is appropriate. Psychological problems usually are not the cause of enuresis, but may result from lack of understanding or insensitivity to the problem. Interventions that punish or shame the child must be avoided.

NOC

Urinary Continence, Knowledge: Enuresis, Family Functioning

Goals

The child will remain dry during the sleep cycle, as evidenced by the following indicator:

- The child and family will be able to list factors that decrease enuresis.

NIC

Urinary Incontinence Care: Enuresis, Urinary Habit Training, Anticipatory Guidance, Family Support

Interventions

Ask About the Pattern of Bedwetting, Including Questions Such as

- How many nights a week does bedwetting occur?
- How many times a night does bedwetting occur?
- Does there seem to be a large amount of urine?
- At what times of night does the bedwetting occur?
- Does the child or young person wake up after bedwetting?

Ask About the Presence of Daytime Symptoms in a Child or Young Person With Bedwetting, Including

- Daytime frequency (that is, passing urine more than seven times a day)
- Daytime urgency
- Daytime wetting
- Passing urine infrequently (fewer than four times a day)
- Abdominal straining or poor urinary stream
- Pain passing urine

Ask About Daytime Toileting Patterns in a Child or Young Person With Bedwetting, Including

- Whether daytime symptoms occur only in some situations
- Avoidance of toilets at school or other settings

- Whether the child or young person goes to the toilet more or less frequently than his or her peers

Assess Whether the Child or Young Person Has Any Comorbidities or There Are Other Factors to Consider, in Particular

- Constipation and/or soiling
- Developmental, attention, or learning difficulties
- Diabetes mellitus
- Behavioral or emotional problems
- Family problems or a vulnerable child or young person or family

Recent Change or Stressor; School, Peers, New Family Member, Relocation, Family Problems (Financial, Illness, Separation, Divorce)

- Consider maltreatment (for the purposes of the child mistreatment guideline, to consider maltreatment means that maltreatment is one possible explanation for the alerting feature or is included in the differential diagnosis) if:
  - A child or young person is reported to be deliberately bedwetting.
  - Parents or caregivers are seen or reported to punish a child or young person for bedwetting despite professional advice that the symptom is involuntary.

Ascertain That Physiologic Causes of Enuresis Have Been Ruled Out

- Examples include infections, meatal stenosis, fistulas, pinworms, epispadias, ectopic ureter, and minor neurologic dysfunction (hyperactivity, cognitive delay).

Determine Contributing Factors

- Refer to Related Factors.

Promote a Positive Parent–Child Relation

- Inform children and young people with bedwetting that it is not their fault. Do not exclude younger children (for example, those under 7 years) from the management of bedwetting on the basis of age alone (National Clinical Guideline Centre, 2010).
- Inform their parents or caregivers that bedwetting is not the child or young person's fault and that punitive measures should not be used in the management of bedwetting (National Clinical Guideline Centre, 2010; Tu, Baskin, & Amhym, 2014).
- Explore with family members if there is a history of bedwetting in the family (e.g., parents, aunts, uncles).

- Explain to the parents and the child the physiologic development of bladder control.
- Explain to parents that disapproval (shaming, punishing) is useless in stopping enuresis but can make child shy, ashamed, and afraid.
- Address excessive or insufficient fluid intake or abnormal toileting patterns before starting other treatment for bedwetting in children and young people.
- Advise parents or caregivers to try a reward system alone (as described above) for the initial treatment of bedwetting in young children who have some dry nights. For example, rewards may be given for (National Clinical Guideline Centre, 2010)
  - Drinking recommended levels of fluid during the day
  - Using the toilet to pass urine before sleep
  - Engaging in management (e.g., taking medication or helping to change sheets)

Reduce Contributing Factors, If Possible

Small Bladder Capacity
- After child drinks fluids, encourage him or her to postpone voiding to help stretch the bladder.

Sound Sleeper
- Have child void before retiring.
- Restrict fluids at bedtime.
- If child is awakened later (about 11 PM) to void, attempt to awaken child fully for positive reinforcement.

Too Busy to Sense a Full Bladder (If Daytime Wetting Occurs)
- Teach child awareness of sensations that occur when it is time to void.
- Teach child the ability to control urination (have him or her start and stop the stream; have him or her "hold" the urine during the day, even if for only a short time).
- Bladder retraining can help control dysfunctional voiding.
- Have child keep a record of how he or she is doing; emphasize dry days or nights (e.g., stars on a calendar).
- If child wets, have him or her explain or write down (if feasible) why he or she thinks it happened.
- With school age children, assess if the child is using the bathroom at school. Do they get sufficient bathroom breaks? Can a reminder device be used (vibrating watch, cell phone)? Ensure teacher understands why the child is requesting access to bathroom, the need for bathroom.

If Indicated Discuss a Bed Alarm System and Refer Them to Their Primary Care Provider (National Clinical Guideline Centre, 2010)

- Encourage children and young people with bedwetting and their parents or caregivers to discuss and agree on their roles and responsibilities for using the alarm and the use of rewards.
- Offer an alarm as the first-line treatment to children and young people whose bedwetting has not responded to advice on fluids, toileting, or an appropriate reward system.
- An alarm is considered inappropriate, particularly if (National Clinical Guideline Centre, 2010):
  - Bedwetting is very infrequent (that is, less than 1 to 2 wet beds per week).
  - The parents or caregivers are having emotional difficulty coping with the burden of bedwetting.
  - The parents or caregivers are expressing anger, negativity, or blame toward the child or young person.
- Continue alarm treatment in children and young people with bedwetting who are showing signs of response until a minimum of 2 weeks' uninterrupted dry nights has been achieved. Stop treatment only if there are no early signs of response.

Initiate Health Teaching and Referrals, as Indicated

- Teach family techniques to control the adverse effects of enuresis (e.g., plastic mattress covers, use of sleeping bag [machine washable] when staying overnight away from home).
- Advise to avoid all caffeine-containing drinks all together. Avoid fluids 2 hours before going to bed.

Functional Urinary Incontinence

NANDA-I Definition

Inability of a usually continent person to reach the toilet in time to avoid unintentional loss of urine

Defining Characteristics

Major (Must Be Present)

Incontinence before or during an attempt to reach the toilet

Related Factors

Pathophysiologic

Related to diminished bladder cues and impaired ability to recognize bladder cues secondary to:

Brain injury/tumor/infection	Demyelinating diseases
Alcoholic neuropathy	Progressive dementia
Cerebrovascular accident	Multiple sclerosis
Parkinsonism	

Treatment Related

Related to decreased bladder tone secondary to:

Antihistamines	Tranquilizers
Immunosuppressant therapy	Sedatives
Epinephrine	Muscle relaxants
Diuretics	Narcotics
Anticholinergics	

Situational (Personal, Environmental)

Related to impaired mobility

Related to decreased attention to bladder cues

Depression	Confusion
Intentional suppression (self-induced deconditioning)	

Related to environmental barriers to using bathroom

Distant toilets/seat height	Side rails
Bed too high	Unfamiliar surroundings
Poor lighting	Clothing

Maturational

Older Adult
Related to motor and sensory losses

 NOC

Tissue Integrity, Urinary Continence, Urinary Elimination

Goals

The individual will report no or decreased episodes of incontinence, as evidenced by the following indicators:

- Remove or minimize environmental barriers at home

- Use proper adaptive equipment to assist with voiding, transfers, and dressing
- Describe causative factors for incontinence

NIC

Perineal Care, Urinary Incontinence Care, Prompted Voiding, Urinary Habit Training, Urinary Elimination Management, Teaching: Procedure/Treatment

Interventions

Explain Age-Related Effects on Bladder Function and That Urgency and Nocturia Do Not Necessarily Lead to Incontinence

Assess Causative or Contributing Factors

Obstacles to Toilet
- Poor lighting, slippery floor, misplaced furniture and rugs, inadequate footwear, toilet too far, bed too high, side rails up
- Inadequate toilet (too small for walkers, wheelchair, seat too low/high, no grab bars)
- Inadequate signal system for requesting help
- Lack of privacy

Sensory/Cognitive Deficits
- Visual deficits (blindness, field cuts, poor depth perception)
- Cognitive deficits as a result of aging, trauma, stroke, tumor, infection

Motor/Mobility Deficits
- Limited upper and/or lower extremity movement/strength (inability to remove clothing)
- Barriers to ambulation (e.g., vertigo, fatigue, altered gait, hypertension)

Urgency

Factors that increase urgency
- Caffeine, carbonated beverages, overhydration, artificial sweeteners, tobacco use

Reduce or Eliminate Contributing Factors, If Possible

Environmental Barriers
- Assess path to bathroom for obstacles, lighting, and distance.
- Assess adequacy of toilet height and need for grab bars.
- Assess adequacy of room size.

- Assess if individual can remove clothing easily.
- Provide a commode between bathroom and bed, if necessary.

Sensory/Cognitive Deficits
- For an individual with diminished vision:
  - Ensure adequate lighting.
  - Encourage individual to wear prescribed corrective lens.
  - Provide clear, safe pathway to bathroom.
  - Keep call bell easily accessible.
  - If bedpan or urinal is used, make sure it is within easy reach in the same location at all times.
  - Assess individual for safety in bathroom.
- For an individual with cognitive deficits:
  - Offer toileting reminders every 2 hours, after meals, and before bedtime.
  - Establish appropriate means to communicate need to void.
  - Provide a normal environment for elimination (use bathroom, if possible).
  - Allow for privacy while maintaining safety.
  - Allow sufficient time for task.
  - Give consistent, simple step-by-step instructions; use verbal and nonverbal cues.
  - Assess need for adaptive devices on clothing to make dressing and undressing easier.
  - Assess individual's ability to provide self-hygiene.

Provide for Factors That Promote Continence

Maintain Optimal Hydration
- Increase fluid intake to 2,000 to 3,000 mL/day, unless contraindicated.
- Teach older adults not to depend on thirst sensations but to drink liquids even when not thirsty.
- Space fluids every 2 hours.
- Decrease fluid intake after 7 PM; provide only minimal fluids during the night.
- Avoid large amounts of tomato and orange juice.
- Avoid bladder irritants, such as alcohol, caffeine, and aspartame (Smeltzer, Bare, Hinkle, & Cheever, 2010).
- Encourage intake of cranberry juice.

Promote Personal Integrity and Provide Motivation to Increase Bladder Control

- Encourage to share feelings about incontinence and determine its effect on his or her social patterns.
- Convey that incontinence can be cured or at least controlled to maintain dignity.

- Work to achieve daytime continence before expecting night-time continence.
  - Discourage the use of bedpans.
  - Encourage and assist individual to groom self.
  - If hospitalized, provide opportunities to eat meals outside bedroom (day room, lounge).

Promote Skin Integrity

- Refer to *Risk for Pressure Ulcers* for specific interventions.

Explain Foods/Fluids That Increase Bladder Irritation and/or Volume, Increasing Urgency as (Davis et al., 2013; Derrer, 2014; Gleason et al., 2013; Lukacz, et al., 2015)

- Caffeinated beverages/foods (e.g., coffee, tea, chocolate), alcohol, red wine, highly acidic foods, and foods high in potassium
  - Excessive fluid intake > overfills bladder
  - Insufficient fluid intake > irritates the bladder
  - Spicy foods > irritates the bladder
  - Artificial sweeteners > irritates the bladder
- Encourage intake of 16 oz of unsweetened/or reduced sugar blueberry or cranberry juice.
- Carbonated beverages should be eliminated or decreased because they may increase bladder activity and urgency (Wilson et al., 2005).
- Teach individual/family to recognize abnormal changes in urine properties.
  - Increased mucus and sediment
  - Blood in urine (hematuria)
  - Change in color (from normal straw colored to cloudy) or foul odor
- Advise family/caregivers to monitor for cognitive changes (new onset or worsening)
- Teach individual/family to monitor for signs and symptoms of infection:
  - Elevated temperature, chills, and shaking
  - A change in baseline cognitive status
    ○ Suprapubic pain
    ○ Painful urination
    ○ Urgency
    ○ Frequent small voids or frequent small incontinences
    ○ Lower back, flank pain, or both

Initiate Health Teaching Referral, When Indicated

- Refer to home health nurse (occupational therapy department) for a home assessment.

Reflex Urinary Incontinence

NANDA-I Definition

Involuntary loss of urine at somewhat predictable intervals when a specific bladder volume is reached

Defining Characteristics

Major (Must Be Present)*

Inability to voluntarily inhibit voiding or imitate voiding
Incomplete emptying with lesion above pontine micturition center
Incomplete emptying with lesion above sacral micturition
Predictable pattern of voiding
Sensation of urgency without voluntary inhibition of bladder contraction
Sensations associated with full bladder (e.g., sweating, restlessness, abdominal discomfort)
No sensation of bladder fullness, urge to void or voiding

Related Factors

Pathophysiologic

Related to impaired conduction of impulses above the reflex arc level secondary to:
Cord injury/tumor/infection

Related to postoperative dribbling and incontinence secondary to:
Transurethral resection of the prostate
Prostate surgery

 NOC
See *Functional Urinary Incontinence.*

Goals

The individual will report a state of dryness that meets personal satisfaction, as evidenced by the following indicators:

• Have a residual urine volume of less than 50 mL
• Use triggering mechanisms to initiate reflex voiding

See also *Functional Urinary Incontinence*, Pelvic Muscle Exercises, Weight Management

Interventions

Assess for Causative and Contributing Conditions

- Refer to Related Factors.
- Explain rationale for treatment(s).

Develop a Bladder-Retraining or Reconditioning Program

- See Interventions under *Continuous Incontinence*.

Teach Techniques to Stimulate Reflex Voiding

- Cutaneous triggering mechanisms
- Repeated deep, sharp suprapubic tapping (most effective)
- Instruct individual to:
  - Place self in a half-sitting position
  - Tap directly at bladder wall at a rate of seven or eight times for 5 seconds (35 to 40 single blows)
  - Use only one hand
  - Shift site of stimulation over bladder to find most successful site
  - Continue stimulation until a good stream starts
  - Wait approximately 1 minute; repeat stimulation until bladder is empty
  - One or two series of stimulations without response signifies that nothing more will be expelled
- If the preceding measures are ineffective, instruct individual to perform each of the following for 2 to 3 minutes, waiting 1 minute between attempts:
  - Stroking glans penis
  - Lightly punching abdomen above inguinal ligaments
  - Stroking inner thigh
- Encourage individual to void or trigger at least every 3 hours.
- Indicate on intake and output sheet which mechanism was used to induce voiding.
- People with abdominal muscle control should use the Valsalva maneuver during triggered voiding.
- Teach individual that if he or she increases fluid intake, he or she also needs to increase the frequency of triggering to prevent overdistention.
- Schedule intermittent catheterization program (see *Continuous Incontinence*).

Initiate Health Teaching, as Indicated

Arrange an At-Home Assessment by a Home Health Nurse
- Teach bladder reconditioning program (see *Continuous Incontinence*).
- Teach intermittent catheterization (see *Continuous Incontinence*).
- Teach prevention of urinary tract infections (see *Continuous Incontinence*).
- If individual is at high risk for dysreflexia, refer to *Dysreflexia*.

Stress Urinary Incontinence

NANDA-I Definition

Sudden leakage of urine with activities that increase intra-abdominal pressure

Defining Characteristics*

Observed or reported involuntary leakage of small amounts of urine:
In the absence of detrusor contraction
In the absence of an overactive bladder
On exertion
With coughing, laughing, sneezing, or all of these

Related Factors

Pathophysiologic

Related to incompetent bladder outlet secondary to:
Congenital urinary tract anomalies

Related to degenerative changes in pelvic muscles and structural supports secondary to:*
Estrogen deficiency

*Related to intrinsic urethral sphincter**

Situational (Personal, Environmental)

Related to high intra-abdominal pressure* and weak pelvic muscles* secondary to:

Obesity	Poor personal hygiene
Sex	Smoking
Pregnancy	

Related to weak pelvic muscles and structural supports secondary to:
Recent substantial weight loss
Childbirth

Maturational

Older Adult
Related to loss of muscle tone

NOC

Refer to *Functional Urinary Incontinence.*

Goals

The individual will report a reduction or elimination of stress incontinence, as evidenced by the following indicators:

• Be able to explain the cause of incontinence and rationale for treatments

NIC

See also *Functional Incontinence,* Pelvic Muscle Exercise, Weight Management

Interventions

Routinely Assess Women of All Ages for Their Knowledge of Pelvic Floor Health and Stress Incontinence

• "Specifically ask if they experience leaking of urine during their sports, 13% beginning in junior high" (*Nygaard et al., 1994). "Gymnastic athletes had the highest incidence of urinary leakage at 67%, with basketball close behind at 66%, and tennis at 50%" (*Nygaard et al., 1994, *Smith 2004).

Determine Contributing Factors That Can Be Reduced as (*Smith, 2004)

• Obesity refers also to the nursing diagnosis *Obesity* or *Overweight.*

- Lack of knowledge of pelvic muscle structures and effects of weakness caused by, for example, obesity, vaginal childbirth, sports, loss of estrogen (perimenopause, menopause)
- With aging, a stretching or sagging of the pelvic floor may result in hernia-like positions of the bladder, the uterus, or the rectum.
- Chronic constipation—frequent straining and bearing down to have a bowel movement stretches the pelvic muscles
- Hysterectomy—the removal of the uterus removes one of the support structures for the other pelvic organ
- Situational—prolonged standing, lifting, or carrying weight for a job or exercise
- Smoking and chronic coughing add extra stress to the pelvic floor muscles and ligaments.

Teach Pelvic Muscle Exercises

- Explain it will take 4 to 6 months before results can be noted (*Smith 2004; Mayo Clinic, 2012).
- Consult an incontinence specialist for use of vaginal weights for pelvic floor strengthening if indicated.

Provide Instructions for Pelvic Muscle Exercises (Kegel Exercises)

Explain
- Learn which muscles to tighten to stop urination; this includes tightening the rectal muscles
- Empty your bladder before doing Kegel exercises
- Hold the contractions for 5 to 10 seconds and release. Relax between contractions taking care to keep contraction and relaxation times equal. Gradually increase the time of contracting from 2 seconds to 10 seconds. If you contract for 10 seconds, relax for 10 seconds before next contraction.
- Perform 40 to 60 contractions divided in 2 to 4 sessions each time. These should be spread out through the day and incorporate different positions (sitting, standing, and lying).
- For best results, focus on tightening only your pelvic floor muscles. Be careful not to flex the muscles in your abdomen, thighs, or buttocks. Avoid holding your breath. Instead, breathe freely during the exercises (Mayo Clinic, 2012).
- Advise a good way to help to remember to do exercises is to incorporate them into daily routine, such as stopping at a traffic light or washing dishes (Wilkinson & Van Leuven, 2007)
- Refer individuals to the Mayo Clinic website for the article, "How to do Kegel Exercises"

Maternal Interventions

- For increased abdominal pressure during pregnancy:
  - Teach to avoid prolonged standing.

- Teach to the benefit of frequent voiding (at least every 2 hours).
- Teach pelvic muscle exercises after delivery.

Continuous Urinary Incontinence[54]

Definition

State in which an individual experiences continuous, unpredictable loss of urine*, without distention or awareness of bladder fullness

Defining Characteristics

Constant flow of urine at unpredictable times without uninhibited bladder contractions/spasm or distention
Lack of bladder filling or perineal filling
Nocturia
Unawareness of incontinence
Incontinence refractory to other treatments

Related Factors

Refer to *Impaired Urinary Elimination*.

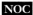

Refer to Functional Urinary Incontinence.

Goals

The individual will be continent (specify during day, night, 24 hours), as evidenced by the following indicators:

- Identify the cause of incontinence and rationale for treatments
- Identify daily goal for fluid intake

NIC

See also *Functional Incontinence*, Environmental Management, Urinary Catheterization, Teaching: Procedure/Treatment, Tube Care: Urinary, Urinary Bladder Training

---

[54]This diagnosis is not presently on the NANDA-I list but has been included for clarity and usefulness.

Interventions

Develop a Bladder-Retraining or Reconditioning Program, Which Should Include Communication, Assessment of Voiding Pattern, Scheduled Fluid Intake, and Scheduled Voiding Times

Promote Communication Among All Staff Members and Among Individual, Family, and Staff

- Provide all staff with sufficient knowledge concerning the program planned.
- Assess staff's response to program.

Assess the Individual's Potential for Participation in a Bladder-Retraining Program

- Cognition
- Desire to change behavior
- Ability to cooperate
- Willingness to participate

Provide Rationale for Plan and Acquire Individual's Informed Consent

Encourage Individual to Continue Program by Providing Accurate Information Concerning Reasons for Success or Failure

Assess Voiding Pattern

- Monitor and record:
  - Intake and output
  - Time and amount of fluid intake
  - Type of fluid
  - Amount of incontinence; measure if possible or estimate amount as small, moderate, or large
  - Amount of void, whether it was voluntary or involuntary
  - Presence of sensation of need to void
  - Amount of retention (amount of urine left in the bladder after an unsuccessful attempt at manual triggering or voiding)
  - Amount of residual (amount of urine left in the bladder after either a voluntary or manual triggered voiding; also called a *postvoid residual*)
  - Amount of triggered urine (urine expelled after manual triggering [e.g., tapping, Credé's method])
- Identify certain activities that precede voiding (e.g., restlessness, yelling, exercise).
- Record in appropriate column.

Schedule Fluid Intake and Voiding Times

- Provide fluid intake of 2,000 mL each day unless contraindicated.

- Discourage fluids after 7 PM.
- Initially, bladder emptying is done at least every 2 hours and at least twice during the night; goal is 2- to 4-hour intervals.
- If the individual is incontinent before scheduled voids, shorten the time between voids.
- If the individual has a postvoid residual greater than 100 to 150 mL, schedule intermittent catheterization.

Initiate Health Teaching

- Instruct in prevention of urinary tract infection.
- For people living in the community, initiate a referral to the home health nurse for follow-up.

Urge Urinary Incontinence

NANDA-I Definition

Involuntary passage of urine occurring soon after a strong sense of urgency to void

Defining Characteristics*

Observed or reported inability to reach toilet in time to avoid urine loss
Reports urinary urgency
Reports involuntary loss of urine with bladder contractions or bladder spasms

Related Factors

Pathophysiologic

Related to decreased bladder capacity secondary to:

Infection
Cerebrovascular accident
Trauma
Demyelinating diseases
Urethritis

Diabetic neuropathy
Neurogenic disorders or injury/tumor/infection injury
Alcoholic neuropathy
Brain Parkinsonism

Treatment Related

Related to decreased bladder capacity secondary to:
Abdominal surgery
After use of indwelling catheters

Situational (Personal, Environmental)

Related to irritation of bladder stretch receptors secondary to:
Alcohol   Excess fluid intake
Caffeine

Related to decreased bladder capacity* secondary to:
Frequent voiding

Maturational

Child
Related to small bladder capacity

Older Adult
Related to decreased bladder capacity

 NOC
Refer to *Functional Urinary Incontinence.*

Goals

The individual will report no or decreased episodes of incontinence (specify), as evidenced by the following indicators:

* Explain causes of incontinence
* Describe bladder irritants

 NIC
Refer to *Functional Urinary Incontinence.*

Interventions

Assess for Causative or Contributing Factors

* Refer to Related Factors.
* Weight loss: recommended as noninvasive therapy. Outcomes were better when looking at stress versus urge incontinence, and obese versus overweight, but still effective. Formerly, obese patients were shown to have improved outcomes after weight

loss (Grade A, Evidence Fair) (DuBeau, 2015; Holroyd-Leduc & Straus, 2004; *Morant, 2005.

- Dietary changes: recommended as noninvasive therapy. The elimination of bladder irritants from the diet has not been rigorously evaluated (Grade A, Evidence Fair) (DuBeau, 2014, 2015; *Morant, 2005).

Assess Pattern of Voiding/Incontinence and Fluid Intake

- Maintain optimal hydration (see *Continuous Incontinence*).
- Assess voiding pattern (see *Continuous Incontinence*).

Reduce or Eliminate Causative and Contributing Factors, When Possible

Bladder Irritants
- Explain foods/fluids that increase bladder irritation and/or volume increasing urgency as (Davis et al., 2013; Derrer, 2014; Gleason et al., 2013; Lukacz, 2015):
  - Caffeinated beverages/foods (e.g., coffee, tea, chocolate), alcohol, red wine, highly acidic foods, and foods high in potassium
    ○ Excessive fluid intake > overfills bladder
    ○ Insufficient fluid intake > irritates the bladder
    ○ Spicy foods > irritates the bladder
    ○ Artificial sweeteners > irritates the bladder
- Encourage intake of 16 oz of unsweetened/or reduced sugar blueberry or cranberry juice.
- Carbonated beverages should be eliminated or decreased because they may increase bladder activity and urgency (Wilson et al., 2005).
- Smoking cessation is recommended. Explain tobacco is a bladder irritant.
- Understand and explain the risk of insufficient fluid intake and its relation to infection and concentrated urine.

Diminished Bladder Capacity
- Determine time between urge to void and need to void (record how long individual can delay urination).
- For an individual with difficulty prolonging waiting time, communicate to personnel the need to respond rapidly to his or her request for assistance for toileting (note on care plan).
- Teach individual to increase waiting time by increasing bladder capacity.
  - Determine volume of each void.
  - Ask to "hold off" urinating as long as possible.
  - Develop bladder reconditioning program (see *Continuous Incontinence*).

Overdistended Bladder
- Explain that diuretics are given to help reduce the water in the body; they work by acting on the kidneys to increase the flow of urine.
- Explain that in diabetes mellitus, insulin deficiency causes high levels of blood sugar. The high level of blood glucose pulls fluid from body tissues, causing osmotic diuresis and increased urination (polyuria).
- Explain that because of the increased urine flow, regular voiding is needed to prevent overdistention of the bladder.
- Assess voiding pattern (see *Continuous Incontinence*).
- Check postvoid residual; if greater than 100 mL, include intermittent catheterization in bladder reconditioning program.
- Initiate bladder reconditioning program (see *Continuous Incontinence*).

Uninhibited Bladder Contractions
- Assess voiding pattern (see *Continuous Incontinence*).
- Establish method to communicate urge to void (document on care plan).
- Communicate to personnel the need to respond rapidly to a request to void.
- Establish a planned-voiding pattern.
  - Provide an opportunity to void on awakening; after meals, physical exercise, bathing, and drinking coffee or tea; and before going to sleep.
  - Begin by offering use of bedpan, commode, or toilet every half hour initially, and gradually lengthen the time to at least every 2 hours.
  - If individual has incontinent episode, reduce the time between scheduled voidings.
  - Document behavior/activity that occurs with void or incontinence (see *Continuous Incontinence*).
- Encourage individual to try to "hold" urine until time to void, if possible.
- Consult primary care professional for pharmacologic interventions.
- Refer to *Continuous Incontinence* for additional information on developing a bladder reconditioning program.

Initiate Health Teaching

- Instruct individual about prevention of urinary tract infections (refer to *Functional Incontinence*).

Risk for Urge Urinary Incontinence

NANDA-I Definition

Vulnerable for involuntary passage of urine occurring soon after a strong sense of urgency to void, which may compromise health

Risk Factors

Refer to Related Factors in *Urge Urinary Incontinence*.

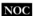

Refer to *Functional Urinary Incontinence*.

Goals

The individual will report continued continence comfort, as evidenced by the following indicators:

- Explain causes of incontinence
- Explain strategies to maintain continence

NOC

Refer to *Functional Urinary Incontinence*.

Interventions

Refer to *Urge Urinary Incontinence*.

Overflow Urinary Incontinence[55]

NANDA-I Definition

Involuntary loss of urine associated with overdistention of the bladder

---

[55]Previously called *Urinary Retention*.

Defining Characteristics*

Bladder distention
High residual volume observed after void
Observed or reported involuntary leakage of small volumes of
   urine
Nocturia

Related Factors

Pathophysiologic

Related to sphincter blockage secondary to:

Strictures	Prostatic enlargement
Ureterocele	Perineal swelling
Bladder neck contractures	Severe pelvic prolapse

Related to impaired afferent pathways or inadequacy secondary to:

Cord injury/tumor/infection	Multiple sclerosis
Brain injury/tumor/infection	Diabetic neuropathy
Cerebrovascular accident	Alcoholic neuropathy
Demyelinating diseases	Tabes dorsalis

Treatment Related

Related to bladder outlet obstruction or impaired afferent pathways
secondary to drug therapy (iatrogenic)*

Antihistamines	Decongestants*
Theophylline	Anticholinergics*
Epinephrine	Calcium channel blockers*
Isoproterenol	

Situational (Personal, Environmental)

Related to bladder outlet obstruction secondary to:
Fecal impaction*

Related to detrusor hypocontractility secondary to:*
Deconditioned voiding
Association with stress or discomfort

Refer to *Functional Urinary Incontinence.*

Goals

The individual will achieve a state of dryness that meets personal satisfaction, as evidenced by the following indicators:

- Empty the bladder using Créde's or Valsalva maneuver with a residual urine of less than 50 mL if indicated
- Void voluntarily

NIC

See also *Functional Urinary Incontinence*, Overflow Retention Care, Urinary Bladder Training

Interventions

- Refer to Related Factors.

Causes of Overflow Incontinence

- Bladder outlet obstruction
- Detrusor inadequacy implies insufficient detrusor tone to overcome normal intraurethral resistance. One cause of detrusor inadequacy is deconditioned voiding reflexes characterized by anxiety or discomfort associated with voiding. Another cause is central nervous system diseases.
- Impaired afferent pathways occur when both the sensory and motor branches of the simple reflex arc are damaged. There are no sensations to tell the individual the bladder is full and no motor impulses for emptying the bladder. It develops into a neurogenic bladder (autonomous).

Develop a Bladder-Retraining or Reconditioning Program (See *Continuous Incontinence*)

- Consult with Institution's Expert Professional and/or Protocol.

Indicate on the Intake and Output Record Which Technique Was Used to Induce Voiding

Obtain Postvoid Residuals After Attempts at Emptying Bladder

- If residual urine volumes are greater than 100 mL, schedule intermittent catheterization program (see *Continuous Incontinence*).

Initiate Health Teaching

- Teach bladder reconditioning program (refer to *Continuous Incontinence*).
- Teach intermittent catheterization (refer to *Continuous Incontinence*).
- Instruct individual about prevention of urinary tract infections (refer to *Continuous Incontinence*).

RISK FOR VASCULAR TRAUMA

NANDA-I Definition

Vulnerable for damage to a vein and its surrounding tissues related to the presence of a catheter and/or infused solutions, which may compromise health

Risk Factors*

Treatment Related

Catheter type[56]
Catheter width[56]
Impaired ability to visualize the insertion site
Inadequate catheter fixation[56]

Infusion rate[56]
Insertions site[56]
Length of insertion time
Nature of solution (e.g., concentration, chemical irritant, temperature, pH)

 Author's Note

This NANDA-I diagnosis represents a risk for all individuals with intravenous catheters. Procedure manuals on the clinical unit should contain the correct placement, fixation, and monitoring of all intravenous sites. Nurses needing these guidelines should refer to the procedure manual. Practicing nurses do not need to have this diagnosis on the care plan.

---

[56]May indicate poor clinical practice.

Students should refer to their fundamentals of nursing text for specific techniques to start, secure, and monitor intravenous therapy. Consult with your faculty to determine if this should be written on your assigned individual's care plan.

Clinically, certain intravenous medications (e.g., chemotherapy, vesicant medications) are extremely toxic and therefore require specific interventions to prevent occurrence and tissue necrosis. Interventions and goals for preventing and responding to extravasation of the intravenous vesicant medications will be outlined for this diagnosis. These interventions are usually also found in a procedure manual.

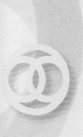

Section 2

Health-Promotion Nursing Diagnoses

This section organizes all the health-promotion nursing diagnoses for individuals/groups.

Health-promotion nursing diagnosis "is a clinical judgement concerning motivation and desire to increase well-being and to actualize human health potential" (Herdman & Kamitsuro, 2014). A valid health promotion nursing diagnosis has two requirements: (1) the individual has a desire for better health in a particular area and (2) the individual is currently functioning effectively in a particular area.

Health promotion nursing diagnoses are one-part statements with no related factors. The goals established by the individual or group will direct their actions to enhance their health.

There is still confusion about the clinical usefulness of this type of diagnoses. Some of the diagnoses included in this section represent unhealthy lifestyles. They have been included with a health-promotion focus, for example, *Stress Overload*, *Sedentary Lifestyle*, *Risk-Prone Health Behavior*. The author believes that some of these diagnoses can be strengthened and are clinically useful, such as *Readiness for Enhanced Parenting* or *Readiness for Enhanced Community Coping*; whereas others, such as *Readiness for Enhanced Power*, *Readiness for Enhanced Urinary Elimination*, and other similar diagnoses, are questionable relative to clinical usefulness. Under each diagnosis, Author's Notes will elaborate on the clinical usefulness of the diagnosis.

Clinically, data that represent strengths are important for nurses to know. The strengths of individuals/families/communities are critical to coping with challenges to their health and relationships. These strengths can assist the nurse in selecting interventions to reduce or prevent a problem in another health pattern. If nurses want to designate strength, it should be documented as strength on the assessment form or care plan. If the individual desires assistance in promoting a higher level of function, *Readiness for Enhanced (specify)* would be useful in certain settings, such as schools, community centers, and assisted living facilities. Interested clinicians who use these health-promotion/nursing diagnoses are invited to share their work with NANDA-I as well as the author (juall46@msn.com).

Health-Promotion Assessment
(Carpenito-Moyet, 2007; Edelman, Kudzma, & Mandle, 2014; *Gordon, 2002)

Subjective Data

Health Perception–Health Management Pattern
Ask the individual to place one check next to the category in which they usually practice; place two checks for those they practice daily (*Breslow & Hron, 2004):

- Three meals a day at regular times and no snacking
- Breakfast every day
- Moderate exercise two or three times a week
- 7 to 8 hours of sleep, not more or less
- No smoking
- Moderate weight
- No alcohol or in moderation

What Is the Individual's/Family's Perception of Their Overall Health?
- What personal practices maintain their health?
- What sources does the individual or family access to maintain or improve their healthy lifestyle?
- How could the individual be healthier?

Nutrition–Metabolic Pattern
- What is the individual's body mass index?
- Typical daily fluid intake
- Supplements (vitamins, types of snacks)
- Daily intake of whole grain or enriched breads, cereals, rice, or pasta
- Three servings of fruit/fruit juice daily
- Unlimited raw or 5 to 8 servings of cooked nonstarch vegetables daily
- Skim or low-fat dairy products
- Meats and poultry trimmed of fat and skin
- No fried foods/snacks
- No or limited (fewer than two) sugar drinks (e.g., soda, ice tea, juices)
- Do you see a relationship among stress and tension, emotional upsets, and your eating habits?

Elimination Pattern
- Bowel elimination pattern? (Describe.)
  - Frequency (every 2 to 3 days), character (soft, bulky)
- Urinary elimination pattern? (Describe.)
  - Character (amber, yellow, straw-colored)

Activity–Exercise Pattern
- Exercise pattern? (Type, frequency)
- Leisure activities? (Frequency)
- Energy level? (High, moderate, adequate, low)
- Are there barriers to exercising?
- What are five things that you do to play?
- What things do you do that make you feel good?

Sleep–Rest Pattern
* Satisfied and rested?
* Average hours of sleep per night
* Relaxation periods? (How often, how long?)

Cognitive–Perceptual Pattern
* Satisfied with:
  * Decision making?
  * Memory?
  * Ability to learn?
* Describe briefly your educational background.

Self-Perception–Self-Concept Pattern
* Describe how you feel about:
  * Yourself
  * Your body? Changes?
* Do you have trouble expressing anger, sadness, happiness, love, and/or sexuality?
* What are your major strengths or personal qualities?
* What are your weaknesses or negative aspects?
* In your life right now, what is your most meaningful activity?
* How many more years do you expect to live, and how do you think you will die?
* How do you imagine your future?
* What would you like to accomplish in your future? Are there changes you need to make to accomplish this?

List the Most Important Events, Crises, Transitions, and/or Changes (Positive or Negative) in Your Life
* Take time to reflect on how they affected you. Place an asterisk in front of one or two that were especially important.

Roles–Relationships Pattern
* Satisfied with job? Need a change?
* Satisfied with role responsibilities?
* Describe your relationship with your family/partner.
* Describe your friendships (close, casual).
* List the most important people in your life right now and why they are important.

Sexuality–Reproductive Pattern
* Is sex an important aspect of your life?
* Are you currently in a sexual relationship?
* What would you want to change about your current sexual relationship?

Coping–Stress Tolerance Pattern
* List the most regular sources of stress in your life. How could you make them less stressful?

- How do you usually respond to stressful situations (get angry, withdraw, take it out on others, get sick, drink, eat)?
- What situations make you feel calm or relaxed?
- What situations make you feel anxious or upset? What can you do to make yourself feel better?

Values–Beliefs Pattern
- Write 10 things you most value in life.
- Would you describe yourself as a religious or spiritual person?
- How do your beliefs help you?

READINESS FOR ENHANCED BREASTFEEDING

NANDA-I Definition

A pattern of providing milk to an infant or young child directly from the breasts which may be strengthened

Defining Characteristics

Mother expresses desire to enhance ability to provide breast milk for child's nutritional needs.
Mother expresses desire to enhance ability to exclusively breast-feed.

NOC
Knowledge: Breastfeeding

Goal

The mother will report an increase in confidence and satisfaction with breastfeeding, as evidenced by the following indicator:

- Identify two new strategies (specify) to enhance breastfeeding

NIC
Breastfeeding Assistance, Lactation Counseling

Interventions

- Refer to the Internet sites for resources and information on breastfeeding.
- Refer to *Ineffective Breastfeeding* for interventions to enhance breastfeeding.

READINESS FOR ENHANCED CHILDBEARING PROCESS

NANDA-I Definition

A pattern of preparing for and maintaining a healthy pregnancy, childbirth process, and care of the newborn that is sufficient for ensuring well-being and which can be strengthened

Defining Characteristics*

During Pregnancy
Expresses desire to enhance knowledge of childbearing process
Expresses a desire to enhance management of unpleasant symptoms in pregnancy
Expresses desire to enhance lifestyle (e.g., nutrition, elimination, sleep, body movement, exercise, personal hygiene)
Expresses desire to enhance preparation for newborn

During Labor and Delivery
Expresses desire to enhance lifestyle (e.g., diet, elimination, sleep, body movement, personal hygiene) that is appropriate for the stage of labor
Expresses desire to enhance proactivity during labor and delivery

After Birth
Expresses desire to enhance attachment behaviors
Expresses desire to enhance baby care techniques
Expresses desire to enhance baby feeding techniques
Expresses desire to enhance breast care
Expresses desire to enhance environmental safety for the baby
Expresses desire to enhance postpartum lifestyle (e.g., diet, elimination, sleep, body movement, exercise, personal hygiene)
Expresses desire to enhance use of support system

Author's Note

This NANDA-I nursing diagnosis represents the comprehensive care that is needed to promote the following: healthy pregnancy, childbirth and the postpartum process, enhanced relationships (mother, father, infant, and siblings), and optimal care of the newborn. This care is beyond the scope possible in this text. Refer to a text about maternal–child health for the specific interventions for this diagnosis.

READINESS FOR ENHANCED COMFORT

NANDA-I Definition

A pattern of ease, relief, and transcendence in physical, psycho-spiritual, environmental, and/or social dimensions that is sufficient for well-being, which can be strengthened

Defining Characteristics*

Expresses desire to enhance comfort
Expresses desire to enhance feeling of contentment
Expresses desire to enhance relaxation
Expresses desire to enhance resolution of complaints

 Author's Note

This diagnosis is too general and therefore does not direct specific interventions. It encompasses physical, psychological, spiritual, environmental, and social dimensions. It would be more clinically useful to focus on a particular dimension, such as *Readiness for Enhanced Spiritual Well-Being*.

READINESS FOR ENHANCED COMMUNICATION

NANDA-I Definition

A pattern of exchanging information and ideas with others which can be strengthened

Defining Characteristics*

Able to speak and/or write a language
Expresses feelings
Expresses satisfaction with ability to share ideas with others
Expresses satisfaction with ability to share information with
    others
Expresses willingness to enhance communication
Forms phrases
Forms sentences
Forms words
Interprets nonverbal cures appropriately
Uses nonverbal cues appropriately

 Author's Note

This diagnosis represents an individual with good communications skills.
Interventions to enhance communication skills can be found in Section 1 in
Impaired Communication and *Impaired Verbal Communication*.

READINESS FOR ENHANCED COPING

NANDA-I Definition

A pattern of cognitive and behavioral efforts to manage demands
related to well-being which can be strengthened

Defining Characteristics*

Acknowledges power
Awareness of possible environmental changes
Expresses a desire to enhance knowledge of stress
Expresses a desire to enhance management of stressors
Expresses a desire to enhance social support
Expresses a desire to enhance use of emotion-oriented strategies
Expresses a desire to enhance use of problem-oriented strategies
Expresses a desire to enhance use of spiritual resources

NOC
Family Coping, Family Environment: Internal, Family Normalization, Parenting

Goal

The individual will report increased satisfaction with coping with stressors, as evidenced by the following indicator:

- Identify two new strategies (specify) to enhance coping with stressors

NIC
Family Involvement Promotion, Coping Enhancement, Family Integrity Promotion, Family Therapy, Counseling, Referral

Interventions

If Anxiety Diminishes One's Effective Coping, Teach

- Abdominal relaxation breathing
- Abdominal breathing while imagining a peaceful scene (e.g., ocean, woods, mountains)
- To imagine the feel of the warm sand on your feet, sun on your face, the sound of water.

R: *Relaxation techniques provide an opportunity to regroup prior to reacting.*

Explain Reframing (Halter, 2014; Varcarolis, 2011)

- Reassess the situation; ask yourself:
  - What positive thing can come out of the situation?
  - What did I learn?
  - What would I do differently next time?
  - What might be going on with my (boss, partner, sister friend) that would cause him or her to say or do that?
  - Is she or he stressed out or having problems?

R: *Reframing provides one with the opportunity to analyze and consider reasons for behavior and alternative options.*

Acknowledge Stress-Reducing Tips for Living
(Halter, 2014; Varcarolis, 2011)

- Exercise regularly, at least three times weekly
- Reduce caffeine intake
- Engage in meaningful, satisfying work
- Do not let work dominate your life

- Guard your personal freedom
- Choose your friends; associate with gentle people
- Live with and love whom you choose
- Structure your time as you see fit
- Set your own life goals

R: *The stressors of life are heightened when others decide how one should live his or her life.*

- Refer to the Internet sites for resources and information about stress reduction techniques.

READINESS FOR ENHANCED COMMUNITY COPING

Definition

A pattern of community activities for adaptation and problem solving for meeting the demands or needs of the community, which can be strengthened[1]

Defining Characteristics*

Expresses desire to enhance availability of community recreation programs

Expresses desire to enhance availability of community relaxation programs

Expresses desire to enhance communication among community members

Expresses desire to enhance communication between aggregates and larger community

Expresses desire to enhance community planning for predictable stressors

Expresses desire to enhance community resources for managing stressors

Expresses desire to enhance community responsibility for stress management

Expresses desire to enhance problem solving for identified issue

---

[1]This definition was originally published by L.J Carpenito and has been adapted by NANDA-I.

Author's Note

This diagnosis can be used to describe a community that wishes to improve an already effective pattern of coping. For a community to be assisted to a higher level of functioning, its basic needs for food, shelter, safety, a clean environment, and a supportive network must first be addressed. When these needs are met, programs can focus on higher functioning, such as wellness and self-actualization. Community programs can be designed after a community assessment and because of community requests. They can focus on enhancing health promotion with topics related to optimal nutrition, weight control, regular exercise programs, constructive stress management, social support, and role responsibilities, and preparing for and coping with life events such as retirement, parenting, and pregnancy.

NOC
Community Competence, Community Health Status, Community Risk Control

Goal

The community (specify type of community, e.g., the town of Mullica Hill, the southeast neighborhood of South Tucson) will provide programs to improve (specify type of focus, e.g., nutrition), as evidenced by the following indicators:

- Identify health-promotion needs as (specify: e.g., daily decrease in high-fat foods, increase in fruits and vegetables)
- Access resources needed (specify: e.g., local experts, nutritionist, college students)
- Develop programs (specify: health fair, school cafeteria, printed material) based on needs assessment
- Know the implementation of policies for health (e.g., American Diabetes Association policy for healthy meals)

NIC
Program Development, Risk Identification, Community Health Development, Environmental Risk Protection

Interventions

Conduct Focus Groups to Discuss Programs to Assist Residents With Positive Coping With Developmental Tasks

- Arrange focus groups according to age, including diverse groups.

R: *Focus groups assessments are advantageous because of their efficiency and low cost (Allender, Rector, & Warner, 2014).*

Plan Programs Targeted for a Specific Population

Adolescents (13 to 18 Years)
- Career planning
- Stress management

Young Adults (18 to 35 Years)
- Career selection
- Constructive relationships
- Balancing one's life
- Parenting issues

Middle Age (35 to 65 Years)
- Launching children
- Reciprocal relationships
- Aging parents
- Quality leisure time

Older Adults (65 Years and Older)
- Retirement issues
- Balancing one's life
- Anticipated losses
- Facts and myths of aging

All Ages

- Civic planning
- Meeting needs of all community members
- Crisis intervention
- Grieving
- Community involvement

R: *Life cycle events are predictable developmental tasks of young adults, middle adults, and older adults (refer to Key Concepts for specifics). Programs in the community can be planned to assist individuals with adapting successfully to life events (Clemen-Stone, Eigasti, & McGuire, 2001; Nies & McEwen, 2014).*

Discuss Programs That Promote High-Level Wellness

- Optimal nutrition
- Weight control
- Exercise programs
- Socialization programs
- Effective problem solving

- Injury prevention
- Environmental quality

Define the Target Health-Promotion Needs

- Analyze assessment of community.
- Prioritize the needs:
  - Organize the focus group responses.
  - Probability of success
  - Cost:benefit ratio (e.g., resources available)
  - Potential for policy development

Select a Health-Promotion Program

- Identify target population (e.g., entire community, older adults, adolescents).
- Delineate a timetable for the planning and implementation stages.

Meet With Community Groups (Health Centers, Faith-Based Groups, Government Agencies) to Review Findings of Focus Groups and to Discuss Collaborative Programming

R: *Community building can develop new and existing leadership and strengthen community organizations and interorganizational collaboration (Nies & McEwen, 2014).*

Plan the Program

- Develop detailed program objectives and the evaluation framework to be used.
  - Content
  - Time needed
  - Ideal teaching method for targeting group
  - Teaching aids (e.g., large-print materials)
- Establish resources needed and sources.
  - Space
  - Transportation facilities
  - Optimal day of week
  - Optimal time of year
  - Supplies, audiovisual equipment
  - Financial (budgeted, donations)
- Market the program.
  - Media (e.g., newspaper, TV, radio)
  - Posters (food market, train station)
  - Flyers (distribute via school to home)
  - Word of mouth (religious organizations, community clubs, schools)
  - Guest speaker (community clubs, schools)

R: *As an advocate and community liaison, the community health nurse collaborates with other disciplines and agencies to match resources with community-identified needs for program success (*Edelman & Mandle, 2010).*

Provide Program and Evaluate Whether Desired Results (Objectives) Were Achieved

- Number of participants
- Negative feedback
- Objectives achieved
- Actual expenditures versus budgeted
- Statistics (e.g., bicycle accidents)
- Participant evaluations
- Adequate planning
- Revisions for future planning
- Shared responsibility

R: *Evaluation will determine if the program was completely effective, partly effective, or ineffective in achieving the program objectives (*Edleman & Mandle, 2010).*

Determine the Strengths and Limitations of the Program and Plan a New Approach If Indicated

R: *Community health-promotion programs must demonstrate effectiveness to earn continued community and economic support (*Edelman & Mandle, 2010).*

READINESS FOR ENHANCED DECISION MAKING

NANDA-I Definition

A pattern of choosing a course of action that is sufficient for meeting short- and long-term health-related goals and can be strengthened

Defining Characteristics*

Expresses desire to enhance congruency of decisions with sociocultural goals

Expresses desire to enhance congruency of decisions with sociocultural values

Expresses desire to enhance congruency of decisions with goal

Expresses desire to enhance congruency of decisions with values

Expresses desire to enhance decision making

Expresses desire to enhance risk–benefit analysis of decisions

Expresses desire to enhance understanding of choices and the meaning of the choices

Expresses desire to enhance understanding of meaning of choices

Expresses desire to enhance use of reliable evidence for decisions

NOC
Decision-Making, Information Processing

Goal

The individual/group will report increased satisfaction with decision making, as evidenced by the following indicator:

- Identify two new strategies (specify) to enhance decision making

NIC
Decision-Making Support, Mutual Goal Setting

Interventions

- Refer to Interventions for *Decisional Conflict*.
- Refer to the Internet sites for resources and information about decision making.

READINESS FOR ENHANCED EMANCIPATED DECISION MAKING

Definition

A process of choosing a health-care decision that includes personal knowledge and/or consideration of social norms, which can be strengthened

Defining Characteristics

Expresses desire to enhance ability to choose health-care options that best fit current lifestyle

Expresses desire to enhance ability to enact chosen health-care option

Expresses desire to enhance ability to understand all available health-care options

Expresses desire to enhance ability to verbalize own opinion without constraint

Expresses desire to enhance comfort to verbalize health-care options in the presence of others

Expresses desire to enhance confidence in decision making

Expresses desire to enhance confidence to discuss health-care options openly

Expresses desire to enhance decision making

Expresses desire to enhance privacy to discuss health-care options

NOC

Decision-Making, Information Processing

Goal

The individual/group will report increased satisfaction with decision making, as evidenced by the following indicator:

• Identify two new strategies (specify) to enhance decision making

NIC

Decision-Making Support, Mutual Goal Setting

Interventions

Refer to Interventions for *Emancipated decision making*.

READINESS FOR ENHANCED FAMILY COPING

NANDA-I Definition

A pattern of management of adaptive tasks by primary person (family member, significant other, or close friend) involved with the client's health challenge that is sufficient for health and growth, in regard to self and in relation to the client, and can be strengthened

Defining Characteristics*

Expresses desire to acknowledge growth impact of crisis
Expresses desire to choose experiences that optimize wellness
Expresses desire to enhance connections with others who have
    experienced a similar situation
Expresses desire to enhance enrichment of lifestyle
Expresses desire to enhance health promotion

Related Factors

Refer to *Interrupted Family Processes*.

 Author's Note

This nursing diagnosis describes components found in *Interrupted Family Processes*. Until clinical research differentiates the category from the aforementioned categories, use *Interrupted Family Processes*, depending on the data presented.

READINESS FOR ENHANCED FAMILY PROCESSES

NANDA-I Definition

A pattern of family functioning that is sufficient to support the well-being of family members, which can be strengthened

Defining Characteristics*

Expresses desire to enhance balance between autonomy and
    cohesiveness
Expresses desire to enhance communication patterns
Expresses desire to enhance energy level of family to support
    activities of daily living

Expresses desire to enhance family adaptation to change
Expresses desire to enhance family dynamics
Expresses desire to enhance family resilience
Expresses desire to enhance growth of family members
Expresses desire to enhance interdependence with community
Expresses desire to enhance maintenance of boundaries
Expresses desire to enhance respect for family members
Expresses desire to enhance safety of family members

Family Environment: Internal

Goal

The family will expresses willingness to enhance family dynamics and growth.

Family Involvement Promotion, Family Integrity Promotion

Interventions

Discuss Elements That Influence Health Promotion in a Family
(Kaakinen et al., 2015)

R: *These elements interact with each other and need to be addressed for successful family health-promotion interventions. Suggestions for health promotion that conflict with the family's culture, religion, or spirituality will be rejected (Kaakinen, 2015).*

• Family culture
• Lifestyles patterns/role models
• Family nutrition
• Religion/spirituality
• Family processes
• Encourage the family to examine their patterns of communication (verbal, nonverbal) and family interactions (Kaakinen, 2010).
  • Are they effective?
  • Are all members involved in feeling sharing and decision making?
  • Is there positive, reinforcing interactions?
  • Are parent's role-modeling positive family processes?

R: *Effective, positive interactions enhance family lifestyle and adaption to transitions/stressors. They promote cohesiveness and healthier family lifestyles (Kaakinen, 2010).*

- Convey that the family has the capacity to achieve a higher level of health and has the right to health information to make informed decisions.
- Elicit from family areas for growth and change. Assure the commitment of all family members (e.g., improved nutrition, exercising, family meals, group relaxation activities, family time).

R: *This collaboration promotes family empowerment to make healthier choices.*

- Determine one area for improvement, and write a family self-care contract (Bomar, 2005; Kaakinen et al., 2010).
- Set a goal and time frame for initiating and frequency.
- Develop a plan.
- Assign responsibilities.
- Evaluate outcomes.
- Modify, renegotiate, or terminate.

R: *A written self-care contract represents negotiation and commitment of all members (Kaakinen et al., 2010).*

- Direct family to seek resources independently (e.g., community resources, websites).

R: *Families desire information about developmental issues and health promotion, and seeking information is empowering (Kaakinen et al., 2010).*

- Refer to *Interrupted Family Processes* for additional interventions for strengthening family functioning, promoting family integrity, mutual support, and positive functioning.

READINESS FOR ENHANCED FLUID BALANCE

NANDA-I Definition

A pattern of equilibrium between the fluid volume and the chemical composition of body fluid, which can be strengthened

Defining Characteristics

Expresses a desire to enhance fluid balance

Author's Note

If an individual has a pattern of equilibrium between fluid volume and the chemical composition of body fluids that is sufficient for meeting physical needs, how can this be strengthened? Would it be more useful to focus on education under the diagnosis *Risk for Deficient Fluid Volume*?

NOC

Fluid Balance, Hydration, Electrolyte Balance

Goal

The individual will report increased satisfaction with fluid balance, as evidenced by the following indicator:

• Identify two new strategies (specify) to enhance fluid balance

NIC

Fluid/Electrolyte Management

Interventions

Refer to Interventions for *Deficient Fluid Balance*.

READINESS FOR ENHANCED HEALTH MANAGEMENT

NANDA-I Definition

A pattern of regulating and integrating into daily living a therapeutic regimen for the treatment of illness and its sequelae, which can be strengthened

Defining Characteristics*

Expresses desire to enhance choices of daily living for meeting goals
Expresses desire to enhance management of illness
Expresses desire to enhance management of prescribed regimen
Expresses desire to enhance management of risk factors
Expresses desire to enhance management of symptoms

Expresses desire to enhance immunization/vaccination status
Expresses desire to manage the illness (e.g., treatment and
    prevention of sequelae)
Choices of daily living are appropriate for meeting goals
    (e.g., treatment, prevention)
Expresses little difficulty with prescribed regimens
Describes reduction of risk factors
No unexpected acceleration of illness symptoms

 Author's Note

This diagnosis can be used to focus on a personal or lifestyle change in a specific area that is effective and can be enhanced to increase management of an illness.

NOC

Adherence Behavior, Health Beliefs, Health Promoting Behaviors, Well-Being

Goal

The individual will express a desire to move from wellness to a higher level of wellness in management of a disease for condition (specify) (e.g., nutrition, decision making), as evidenced by the following indicators:

- Identify two new strategies (specify) to enhance management of a disease/condition

NIC

Health Education, Risk Identification, Values Classification, Behavior Modification, Coping Enhancement, Knowledge: Health Resources

Interventions

The following interventions are appropriate for any health-promotion/wellness nursing diagnosis that focuses on lifestyle changes and choices, for example, *Readiness for Enhanced Nutrition*, *Parenting*, *Sleep*, *Breastfeeding*, *Family Coping*, and *Family Processes*. These areas of wellness and health promotion can be found readily in Section 1 with health-promoting interventions under nursing diagnoses such as *Sedentary Lifestyle*, *Risk for Ineffective Health Management*, and *Imbalanced Nutrition*. Some of the interventions for the wellness nursing diagnoses, such as *Readiness for Enhanced Grieving*, *Readiness for Enhanced Coping*, or *Readiness for Enhanced*

Decision Making can be found in Section 1, under the individual nursing diagnosis. For example, in *Decisional Conflict* there are interventions that can promote better decision making even for someone already making good decisions.

Engage in Collaborative Negotiation

• Ask: How can you be healthier? Focus on the area the individual chooses.

R: *Motivational interviewing involves helping the person identify the discrepancy between present behaviors and future health goals. Asking someone to identify an unhealthy lifestyle versus telling him or her that he or she needs to lose weight, stop smoking, exercise, eat better, and so on, starts a mutual conversation versus a one-direction dictum.*

Evaluate

• Primary language: ability to read and write in primary language
• English as a second language
• English as primary language; ability to read, write

 Carp's Cues

For successful outcomes for self-heath management at home, specific teaching techniques have proven to be effective. Refer to Appendix A for techniques to improve health literacy at the bedside and in the community.

Complete Assessment of One or More or All Functional Health Patterns as the Individual Desires

Renew Data With Individual or Group

• Does the individual/group report good or excellent health?
• Does the individual desire to learn a behavior to maximize health in a specific pattern?

R: *Every day individuals decide what they are going to eat, whether they will exercise, and other lifestyle choices (*Bodenheimer, MacGregor, & Sharifi, 2005).*

Focus on the Wellness Focus That the Individual Selected

Encourage the Individual to Select Only One Wellness Focus at a Time (e.g., Exercise, Decrease Intake of Carbohydrates, Increase Intake of Water)

R: *Addressing multiple behavioral changes at once is time consuming, which may discourage the change (*Bodenheimer et al., 2005).*

Determine With the Individual Three New Behaviors That Are Doable as

- Will not skip any meals
- Will reduce or eliminate sugar drinks (e.g., soda, juice)
- Will eat at least three servings of vegetables (e.g., carrot stick snacks)
- Will move more as use down steps, park farther from destination, or walk with a buddy

Refer to *Risk for Overweight* for Healthy Eating Guidelines

Refer to Educational Resources About a Particular Focus (Print, Online); Examples of Generic Databases/Websites Include

- www.seekwellness.com/wellness/
- www.cdc.gov/—Centers for Disease Control and Prevention
- www.agingblueprint.org—focuses on aging well
- www.nhlbi.nih.gov—US Department of Health and Human Services
- www.ahrq.gov—US Preventive Services Task Force
- www.health.gov—various health topics
- www.nih.gov—National Institutes of Health
- www.fda.gov—Food and Drug Administration
- www.mbmi.org—Mind-Body Medical Institute
- www.ahha.org—American Holistic Health Association

Discuss the Strategies or Targeted Behavior Changes; Have the Individual Record Realistic Goals and Time Frames That Are Highly Specific; Avoid Recommendations of "Exercise More" or "Eat Less"

- For example: Goal—I will reduce my daily intake of carbohydrates.
- Indicators—Reduce cookie intake from five to two each day.
- Change pasta to multigrain pasta.
- Reduce potato intake by 50% and replace with 50% root vegetables.

Ask the Individual If You Can Contact Him or Her at Designated Intervals (Every Month, at 4 to 6 Months, at 1 Year); Call or e-Mail Individual to Discuss Progress

Advise the Individual That This Process Can Be Repeated as They Desire in Other Functional Health Patterns

READINESS FOR ENHANCED HOPE

NANDA-I Definition

A pattern of expectations and desires for mobilizing energy on one's own behalf, which can be strengthened

Defining Characteristics*

Expresses desire to enhance congruency of expectations with desires
Expresses desire to enhance ability to set achievable goals
Expresses desire to enhance problem solving to meet goals
Expresses desire to enhance belief in possibilities
Expresses desire to enhance spirituality
Expresses desire to enhance sense of meaning to life
Expresses desire to enhance connectedness with others
Expresses desire to enhance hope

Refer to *Hopelessness.*

Goal

The individual will report increased hope, as evidenced by the following indicator:

• Identify two new strategies (specify) to enhance hope

Refer to *Hopelessness.*

Interventions

Refer to *Hopelessness* for interventions to promote hope.
Refer to Internet sites for resources and information about hope.

READINESS FOR ENHANCED ORGANIZED INFANT BEHAVIOR

NANDA-I Definition

A pattern of modulation of the physiologic and behavioral systems of functioning (i.e., autonomic, motor, state-organization, self-regulatory, and attentional-interactional systems) in an infant, which can be strengthened

Defining Characteristics
(*Blackburn & Vandenberg, 1993)

Impaired motor functioning
Insufficient containment within environment
Invasive procedure
Oral impairment
Pain
Parent expresses desire to enhance environmental conditions
Prematurity
Procedure

 Author's Note

This diagnosis describes an infant who is responding to the environment with stable and predictable autonomic, motor, and state cues. The focus of interventions is to promote continued stable development and to reduce excess environmental stimuli that may stress the infant. Because this is a wellness diagnosis, the use of related factors is not needed. The nurse can write the diagnostic statement as *Readiness for Enhanced Organized Infant Behavior*, as evidenced by ability to regulate autonomic, motor, and state systems to environmental stimuli. However, *Risk for Disorganized Infant Behavior* would be more appropriate.

 NOC
Child Development: Specify Age, Sleep, Comfort Level

Goals

The infant will continue age-appropriate growth and development and not experience excessive environmental stimuli. The parent(s)

will demonstrate handling that promotes stability, as evidenced by the following indicators:

- Describe developmental needs of infant
- Describe early signs of stress of exhaustion
- Demonstrate:
  - Gentle, soothing touch
  - Melodic tone of voice, coos
  - Mutual gazing
  - Rhythmic movements
  - Acknowledgment of all baby's vocalizations
  - Recognition of soothing qualities of actions

NIC

Developmental Care, Infant Care, Sleep Enhancement, Environmental Management: Comfort, Parent Education: Infant Attachment Promotion, Caregiver Support, Calming Technique

Interventions

Explain to Parents the Effects of Excess Environmental Stress on the Infant

Provide a List of Signs of Stress for Their Infant; Refer to *Disorganized Infant Behavior* **for a List of Signs**

Teach Parents to Terminate Stimulation if Infant Shows Signs of Stress

R: *Premature infants must adapt to the extrauterine environment with underdeveloped body systems (*Vandenberg, 1990). These infants can tolerate only one activity at a time (*Blackburn, 1993).*

Model Developmental Interventions

- Offer only when the infant is alert (if possible, show parents examples of alert and not alert).
- Begin with one stimulus at a time (touch, voice).
- Provide intervention for a short time.
- Increase interventions according to infant's cues.
- Provide frequent, short interventions instead of infrequent, long-term ones.
- Provide stimulation (visual, auditory, vestibular, tactile, olfactory, gustatory).
- Check periods of alertness.
- Assess sleep requirements.

R: *Parents need to understand that they must pace the type, amount, intensity, and timing of stimulation. Behavioral cues from the infant should guide these decisions (*Becker, 1997).*

Explain, Model, and Observe Parents Engaging in Developmental Interventions

Visual

- Eye contact
- Face-to-face experiences
- High-contrast colors, geometric shapes (e.g., black and white shapes on paper mobile); up to 4 weeks, simple mobiles of four dessert-size paper plates with stripes, four-square checkerboards, a black dot, and a simple bull's eye hung 10 to 13 inches from baby's eyes.

Auditory

- Use high-pitched vocalizations.
- Play classical music softly.
- Use a variety of voice inflections.
- Avoid loud talking.
- Call infant by name.
- Avoid monotone speech patterns.

Vestibular (Movement)

- Rock baby in chair.
- Place infant in sling and rock.
- Close infant's fist around a soft toy.
- Slowly change position during handling.
- Provide head support.

Tactile

- Use firm, gentle touch as initial approach.
- Use skin-to-skin contact in a warm room.
- Provide alternative textures (e.g., sheepskin, velvet, satin).
- Avoid stroking if responses are disorganized.

Olfactory

- Wear a light perfume.

Gustatory

- Allow nonnutritive sucking (e.g., pacifier, hand in mouth).

R: *Individualized developmental care can improve developmental outcomes, weight gain, sleep, motor function, pain tolerance, and feeding. Parents are helped to understand the infant's needs, which will improve attachment and reduce fears (Als et al., 2003).*

Promote Adjustment and Stability in Caregiving Activities
(*Blackburn & Vandenberg, 1993; Merenstein & Gardner, 1998)

Waking
- Enter room slowly.
- Turn on light and open curtains slowly.
- Avoid walking baby if he or she is asleep.

Changing
- Keep room warm.
- Gently change position; contain limbs during movement.
- Stop changing if infant is irritable.

Feeding
- Time feedings with alert states.
- Hold infant close and, if needed, swaddle in a blanket.

Bathing
- Ventral openness may be stressful.
- Cover body parts not being bathed.
- Proceed slowly; allow for rest.
- Offer pacifier or hand to suck.
- Eliminate unnecessary noise.
- Use a soft, soothing voice.

Explain the Need to Reduce Environmental Stimuli When Taking the Infant Outside

- Shelter eyes from light.
- Swaddle the infant so his or her hands can reach the mouth.
- Protect from loud noises.

Praise Parent(s) for Interaction Patterns; Point Out Infant's Engaging Responses

Initiate Health Teaching and Referrals, as Needed

- Explain that developmental interventions will change with maturity. Refer to *Delayed Growth and Development* for specific age-related developmental needs.
- Provide parent(s) with resources for assistance at home (e.g., community resources).
- Refer to the Internet sites for resources and information about preterm newborns.

READINESS FOR ENHANCED KNOWLEDGE (SPECIFY)

NANDA-I Definition

A pattern of cognitive information related to a specific topic, or its acquisition which can be strengthened

Defining Characteristics*

Expresses an interest in learning

 Author's Note

Readiness for Enhanced Knowledge is too broad. All nursing diagnoses— actual, risk, and wellness—seek to enhance knowledge. Once the specific area of enhanced knowledge is identified, refer to that specific diagnosis, for example, *Readiness for Enhanced Nutrition*, *Grieving*, *Risk for Ineffective Parenting*, *Deficient Health Behavior*, or *Ineffective Health Management*. *Readiness for Enhanced Knowledge* is not needed because it lacks the reason for the desired or needed knowledge.

READINESS FOR ENHANCED NUTRITION

NANDA-I Definition

A pattern of nutrient intake, which can be strengthened

Defining Characteristics*

Expresses willingness to enhance nutrition

Nutritional Status, Teaching Nutrition

Goal

The individual/group will report an increase in balanced nutrition, as evidenced by the following indicator:

- Identify two new strategies (specify) to enhance nutrition

Nutrition Management, Nutrition Monitoring

Interventions

- Refer to *Risk for Imbalanced Nutrition* for interventions to promote healthy eating as nutritionally dense foods and fluids.
- Refer to Internet sites for resources and information about nutrition:
  - www.myplate.gov
  - www.health.gov/dietaryguidelines

READINESS FOR ENHANCED PARENTING

NANDA-I Definition

A pattern of providing an environment for children or other dependent/person(s), which can be strengthened

Defining Characteristics*

Children express desire to enhance home environment.
Expresses desire to enhance parenting
Parents express desire to enhance emotional support of children.
Parents express desire to enhance emotional support of other
   dependent person.

 Author's Note

Refer to *Compromised Family Processes* for strategies to support effective family

READINESS FOR ENHANCED POWER

NANDA-I Definition

A pattern of participating knowingly in change for well-being, which can be strengthened

Defining Characteristics*

Expresses a desire to enhance awareness of possible changes to be made

Expresses desire to enhance identification of choices that can be made for change

Expresses desire to enhance involvement in change

Expresses desire to enhance knowledge for participation in change

Expresses desire to enhance participation in choices for daily living and change

Expresses desire to enhance power

Health Beliefs: Perceived Control, Participation: Health Care Decisions

Goal

The individual/group will report increased power, as evidenced by the following indicator:

• Identify two new strategies (specify) to enhance power

NIC
Decision-Making Support, Self-Responsibility Facilitation, Teaching: Individual

Interventions

Refer to *Powerlessness* for strategies to increase power.

READINESS FOR ENHANCED RELATIONSHIP

NANDA-I Definition

A pattern of mutual partnership to provide each other's needs which can be strengthened

Defining Characteristics*

Expresses desire to enhance autonomy between partners
Expresses desire to enhance collaboration between partners
Expresses desire to enhance communication between partners
Expresses desire to enhance emotional need fulfilment for each partner
Expresses desire to enhance mutual respect between partners
Expresses desire to enhance satisfaction with complementary relation between partners
Expresses desire to enhance satisfaction with emotional need fulfilment between partners
Expresses desire to enhance idea sharing between partners
Expresses desire to enhance satisfaction with physical need fulfilment for each partner
Expresses desire to enhance understanding of partner's functional deficit (e.g., physical. psychological, social)

Goal

The individual will report increased satisfaction with partnership, as evidenced by the following indicator:

- Identify two new strategies (specify) to enhance partnership

Interventions

Teach to (*Murray, Zentner, & Yakimo, 2009)

- Talk daily about feelings
- Elicit feelings of partner
- Explore "what if. . ." conversations

R: *Regular sharing of feelings provides opportunities to solve small problems before they escalate.*

Vary Family Responsibilities, Schedule, Chores, and Roles

R: *Each family member should assume assigned chore, with turmoil.*

Engage Each Partner to Discuss Individual Problems and Validate Solutions or Ask Each Partner's Opinion About the Problem

R: *This strategy provides a forum for each partner.*

Establish a Support System That Can Help When Needed; Provide Such Support to Other Families or Individuals in Need

During Times of High Stress or Crises, Encourage Sharing Feelings of Guilt, Anger, or Helplessness. Determine Who Each Partner Seeks Out When They Need Emotional Support

R: *Discussion of feelings about the situation clarifies that the stress is situation related, not about the partner.*

Engage in Activities Together as Partners, Family

R: *An enjoyable activity can bond a family. Isolating behaviors can increase fears and anger.*

Refer to *Grieving, Caregiver Role Strain, Compromised Family Process* If Indicated

READINESS FOR ENHANCED RELIGIOSITY

NANDA-I Definition

A pattern of reliance on religious beliefs and/or participation in rituals of a particular faith tradition which can be strengthened

Defining Characteristics

Expresses a desire to enhance religious belief patterns used in
  past
Expresses a desire to enhance connection with a religious leader
Expresses a desire to enhance forgiveness

Expresses a desire to enhance participation in religious experiences

Expresses a desire to enhance participation in religious practices (e.g., ceremonies, regulations, clothing, prayer, services, and holiday observances)

Expresses a desire to enhance religious customs used in the past

Expresses a desire to enhance religious options

Expresses a desire to enhance use of religious material

READINESS FOR ENHANCED RESILIENCE

NANDA-I Definition

A pattern of positive responses to an adverse situation or crisis, which can be strengthened

Defining Characteristics*

Demonstrates positive outlook

Exposure to crisis

Expresses desire to enhance available resources

Expresses desire to enhance communication skills

Expresses desire to enhance environmental safety

Expresses desire to enhance goal-setting

Expresses desire to enhance involvement in activities

Expresses desire to enhance own responsibility for action

Expresses desire to enhance progress toward goals

Expresses desire to enhance relationship with others

Expresses desire to enhance resilience

Expresses desire to enhance self-esteem

Expresses desire to enhance sense of control

Expresses desire to enhance support system

Expresses desire to enhance use of conflict-management strategies

Expresses desire to enhance use of coping skills

Expresses desire to enhance use of resources

Exhibits effective use of conflict-management strategies

Enhances personal coping skills

Expresses desire to enhance resilience

Identifies support systems

Increases positive relationships with others
Exhibits involvement in activities
Makes progress toward goals
Identifies presence of a crisis
Maintains safe environment
Sets goals
Takes responsibilities for actions
Uses effective communication skills
Verbalizes an enhanced sense of control
Verbalizes self-control

Related Factors

Demographics that increase chance of maladjustment

Drug used	Parental mental illness
Gender	Poor impulse control
Inconsistent parenting	Poverty
Low intelligence	Psychological disorders
Low maternal education	Condition
Large family size	Violence
Minority status	Vulnerability factors that encompass indices that exacerbate the negative reflects of the risk

 Author's Note

This NANDA-I diagnosis focuses on the concept of resilience. Resilience is a strength that allows one to persevere and overcome difficulties. When faced with a crisis or problem, resilient people respond constructively with solutions or effective adaptation. Resilience is not a nursing diagnosis. It is an important and vital characteristic that can be nurtured and taught to children to assist them to cope with problematic life events.

The Defining Characteristics describe enhanced or effective coping. In contrast, the Related Factors are contributing factors for ineffective coping.

This author recommends the following:

- Use *Risk for Ineffective Coping* or *Risk for Compromised Family Coping* related to the Related Factors listed above to assist someone to which are preventing effective coping.
- Use *Ineffective Coping* related to the above Related Factors if Defining Characteristics of *Ineffective Coping* exist.

(Refer to Section 1 under *Ineffective Coping* for specific defining characteristics.)
• Refer to the interventions for promoting resiliency in children and adults. (Refer to Index under resiliency for specific pages.)

READINESS FOR ENHANCED SELF-CARE

NANDA-I Definition

A pattern of performing activities for oneself that helps to meet health-related goals and which can be strengthened

Defining Characteristics*

Expresses a desire to enhance independence in maintaining life
Expresses desire to enhance independence with health
Expresses desire to enhance independence with life
Expresses desire to enhance independence with personal development
Expresses desire to enhance independence with well-being
Expresses desire to enhance knowledge of self-care
Expresses desire to enhance self-care

 Author's Note

This diagnosis focuses more on improving self-care activities. Refer to *Self-Care Deficits* for interventions to improve self-care.

READINESS FOR ENHANCED SELF-CONCEPT

NANDA-I Definition

A pattern of perceptions or ideas about the self, which can be strengthened

Defining Characteristics*

Acceptance of limitations
Acceptance of strengths
Actions congruent with verbal expression
Confidence in abilities
Expresses a desire to enhance role performance
Expresses a desire to enhance self-concept
Satisfaction with body image
Satisfaction with personal identity
Satisfaction with sense of worth
Satisfaction with thoughts about self

Quality of Life, Self-Esteem, Coping

Goal

The individual will report increased self-concept in (specify situation), as evidenced by the following indicator:

• Identify two new strategies (specify) to enhance self-concept

NIC
Hope Instillation, Values Clarification, Coping Enhancement

Interventions

Refer to *Disturbed Self-Concept* for interventions to improve self-concept.

READINESS FOR ENHANCED SLEEP

NANDA-I Definition

A pattern of natural, periodic suspension of relative consciousness that provides rest, sustains a desired lifestyle, which can be strengthened

Defining Characteristics*

Expresses desire to enhance sleep

Goal

The individual will report satisfactory sleep pattern, as evidenced by the following indicator:

• Identify two new strategies (specify) to enhance sleep

Interventions

Refer to *Disturbed Sleep Patterns* for strategies to promote sleep.

READINESS FOR ENHANCED SPIRITUAL WELL-BEING

NANDA-I Definition

A pattern of experiencing and integrating meaning and purpose in life through connectedness with self, others, art, music, literature, nature, and/or a power greater than oneself, which can be strengthened

Defining Characteristics*

Connections to Self
Expresses desire to enhance acceptance
Expresses desire to enhance coping
Expresses desire to enhance courage
Expresses desire to enhance hope
Expresses desire to enhance joy
Expresses desire to enhance love
Expresses desire to enhance meaning in life
Expresses desire to enhance meditative practice
Expresses desire to enhance purpose in life

Expresses desire to enhance satisfaction with philosophy of life
Expresses desire to enhance self-forgiveness
Expresses desire to enhance serenity (e.g., peace)
Expresses desire to enhance surrender

Connections With Others
Expresses desire to enhance forgiveness from others
Expresses desire to enhance interaction with significant others
Expresses desire to enhance interaction with spiritual leaders
Expresses desire to enhance service to others

Connections With Art, Music, Literature, and Nature
Expresses desire to enhance creative energy (e.g., writing, poetry, music)
Expresses desire to enhance spiritual reading
Expresses desire to enhance time outdoors

Connections With Power Greater Than Self
Expresses desire to enhance mystical experiences
Expresses desire to enhance participation in religious activity
Expresses desire to enhance prayerfulness
Expresses desire to enhance reverence

NOC
Hope, Spiritual Well-Being

Goals

The individual will express enhanced spiritual harmony and wholeness, as evidenced by the following indicators:

- Maintain previous relationship with higher being
- Continue spiritual practices not detrimental to health

NIC
Spiritual Growth Facilitation, Spiritual Support, Hope

Interventions

Refer to the Internet sites for resources and information about spiritual health

READINESS FOR ENHANCED URINARY ELIMINATION

NANDA-I Definition

A pattern of urinary functions that is sufficient for meeting eliminatory needs, which can be strengthened

Defining Characteristics*

Expresses willingness to enhance urinary elimination

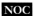 **NOC**

Fluid balance, hydration, electrolyte balance

Goal

The individual will report an increased balance in urinary elimination, as evidenced by the following indicator:

- Identify two new strategies (specify) to enhance urinary elimination

 NIC

Education: fluid/electrolyte

Interventions

- Refer to the Internet sites for resources and information about fluid balance:
  - www.health.gov/dietaryguidelines

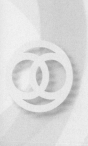

Section 3

Manual of Collaborative Problems[1]

This section contains 14 specific collaborative problems. (Collaborative problems were labeled as *Potential Complication: (specify)* or *PC (specify)* in earlier editions of this book.) These 14 collaborative problems have been selected because of their high incidence of occurrence in most clinical settings. One generic collaborative problem, *Risk for Complications of Cardiac/Vascular/Respiratory Dysfunction*, represents the general monitoring that is done for all individuals under nursing care. If the individual is at more risk for a specific complication, then that collaborative problem can be identified; for example, *Risk for Complications of Deep Vein Thrombosis*.

Carpenito (1999) defines collaborative problems as

> Certain physiologic complications that nurses monitor to detect onset or changes in status. Nurses manage collaborative problems using physician-prescribed and nursing-prescribed interventions to minimize the complications of the event.

[1]Some of the content for this section is derived from Carpenito, L. J. (2016). *Nursing Diagnoses: Application to Clinical Practice* (15th ed.). Philadelphia: Wolters Kluwer, and Carpenito, L. J. (2014). *Nursing Care Plans: Transitional Patient & Family Centered Care* (6th ed.). Philadelphia: Wolters Kluwer Health.

693

Key Concepts

- Not all physiologic complications are collaborative problems; some are nursing diagnoses. For example, *Risk for Infection* and *Risk for Pressure Ulcers* are nursing diagnoses because nurses prescribe preventive measures.
- Nurses cannot prevent, for example, seizures, bleeding, hepatic dysfunction, or arrhythmias, but nursing monitoring is critical to early detection of onset of the condition or worsening of physiologic complications. Nurses provide both nursing-prescribed interventions and medical provider–prescribed interventions, such as protocols in response to the onset or worsening of a physiologic complication, because nurses prescribe preventive measures.
- Physicians, nurse practitioners, and physician assistants cannot treat collaborative problems without nursing knowledge, vigilance, and judgment.
- Priority diagnoses (nursing diagnoses or collaborative problems) are those that take precedence over others. For example, if someone is short of breath, the nurse would address *Anxiety* and *Risk for Complications of Hypoxemia*.
- Individuals who are stable physiologically will have priorities of nursing diagnoses.
- All individuals will have a set of priority diagnoses; nursing diagnoses will always be present in this set. The number of nursing diagnoses versus collaborative problems will depend on the individual's present vulnerability for physiologic instability.

Information on each generic collaborative problem is presented under the following subheads:

- Definition
- Author's Note: Discussion of the problem to clarify its clinical use
- Significant Laboratory/Diagnostic Assessment Criteria: Laboratory findings useful in monitoring

Discussions of the specific collaborative problems cover the following information:

- Definition
- High-Risk Populations
- Collaborative Goals: A statement specifying the nursing accountability for monitoring for physiologic instability and for providing interventions (nursing and medical) to maintain or

restore stability. Indicators of physiologic stability have been added to evaluate the individual's condition.

- General Interventions and Rationales: These specifically direct the nurse to
  - Monitor for onset or early changes in status
  - Initiate physician-, physician assistant-, or advanced practice nurse-prescribed interventions as indicated
  - Initiate nurse-prescribed interventions as indicated
  - Evaluate the effectiveness of these interventions

Keep in mind that for many of the collaborative problems covered here, associated nursing diagnoses also can be predicted to be present. For example, an individual with diabetes mellitus would receive care under the collaborative problem *Risk for Complications of Hypo/Hyperglycemia*, along with the nursing diagnosis *Risk for Ineffective Health Maintenance related to insufficient knowledge of (specify)*; an individual with renal calculi would be under the collaborative problem *Risk for Complications of Renal Calculi* and also the nursing diagnosis *Risk for Ineffective Health Management related to insufficient knowledge of prevention of recurrence, dietary restrictions, and fluid requirements.*

Special Text Features

Clinical Alerts

Clinical Alerts are found in the intervention section to advise the student or nurse to take an immediate action because of a serious event or a change in the individual's physiologic status. An example is, Notify Rapid Response Team.

Rationale

A rationale statement, noted with an "**R:**" and italics, explains why a sign or symptom is present or gives the scientific explanation for why an intervention is recommended to achieve the desired response.

Carp's Cues

This feature provides additional information to challenge the reader to consider other options or to emphasize the severity of an event.

RISK FOR COMPLICATIONS OF CARDIAC/VASCULAR/RESPIRATORY DYSFUNCTION

Risk for Complications of Cardiac/Vascular/ Respiratory Dysfunction

Risk for Complications of Arrhythmias

Risk for Complications of Bleeding

Risk for Complications of Decreased Cardiac Output

Risk for Complications of Compartment Syndrome

Risk for Complications of Deep Vein Thrombosis/Pulmonary Embolism/Fat Embolism

Risk for Complications of Hypovolemia

Definition

Describes a person experiencing or at high risk to experience various cardiac and/or vascular dysfunctions

 Author's Note

The nurse can use this generic collaborative problem to describe a person at risk for several types of cardiovascular problems. For example, all individuals in critical care units are vulnerable to cardiovascular dysfunction. Using *Risk for Complications of Cardiac/Vascular Dysfunction* would direct nurses to monitor cardiovascular status for various problems, based on focus assessment findings. Nursing interventions for such individuals would focus on detecting abnormal functioning and providing the appropriate response or interventions.

For an individual with a specific cardiovascular complication, the nurse would add the applicable collaborative problem to the individual's problem list, along with specific nursing interventions for that problem. For example, a Standard of Care for an individual after myocardial infarction could contain the collaborative problem *Risk for Complications of Cardiac/ Vascular Dysfunction*, directing nurses to monitor cardiovascular status. If this individual later experienced a dysrhythmia, the nurse would add *Risk for Complications of Risk for Arrhythmias* to the problem list, along with specific nursing management information (e.g., *Risk for Complications of Risk for Arrhythmias related to myocardial infarction*). When the risk factors or etiology is not directly related to the primary medical diagnosis, the nurse still should add them, if known (e.g., *Risk for Complications of Hypo/Hyperglycemia related to diabetes mellitus* in an individual who has sustained myocardial infarction).

Significant Laboratory/Diagnostic Assessment Criteria

Screening for Risk of Cardiovascular Disease (Labs on Line, 2014)

- Lipid profile (LDL-C, HDL-C, cholesterol, triglycerides)
- hs-CRP—detects low concentrations of C-reactive protein, a marker of inflammation that is associated with atherosclerosis, among other conditions
- Lp(a)—an additional lipid test that may be used to identify an elevated level of lipoprotein (a), a modification to LDL-C that increases risk of atherosclerosis

Cardiac Biomarkers (Labs on Line, 2014)

- Troponin—elevated within a few hours of heart damage and remain elevated for up to 2 weeks
- CK-MB—elevated when there is damage to the heart muscle cells
- Brain-type natriuretic peptide (BNP) or NT-proBNP—released by the body as a natural response to heart failure; increased levels of BNP, while not diagnostic for a heart attack, indicate an increased risk of cardiac complications in persons with ACS
- Cardiac enzymes and proteins—currently, the gross total values of CK, LDH, SGOT, and/or SGPT in the evaluation of cardiac injury are relatively low. Isoenzymes or bands as well as troponins are the only ones usually used; elevated with cardiac tissue damage (e.g., in myocardial infarction)
- Creatinine kinase (CK)
- Creatinine phosphokinase, isoenzymes (e.g., CK-MB, CK-BB, CK-MM)
- Creatinine kinase isoforms (CK-MB, CK-MM subforms)
- Lactic dehydrogenase (LDH), isoenzymes
- Myoglobin (troponin)
- BNP (hormones released as a peripheral response to cardiac impairment) (e.g., heart failure)

- C-reactive protein, P-selectin (markers of inflammation and necrosis)
- Serum potassium (fluctuates with diuretic therapy, parenteral fluid replacement)
- Serum calcium, magnesium, phosphate
- White blood cell count (elevated with inflammation)
- Erythrocyte sedimentation rate (elevated with inflammation, tissue injury)
- Arterial blood gas (ABG) values (lowered SaO_2 indicates hypoxemia; elevated pH, alkalosis; lowered pH, acidosis)
- Coagulation studies (elevated with anticoagulant and/or thrombolytic therapy or coagulopathies)
- Hemoglobin and hematocrit (elevated with polycythemia, lowered with anemia)
- Electrocardiograph with or without stress test
- Doppler ultrasonic flow meter
- Cardiac catheterization
- Intravascular ultrasonography (IVU)
- Electrophysiology studies
- Computed tomography (CT), ultrafast CT
- Magnetic resonance imaging
- Signal-averaged electrocardiography
- Echocardiography with or without stress test
- Phonocardiography
- Exercise electrocardiography (ECG)
- Perfusion imaging
- Infarct imaging
- Angiocardiography
- Holter monitoring
- Inflatable loop monitor
- Deep vein thrombosis (DVT) diagnostic work-up:
  - D-dimer—D-dimer is a substance in the blood that is often increased in people with DVT or pulmonary embolism (PE).
  - Compression ultrasonography—Compression ultrasonography uses sound waves to generate pictures of the structures inside the leg.
  - Contrast venography
  - Magnetic resonance imaging (MRI)

Collaborative Outcomes

The individual will be monitored for early signs and symptoms of (a) cardiovascular dysfunction and (b) respiratory insufficiency, and will receive collaborative interventions if indicated to restore physiologic stability.

Indicators of Physiologic Stability

- Calm, alert, oriented (a, b)
- Respiration 16 to 20 breaths/min, relaxed and rhythmic (b)
- Breath sounds present all lobes, no rales or wheezing (b)
- Pulse 60 to 100 beats/min (a, b)
- BP >90/60, <140/90 mm Hg (a, b)
- Capillary refill <3 seconds; skin warm and dry (a, b)
- Peripheral pulses full, equal (a)
- Temperature 98.5° F to 99° F (a, b)
- Pulse oximetry >90 to 100%
- $PaCO_2$ 35 to 45
- PaO_2 80 to 100
- Urine output >0.5 mL/kg/hour

Interventions With Rationale

Closely Monitor Risk Individuals for Hospital-Acquired (Nosocomial) Pneumonia as

- The elderly and very young
- Those with chronic or severe medical conditions, such as lung problems, heart disease, nervous system (neurologic) disorders, and immune compromised (AIDS, cancer)
- Those postsurgery as over age 80 post splenectomy, abdominal aortic aneurysm repair, or any factor that impairs coughing, e.g., fractured ribs
- Those in the intensive care unit (ICU), in prolonged prone positions, on mechanical ventilators
- Those sedated

Monitor Cardiovascular Status

- Radial pulse (rate and rhythm)
- Apical pulse (rate and rhythm)
- Blood pressure
- Skin (color, temperature, moisture) and temperature
- Pulse oximetry

R: *Physiologic mechanisms governing cardiovascular function are very sensitive to any change in body function, making changes in cardiovascular status important clinical indicators.*

a. *Pulse monitoring provides data to detect cardiac dysrhythmia, blood volume changes, and circulatory impairment.*
b. *Apical pulse monitoring is indicated if the individual's peripheral pulses are irregular, weak, or extremely rapid.*
c. *Blood pressure represents the force that the blood exerts against the arterial walls. Hypertension (systolic pressure >140 mm Hg, diastolic*

pressure >85 mm Hg) may indicate increased peripheral resistance, cardiac output, blood volume, or blood viscosity. Hypotension can result from significant blood or fluid loss, decreased cardiac output, and certain medications.

d. *Skin assessment provides information evaluating circulation, body temperature, and hydration status.*

e. *Pulse oximetry is a noninvasive method (probe sensor on fingertip) for continuous monitoring of oxygen saturation of hemoglobin.*

Monitor for Signs and Symptoms of Hypoxemia

- Increased pulse rate with normal or slightly decreased blood pressure, narrowing pulse pressure; decreased mean arterial pressure (MAP)
- Urine output <0.5 mL/kg/hr
- Restlessness, agitation, decreased mentation
- Increased respiratory rate, thirst
- Diminished peripheral pulses
- Cool, pale, moist, or cyanotic skin
- Decreased oxygenation saturation (SaO_2, SvO_2), pulmonary artery pressures
- Decreased hemoglobin/hematocrit, decreased cardiac output/index

R: *The compensatory response to decreased circulatory volume aims to increase oxygen delivery through increased heart and respiratory rates and decreased peripheral circulation (manifested by diminished peripheral pulses and cool skin). Decreased oxygen to the brain alters mentation. Decreased circulation to the kidneys leads to decreased urine output. Hemoglobin and hematocrit values decline if bleeding is significant.*

Monitor for Decreased Urine Output (<0.5 mL/hr); Cool, Pale, or Cyanotic Skin

R: *The compensatory response to decreased circulatory oxygen aims to increase blood oxygen by increasing heart and respiratory rates and to decrease circulation to the kidneys and extremities (marked by decreased pulses and skin changes).*

Administer Low-Flow (2 L/min) Oxygen as Needed Through Nasal Cannula, Titrate up per Protocol to Keep Pulse Oximetry Between 90% and 92%

R: *Oxygen therapy increases circulating oxygen levels. Using a cannula rather than a mask may help reduce the individual's fears of suffocation.*

Monitor for Signs and Symptoms of Heart Failure

R: *Heart failure plays a huge role in derangement in autoregulation of circulation. The end stages of heart failure leads to fluid overload of one or more organs. Changes in both systolic and diastolic ventricular performance occur with heart failure (Lloyd-Jones et al., 2010).*

a. *Circulatory overload is very common and generally are early signs that the individual is getting into trouble.*
b. *Circulatory shock tends to contribute to multiple organ failure. This is due to the inadequate global oxygen delivery.*

Weigh Individual Daily

- Ensure accuracy by weighing at the same time every day on the same scale and with the individual wearing the same amount of clothing.

 Carp's Cues

If heart failure occurs, add a new collaborative problem of *Risk for Complications of Heart Failure.*

R: *Daily weights and strict input and output are vital in determining the effects of treatment and for early detections of fluid retention.*

Monitor for Signs and Symptoms of Acute Pulmonary Edema

Dyspnea, cyanosis
- Tachypnea, labored breathing
- Adventitious breath sounds, crackles
- Persistent cough or productive cough with frothy, pink-tinged sputum
- Abnormal ABGs
- Decreased O_2 saturation by pulse oximetry
- Decreased cardiac output/cardiac index
- Elevated pulmonary artery pressure
- Tachycardia
- Abnormal heart sounds (S_3)

Jugular vein distention (JVD)
- Persistent cough
- Productive cough with frothy sputum
- Cyanosis
- Diaphoresis

R: *Impaired pumping of left ventricle accompanied by decreased cardiac output and increased pulmonary artery pressure produce pulmonary edema. Hypoxia produces increased capillary congestion, causing fluid* *to enter pulmonary tissue and triggering signs and symptoms. (Venous pressure and pulmonary lungs become so congested with fluid that it affects the exchange of oxygen, which is considered pulmonary edema.) Diuretics help the body to rid itself of excess fluids and sodium through urination. Helps to relieve the heart's workload (AHA, 2010).*

a. *Decreased cardiac output leads to insufficient oxygenated blood to meet the tissues' metabolic needs. Decreased circulating volume/cardiac output can cause hypoperfusion of the kidneys and decreased tissue perfusion with a compensatory response of decreased circulation to the extremities and increased pulse and respiratory rates. Changes in mentation may result from cerebral hypoperfusion. Vasoconstriction and venous congestion in dependent areas (e.g., limbs) produce changes in skin and pulses.*

b. *Circulatory overload can result from the reduced size of the pulmonary vascular bed. Hypoxia causes increased capillary permeability that, in turn, causes fluid to enter pulmonary tissue, producing the signs and symptoms of pulmonary edema.*

Monitor With Pulse Oximetry

• Monitor for signs and symptoms of acute pulmonary edema:
  • Severe dyspnea with use of accessory muscles
  • Tachycardia
  • Adventitious breath sounds

R: *The pulse oximeter is an accurate, noninvasive monitor of oxygen concentrations.*

Cautiously Administer Intravenous (IV) Fluids

• Consult with the physician/NP if the ordered rate plus the PO intake exceeds 2 to 2.5 L/24 hr. Be sure to include additional IV fluids (e.g., antibiotics) when calculating the hourly allocation. Oral fluid intake must also be monitored and, if indicated, possibly restricted.

R: *Failure to regulate IV fluids carefully can cause circulatory overload.*

Assist With Measures to Conserve Strength, Such as Resting Before and After Activities (e.g., Meals)

R: *Adequate rest reduces oxygen consumption and decreases the risk of hypoxia.*

Monitor for Signs for Renal Insufficiency

• Refer to Renal Insufficiency for interventions.

R: *Hypoxemia will compromise renal function, and decreased urine output can be the first sign.*

Risk for Complications of Arrhythmias

Definition

Describes a person experiencing or at high risk to experience a disorder of the heart's conduction system that results in an abnormal heart rate, abnormal rhythm, or a combination of both

High-Risk Populations

- A-type coronary artery disease (CAD):
  - Angina
  - Myocardial infarction (acute coronary syndrome [ACS])
  - Congestive heart failure
  - Significant hypoglycemia (Chow et al., 2014)
  - Accidental hypothermia
    - Mild hypothermia, leading to tachycardia
    - Moderate hypothermia, leading to atrial fibrillation, junctional bradycardia
    - Severe hypothermia, leading to bradycardia, ventricular arrhythmias (including ventricular fibrillation), and asystole (Zafren & Mechem, 2014)
  - Sepsis
  - Increased intracranial pressure
  - Electrolyte imbalance (calcium, potassium, magnesium, phosphorus)
  - Atherosclerotic heart disease
- Medication side effects (e.g., aminophylline, dopamine, stimulants, digoxin, beta blockers, calcium-channel blockers, dobutamine, lidocaine, procainamide, quinidine, diuretics, class 1C antiarrhythmic drugs, anticonvulsants such as phenytoin, tricyclic antidepressants, and some agents used to treat neuropathic pain and immunomodulators (Heist & Ruskin, 2010)
  - COPD
  - Cardiomyopathy, valvular heart disease
  - Anemia
  - Postoperative cardiac surgery
  - Postoperative, after any major anesthesia
  - Trauma
  - Sleep apnea
  - Hypoxia

Collaborative Outcomes

The individual will be monitored for early signs and symptoms of arrhythmias and decreased cardiac output and will receive collaborative interventions if indicated to restore physiologic stability.

Indicators of Physiologic Stability

Normal sinus rhythm

Refer also to *Decreased Cardiac Output* indicators of physiologic stability.

Interventions and Rationales

Monitor for Signs and Symptoms of Arrhythmias[2]

- Abnormal rate, rhythm
- Palpitations, chest pain, syncope, fatigue
- Decreased SaO_2
- Hypotension
- Change in level of consciousness

R: *Ischemic tissue is electrically unstable, causing arrhythmias. Certain congenital cardiac conditions fibrosis or scar tissue of conduction system, inflammatory disease, cardiac surgery, infection, cancer, electrolyte imbalances, and medications also can cause disturbances in cardiac conduction.*

Monitor ECG Patterns and Changes as[2]

- ACS (ST-segment elevation, prolongation of Q wave, inversion of T wave)

R: *The above ECG changes may not be present immediately. The first ECG change seen clinically is usually ST-segment elevation, which indicates myocardial injury in tissue underlying the electrodes. ECG changes of infarction include ST elevation (indicating injury), Q waves (indicating necrosis), and T-wave inversion (indicating ischemia and evolution of the infarction). These signs of ischemia can be isolated to ECG leads overlying the involved myocardium and indicating localized ischemia. If they are present in many ECG leads, more widespread ischemia is suspected (Grossman & Porth, 2014).*

---

[2]Notify physician, physician assistant, or nurse practitioner of ST elevation and of other serious EKG changes.

CLINICAL ALERT "If the initial ECG is normal or inconclusive, additional recordings should be obtained if the individual develops symptoms. These should be compared with recordings obtained in an asymptomatic state. The standard ECG at rest does not adequately reflect the dynamic nature of coronary thrombosis and myocardial ischemia. Almost two-thirds of all ischemic episodes in the phase of instability are clinically silent, and hence are unlikely to be detected by a conventional ECG. Accordingly, online continuous computer-assisted 12-lead ST-segment monitoring is also a valuable diagnostic tool".

CLINICAL ALERT This is termed ST-elevation ACS (STE-ACS) and generally reflects an acute total coronary occlusion. Most of these individuals will ultimately develop an ST-elevation myocardial infarction (STEMI). The therapeutic objective is to achieve rapid, complete, and sustained reperfusion by primary angioplasty or fibrinolytic therapy.

- Sinus node arrhythmias (sinus tachycardia, sinus bradycardia, sinus block, sinus pause or arrest, sick sinus syndrome)

R: *Alterations in SA node function leads to changes in rate or rhythm of the heartbeat (Grossman & Porth, 2014).*

- Atrial origin arrhythmias (premature atrial contractions (PAC), multifocal/focal atrial tachycardia, atrial flutter, atrial fibrillation, paroxysmal supraventricular tachycardia)

R: *PAC's and tachycardia can be caused by stress, caffeine, alcohol, tobacco, cardiac ischemia, digitalis toxicity, hypokalemia, hypomagnesemia, and hypoxia. Atrial flutter rarely occurs in healthy persons and is usually seen in children and young adults, who have had surgery for complex congenital heart disease (Grossman & Porth, 2014).*

- Junctional arrhythmias (bradycardia, nonparoxysmal, junctional tachycardia)
- Ventricular arrhythmias (premature ventricular contractions, ventricular tachycardia, ventricular flutter, ventricular fibrillation)

R: *Ventricular arrhythmias are considered more serious than those in the atria because the pumping action of the heart can be impaired causing decreased cardiac output (Grossman & Porth, 2014).*

- Disorders of atrioventricular conduction (first-degree AV block, second-degree block, third-degree AV block)

R: *Heart block is caused by abnormal impulse conduction. It may be normal, physiologic (vagal tone), or pathologic. Causes can be scar tissue, certain medications, electrolyte imbalances, acute myocardial infarction, inflammatory diseases, or cardiac surgery (Grossman & Porth, 2014).*

Initiate Appropriate Protocols Depending on the Type of Arrhythmia

- Administer supplemental oxygen.

R: *It increases circulating oxygen levels and decreases cardiac workload.*

- Monitor oxygen saturation (SaO_2) with pulse oximetry and ABG as necessary.
- Monitor serum electrolyte levels (e.g., sodium, potassium, calcium, magnesium).

R: *High or low electrolyte levels may exacerbate a dysrhythmia.*

Risk for Complications of Bleeding

Definition

Describes a person experiencing or at high risk to experience a decrease in blood volume

High-Risk Populations

- Intraoperative status
- Postoperative status
- Post procedural cannulation of any arterial vessel but particularly those at risk for retroperitoneal bleed due to cannulation of femoral vessel
- Anaphylactic shock
- Trauma
- A history of bleeding disease or dysfunction

- Anticoagulant use, including over-the-counter use of aspirin or NSAIDs (nonsteroidal anti-inflammatory drugs)
- Chronic steroid use
- Acetaminophen use with associated liver dysfunction
- Anemia
- Liver disease
- Disseminated intravascular coagulation (DIC)
- Rupture of esophageal varices
- Dissecting aneurysms
- Trauma in pregnancy
- Pregnancy-related complications (placenta previa, molar pregnancy, abruption placenta)
- Thrombolytic therapy

Collaborative Outcomes

The individual will be monitored for early signs and symptoms of bleeding and will receive collaborative interventions if indicated to restore physiologic stability.

Indicators of Physiologic Stability

- Alert, oriented, calm
- Urine output >0.5 mL/kg/hr
- Neutrophils 60% to 70%
- Red blood cells
  - Male: 4.6 to 5.9 million/mm^3
  - Female: 4.2 to 5.4 million/mm^3
- Platelets 150,000 to 400,000/mm^3
- No petechiae or purpura
- No gum or nasal bleeding
- Regular menses
- No headache
- Clear vision
- Intact coordination, facial symmetry, and muscle strength
- No splenomegaly
- Identify risk factors that can be reduced.
- Relate early signs and symptoms of infection.
  - Oxygen saturation >95%
  - Normal sinus rhythm
  - No chest pain
  - No life-threatening dysrhythmias
  - Skin warm and dry, usual skin color (appropriate for race)
  - Pulse: regular rhythm, rate 60 to 100 beats/min
  - Respirations 16 to 20 breaths/min

- Blood pressure >90/60, <140/90 mm Hg, MAP >70, or central venous pressure (CVP) >11
- Urine output >0.5 mL/kg/hr
- Serum pH 7.35 to 7.45
- Serum RCO_2 35 to 45 mm Hg
- SpO_2 goals >95% for those without history of lung disease
- Breath sounds without evidence of new, abnormal sounds (rales)
- No presence of distended neck veins (JVD)

Interventions and Rationales

Monitor Fluid Status, Evaluate

- Intake (parenteral and oral)
- Output and other losses (urine, drainage, and vomiting); nasogastric tube
- Increase monitoring of urine output to hourly.

R: *Decreased blood volume reduces blood to kidneys, which decreases the glomerular filtration rate (GFR), causing a decrease in urine output. When blood flow to the kidneys is less than 20% to 25% of normal, ischemic damage occurs (Grossman & Porth, 2014). Decreased urine output is an early sign of bleeding/hypovolemia.*

Monitor for Signs and Symptoms of Bleeding Dependent on Site

- Integumentary system:
  - Petechiae
  - Ecchymoses
  - Hematomas
  - Oozing from venipuncture sites
  - Cyanotic patches on arms/legs
- Increase in bleeding from surgical wound
- Eyes and ears:
  - Visual disturbances
  - Periorbital edema
  - Subconjunctival hemorrhage
  - Ear pain
- Nose, mouth, and throat:
  - Petechiae
  - Epistaxis
  - Tender or bleeding gums
- Cardiopulmonary system:
  - Crackles and wheezes
  - Stridor and dyspnea

- Tachypnea and cyanosis
- Hemoptysis
- Gastrointestinal (GI) system:
  - Pain
  - Blood streaks in stool/emesis
  - Bleeding around rectum
  - Occult blood in stools
  - Dark stools
- Genitourinary system:
  - Increased menses
  - Decreased urine output
- Musculoskeletal system:
  - Painful joints
- Central nervous system:
  - Mental status changes
  - Vertigo
  - Seizures
  - Restlessness

Monitor for Signs and Symptoms of Shock

- Increased pulse rate with normal or slightly decreased blood pressure, narrowing pulse pressure; decreased MAP
- Urine output <5 mL/kg/hr
- Restlessness, agitation, decreased mentation
- Increased respiratory rate, thirst
- Diminished peripheral pulses
- Cool, pale, moist, or cyanotic skin
- Decreased oxygenation saturation (SaO_2, SvO_2); pulmonary artery pressures, right atrial pressure, wedge/occlusion pressure, cardiac output/index
- Decreased hemoglobin/hematocrit
- Decreased CVP
- Capillary refill >3 seconds (indicates poor tissue perfusion)

R: *The compensatory response to decreased circulatory volume aims to increase oxygen delivery through increased heart and respiratory rates and decreased peripheral circulation (manifested by diminished peripheral pulses and cool skin). Decreased oxygen to the brain alters mentation. Decreased circulation to the kidneys leads to decreased urine output. Hemoglobin and hematocrit values decline if bleeding is significant (Grossman & Porth, 2014).*

If Shock Occurs, Place the Individual in the Supine Position Unless Contraindicated (e.g., Head Injury)

R: *This position increases blood return (preload) to the heart.*

- Insert an IV line; use a large-bore catheter if blood or large-volume fluid replacement is anticipated. Initiate appropriate protocols for shock (e.g., vasopressor therapy). Refer also to *Risk for Complications of Acidosis* or *Risk for Complications of Alkalosis*, if indicated, for more information.

R: *Protocols aim to increase peripheral resistance and elevate blood pressure.*

- Contact physician, physician assistant, or advanced practice nurse with assessment data that may indicate bleeding and to replace fluid losses at a rate sufficient to maintain urine output >0.5 mL/kg/hr (e.g., saline or Ringer's lactate).

R: *This measure promotes optimal renal tissue perfusion.*

Monitor the Surgical Site for Bleeding, Dehiscence, and Evisceration

R: *Careful monitoring allows early detection of complications.*

Teach the Individual to Splint the Surgical Wound With a Pillow When Coughing, Sneezing, or Vomiting

R: *Splinting reduces stress on suture line by equalizing pressure across the wound.*

If Anticoagulant or Thrombolytic Therapy, Monitor for

- Bruises, nosebleeds
- Bleeding gums
- Hematuria
- Severe headaches
- Red or black stools

R: *The prolonged clotting time of anticoagulants by anticoagulant therapy can cause spontaneous bleeding anywhere in the body. Hematuria is a common early sign.*

Monitor for Signs of Bleeding From Venous Access Devices (e.g., IVs, Long-Term Venous Access Devices)

- Hematoma at site
- Bleeding at site

R: *Bleeding can occur several hours after insertion after blood pressure returns to normal and puts increased pressure on newly formed clot at the insertion site. It can also develop later, secondary to vascular erosion due to infection.*

Minimize Movement and Activity

R: *This helps decrease tissue demands for oxygen.*

Provide Reassurance, Simple Explanations, and Emotional Support to Help Reduce Anxiety

R: *High anxiety increases metabolic demands for oxygen.*

Administer Oxygen as Ordered

R: *Diminished blood volume causes decreased circulating oxygen levels.*

Risk for Complications of Decreased Cardiac Output

Definition

Describes a person experiencing or at high risk to experience inadequate blood supply for tissue and organ needs because of insufficient blood pumping by the heart.

Deceased cardiac output is a phenomenon that is not restricted to individuals or environments that specifically focus on cardiovascular care. It is not only prevalent in cardiovascular care units, but also in postanesthetic units and noncardiac care units among individuals with noncardiogenic disorders. A significant decrease in cardiac output is a life-threatening situation, demonstrating the need for developing a risk nursing diagnosis for early intervention (Pereira de Melo et al., 2011).

High-Risk Populations

- ACS
- Congestive heart failure
- Cardiogenic shock
- Hypertension
- Valvular heart disease
- Cardiomyopathy
- Cardiac tamponade
- Hypothermia
- Anaphylaxis
- Dilated cardiomyopathy
- Streptococcal toxic shock syndrome
- Severe diarrhea

- Systemic inflammatory response syndrome (SIRS)
- Coarctation of the aorta
- Chronic obstructive pulmonary disease (COPD)
- Pheochromocytoma
- Chronic renal failure
- Adult respiratory distress syndrome
- Hypotension/hypovolemia (e.g., postsurgery, severe bleeding, or burns)
- Bradycardia
- Tachycardia

Collaborative Outcomes

The individual will be monitored for early signs and symptoms of *Decreased Cardiac Output* and will receive collaborative interventions if indicated to restore physiologic stability.

Indicators of Physiologic Stability

- Calm, alert, oriented
- Oxygen saturation >95%
- Normal sinus rhythm
- No chest pain
- No life-threatening dysrhythmias
- Skin warm and dry
- Usual skin color (appropriate for race)
- Pulse: regular rhythm, rate 60 to 100 beats/minute
- Respirations 16 to 20 breaths/minute
- Blood pressure >90/60, <140/90 mm Hg, MAP >70, or CVP >11
- Urine output >0.5 mL/kg/hr

Interventions and Rationales

Monitor for Signs and Symptoms of Decreased Cardiac Output/ Index

- Increased, decreased, and/or irregular pulse rate
- Increased respiratory rate
- Decreased blood pressure, increased blood pressure
- Abnormal heart sounds
- Abnormal lung sounds (crackles, rales)
- Decreased urine output (<0.5 mL/kg/hr)
- Changes in mentation

- Cool, moist, cyanotic, mottled skin
- Delayed capillary refill time
- Neck vein distention
- Weak peripheral pulses
- Abnormal pulmonary artery pressures
- Abnormal renal artery pressures
- Decreased mixed venous oxygen saturation
- Electrocardiogram (ECG) changes
- Dysrhythmias
- Decreased SaO_2
- Decreased ($ScvO_2$)

R: *Decreased cardiac output/index leads to insufficient oxygenated blood to meet the metabolic needs of tissues. Decreased circulating volume can result in hypoperfusion of the kidneys and decreased tissue perfusion with a compensatory response of decreased circulation to extremities and increased pulse and respiratory rates (Grossman & Porth, 2014). Changes in mentation may result from cerebral hypoperfusion. Vasoconstriction and venous congestion in dependent areas (e.g., limbs) produce changes in skin and pulses.*

Closely Monitor Urine Output Hourly

R: *Decreased blood volume reduces blood to kidneys, which decreases the GFR, causing a decreased urine output. When blood flow to the kidneys is less than 20 to 25% of normal, ischemic damage occurs (Grossman & Porth, 2014). Decreased urine output is an early sign of bleeding/hypovolemia.*

Initiate Appropriate Protocols or Standing Orders, Depending on the Underlying Etiology of the Problem Affecting Ventricular Function

R: *Nursing management differs based on etiology (e.g., measures to help increase preload for hypovolemia and to decrease preload for impaired ventricular contractility).*

Position With the Legs Elevated, Unless Ventricular Function is Impaired

R: *This position can help increase preload and enhance cardiac output.*

Assist With Measures to Conserve Strength, Such as Resting Before and After Activities (e.g., Meals, Baths)

R: *Adequate rest reduces oxygen consumption and decreases the risk of hypoxia.*

If Decreased Cardiac Output Results From Hypovolemia, Septic Shock, or Dysrhythmia

• Refer to the specific collaborative problem in this section.

Risk for Complications of Compartment Syndrome

Definition

Describes a person experiencing increased pressure in a limited space, such as a fascial envelope, which compromises circulation and function, usually in the forearm or leg. ACS is a surgical emergency. Compartment syndrome can also occur in the abdomen (*Intra-Abdominal Hypertension*) when there is a sustained or repeated elevation of 12 mm Hg or greater (Stracciolini & Hammerberg, 2014).

High-Risk Populations

A prerequisite for the development of increased compartment pressure is a fascial structure that prevents adequate expansion of tissue volume to compensate for an increase in fluid.

Internal Factors

• Fractures
• Musculoskeletal surgery
• Injuries (crush, electrical, vascular)
• Allergic response (snake, insect bites)
• Excessive edema
• Thermal injuries
• Vascular obstruction
• Intramuscular bleeding
• Extremely vigorous exercise, especially eccentric movements (extension under pressure)
• Anabolic steroids

External Factors

• Extravasation of IV fluids
• Procedural cannulation of vessel for diagnostic or interventional reasons:

- Casts
- Prolonged use of tourniquet
- Tight dressings
- Tight closure of fascial detects
- Positioning during surgery
- Lying on limb for extended periods
- Drug abuse (arterial injection; Stracciolini & Hammerberg, 2014)

Collaborative Outcomes

The individual will be monitored for early signs and symptoms of compartment syndrome and will receive collaborative interventions if indicated to restore physiologic stability.

Indicators of Physiologic Stability

- Pedal pulses 2+, equal
- Capillary refill <3 seconds
- Warm extremities
- No complaints of paresthesia (numbness), tingling
- Minimal swelling
- Ability to move toes or fingers

Interventions and Rationales

Explain to Individual/Family the Reason for the Specific Questions and Examinations

R: *Diagnosing changes in neurovascular function in individuals with trauma is difficult; thus, cooperation of involved persons can be useful.*

Assess for Specific Signs of Compartment Syndrome (Shadgan et al., 2010; Stracciolini & Hammerberg, 2014)

- Complaints of tingling or burning sensations—numbness

R: *Sensory deficits typically precede motor deficits and manifest distal to the involved compartment.*

- Pain is out of proportion to the injury, unrelieved by narcotics
- Pain with passive stretch of muscles in the affected compartment or hyperextension of digits (toes or fingers) (early finding)

R: *Passive stretching of muscles decreases muscle compartment, thus increasing pain. Pain in response to passive stretching of muscles within the affected compartment is widely described as a sensitive early sign of ACS (Stracciolini & Hammerberg, 2014).*

* A new and persistent deep ache in an arm or leg
* Electricity-like pain in the limb

R: *Pain and paresthesia indicate compression of nerves and increasing pressure within muscle compartment.*

* Increases with the elevation of the extremity

R: *This increases the pressure in the compartment.*

* Involved compartment or limb will feel tense and warm on palpation.
* Skin is tight and shiny.
* Late signs/symptoms:
  * Diminished or absent pulse
  * Pallor, cool skin
  * Pale, grayish, or whitish tone to skin

R: *Arterial occlusion produces these late signs.*

* Prolonged capillary refill (>3 seconds)

R: *Delayed capillary refill or pale, mottled, or cyanotic skin indicates obstructed capillary blood flow.*

* Complaints of weakness when moving affected limb
* Progresses to inability to move joint or fingers/toes
* Pulselessness

R: *Decreased arterial perfusion results in pulselessness.*

Examine Laboratory Findings of Compartment Syndrome

* Elevated WBC (white blood cell count) and ESR (erythrocyte sedimentation rate)

R: *These elevations are a result of the severe inflammatory response.*

* Lowered serum pH

R: *This reflects tissue damage with acidosis.*

* Elevated temperature

R: *This is due to necrosis of tissue.*

* Elevated serum potassium

R: *Cellular damage releases potassium.*

Assess Neurovascular Function at Least Every Hour for First 24 Hours

R: *A delay in diagnosis is the most important determinant of a poor individual outcome.*

Instruct to Report Unusual, New, or Different Sensations (e.g., Tingling, Numbness, and/or Decreased Ability to Move Toes or Fingers)

R: *Early detection of compromise can prevent tissue necrosis and permanent damage*

When the Individual is Unconscious or Heavily Sedated and Unable to Complain or Report Sensations, Intensive Assessment is Required

R: *Permanent nerve injury can occur 12 to 24 hours of nerve compression.*

If Pain Medications Become Ineffective (e.g., Individual Reports "Pain Medications Are Not Working Anymore," Consider Compartmental Syndrome)

R: *Opioids are ineffective for neurovascular pain (Pasero & McCaffery, 2011).*

If Signs of Compartment Syndrome Occur

- Discontinue excessive elevation and ice applications.
- Keep the body part below the level of the heart.

R: *This will improve blood flow into the compartment.*

- Remove restrictive dressings, splints.

R: *Elevation and external devices will impede perfusion.*

Initiate Nasal Oxygen per Protocol

R: *This will improve oxygenation to compromised tissue.*

R: *Immediate medical assessment will determine what specific interventions are needed (e.g., measurement of compartment pressures,*

CLINICAL ALERT (Stracciolini & Hammerberg, 2014)
Immediately advise physician, physician assistant, and nurse practitioner of the need for the evaluation of the neurovascular changes assessed or reported by the individual.

emergency surgery [fasciotomy], removal of cast, splints). Measurement of compartment pressures can be done with a handheld manometer (e.g., Stryker device), a simple needle manometer system, or the wick or slit catheter technique.

Monitor and Document Compartment Pressures According to Protocol; Report Elevated Pressures Promptly

R: *"The normal pressure of a tissue compartment falls between 0 and 8 mm Hg. Clinical findings associated with ACS generally correlate with the degree to which tissue pressure within the affected compartment approaches systemic blood pressures. Capillary blood flow becomes compromised when tissue pressure increases to within 25 to 30 mm Hg of mean arterial pressure"* (Stracciolini, & Hammerberg, 2014).

CLINICAL ALERT "Many surgeons involved in trauma care use a threshold based on the difference between systemic blood pressures and compartment pressures to confirm the presence of ACS. These authors concur with this approach and suggest that a difference between the diastolic blood pressure and the compartment pressure (delta pressure) of 30 mm Hg or less be used as the threshold for diagnosing ACS. The delta pressure is found by subtracting the compartment pressure from the diastolic pressure. Many clinicians use the delta pressure of 30 mm Hg to determine the need for fasciotomy, while others use a difference of 20 mm Hg" (Stracciolini & Hammerberg, 2014).

Carefully Maintain Hydration With at Least 0.5 mL/kg

R: *Muscle necrosis or rhabdomyolysis may lead to the accumulation of myoglobin in the kidneys, causing acute renal failure in up to 50% of individuals with rhabdomyolysis (Mabvuure, Malahias, Hindocha, Khan, & Juma, 2012).*

Continue to Monitor Cardiovascular and Renal Status: Pulse, Respiration, Blood Pressure, and Urine Output

R: *Eight liters of fluid can extravasate into a limb, causing hypovolemia, decreased renal function, and shock.*

Risk for Complications of Deep Vein Thrombosis

Definition

Describes a person experiencing venous clot formation because of blood stasis, vessel wall injury, or altered coagulation and/or experiencing or at high risk to experience obstruction of one or more pulmonary arteries from a blood clot, air, or fat embolus

High-Risk Populations
(Barbar et al., 2010; Lip & Hull, 2014)

- Active cancer (3)
- History of DVT or PE (3)
- Reduced mobility >72 hours (3)
- Known thrombophilic condition (3) (e.g., polycythemia, blood dyscrasias)
- High levels of factor VIII in white people (Payne, Miller, Hooper, Lally, & Austin, 2014)
- High levels of factor VIII and von Willebrand factor in black people (Payne et al., 2014)
- Recent trauma/surgery (2)
- Over 70 years old (1)
- Obesity >30 BMI (1)
- Acute coronary or ischemic stroke (1)
- Acute infection and/or rheumatologic disorder (1)
- Ongoing hormonal therapy (1)
- Heart/respiratory failure (1)
- Age (risk rises steadily from age 40)
- Fractures (especially hip, pelvis, and leg)
- Chemical irritation of vein
- All major surgeries that involve general anesthesia and immobility (over 30 minutes) in the operative course (preop, periop, and postop combined), especially surgeries involving abdomen, pelvis, and lower extremities
- Orthopedic (hips/knees), urologic, or gynecologic surgery
- History of venous insufficiency
- Varicose veins
- Inflammatory bowel disease
- Pregnancy
- Surgery greater than 30 minutes (2)
- Over 40 years of age
- Valve malfunction

- Systemic lupus erythematosus
- Central venous catheters
- Nephrotic syndrome

These risk factors have been identified in the Padua Prediction risk assessment for venous thrombolytic events. A score of > or = 4 is a high-risk individual (Barbar et al., 2010).

Air Embolism

- Central line insertion or removal, sheath central line tubing changes, manipulation, or disconnection

Fat Embolism (Eriksson, Schultz, Cohle, & Post, 2011)

- Fractures—closed fractures produce more emboli than open fractures. Long bones, pelvis, and ribs cause more emboli. Sternum and clavicle furnish less. Multiple fractures produce more emboli.
- Orthopedic procedures—most commonly, intramedullary nailing of the long bones, hip, or knee replacements
- Massive soft tissue injury
- CPR is associated with a high incidence of PFE regardless of cause of death (Eriksson, 2011).
- Severe burns
- Bone marrow biopsy

Nontraumatic settings occasionally lead to fat embolism. These include conditions associated with:

- Liposuction
- Fatty liver
- Prolonged corticosteroid therapy
- Acute pancreatitis
- Osteomyelitis
- Conditions causing bone infarcts, especially sickle cell disease

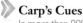 **Carp's Cues**

In more than 90% of cases of PE, the thrombosis originates in the deep veins of the legs. DVT is a distressing but often avoidable condition that leads to long-term complications such as the postphlebitic syndrome and chronic leg ulcers in a large proportion of individuals who have proximal vein thrombosis. PE remains the most common preventable cause of death in hospital (Lip & Hull, 2014).

The incidence of fat embolism syndrome (FES) varies from 1% to 29%. Fat emboli occur in all individuals with long-bone fractures, but only few patients develop systemic dysfunction, particularly the triad of skin, brain, and lung dysfunction known as FES (Eriksson, 2011).

Collaborative Outcomes

The individual will be monitored for early signs and symptoms of (a) DVT and (b) PE, and the individual will receive collaborative interventions if indicated to restore physiologic stability.

Indicators of Physiologic Stability

- No leg pain (a)
- No leg edema (a)
- No change in skin temperature or color (a, b)
- No acute dyspnea, restlessness, decreased mental status, or anxiety (b)
- No acute, sharp chest pain (b)
- Pulse: regular rhythm, rate 60 to 100 beats/min (b)
- Respirations 16 to 20 breaths/min (b)
- Blood pressure >90/60, <140/90 mm Hg, MAP >70, or CVP >11
- Breath sounds without evidence of new, abnormal sounds (rales, crackles) (b)
- No presence of distended neck veins (JVD) (b)

Interventions and Rationales

Screen for Prevention and Institute Prophylaxis per Protocol

- Consult with physician or advanced practice nurse for low-dose heparin/anticoagulant therapy for a high-risk individual. (See Anticoagulant Therapy in *Risk for Complications of Medication Therapy Adverse Effects*.)

R: *Heparin therapy decreases platelet adhesiveness, reducing the risk of embolism. In the presence of thrombosis, treatment goals are preventing the clot from becoming larger, preventing the formation of new blood clots.*

Monitor for Onset or Status of Venous Thrombosis, Noting

- Diminished or absent peripheral pulses

R: *Insufficient circulation causes pain and diminished peripheral pulses.*

- Unusual warmth and redness or coolness and cyanosis; increased leg swelling

R: *Unusual warmth and redness point to inflammation; coolness and cyanosis indicate vascular obstruction.*

* Increasing leg pain

R: *Leg pain results from tissue hypoxia.*

* A rapid heart rate and/or a feeling of passing out
* New chest pain with difficulty breathing

R: *These findings may indicate mobilization of thrombi to the lungs (PE).*

> **CLINICAL ALERT** Stay with person and call for Rapid Response Team.

Continue Use of Elastic Graduated Compression Stockings (GCS) If Prescribed

R: *These devices apply gentle pressure to improve circulation and help prevent clots. They should be used prior to surgery and before anticoagulant therapy (Lip & Hull, 2014).*

All Individuals Should Receive Venous Thromboembolism (VTE) Risk Assessment on Admission (Institute for Clinical System Improvement [ICSI], 2008; Partnership for Patient Care, 2007)

R: *In all individuals, the decision to anticoagulate should be individualized and the benefits of VTE prevention carefully weighed against the risk of bleeding.*

Assess for Contraindications to Anticoagulation (Lip & Hull, 2014)

* Absolute contraindications
  * Active bleeding, severe bleeding diathesis
  * Platelet count <50,000/µL
  * Recent, planned, or emergent surgery/procedure
  * Major trauma
  * A history of intracranial hemorrhage
* Relative contraindications
  * Recurrent bleeding from multiple gastrointestinal telangiectasias
  * Intracranial or spinal tumors
  * Platelet count <150,000/µL
  * Large abdominal aortic aneurysm with concurrent severe hypertension, and stable aortic dissection
* Additional relative contraindications in older patients (e.g., >65 years)

- Include a history of multiple falls and the presence of more than one factor that elevates the bleeding risk

R: *"Such patients are at high risk of bleeding or have a high risk of a catastrophic result should a bleed occur. Consequently, the decision to anticoagulate in this population should be even more cautious to allow the benefits of VTE prevention to be carefully weighed against the risk of bleeding"* (Lip & Hull, 2014).

Monitor for Signs and Symptoms of Pulmonary Embolism (Grossman & Porth, 2014)

- Acute, sharp chest pain
- Dyspnea, restlessness, cyanosis, decreased mental status, or anxiety
- Decreased oxygen saturation (SaO$_2$, SvO$_2$)
- Tachycardia
- Tachypnea (Shaughnessy, 2007)
- Neck vein distention
- Hypotension
- Acute right ventricular dilation without parenchymal disease (on chest X-ray)
- Confusion
- Cardiac dysrhythmias (can be lethal)
- Low-grade fever
- Productive cough with blood-tinged sputum
- Pleural friction rub or new murmur (Shaughnessy, 2007)
- Crackles

R: *Occlusion of pulmonary arteries impedes blood flow to the distal lung, producing a hypoxic state.*

If These Manifestations Occur, Promptly Initiate Protocols for Shock

- Establish an IV line (for medication and fluid administration).
- Administer fluid replacement therapy according to protocol.
- Insert indwelling urinary (Foley) catheter (to monitor circulatory volume through urine output).
- Initiate ECG monitoring and invasive hemodynamic monitoring (to detect dysrhythmias and guide therapy).
- Initiate unit protocols.
- Refer to *Risk for Complications of Hypovolemic* for additional interventions.
- Prepare for angiography and/or perfusion lung scans (to confirm diagnosis and detect the extent of atelectasis).

R: *Because death from massive PE commonly occurs in the first 2 hours after onset, prompt intervention is crucial.*

Initiate Oxygen Therapy; Monitor Oxygen Saturation

R: *This measure rapidly increases circulating oxygen levels.*

Provide Measures to Prevent Thrombosis

- Evaluate hydration status based on urine specific gravity, intake/output, weights, and serum osmolality. Take steps to ensure adequate hydration.

R: *Increased blood viscosity and coagulability and decreased cardiac output may contribute to thrombus formation.*

- Instruct to perform isotonic leg exercises, flexing knees and ankles hourly

R: *They promote venous return.*

- Ambulate as soon as possible with at least 5 minutes of walking each waking hour. Avoid prolonged chair sitting with legs dependent.

R: *Walking contracts leg muscles, stimulates the venous pump, and reduces stasis (ICSI, 2008; Lip & Hull, 2014).*

- Elevate the affected extremity above the level of the heart.

R: *This positioning can help reduce interstitial swelling by promoting venous return.*

- Stop smoking.

R: *Nicotine can cause vasospasms.*

 Carp's Cues

In 2002, the National Quality Forum created and endorsed a list of Serious Reportable Events (SREs), which was updated in 2006. There are 28 events that have been labeled as SREs; also called never events. "The 28 events on the list are largely preventable, grave errors and events that are of concern to the public and health-care providers and that warrant careful investigation and should be targeted for mandatory public reporting" (National Quality Forum, 2006). One of the 28 events is patient death or serious disability, associated with intravascular air embolism that occurs while being cared for in a health-care facility.

For Prevention of Air Emboli (Weinhouse, 2016)

- Explain to the individual what is going to happen and why it is important to follow the specific instructions.

R: *Positioning during central line removal is a critical intervention to prevent air embolism.*

- Perform hand hygiene and put on clean gloves. Remove the dressing carefully and discard it with your gloves. Repeat hand hygiene and put on sterile gloves.
- Assess the catheter insertion site for evidence of complications such as redness, swelling, or drainage. Notify the physician if you see any of these signs, he or she may order a culture. Clean the site according to facility policy, preferably with chlorhexidine.
- Never use scissors near the venous access device, as this could result in accidental severing of the catheter.
- Remove the catheter-securing device.
- Before central line catheter insertion and tubing changes, place the individual in supine or Trendelenburg's position and instruct him or her to perform Valsalva maneuver during the procedure. Instruct to take a deep breath and bear down, simulating applying downward pressure as if having a bowel movement. Have person demonstrate it. Remove the catheter as the person bears down.
- If the individual is unable to cooperate with procedure, perform during positive pressure portion of respiratory cycle (Luettel, 2011; *Lynn-McHale Wiegand, & Carlson, 2005).
  - Spontaneous breathing—during exhalation
  - Mechanical ventilation—during inhalation

R: *These measures increase intrathoracic pressure and help prevent air from entering the catheter.*

Follow Protocol to Remove Central Line Catheter

- After you have removed the catheter, tell the person to breathe normally. Apply pressure with the sterile gauze until bleeding stops (O'Dowd & Kelle, 2015).
- Apply a sterile air-occlusive dressing over the insertion site to prevent a delayed air embolism.
- Assess the length and integrity of the catheter and visually inspect the tip for smoothness. Remove your gloves and perform hand hygiene (O'Dowd & Kelle, 2015).
- Instruct individual to remain supine for 30 minutes after removal (O'Dowd & Kelle, 2015).

- Document the date and time of CVC removal, noting the CVC's length and integrity, the site assessment, patient response, and nursing interventions (O'Dowd & Kelle, 2015).
- Do not pull harder if resistance is met while removing a CVC (O'Dowd & Kelle, 2015).
- Do not remove it when the person is inhaling. Do not apply any dressing that is not air-occlusive, as this would increase the risk of a delayed air embolism (O'Dowd & Kelle, 2015).

R: *These measures help prevent air entry and infection at insertion site.*

Monitor for Signs and Symptoms of Air Embolism During Dressing and IV Tubing Changes and After Any Accidental Separation of IV Connections

- Sucking sound on insertion
- Dyspnea
- Tachypnea
- Wheezing
- Substernal chest pain
- Anxiety

R: *Air embolism can occur with IV tubing changes, with accidental tubing separation, and during catheter insertion, removal, and disconnection (e.g., an individual can aspirate as much as 200 mL of air from a deep breath during subclavian line disconnection). Entry of air into the pulmonary arterial system can obstruct blood flow, causing broncho-constriction of the affected lung area. Use lure lock connections to help prevent accidental disconnection.*

If Air Embolism Is Suspected, Call the Rapid Response Team or Call 911, Do Not Leave the Person

- Administer 100% oxygen.

R: *This promotes diffusion of nitrogen, which compresses an air embolism in about 80% of cases.*

- Place person flat or in Trendelenburg position and turn on to left side.

R: *This position displaces air away from pulmonary valve and traps it in the ventricle for radiologic aspiration.*

- Initiate protocols for respiratory or cardiac arrest if indicated.

For Risk for Complications of Fat Embolism

 Carp's Cues

Although fat emboli occur in all individuals with long-bone fractures, only few individuals develop systemic dysfunction of the skin, brain, and lung dysfunction known as FES. FES typically manifests 24 to 72 hours after the initial insult, but may rarely occur as early as 12 hours or as late as 2 weeks after the inciting event. Affected patients develop a classic triad—hypoxemia, neurologic abnormalities, and a petechial rash (Weinhouse, 2016).

Monitor for Signs and Symptoms of Fat Embolism

R: *FES typically manifests 24 to 72 hours after the initial insult, but may rarely occur as early as 12 hours or as late as 2 weeks after the inciting event. Affected individuals develop a classic triad—hypoxemia, neurologic abnormalities, and a petechial rash.*

- Hypoxemia, dyspnea, and tachypnea are the most frequent early findings. A syndrome indistinguishable from acute lung injury (ALI) or respiratory distress syndrome (ARDS) may develop. Approximately, one-half of individuals with FES caused by long-bone fractures develop severe hypoxemia and require mechanical ventilation.
- Breathlessness with or without vague pains in the chest. Depending on severity, this can progress to respiratory failure with tachypnea, increasing breathlessness and hypoxia.
- Fever—often in excess of 38.3° C with a disproportionately high pulse rate
- Petechial rash—commonly over the upper anterior part of the trunk, arm and neck, buccal mucosa, and conjunctivae. The rash may be transient, disappearing after 24 hours.
- Central nervous system symptoms, varying from a mild headache to significant cerebral dysfunction (restlessness, disorientation, confusion, seizures, stupor, or coma)
- Renal—oliguria, hematuria, anuria
- Tachypnea more than 30 per minute
- Sudden onset of chest pain or dyspnea
- Restlessness, apprehension
- Confusion

R: *Drowsiness with diminished urine output (oliguria) is almost diagnostic. Neurologic abnormalities develop in the majority of patients* *with FES. They typically occur after the development of respiratory distress, with affected patients developing a confusional state, followed by an altered level of consciousness (Weinhouse, 2016).*

- Elevated temperature above 103° F
- Increased pulse rate more than 140 per minute
- Petechial skin rash (12 to 96 hours postoperative)

R: *These changes are the result of hypoxemia. Fatty acids attack red blood cells and platelets to form microaggregates, which impair circulation to vital organs, such as the brain. Fatty globules passing through the pulmonary vasculature cause a chemical reaction that decreases lung compliance and ventilation/perfusion ratio and raises body temperature. Rash results from capillary fragility. Common sites are conjunctiva, axilla, chest, and neck (Weinhouse, 2016).*

- Minimize movement of a fractured extremity for the first 3 days after the injury.

R: *Immobilization minimizes further tissue trauma and reduces the risk of embolism dislodgement (Weinhouse, 2016).*

- Ensure adequate hydration.

R: *Optimal hydration dilutes the irritating fatty acids through the system (Weinhouse, 2016).*

- Monitor intake/output, urine color, and specific gravity.

R: *These data reflect hydration status.*

Risk for Complications of Hypovolemia

Definition

Describes a person experiencing or at high risk to experience inadequate cellular oxygenation and inability to excrete waste products of metabolism secondary to decreased fluid volume (e.g., from bleeding, plasma loss, prolonged vomiting, or diarrhea)

Hypovolemic shock refers to rapid fluid loss, resulting in multiple organ failure due to inadequate circulating volume and subsequent inadequate perfusion; most often caused by rapid blood loss due to a medical or surgical condition. Refer to *Risk for Complications of Bleeding* if indicated.

High-Risk Populations
(Grossman & Porth, 2014)

- Intraoperative status
- Postoperative status
- Postprocedural cannulation of any arterial vessel, but particularly those at risk for retroperitoneal bleed due to cannulation of femoral vessel
- Anaphylactic shock
- Trauma
- Bleeding (e.g., external [laceration, gunshot wound], internal [gastrointestinal, surgical site]
- Diabetic ketoacidosis (DKA) or hyperosmolar hyperglycemic state (HHS)
- Excessive gastrointestinal (GI) fluid losses (vomiting, diarrhea, gastrointestinal suctioning, draining GI fistula)
- Excessive renal losses (diuretic therapy, osmotic diuresis related to hyperglycemia)
- Excessive skin losses (fever, exposure to hot environment, loss of skin due to burns, wounds)
- Infants, children, older persons
- Acute pancreatitis
- Major burns
- Disseminated intravascular coagulation (DIC)
- Diabetes insipidus
- Ascites
- Peritonitis
- Intestinal obstruction
- SIRS/sepsis
- Hyponatremia

Collaborative Outcomes

The individual will be monitored for early signs and symptoms of hypovolemia and will receive collaborative interventions if indicated to restore physiologic stability.

Indicators of Physiologic Stability

Refer to *Risk for Complications of Decreased Cardiac Output* for indicators.

Interventions and Rationales

Monitor Fluid Status Hourly If Indicated; Evaluate

- Intake (parenteral and oral)
- Output and other losses (urine, drainage, and vomiting), naso-gastric tube

R: *Decreased blood volume reduces blood to kidneys, which decreases the GFR, causing a decreased urine output. When blood flow to the kidneys is less than 20% to 25% of normal, ischemic damage occurs (Grossman & Porth, 2014). Decreased urine output is an early sign of bleeding/hypovolemia.*

Monitor the Surgical Site for Bleeding, Dehiscence, and Evisceration

R: *Careful monitoring allows early detection of complications.*

Teach to Splint the Surgical Wound With a Pillow When Coughing, Sneezing, or Vomiting

R: *Splinting reduces stress on suture line by equalizing pressure across the wound.*

Monitor for Signs and Symptoms of Shock

- Increased pulse rate with normal or slightly decreased blood pressure, narrowing pulse pressure; decreased MAP
- Urine output <0.5 mL/kg/hr (early sign)
- Restlessness, agitation, decreased mentation
- Increased respiratory rate, thirst
- Diminished peripheral pulses
- Cool, pale, moist, or cyanotic skin
- Decreased oxygenation saturation (SaO_2, SvO_2), pulmonary artery pressures, cardiac output/index, right atrial pressure, wedge/occlusion pressure
- Decreased hemoglobin/hematocrit, decreased cardiac output/index
- Decreased CVP

R: *The compensatory response to decreased circulatory volume aims to increase oxygen delivery through increased heart and respiratory rates and decreased peripheral circulation (manifested by diminished peripheral pulses and cool skin). Decreased oxygen to the brain alters mentation. Decreased circulation to the kidneys leads to decreased urine output. Hemoglobin and hematocrit values decline if bleeding is significant (Grossman & Porth, 2014).*

If Shock Occurs, Place Individual in the Supine Position Unless Contraindicated (e.g., Head Injury)

R: *This position increases blood return (preload) to the heart.*

Per Protocol, Insert an IV Line; Use a Large-Bore Catheter for Blood or Large-Volume Fluid Replacement

- Initiate appropriate protocols for shock (e.g., vasopressor therapy oxygen therapy).

R: *Protocols aim to increase peripheral resistance and elevate blood pressure.*

Collaborate With Physician, Physician Assistant, or Advanced Practice Nurse to Replace Fluid Losses at a Rate Sufficient to Maintain Urine Output >0.5 mL/kg/hr (e.g., Saline or Ringer's Lactate)

R: *This measure promotes optimal renal tissue perfusion.*

Restrict Individual's Movement and Activity

R: *This helps decrease tissue demands for oxygen.*

Provide Reassurance, Simple Explanations, and Emotional Support to Help Reduce Anxiety

R: *High anxiety increases metabolic demands for oxygen.*

Risk for Complications of Systemic Inflammatory Response Syndrome (SIRS)/Sepsis

 Carp's Cues

"The primary treatment for all shock syndromes is early recognition of factors that may place the client at risk for developing shock." Allergic response can progress to anaphylactic shock. Invasive lines can be sources of infection.

SIRS has replaced the terminology septic syndrome. Sepsis is one contributing factor to SIRS; SIRS is a life-threatening condition related to systemic inflammation, organ dysfunction, and organ failure.

Definition of Risk for Complications of Systemic Inflammatory Response Syndrome (SIRS)

Describes a person experiencing or at high risk to experience a life-threatening condition related to systemic inflammation, organ dysfunction, and organ failure in response to the presence of pathogenic bacteria, viruses, fungi, or their toxins. The microorganisms may or may not be present in the bloodstream. SIRS has replaced the terminology *septic syndrome*. Sepsis is one contributing factor to SIRS.

Definition of Risk for Complications of Septic Shock

Describes a person experiencing or at risk for experiencing a loss of circulatory volume (hypovolemia) and impaired perfusion caused by an infectious agent (bacterial, viral), resulting in compromised tissue perfusion and cellular dysfunction

High-Risk Populations

Individuals with

- Bacterial infection (urinary, respiratory, wound)
- Viral infection
- Complication of surgery (GI, thoracic)
- Drug overdose
  - Burns, multiple trauma
  - Immunosuppression, AIDS
- Invasive lines (urinary, arterial, endotracheal, or central venous catheter)
- Pressure ulcers
  - Extensive slow-healing wounds
  - Immunocompromised (transplants, cancer, chemotherapy, AIDS, cirrhosis, pancreatitis)
- Diabetes mellitus
- Extreme age (<1 year and >65 years)

Collaborative Outcomes

The individual will be monitored for early signs and symptoms of septic shock and will receive collaborative interventions if indicated to restore physiologic stability.

Indicators of Physiologic Stability

- Temperature 98° F to 99.5° F
- Pulse 60 to 100 beats/min
- Capillary refill <2 seconds
- Urine output >0.5/mL/kg/hr
- Urine specific gravity 1.005 to 1.030
- White blood count greater than 4,000 cells/mm^3 or less than 12,000 cells/mm^3
- Less than 10% immature neutrophils (band forms)
- Activated protein C (APC) 65 to 135 International Units/dL
- Platelets 150 to 400
- Prothrombin time 11 to 13.5 seconds
- INR 1.5 to 2.5
- Partial thromboplastin time (PTT) 30 to 45 seconds
- Serum potassium 3.5 to 5.0 mEq/L
- Serum sodium 135 to 145 mEq/L
- Blood glucose (fasting) <100 mg/dL
- Serum lactate levels 1.0 to 2.5 mmol/L

Interventions and Rationales

Monitor for Septic Shock and SIRS (Halloran, 2009)

- Urine output <0.5 mL/kg/hr

R: *Urine output is decreased when sodium shifts into the cells, which pulls water into cells. Decreased circulation to kidneys reduces their ability to detoxify the toxins that result from anaerobic metabolism.*

- Body temperature greater than 38° C or less than 36° C
- Heart rate greater than 90 per minute

R: *High heart rate decreases blood flow to brain, heart, and kidneys.*

- Triggers baroreceptors and release of catecholamines, increasing heart rate/cardiac output and further increasing vasoconstriction
- Hyperkalemia

R: *Potassium moves into the cell with the sodium, impairing nervous, cardiovascular, and muscle cell function.*

- Decreasing blood pressure

R: *Movement of water into the cell causes hypovolemia.*

- Respiratory rate greater than 20 per minute

R: *Anaerobic metabolism decreases circulating oxygen. The body attempts to increase oxygenation by increasing respiratory rate.*

• Hyperglycemia

R: *The liver and kidneys produce more glucose in response to the release of epinephrine, norepinephrine, cortisol, and glucagon. Anaerobic metabolism reduces the effects of insulin. Insulin resistance contributes to multiple organ failure, nosocomial infection, and renal injury (Grossman & Porth, 2014).*

• WBC greater than 12,000 per microliter or less than 4,000 per microliter or presence of 10% immature neutrophils

R: *Increased white cells indicate an infectious process.*

Ensure That Blood Culture is Done Prior to the Start of Any Antibiotic

• Culture any suspected infection sites (e.g., urine, sputum, invasive lines).

R: *"Poor outcomes are associated with inadequate or inappropriate antimicrobial therapy (i.e., treatment with antibiotics to which the pathogen was later shown to be resistant in vitro). They are also associated with delays in initiating antimicrobial therapy, even short delays (e.g., an hour)" (Schmidt & Mandel, 2012).*

• Blood culture obtained after antibiotic therapy has been initiated can be inaccurate. Research of individuals with septic shock demonstrated that the time to initiation of appropriate antimicrobial therapy was the strongest predictor of mortality (Schmidt & Mandel, 2012).

Assess Fluid Status

• Monitor CVP and follow protocol for fluid replacement. Early goal-directed therapy (EGDT) with fluid replacement improves cardiac output, tissue perfusion, and oxygen delivery, improving mortality and morbidity.

R: *Sepsis causes vasodilation and capillary leak, resulting in hypovolemia.*

Monitor Blood Pressure

• Administer replacement fluids and vasopressors (especially norepinephrine) to maintain MAP >65.

R: *In EGDT, maintaining MAP >65 improves tissue perfusion and outcomes (Neviere, 2015).*

Assess for Evidence of Adequate Tissue Perfusion: Heart Rate, Respirations, Urine Output, Mentation, ScvO$_2$/SvO$_2$

R: *Close monitoring detects early changes, with immediate interventions.*

Evaluate Skin Integrity and Protect From Injury and Hypothermia

R: *Decreased perfusion to skin will result in pale, cool, fragile skin. The tissue is more prone to injury and hypothermia.*

Monitor Serum Glucose Levels

- Use insulin (IV) per protocol to maintain tight glycemic control <150mg/dL.

R: *Tight glycemic control improves individual outcomes (Picard et al., 2006).*

Implement Strategies to Prevent Thromboembolic Events

R: *Endothelial injury activates Factor XII, which stimulates the clotting factors. In sepsis, coagulation produces thrombi and emboli, which block microvasculature. Activated protein C (APC) is lowered in sepsis, which results in increased coagulation and fibrinolysis (Halloran, 2009).*

Monitor Older Adults for Changes in Mentation; Weakness, Malaise; Normothermia or Hypothermia; and Anorexia

Risk for Complications of Acute Urinary Retention

Definition

Describes a person experiencing or at high risk to experience an acute abnormal accumulation of urine in the bladder and the inability to void due to a temporary situation (e.g., postoperative status) or to a condition reversible with surgery (e.g., prostatectomy) or medications

High-Risk Populations
(Barrisford & Steele 2014; Selius & Subedi, 2008)

Acute urinary retention is most often secondary to obstruction, but may also be related to trauma, medication, neurologic disease, infection, and occasionally psychologic issues

- Postoperative status (e.g., surgery of the perineal area, lower abdomen)
- Postpartum status
- Benign masses (e.g., fibroids)
- Malignant tumors of the pelvis, urethra, or vagina
- Postpartum vulvar edema
- Anxiety
- Prostate enlargement, prostatitis, prostate cancer
- Medication side effects (e.g., atropine, antidepressants, antihistamines)
- Postarteriography status
- Bladder outlet obstruction (infection, tumor, calculi/stone, constipation, urethral stricture, perianal abscess)
  - Impaired detrusor contractility (spinal cord injuries, progressive neurologic diseases, diabetic neuropathy, cerebrovascular accidents)
  - Malignancy—bladder neoplasm, other tumors causing spinal cord compression
  - Other infections—genital herpes, varicella zoster, infected foreign bodies

Collaborative Outcomes

The individual will be monitored for early signs and symptoms of acute urinary retention and receive collaborative intervention to restore physiologic stability.

Indicators of Physiologic Stability

- Urinary output >1,500 mL/24 hours
- Can verbalize bladder fullness
- No complaints of lower abdominal pressure

Interventions and Rationales

Monitor a Postoperative Individual for Urinary Retention

R: *Trauma to the detrusor muscle and injury to the pelvic nerves during surgery can inhibit bladder function. Anxiety and pain can cause spasms of the reflex sphincters. Bladder neck edema can cause retention.*

Sedatives and narcotics can affect the CNS and effectiveness of smooth muscles (Grossman & Porth, 2014; Urinary Retention, 2012).

Monitor for Urinary Retention by Palpating and Percussing the Suprapubic Area for Signs of Bladder Distention (Overdistension, etc.)

- Instruct individual to report bladder discomfort or inability to void.

R: *These problems may be early signs of urinary retention.*

If an Individual Does Not Void Within 8 to 10 Hours After Surgery or Complains of Bladder Discomfort, Take the Following Steps

- Warm the bedpan.
- Encourage individual to get out of bed to use the bathroom, if possible.
- Instruct the individual to stand when urinating, if possible. If unable to stand, even sitting at the side of the bed helps.
- Run water in the sink as individual attempts to void.
- Pour warm water over individual's perineum.

R: *These measures help promote relaxation of the urinary sphincter and facilitate voiding.*

After the First Voiding Postsurgery, Continue to Monitor and to Encourage Individual to Void Again in 1 Hour or So

R: *The first voiding usually does not empty the bladder completely.*

If the Individual Still Cannot Void After 10 Hours, Follow Protocols for Straight Catheterization, as Ordered by Physician, Physician Assistant, or Advanced Practice Nurse

- Consider bladder scanning to determine if the amount of urine in the bladder necessitates catheterization.

R: *Straight catheterization is preferable to indwelling catheterization because it carries less risk of urinary tract infection from ascending pathogens. Bladder scanning is not a risk for infection.*

If Person is Voiding Small Amounts, Use Straight Catheterization; If Postvoid Residual is >200 mL, Leave Catheter Indwelling

- Notify physician, physician assistant, or advanced practice nurse.

Risk for Complications of Renal Insufficiency/Failure

Definition

Renal insufficiency is an early sign of poor function of the kidneys that may be due to a reduction in blood flow to the kidneys caused by renal artery disease. Proper kidney function may be disrupted, however, when the arteries that provide the kidneys with blood become narrowed, a condition called renal artery stenosis. Some patients with renal insufficiency experience no symptoms or only mild symptoms. Others develop dangerously high blood pressure, poor kidney function, or kidney failure that requires dialysis (Kovesdy, Kopple, & Kalantar-Zadeh, 2015).

Stages of Renal Failure
(Kovesdy et al., 2015)

Stage 1

GFR >90+
Normal kidney function, but urine findings or structural abnormalities or genetic trait points to kidney disease; observation; control of blood pressure

Stage 2

GFR >60 to 89
Mildly reduced kidney function and other findings (as for stage 1) point to kidney disease; observation; control of blood pressure and risk factors

Stage 3A

GFR > 45 to 59
Moderately reduced kidney function; observation, control of blood pressure and risk factors

Stage 3B

GFR >30 to 44
Moderately reduced kidney function; observation, control of blood pressure and risk factors

Stage 4

GFR >15 to 29
Severely reduced kidney function; planning for end-stage renal failure

Stage 5

GFR <15 or on dialysis
Very severe, or end-stage kidney failure (sometimes called established renal failure)

High-Risk Populations
(Grossman & Porth, 2014; Kovesdy et al., 2015)

- High-risk individuals
  - Older persons
  - Postsurgical
  - Major trauma
  - Underlying chronic kidney disease
- Renal tubular necrosis from ischemic causes
  - Excessive diuretic use
  - PE
  - Burns
  - Intrarenal thrombosis
  - Rhabdomyolysis
  - Renal infections
  - Renal artery stenosis/thrombosis
  - Peritonitis
  - Sepsis
  - Hypovolemia
  - Hypotension
  - Congestive heart failure
  - Myocardial infarction
  - Aneurysm
  - Aneurysm repair
- Renal tubular necrosis from toxicity
- Nonsteroidal anti-inflammatory drugs
  - Gout (hyperuricemia)
  - Hypercalcemia
  - Certain street drugs (e.g., PCP)
  - Gram-negative infection
  - Radiocontrast media
  - Aminoglycoside antibiotics

- Antineoplastic agents
- Methanol, carbon tetrachloride
- Snake venom, poison mushroom
- Phenacetin-type analgesics
- Heavy metals
- Insecticides, fungicides
- Diabetes mellitus
- Malignant hypertension
- Hemolysis (e.g., from transfusion reaction)

Collaborative Outcomes

The individual will be monitored for early signs and symptoms of renal insufficiency with a goal of preventing or minimizing chronic damage. The individual will receive collaborative interventions as indicated to restore and/or maintain physiologic stability.

Indicators of Physiologic Stability

- Blood pressure: Less than 120 systolic and less than 80 diastolic
- Urine specific gravity 1.005 to 1.030
- Urine output >0.5 mL/hr
- Urine sodium 40 to 220 mEq/L/24 hr (varies by dietary intake, medications)
- Blood urea nitrogen 10 to 20 mg/dL
- Serum potassium 3.8 to 5 mEq/L
- Serum sodium 135 to 145 mEq/L
- Serum phosphorus 2.5 to 4.5 mg/dL
- Serum creatinine clearance 100 to 150 mL/min (varies by age, gender, and race)
- GFR over 90 in individuals with no renal failure or in Stage I

Interventions and Rationales

Monitor for Early Signs and Symptoms of Renal Insufficiency

- Sustained elevated urine specific gravity, elevated urine sodium levels
- Sustained insufficient urine output (<30 mL/hr), elevated blood pressure
- Elevated blood urea nitrogen (BUN), serum creatinine, potassium, phosphorus, and decreased bicarbonate (CO_2); decreased creatinine clearance
- Dependent edema (periorbital, pedal, pretibial, sacral)

- Nocturia
- Lethargy
- Itching
- Nausea/vomiting

R: *Hypovolemia and hypotension activate the renin–angiotensin system, which causes peripheral vasoconstriction and increases glomerular blood flow. The result is increased sodium and water reabsorption with decreased urine output. BUN is also reabsorbed. If this adaptive mechanism is inadequate, acute kidney injury from ischemia develops. Urine output remains low or diminishes and blood pressure is elevated (Fazia, Lin, & Staros, 2012). Decreased excretion of urea and creatinine in the urine elevates BUN and creatinine levels. Dependent edema results from increased plasma hydrostatic pressure, salt, and water retention, and/or decreased colloid osmotic pressure from plasma protein losses (Grossman & Porth, 2014).*

Notify Physician/NP/PA of Changes in Condition or Laboratory Results, Which Reflect Increasing Renal Insufficiency

Weigh Daily at a Minimum; More Often, If Indicated

- Ensure accurate findings by weighing at the same time each day, on the same scale, and with the individual wearing the same amount of clothing.

R: *Daily weights and intake and output records help evaluate fluid balance and guide fluid intake recommendations.*

- Maintain strict intake and output records; determine the net fluid balance and compare with daily weight loss or gain for correlation. (A 1-kg [2.2-lb] weight gain correlates with excess intake of 1 L.)
- Administer oral medications with meals whenever possible. If medications must be administered between meals, give with the smallest amount of fluid necessary.

R: *This measure avoids using parts of the fluid allowance unnecessarily.*

- Explain prescribed fluid management goals.

R: *Individual and family understanding may enhance cooperation.*

- Adjust daily fluid intake so it approximates fluid loss plus 300 to 500 mL/day.

R: *Careful replacement therapy is necessary to prevent fluid overload.*

- Distribute fluid intake fairly evenly throughout the entire day and night. It may be necessary to match fluid intake with loss every 8 hours or even every hour if the individual is critically imbalanced.

R: *Maintaining a constant fluid balance, without major fluctuations, is essential. Allowing toxins to accumulate because of poor hydration can cause complications such as nausea and sensorium changes.*

• Encourage to express feelings; give positive feedback.

R: *Fluid and diet restrictions can be extremely frustrating. Emotional support can help reduce anxiety and may improve compliance with the treatment regimen.*

• Consult with a dietitian regarding the fluid and diet plan.

R: *Important considerations in fluid management, requiring a specialist's attention, include the fluid content of nonliquid food, appropriate amount and type of liquids, liquid preferences, and sodium content.*

For Renal Failure

Monitor for Hematuria and Proteinuria (The Renal Association, 2013)

Visible (macroscopic) hematuria (usually referred immediately to urology or to nephrology if acute renal pathology is suspected)

Invisible (microscopic) hematuria without proteinuria, GFR >60 mL/min/1.73m^2

• Age >40, usually refer to Urology (recommended age may vary locally)
• Age <40 or >40 with negative urologic investigations. Refer to nephrology.

Microscopic hematuria with protein/creatinine ratio >50 mg/mmol

• Refer to nephrology if urologic investigations negative.
• Refer to nephrology.

CLINICAL ALERT GFR is usually based on serum creatinine level, age, sex, and race. For Afro-Caribbean black individuals, estimated GFR was 21% higher for any given creatinine.

Most laboratory reports indicate a normal range for white and black individuals (The Renal Association, 2013).

Monitor for Signs and Symptoms of Increasing Renal Failure

• GFR over 90
• Sustained elevated urine specific gravity, elevated urine sodium levels
• Sustained insufficient urine output (<30 mL/hr), elevated blood pressure

Risk for Complications of Cardiac/Vascular/Respiratory Dysfunction 743

- Elevated BUN, serum creatinine, potassium, phosphorus, and decreased bicarbonate (CO_2); decreased creatinine clearance
- Dependent edema (periorbital, pedal, pretibial, sacral)
- Nocturia
- Lethargy
- Itching
- Nausea/vomiting

R: *Hypovolemia and hypotension activate the renin–angiotensin system, which causes peripheral vasoconstriction and decreases GFR (blood flow). The result is increased sodium and water reabsorption with decreased urine output. BUN is also reabsorbed. If this adaptive mechanism is inadequate, acute kidney injury from ischemia develops. Urine output remains low or diminishes and blood pressure is elevated (Fazia et al., 2012). Decreased excretion of urea and creatinine in the urine elevates BUN and creatinine levels. Dependent edema results from increased plasma hydrostatic pressure, salt, and water retention, and/or decreased colloid osmotic pressure from plasma protein losses (Grossman & Porth, 2014).*

Notify Physician, Physician Assistant, or Nurse Practitioner of Changes in Condition or Laboratory Results, Which Reflect Increasing Renal Insufficiency/Failure

Weigh Daily at a Minimum

- Ensure accurate findings by weighing at the same time each day, on the same scale, and with the person wearing the same amount of clothing.

Avoid Continuous IV Fluid Infusion Whenever Possible

- Dilute all necessary IV drugs in the smallest amount of fluid that is safe for IV administration. Use small IV bags and an IV controller or pump, if possible, to prevent accidental infusion of a large volume of fluid.

R: *Extremely accurate fluid infusion is necessary to prevent fluid overload.*

Monitor for Signs and Symptoms of Metabolic Acidosis

- Rapid, shallow respirations
- Headaches
- Nausea and vomiting
- Low plasma pH
- Behavioral changes, drowsiness, lethargy

R: *Acidosis results from the kidney's inability to excrete hydrogen ions, phosphates, sulfates, and ketone bodies. Bicarbonate loss results from decreased renal resorption. Hyperkalemia, hyperphosphatemia, and*

*decreased bicarbonate levels aggravate metabolic acidosis. Excessive
ketone bodies cause headaches, nausea, vomiting, and abdominal pain.
Respiratory rate and depth increase in an attempt to increase CO_2
excretion and thus reduce acidosis. Acidosis affects the CNS and can
increase neuromuscular irritability because of the cellular exchange of
hydrogen and potassium.*

**Assess for Signs and Symptoms of Hypocalcemia, Hypokalemia, and
Alkalosis as Acidosis is Corrected**

R: *Rapid correction of acidosis may cause rapid excretion of calcium and
potassium and result in rebound alkalosis.*

Monitor for Signs and Symptoms of Hypernatremia With Fluid Overload

- Extreme thirst
- CNS effects ranging from agitation to convulsion

R: *Hypernatremia results from excessive sodium intake or increased
aldosterone output. Water is pulled from the cells, causing cellular
dehydration and producing CNS symptoms. Thirst is a compensatory
response aimed at diluting sodium.*

Maintain Prescribed Sodium Restrictions

R: *Hypernatremia must be corrected slowly to minimize CNS deterioration.*

Monitor for Electrolyte Imbalances

- Potassium
- Calcium
- Phosphorus
- Sodium
- Magnesium

Monitor for GI Bleeding

- Refer to *Risk for Complications of GI Bleeding* for specific
  interventions.

R: *The poor platelet aggregation and capillary fragility associated
with high serum levels of nitrogenous wastes may aggravate bleeding.
Heparinization required during dialysis in cases of gastric ulcer disease
also may precipitate GI bleeding.*

Monitor for Manifestations of Anemia

- Dyspnea
- Fatigue
- Tachycardia, palpitations
- Cold intolerance
- Pallor of nail beds and mucous membranes

- Low hemoglobin and hematocrit levels
- Easy bruising

R: *Chronic renal failure results in decreased red blood cell production because of decreased erythropoietin production and decreased survival time because of elevated uremic toxins.*

Instruct Individual to Use a Soft Toothbrush and to Avoid Vigorous Nose Blowing, Constipation, and Contact Sports

R: *Trauma prevention reduces the risk of bleeding and infection.*

Demonstrate the Pressure Method to Control Bleeding Should It Occurs

R: *Applying direct, constant pressure on a bleeding site can help prevent excessive blood loss.*

Monitor for Manifestations of Hypoalbuminemia (Deegens & Wetzels, 2011)

- Serum albumin level <3.5 g/dL; proteinuria (>150 mg/24 hr)
- Edema formation: pedal, facial, sacral
- Hypovolemia (more common in very low [<1 m/dL] serum albumin levels)
- Decreased hematocrit and hemoglobin levels in advancing disease
- Hyperlipidemia

R: *When albumin leaks into the urine because of changes in the glomerular electrostatic barrier or because of peritoneal dialysis, the liver responds by increasing production of plasma proteins. When the loss is great, the liver cannot compensate, and hypoalbuminemia results.*

Monitor for Hypervolemia

- Evaluate daily
  - Weight
  - Fluid intake and output records
  - Rales in lungs
  - Circumference of the edematous parts
  - Laboratory data: hematocrit, serum sodium, and plasma protein in specific serum albumin

R: *As GFR decreases and the functioning nephron mass continues to diminish, the kidneys lose the ability to concentrate urine and to excrete sodium and water, resulting in hypervolemia.*

Monitor for Signs and Symptoms of Congestive Heart Failure and Decreased Cardiac Output

- Refer to *RC of Decreased Cardiac Output.*

Risk for Complications of GI Bleeding

Definition

Describes a person experiencing or at high risk to experience GI bleeding

 Carp's Cues

The three nonsurgical modalities used to diagnose lower gastrointestinal bleeding (LGIB) are colonoscopy, radionuclide scans, and angiography. Apart from colonoscopy, endoscopic procedures such as esophagogastroduodenoscopy (EGD), wireless capsule endoscopy (WCE), push enteroscopy, and double-balloon enteroscopy are used depending on the clinical circumstance. The sequence of using various modalities depends on such factors as rate of bleeding, hemodynamic status of the individual, and inability to localize bleeding with the initial modality.

High-Risk Populations

Upper GI Bleeding (Rockey, 2015)

- Miscellaneous causes
  - Older persons
  - Daily use of aspirin or nonsteroidal anti-inflammatory drugs (NSAIDs)
  - Antiplatelet therapy and proton pump inhibitor cotherapy
  - Selective serotonin reuptake inhibitors or serotonin-specific reuptake inhibitors (SSRIs)
  - Prolonged mechanical ventilation >48 hours
  - Recent stress (e.g., trauma, sepsis)
  - Platelet deficiency
  - Coagulopathy
  - Shock, hypotension
  - Major surgery (>3 hours)
  - Head injury
  - Severe vascular disease
  - Disorders of GI, hepatic, and biliary systems
  - Transfusion of 5 units (or more) of blood
  - Burns (>35% of body)
  - Hematobilia, or bleeding from the biliary tree

- Hemosuccus pancreaticus, or bleeding from the pancreatic duct
- Severe superior mesenteric artery syndrome
- Esophageal causes
  - Esophageal varices
  - Esophagitis
  - Esophageal cancer
  - Esophageal ulcers
  - Mallory-Weiss tear
- Gastric causes
  - Gastric ulcer
  - Gastric cancer
  - Gastritis
  - Gastric varices
  - Gastric antral vascular ectasia
  - Dieulafoy's lesions
- Duodenal causes
  - Duodenal ulcer
  - Vascular malformation
  - Antithrombotic therapy

Lower GI Bleeding in Adults/Percentage (Strate, 2015)

- Diverticular disease (60%)
  - Diverticulosis/diverticulitis of small intestine
  - Diverticulosis/diverticulitis of colon
- Inflammatory bowel disease (13%)
  - Crohn's disease of small bowel, colon, or both
  - Ulcerative colitis
  - Noninfectious gastroenteritis and colitis
- Benign anorectal diseases (11%)
  - Hemorrhoids
  - Anal fissure
  - Fistula-in-ano
- Neoplasia (9%)
  - Malignant neoplasia of small intestine
  - Malignant neoplasia of colon, rectum, and anus
- Coagulopathy (4%)
- Arteriovenous malformations (3%)

Collaborative Outcomes

The individual will be monitored for early signs and symptoms of GI bleeding and will receive collaborative interventions if indicated to restore physiologic stability.

Indicators of Physiologic Stability

- Negative stool occult blood
- Calm, oriented
- Hemodynamic stability (BP, pulse, urine output)
- Refer to *Risk for Complications of Hypovolemia.*

Interventions and Rationales

Monitor Heart Rate and Blood Pressure for Signs of Hypovolemia as (Strate, 2015)

- Mild to moderate hypovolemia: Resting tachycardia
- Blood volume loss of at least 15%: orthostatic hypotension (a decrease in the systolic blood pressure of more than 20 mm Hg and/or an increase in heart rate of 20 beats/min when moving from recumbency to standing)
- Blood volume loss of at least 40%: supine hypotension

R: *Small changes in pulse and blood pressure findings can be significant for early detection.*

Monitor Hemoglobin Level Every 2 to 8 Hours, Depending on the Severity of the Bleed

- Determine the individual's baseline prior to GI bleeding.

R: *The individual may have a lower baseline due to chronic anemia (Strate, 2015).*

Monitor for Signs and Symptoms of Acute Upper GI Bleeding

- Hematemesis (vomiting blood)
- Melena (dark stool)
- Dysphasia, dyspepsia
- Epigastric pain
- Heartburn
- Diffuse abdominal pain
- Weight loss
- Presyncope, syncope

R: *Clinical manifestations depend on the amount and duration of upper GI bleeding. Early detection enables prompt intervention to minimize complications.*

Monitor for Lower GI Bleeding

- Maroon-colored stools
- Bright red blood
- Blood clots in rectum

R: *LGIB ranges from trivial hematochezia (blood in stool) to massive hemorrhage with shock and accounts for up to 24% of all cases of GI bleeding. This condition is associated with significant morbidity and mortality (10% to 20%). LGIB is one of the most common gastrointestinal indications for hospital admission, particularly in older persons. Diverticulitis accounts for up to 50% of cases, followed by ischemic colitis and anorectal lesions (Strate, 2015).*

Monitor for Occult Blood in Gastric Aspirates and Bowel Movements

R: *An individual can lose 100 mL of blood in stool and may have normal appearing stools. Testing stool for occult blood is more accurate.*

• Test nasogastric aspirate with Gastroccult.

R: *The Hemoccult test's sensitivity is reduced by the acidic environment, and the Gastroccult test is the most accurate.*

• Test stool for occult blood with FOBT (fecal occult blood test).

R: *The Gastroccult test is not recommended for use with fecal samples.*

CLINICAL ALERT Massive LGIB is a life-threatening condition; although this condition manifests as maroon stools or bright red blood from the rectum, individuals with massive upper gastrointestinal bleeding (UGIB) may also present with similar findings. Regardless of the level of the bleeding, one of the most important elements of the management of individuals with massive UGIB or LGIB is restoring hemodynamic stability (Strate, 2015).

Institute Protocols for Volume Replacement (e.g., Two Large-Bore Intravenous (IV) Catheters and Isotonic Crystalloid Infusions)

R: *Orthostatic hypotension (i.e., a blood pressure fall of >10 mm Hg) is usually indicative of blood loss of more than 1,000 mL (Grossman & Porth, 2014).*

Prepare for Transfusion per Physician/Physician Assistant/Advanced Practice Nurse Orders and Protocol

R: *The goal is to increase blood volume and treat or prevent hypovolemic shock.*

Monitor Hemoglobin, Hematocrit, Red Blood Cell Count, Platelets, Prothrombin Time, Partial Thromboplastin Time, Type Blood and Cross Match, and BUN Values

R: *These values reflect the effectiveness of therapy.*

- Initiate prophylaxis stress ulcers protocol for persons on mechanical ventilation (e.g., oral proton pump inhibitor or intravenous histamine-2 receptor antagonist [H_2 blocker] or intravenous PPI; Weinhouse, 2016).

R: *Researchers have reported an incidence of 46.7% of GI bleeding in individuals on mechanical ventilation (Chu et al., 2010, p. 34). Critically ill individuals experience a decrease in the protective mucous layer in the stomach, hyper secretion of acid due to excessive gastrin stimulation, and inadequate perfusion to stomach secondary to shock, infection, or trauma (Weinhouse, 2016).*

CLINICAL ALERT Acute respiratory failure requiring mechanical ventilation for more than 48 hours has been shown to be one of the two strongest independent risk factors for clinically important GI bleeding in the ICU (Chu et al., 2010).

Monitor for Complications Associated with Mechanical Ventilation, Such as Stress Ulcer and GI Hypomotility

R: *Mechanical ventilation, with increased positive end expiratory pressure (PEEP), increases intrathoracic pressure. This decreases perfusion to GI tract (Weinhouse, 2016).*

- Diarrhea
- Decreased bowel sounds
- High gastric residuals
- Constipation
- Ileus

If hypovolemia occurs, refer to *Risk for Complications of Hypovolemia* for more information and specific interventions.

Risk for Complications of Paralytic Ileus

Definition

Describes a person experiencing or at high risk to experience neurogenic or functional bowel obstruction

High-Risk Populations

- Bacteria or viruses that cause intestinal infections (gastroenteritis)
- Thrombosis or embolus to mesenteric vessels
- Any major surgery with use of general anesthesia and subsequent limitation of mobility, as well as minor surgery of the abdomen
- Postoperative status (bowel, retroperitoneal, or spinal cord surgery)
- Kidney or lung disease
- Use of certain medications, especially narcotics
- Decreased blood supply to the intestines (mesenteric ischemia)
- Postshock status
- Hypovolemia
- Infections inside the abdomen, such as appendicitis
- Chemical, electrolyte, mineral imbalances (e.g., hypokalemia)
- Posttrauma (e.g., spinal cord injury)
- Uremia
- Spinal cord lesion
- Mechanical causes of intestinal obstruction may include (Bordeianou & Yeh, 2015):
  - Adhesions or scar tissue that forms after surgery
  - Foreign bodies that block the intestines
  - Gallstones (rare)
  - Hernias
  - Impacted stool
  - Intussusception (telescoping of one segment of bowel into another)
  - Tumors blocking the intestines
  - Volvulus (twisted intestine)

Collaborative Outcomes

The individual will be monitored for early signs and symptoms of paralytic ileus and will receive collaborative interventions, if indicated, to restore physiologic stability.

Indicators of Physiologic Stability

- Bowel sounds present
- No nausea and vomiting
- No abdominal distention
- No change in bowel function
- Evidence of flatus

Interventions and Rationales

Auscultate Each of the Four Abdominal Quadrants to Evaluate the Specific Function of Large (Colon) and Small Intestines as

- The right upper quadrant contains lower margin of the liver, the gallbladder, part of the large intestine, a few loops of the small intestine.
- The right lower quadrant contains the appendix, the connection between the large and small intestines, loops of bowel.
- The left upper quadrant contains the lower margin of the spleen, part of the pancreas, some of the stomach and duodenum.
- The left lower quadrant contains bowel loops and the descending colon.

R: *Knowing the structures under the stethoscope will help to determine the nature of the bowel sounds. Large intestines (colon) function can be auscultated at the outer (distal) aspects of each quadrant. Small intestine function can be auscultated in the inner aspect of each quadrant.*

In a Postoperative Individual, Monitor Bowel Function, Looking for

- Bowel sounds in small intestines can return within 24 to 48 hours of surgery.
- Bowel sounds in large intestines can return within 3 to 5 days of surgery.
- Flatus and defecation resuming by the second or third postoperative day.

R: *Resolution of normal bowel function starts in the proximal or right colon and progresses to the distal or left colon. Normally the small bowel regains function within hours, whereas it may take 3 to 5 days for the colon to regain function. Bowel sounds should be auscultated to help differentiate paralytic ileus from a mechanical ileus. Continued absence of bowel sounds suggests paralytic ileus, whereas hyperactive bowel sounds may indicate a mechanical ileus (McCutcheon, 2013).*

Monitor for Signs and Symptoms of Paralytic Ileus (McCutcheon, 2013)

- Mild abdominal pain and bloating
- Nausea, vomiting, poor appetite
- Distended and tympanic abdomen
- Constipation, obstipation
- Absent or hypoactive bowel sounds, passing flatus or stool

R: *Intraoperative manipulation of abdominal organs and the depressive effects of narcotics and anesthetics on peristalsis reduce bowel motility. The physiologic postoperative ileus that usually follows surgery has a benign and self-limited course. However, when ileus is prolonged, it leads to increasing discomfort and must be differentiated from other potential complications (e.g., bowel obstruction, intra-abdominal abscess) (McCutcheon, 2013).*

Differentiated Between Paralytic Ileus and Mechanical Bowel Obstruction

> **CLINICAL ALERT** "It is useful to note that nearly all individuals with early postoperative bowel obstruction have an initial return of bowel function and oral intake, which is then followed by nausea, vomiting, abdominal pain, and distention, whereas patients with ileus generally do not experience return of bowel function" (Bordeianou & Yeh, 2015).

- Abdominal distention, vomiting, obstipation: may be present
- Bowel sounds: paralytic ileus—usually quiet or absent
  - Bowel obstruction: may be high-pitched, may be absent
- Pain: paralytic ileus—mild and diffuse
  - Bowel obstruction: moderate to severe, colicky
- Fever, tachycardia: paralytic ileus—absent
  - Bowel obstruction: should raise suspicion

R: *Localized tenderness, fever, tachycardia, and peritoneal signs suggest bowel ischemia or perforation, which indicate the need for emergent surgical intervention.*

> **CLINICAL ALERT** Notify physician/nurse practitioner with new onset or increasing signs and symptoms of paralytic ileus. If the obstruction blocks the blood supply to the intestine, it may cause infection and tissue death (gangrene). The risk for tissue death is increased the longer the duration of the blockage. Hernias, volvulus, and intussusception carry a higher gangrene risk (Bordeianou & Yeh, 2015).

When Bowel Obstruction is Suspected, a Plain Abdominal X-ray or CT With Contrast Is Indicated

R: *Small bowel obstruction can be diagnosed on X-ray if the more proximal small bowel is dilated and the more distal small bowel is not dilated. The stomach may also be dilated. However, if there remains any suspicion for small bowel obstruction or another diagnosis, we suggest CT of the abdomen (Bordeianou & Yeh, 2015).*

Restrict Fluids Until Bowel Sounds are Present. When Indicated, Begin With Small Amounts of Clear Liquids Only

- Monitor individual's response to resumption of fluid and food intake, and note the nature and amount of any emesis or stools.

R: *The individual will not tolerate fluids until bowel sounds resume.*

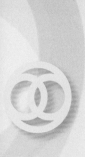

Section 4

Diagnostic Clusters

This section presents a sampling of medical conditions or clinical situations with associated nursing diagnoses and collaborative problems. Included are one example each of a medical condition, a surgical procedure, an obstetric/gynecologic condition, a neonatal condition, a pediatric/adolescent disorder, a mental health disorder, and a diagnostic and therapeutic procedure. A wider array of conditions and situations in each of these categories is presented on thePoint'.

Medical Conditions

CARDIOVASCULAR/HEMATOLOGIC/ PERIPHERAL VASCULAR DISORDERS

Cardiac Conditions

Angina Pectoris

Collaborative Problems

Refer to *Heart Failure*.
- RC of Acute Coronary Syndrome
- RC of Arrhythmias

Nursing Diagnoses[1]

- Anxiety related to chest pain secondary to effects of hypoxia
- Fear related to present status and unknown future
- Disturbed Sleep Pattern related to treatments and environment
- Risk for Constipation related to bed rest, change in lifestyle, and medications
- Activity Intolerance related to deconditioning secondary to fear of recurrent angina
- Risk for Interrupted Family Processes related to impaired ability of person to assume role responsibilities
- Risk for Ineffective Health Management related to insufficient knowledge of condition, home activities, diet, and medications

Go to thePoint* *for an expanded list of Diagnostic Clusters for medical conditions.*

---

[1]List includes nursing diagnoses that may be associated with the medical diagnosis.

2
Surgical Procedures

General Surgery

Preoperative Period

Nursing Diagnoses

- Anxiety related to loss of control, unpredictable outcome, pre-operative procedures (surgical permit, diagnostic studies, Foley catheter, diet and fluid restrictions, medications, skin preparation, waiting area for family), and postoperative procedures (disposition [recovery room, intensive care unit], medications for pain, coughing/turning/leg exercises, tube/drain placement, nothing by mouth [NPO]/diet restrictions, bed rest)

Postoperative Period

Collaborative Problems

- RC of Urinary Retention
- RC of Bleeding
- RC of Hypovolemia/Shock
- RC of Pneumonia
- RC of Peritonitis
- RC of Thrombophlebitis
- RC of Paralytic ileus
- RC of Evisceration/Dehiscence

Nursing Diagnoses

- Risk for Infection related to site for bacterial invasion
- Risk for Ineffective Respiratory Function related to postanesthesia state, postoperative immobility, and pain
- Acute Pain related to incision, flatus, and immobility
- Risk for Constipation related to decreased peristalsis secondary to the effects of anesthesia, immobility, and pain medication

- Risk for Imbalanced Nutrition: related to increased protein/vitamin requirements for wound healing and decreased intake secondary to pain, nausea, vomiting, and diet restrictions
- Risk for Ineffective Health Management related to insufficient knowledge of home care, incisional care, signs and symptoms of complications, activity restriction, and follow-up care

Go to thePoint° *for an expanded list of Diagnostic Clusters for surgical procedures.*

3
Obstetric/Gynecologic Conditions

PRENATAL PERIOD (GENERAL)

Nursing Diagnoses

- Nausea related to elevated estrogen levels, decreased blood sugar, or decreased gastric motility and pressure on cardiac sphincter from enlarged uterus
- Risk for Constipation related to decreased gastric motility and pressure of uterus on lower colon
- Activity Intolerance related to fatigue and dyspnea secondary to pressure of enlarging uterus on diaphragm and increased blood volume
- Risk for Injury related to syncope/hypotension secondary to peripheral venous pooling secondary to peripheral venous pooling
- Risk for Ineffective Health Management related to insufficient knowledge of (examples) effects of pregnancy on body systems (cardiovascular, integumentary, gastrointestinal, urinary, pulmonary, musculoskeletal), psychosocial domain, sexuality/sexual function, family unit (spouse, children), fetal growth and development, nutritional requirements, hazards of smoking, excessive alcohol intake, drug abuse, excessive caffeine intake, excessive weight gain, signs and symptoms of complications (vaginal bleeding, cramping, gestational diabetes, excessive edema, preeclampsia), preparation for childbirth (classes, printed references)

Abortion, Induced

Preprocedure Period

Nursing Diagnosis

- Anxiety related to significance of decision, procedure, and postprocedure care

Postprocedure Period

Collaborative Problems

- RC of Bleeding
- RC of Infection

Nursing Diagnoses

- Risk for Ineffective Coping related to unresolved emotional responses (guilt) to societal, moral, religious, and familial opposition
- Risk for Interrupted Family Processes related to effects of procedure on relationships (disagreement about decisions, previous conflicts [personal, marital], or adolescent identity problems)
- Risk for Ineffective Care Management related to insufficient knowledge of self-care (hygiene, breast care), nutritional needs, expected bleeding, cramping, signs and symptoms of complications, resumption of sexual activity, contraception, sex education as indicated, comfort measures, expected emotional responses, follow-up appointment, and community resources

*Go to the*Point® *for an expanded list of Diagnostic Clusters for obstetric/ gynecologic conditions.*

4
Neonatal Conditions

Neonate, Normal

Collaborative Problems

- RC of Hypothermia
- RC of Hypoglycemia
- RC of Hyperbilirubinemia
- RC of Bradycardia

Nursing Diagnoses

- Risk for Infection related to vulnerability of infant, lack of normal flora, environmental hazards, and open wound (umbilical cord, circumcision)
- Risk for Ineffective Airway Clearance related to oropharynx secretions
- Risk for Impaired Skin Integrity related to susceptibility to nosocomial infection and lack of normal skin flora
- Ineffective Thermoregulation related to newborn extrauterine transition
- Risk for Ineffective Infant's Health Management related to insufficient knowledge of (specify) (see *Postpartum Period*)

Go to thePoint* *for an expanded list of Diagnostic Clusters for neonatal conditions.*

5
Pediatric/Adolescent Disorders

Developmental Problems/Needs Related to Chronic Illness
(Permanent Disability, Multiple Handicaps, Developmental Disability [Mental/Physical], Life-Threatening Illness)

Nursing Diagnoses[2]

- Chronic Sorrow (parental) related to anticipated losses secondary to condition
  - Diabetes mellitus
  - Anorexia nervosa (psychiatric disorders)
  - Spinal cord injury
  - Head trauma
  - Neoplastic disorders
  - Fractures
  - Congestive heart failure
  - Pneumonia
- Compromised Family Processes related to adjustment requirements for situation: (examples) time, energy (emotional, physical), financial, and physical care
- Risk for Impaired Home Maintenance related to inadequate resources, housing, or impaired caregiver(s)
- Risk for Parental Role Conflict related to separations secondary to frequent hospitalizations
- Risk for Loneliness (child/family) related to decreased socialization due to the disability and the requirements of the caregiver(s)
- Risk for Impaired Parenting related to abuse, rejection, overprotection secondary to inadequate resources, or coping mechanisms
- Decisional Conflict related to illness, health-care interventions, and parent–child separation

---

[2]For additional pediatric medical diagnoses, see the adult diagnoses and Developmental Problems/Needs.

- (Specify) Self-Care Deficit related to illness limitations or hospitalization
- Risk for Development related to (specify impaired ability) to achieve developmental tasks
- Caregiver Role Strain related to multiple ongoing care needs secondary to restrictions imposed by disease, disability, or treatments
- Ineffective Child's Health Management has been used for clinical usefulness since Ineffective Self-Health Management does not apply when the patient is a child.

Go to thePoint *for an expanded list of Diagnostic Clusters for pediatric/ adolescent disorders.*

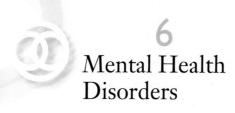

6
Mental Health Disorders

Alcoholism

Collaborative Problems

- RC of Delirium Tremens
- RC of Autonomic Hyperactivity
- RC of Seizures
- RC of Alcoholic Hallucinosis
- RC of Hypertension
- RC of Hypoglycemia

Nursing Diagnoses

- Imbalanced Nutrition: related to anorexia
- Risk for Deficient Fluid Volume related to abnormal fluid loss secondary to vomiting and diarrhea
- Risk for Injury related to disorientation, tremors, or impaired judgment
- Risk for Violence related to chemical withdrawal with impulsive behavior, disorientation, tremors, or impaired judgment
- Disturbed Sleep Pattern related to irritability, tremors, and nightmares
- Anxiety related to loss of control, memory losses, and fear of withdrawal
- Ineffective Coping related to inability to manage stressors constructively without drugs/alcohol
- Impaired Social Interaction related to alcoholic problematic behavior with emotional immaturity, irritability, high anxiety, impulsive behavior, or aggressive responses
- Ineffective Sexuality Patterns related to impotence/loss of libido secondary to altered self-concept and substance abuse
- Ineffective Family Coping related to disruption in marital dyad and inconsistent limit setting

- Disabled Family Coping related to the destructive effects of alcoholic family member on family functioning and each family member
- Risk for Ineffective Health Management related to insufficient knowledge of condition, treatments available, high-risk situations, and community resources

Go to thePoint *for an expanded list of Diagnostic Clusters for mental health disorders.*

7

Diagnostic and Therapeutic Procedures

Angioplasty
(Percutaneous, Transluminal, Coronary, Peripheral)

Preprocedure Period

Nursing Diagnoses

- Anxiety/Fear (individual, family) related to health status, angioplasty procedure, routines, outcome, and possible need for cardiac surgery

Postprocedure Period

Collaborative Problems

- RC of Dysrhythmias
- RC of Acute Coronary Occlusion (clot, spasm, collapse)
- RC of Myocardial Infarction
- RC of Arterial Dissection or Rupture
- RC of Hemorrhage/Hematoma at Angioplasty Site
- RC of Paresthesia Distal to Site
- RC of Arterial Thrombosis
- RC of Embolization (Peripheral)

Nursing Diagnoses

- ▲ Impaired Physical Mobility related to prescribed bed rest and restricted movement of involved extremity
- ▲ Risk for Ineffective Health Management related to insufficient knowledge of care of insertion site, discharge activities, diet, medications, signs and symptoms of complications, exercises, and follow-up care

Go to thePoint® *for an expanded list of Diagnostic Clusters for diagnostic and therapeutic procedures.*

Appendix A

Nursing Diagnoses Grouped by Functional Health Pattern

This Appendix can be found on the**Point**®

Nursing Admission Baseline Assessment

This Appendix can be found on thePoint®

Appendix C

Strategies to Promote Engagement of Individual/Families for Healthier Outcomes

Types of Literacy

Functional illiteracy is when someone who has minimal reading and writing skills does not have the capacity for health literacy to manage ordinary everyday needs and requirements of most employments.

Health literacy is the capacity to obtain, process, and understand basic health information and services needed to

- Make appropriate health decisions (*Ratzan, 2001)
- Follow instructions for treatments and medications (*White & Dillow, 2005)
- Sign a consent form
- Make appointments

 Carp's Cues

Individuals who are illiterate (who cannot read or write) are easier to identify than those who are functionally illiterate.

Do not assume an individual can read and understand health literature even if translated.

R: *The National Assessment of Adult Literacy (NAAL) (*2003) reported that 9 out of 10 English-speaking adults in the United States do not have health literacy (Kutner, Greenberg, Jiny, & Paulson, 2006). A large study on the scope of health literacy at two public hospitals (*Williams et al., 1995) found the following:*

- *Half of English-speaking patients could not read and understand basic health education material.*
- *60% could not understand a routine consent form.*
- *26% could not understand the appointment card.*
- *42% failed to understand directions for taking their medications.*

Assess for the Red Flags of Low Literacy

- Frequently missed appointments
- Incomplete registration forms
- Noncompliance with medication
- Inability to name medications, explain purpose, or describe dosing
- Identification of pills by appearance, not by reading of label
- Inability to give coherent, sequential history
- Few questions asked
- Lack of follow-through on tests or referrals

Strategies to Improve Comprehension

R: *Research shows that individuals remember and understand less than half of what clinicians explain to them (Williams et al., 1995; Roter, Rune, & Comings, 1998). Testing general reading levels does not ensure understanding in the clinical setting (Weiss, 2007).*

- For comprehension to occur, the nurse must accept that there is limited time and that the use of this time is enhanced by
  - Using every contact time to teach something
  - Creating a relaxed encounter
  - Using eye contact
  - Slowing down—break it down into short statements
  - Having limited content—focus on 2 or 3 concepts
  - Using plain language
  - Engaging individual/family in discussion
  - Using graphics
  - Explaining what you are doing to the individual/family and why

- Asking them to tell you about what you taught. Tell them to use their own words.

 Carp's Cues

Health-care professionals must quiet themselves regarding what they *think* a person or family needs to know. The goal is to find what information the individual wants to know; otherwise even the best teaching techniques will "fall on deaf ears." "Making the suggestion to lose 20 pounds, start going to the gym, and regularly take their hypertension medication to a person who has little understanding that they even have a chronic illness, the nature of that illness, or that they must play a part in managing it, is unlikely to result in the desired outcome" (Hibbard & Greene, 2013).

The Teach–Back Method
(DeWalt, Callahan, Hawk et al, 2010)

- This method includes (source: www.teachbacktraining.org/) the following:
  - A way to make sure you—the health-care provider—explained information clearly; it is not a test or quiz of individuals or families.
  - Asking an individual (or family member) to explain—*in their own words*—what they need to know or do, in a caring way.
  - A way to check for understanding and, if needed, re-explain and check again.

Use the Teach-Back Method (see chart)

- Explain/demonstrate
  - Explain one concept (e.g., medication, condition, when to call PCP).
  - Demonstrate one procedure (e.g., dressing charge, use of inhaler).
- Assess
  - I want to make sure, I explained _____ clearly, can you tell me _____.
  - Tell me what I told you.
  - Show me how to _____.
  - Avoid asking, "Do you understand?"

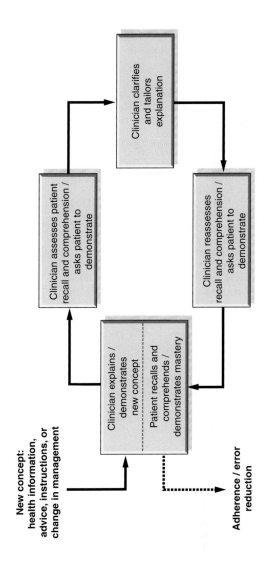

- Clarify
  - Add more explanation if you are not satisfied that the person understands or can perform the activity.
  - If the person cannot report the information, don't repeat the same explanation; rephrase it.

 Carp's Cues

Be careful the person/family does not think you are testing him or her. Assure them it is important that you help them to understand that the teaching method can help you teach and also diagnose educational needs.

- Teach-back questions (examples):
  - When should you call your PCP?
  - How do you know your incision is healing?
  - What foods should you avoid?
  - How often should you test your blood sugar?
  - What should you do for low blood sugar?
  - What weight gain should you report to your PCP?
  - Which inhaler is your rescue inhaler?
  - Is there something you have been told to do that you do not understand?
  - What should you bring to your PCP office?
  - Is there something you have a question about?

 Carp's Cues

Use every opportunity to explain a treatment, a medication, the condition, and/or restrictions. Focus on "need to know" and "need to do."

- For example, as you change a dressing
  - Explain and ask the individual/family member to redress the wound.
  - Point out how the wound is healing and what would indicate signs of infection.

 Carp's Cues

When individual/family do not understand what was said or demonstrated, the teach-back needs to be revised in a manner that will improve understanding. Teach-back has the potential to improve health outcomes, because if done correctly, it forces the nurse to limit the information to need to know. The likelihood of success is increased when the individual is not overwhelmed.

Helping to Activate Individuals/Families to Make Healthier Choices

Take opportunities to activate the individual/family. Ask, "How can you be healthier?" regardless of "Your Agenda" focus on what they said, for example, exercise more, eat better, stop smoking.

R: *"Activation refers to a person's ability and willingness to take on the role of managing their health and health care" (Hibbard & Cunningham 2008).*

* If interested in changing diet;
  * What do you usually have for breakfast?
    o If nothing—why? Explore options—what could you eat if you are in a hurry? Wait for an answer—if none, suggest cereal and granola bar.
    o If unhealthy, ask them what parts of their breakfast could they change, for example, save bacon/sausage for a treat on the weekends or have 1 piece of toast instead of 2 or delete the juice and have a piece of fruit as a snack later.

R: *A breakfast increases the body's metabolism early and can reduce excessive eating as the day continues.*
  * What did you have for dinner last night?
    o 10 Fried wings and a large soda.
    o Do you think eating 1 to 2 pieces of chicken is better than 10 wings? They have less fat and more meat than wings.
    o Give them the diagram of MyPlate from www.choosemyplate.gov/. Ask them what they can add to their plate in each section.

R: *Asking the person to select foods from each type of food section will help to teach the person/family what is a starch e.g., corn, peas, (not vegetables) sources of protein, as beans e.g., legumes not green beans, which are a vegetable.*

    o What vegetable could you include in this meal? Carrots, green beans, salad.

 Carp's Cues
  Have copies of readable educational materials that can be easily accessed (e.g., picture of Choose MyPlate).

* How could you eat healthier?
    o Stress that there are no bad foods but bad amounts. Yes, there are healthier foods/drinks? What are they? Roasted chicken.

- ○ What do you drink during the day? Could you substitute water or diet drinks for soda or sugar drinks? "The body has to burn calories to process the water you drink, and since water has no calories, it burns other calories in your food."
- ○ When you eat out, do you think you are given too much food? If yes, how about asking for a take-out box before you start eating? Share a dessert.
- What three changes can you make to eat better?

R: *Keep it simple so the individual sees it as doable.*

- If interested in exercising more, focus on moving more.

R: *The word "exercise" has images of 1/2 to 1 hour sessions, joining a gym.*

- How do you travel to work? School?
  - ○ If you drive, park further away from the building, the store, etc.
  - ○ If you take the train or bus, get off 1 to 2 blocks or stops from your usual stop.
  - ○ Use stairs. If walking upstairs is a problem, walk down only.
  - ○ Walk your dog.
  - ○ Arrange to walk with someone for the company and to increase the commitment.
- If interested in stopping smoking:
  - Set a date.
  - Be realistic, relapses occur.
  - Print out something for the person to take.
    - ○ Go to thePoint® and print out "Getting Started to Quit Smoking?" for individuals with low health literacy.
    - ○ Go to 5 steps to quitting > http://smokefree.gov/steps-on-quit-day for most individuals.
    - ○ Go to www.helpguide.org/articles/addiction/how-to-quit-smoking.htm for more educated individuals.

R: *"Strategies are needed to ensure that individuals/families are supported to become engaged, at the level they desire, instead of teaching what 'we' think they need" (Frosch & Elwyn. 2014).*

- If the individual does not offer what healthier choices they could choose, focus on 1 or 2 consequences of their unhealthy choices as follows:
  - If weight loss would be helpful:
    - ○ Do your legs swell during the day and return to normal when you wake up?
      - – "Your weight is compressing the tubes/vessels in your legs which prevent the fluid from returning to your

body. At some point the swelling will not go away when you are sleeping. It is permanent! Look at overweight people's feet; many wear slippers as shoes.

- ○ What could you do if you lost 20 lb that you cannot do now?
  - – Pick up 5 pounds of sugar. It is heavy; imagine how your joints or heart would like 5 pounds less of strain. Imagine 2 bags of sugar as 2 pounds of sugar. Focus on 3 pounds at a time as the goal.
- If the person smokes:
  - ○ How much does smoking cost you each month?
  - ○ If respiratory infections or chronic lung diseases are present, acknowledge that smoking will continue to cause deterioration. Ask them if they ever experienced trouble breathing? Gently explore how frightening it was. Continued smoking will cause progression of the breathing difficulties, with no treatments offering a cure.
  - ○ Do you have leg cramps when you walk? If yes, explain that smoking changes their blood vessels that reduce the blood flow when walking. Eventually the pain will prevent them from walking at all.
  - ○ Smoking interferes with circulation, so your body cannot heal well after an injury or surgery. Smokers also get leg ulcers that never heal.
- If a person is reporting not taking medications as prescribed, explore why. Refer to Medication Reconciliation and Barriers to Adherence later in this section. If the reason is "Don't think I need it," ask, "Do you know anyone with diabetes mellitus, heart disease, had a stroke, or kidney failure?" If yes, say, "Tell me about them."
- Try to make a connection with failure to adhere to treatment plan to the unsatisfactory effect on their daily life or death.
- Does he/she think the poor outcome could have been prevented?

R: *Some individuals report "diabetes (or cardiac disease, or strokes, or renal failure) runs in my family." Discussions can focus on what they do to prevent or reduce this from happening to them.*

- Personalized information (paper and electronic) which
  - Determines person's goal in treatment
  - Serves to identify barriers to adherence and solutions.

R: *"Starting with appropriate goals that fit the person's level of activation, and working toward increasing activation step by step, he/she can experience small successes and steadily build up the confidence and skill for effective self-management" (Hibbard & Greene, 2013).*

R: *The potential for individuals to contribute to their safety by speaking up about their concerns depends heavily on the quality of professional interactions and relationships (Entwistle et al., 2010).*

- Offer praise for honesty about problems with compliance and for sharing reasons. For example (Sofaer & Schumann, 2013, p. 19):
  - "I'm glad you told me that you stopped taking Motrin because it made your stomach hurt. Now I understand why your hands still ache. Let's talk about other ways we can get you some comfort."
  - "It's good that you told me about your stopping the blood pressure pills. That explains your headaches and higher pressure today. Let's discuss how those pills made you feel."

R: *Individuals/Families "will only be successful in taking greater responsibility for their health care decisions and actions if they are well-nurtured in this process, consistently protected from making profoundly negative decisions along the way, and kept safe" (Sofaer & Schumann, 2013, p. 19).*

- Suggest self-monitoring is useful to determine positive and negative influences on compliance.
  - Daily records
  - Charts
  - Diary of progress or symptoms, clinical values (e.g., blood pressure), or dietary intake

R: *"Involving the individual/family in decision-making places some responsibility on him or her to make sure the plan works, promoting engagement with treatment/plan" (Sofaer & Schumann 2013).*

> **CLINICAL ALERT** Many persons who are ready to engage believe that they will engage at their peril and that clinicians and others will react negatively if they ask probing questions, disagree, suggest an alternative approach, ask for a second opinion, question an insurance company decision, or indicate dissatisfaction (Frosch, May, Rendle, Tietbohl, & Elwyn, 2012; Sofaer & Schumann, 2013).

Medication Reconciliation and Barriers to Adherence
(Carpenito, 2014)

Medication errors occur 46% of the time during transitions, admission, transfer, or discharge from a clinical unit/hospital.

Almost 60% of individuals have at least one discrepancy in their medication history completed on admission. "The most common error (46.4%) was omission of a regularly used medication. Most (61.4%) of the discrepancies were judged to have no potential to cause serious harm. However, 38.6% of the discrepancies had the potential to cause moderate to severe discomfort or clinical deterioration" (Cornish et al., 2005, p. 424).

Medication reconciliation on admission to the health-care facilities often entails the following:

- Name of medication (prescribed, over-the-counter)
- Prescribed dose
- Frequency (daily, bid, tid, as needed)

A list of medications that have been prescribed by a provider does not represent a process of medication reconciliation. A family member recently took an older relative to the ER with chest pain. A typed list of her medications was given to the ER nurse. No discussion occurred about her medication.

Unfortunately, one of two hypertension medications she regularly took was not entered in the electronic health record. Since her blood pressure was elevated on admission and persisted, another antihypertensive medication was ordered. After two days, another medication was added with good results.

The first medication that was added was the medication she was already taking before admission. So essentially, no new medication was added as a result of the error. She spent three unnecessary days in the hospital with increased costs to Medicare and would have definitely rather been home eating her own food and having a good night's sleep in her own bed.

According to the Joint Commission (p. 1), Medication reconciliation is the process of comparing an individual's medication orders to all of the medications that the patient has been taking. This reconciliation is done to avoid medication errors such as omissions, duplications, dosing errors, or drug interactions. It should be done at every transition of care in which new medications are ordered or existing orders are rewritten. Transitions in care include changes in setting, service, practitioner, or level of care. The process comprises five steps: (1) develop a list of current medications; (2) develop a list of medications to be prescribed; (3) compare the medications on the two lists; (4) make clinical decisions based on the comparison; and (5) communicate the new list to appropriate caregivers to the patient.

Critical to acquiring a list of medications are the additional assessment questions, which are the defining elements for medication reconciliation: "*versus a list of medications reported to be taking.*"

For each medication reported, ask the individual/family member the following questions (DeWalt et al., 2010):

- What is the reason you are taking each medication?
- Are you taking the medication as prescribed? Specify once a day, twice a day, etc.
- Are you skipping any doses? Do you sometimes run out of medications?
- How often are you taking the medication prescribed "if needed as a pain medication"?
- Have you stopped taking any of these medications?
- How much does it cost you to take your medications?
- Are you taking anybody else's medication?

Prepare the Individual/Family for Correctly Taking Medications at Home
- Explain what OTC not to take.
- Finish all the medications like antibiotics.
- Do not to take any medications that are at home unless approved by PCP.
- Ask bring all his or her medications to next visit to PCP (e.g., prescribed, OTC, vitamins, herbal medicines).
- As indicated:
  - Create a list of each medication, what used for, times to take, with food or without food.
  - Create a pill card with columns, pictures of pill.
  - For a printable pill card to use with individuals, refer to thePoint.
  - Have individual or family member fill a weekly pill box with sections for bid and tid slots.
  - Warn that if a pill looks different, check with pharmacy.
- Remember, as a nurse:
  - Create a habit of using every contact time to teach something.
  - The more you do it, the better you get.
  - The better you get, the better it is for those you care for.

High-Risk Assessment Tools for Preventable Hospital-Acquired Conditions

This edition has identified the importance of prevention of eight conditions identified by Centers for Medicare and Medicaid Services.

These eight events or conditions are as follows:

- Pressure ulcer stages III and IV
- Falls and trauma
- Surgical site infection after bariatric surgery for obesity, certain orthopedic procedures, and bypass surgery (mediastinitis)
- Vascular catheter-associated infection
- Catheter-associated urinary tract infection
- Administration of incompatible blood
- Air embolism
- Foreign object unintentionally retained after surgery

Using evidence-based guidelines, the following can be accessed:

- Nursing diagnoses that represent prevention of infection, falls, pressure ulcers, and delayed discharge
- Collaborative problems that identify individuals at high risk for air emboli, deep vein thrombosis, and sepsis
- Medical condition, postsurgical care, and treatment plan specifically identify adverse events that are associated with clinical diagnoses or situations (refer to Section 3: Collaborative Problems)
- Standardized risk assessment tools for falls, infection, and pressure ulcers that are incorporated in every care plan. Refer the following for these tools.

For the assessment tools to identify individuals at high risk for one or more of these condition(s), refer to the table of contents for

- Infection—Risk for Infection
- Risk for Delayed Surgical Healing
- Risk for Complications of Deep Vein Thrombosis
- Risk for Complication of Sepsis

Standardized Risk Assessment Tools for Falls, Infection, and Pressure Ulcer

High Risk for Falls

Fall Risk Assessment

Assess for the following risk factors. Record the number of checks in the fall assessment scores in the ( ) as High Risk for Falls (score), or add the risk factors, for example, as High Risk for Falls related to instability, postural hypotension, and IV equipment.

Assess all individuals for risk factors for falls, using the assessment tool in the institution. The following represents one assessment tool:

Variables Score
History of falling
    No (score as 0)
    Yes (score as 25)

Secondary diagnosis
    No (score as 0)
    Yes (score as 15)

Ambulatory aid
    Bed rest/nurse assistance (score as 0)
    Crutches/cane/walker (score as 15)
    Furniture (score as 30)

IV or IV access
    No (score as 0)
    Yes (score as 20)

Gait
    Normal/bed rest/immobile (score as 0)
    Weak (score as 10)
    Impaired (score as 20)

Mental status
    Knows own limits (score as 0)
    Overestimates or forgets limits (score as 15)

Total Score _____

Risk Level Morse Fall Scale (MFS) Score Action

No risk
    0–24 Good basic nursing care

Low to moderate risk
    25–45 Implement standard fall prevention interventions

High risk
    46+ Implement high-risk fall prevention interventions
Morse Fall Scale (*Morse, 1997). Used with permission.

Timed Up and Go (Podsiadlo & Richardson, 1991)

For individuals who are independent and ambulatory but frail, fatigued, and/or with possible compromised ambulation, assess the person's ability to Timed Up and Go (TUG):

- Have the person wear their usual footwear, and use any assistive device they normally use.
- Have the person sit in the chair with their back to the chair and their arms resting on the arm rests.
- Ask the person to stand up from a standard chair and walk a distance of 10 ft (3 m).
- Have the person turn around, walk back to the chair, and sit down again.
- Timing begins when the person starts to rise from the chair and ends when he or she returns to the chair and sits down.

The person should be given one practice trial and then three actual trials if needed. The times from the three actual trials are averaged.

Predictive Results

Seconds Rating

<10	Freely mobile
10–19	Mostly independent
20–29	Variable mobility
>29	Impaired mobility

Risk Factors for Surgical Site Infection

The risk of surgical site infection is influenced by the amount and virulence of the microorganism and the ability of the individual to resist it (Pear, 2007).

    Assess for the following risk factors. Record the number of risk factors in the ( ) as High Risk for Surgical Site Infection (1–10) or add the risk factors, for example, as High Risk for Surgical Site Infection related to obesity, diabetes mellitus, and tobacco use.

Infection colonization of microorganisms (1)
Preexisting remote body site infection (1)
Preoperative contaminated or dirty wound (e.g., posttrauma) (1)
Glucocorticoid steroids (2)
Tobacco use (3)
Malnutrition (4)
Obesity (5)
Perioperative hyperglycemia (6)
Diabetes mellitus (7)
Altered immune response (8)
Chronic alcohol use/acute alcohol intoxication (9)

1. Preoperative nares colonization with *Staphylococcus aureus* noted in 30% of most healthy populations, and especially methicillin-resistant *Staph. aureus* (MRSA), predisposes individuals to have higher risk of surgical site infection (Price et al., 2008).

2. Systemic glucocorticoids, which are frequently used as anti-inflammatory agents, are well-known to inhibit wound repair via global anti-inflammatory effects and suppression of cellular wound responses, including fibroblast proliferation and collagen synthesis. Systemic steroids cause wounds to heal with incomplete granulation tissue and reduced wound contraction (Franz et al., 2007).

3. Smoking has a transient effect on the tissue microenvironment and a prolonged effect on inflammatory and reparative cell functions, leading to delayed healing and complications. Quit smoking four weeks before surgery; restores tissue oxygenation and metabolism rapidly (Sørensen, 2012).

4. Malnourished individuals have been found to have less competent immune response to infection and decreased nutritional stores which will impair wound healing (Speaar, 2008).

5. An obese individual may experience a compromise in wound healing due to poor blood supply to adipose tissue. In addition, antibiotics are not absorbed well by adipose tissue. Despite excessive food intake, many obese individuals have protein malnutrition, which further impedes the healing (Cheadle, 2006).

6. There are two primary mechanisms that place individuals experiencing acute perioperative hyperglycemia at increased risk for surgical site infection. The first mechanism is the decreased vascular circulation, reducing tissue perfusion and impairing cellular-level functions. A clinical study by Akbari et al. (1998) noted that when healthy, nondiabetic subjects

ingested a glucose load, the endothelial-dependent vasodilatation in both the micro and macro circulations were impaired similar to that seen in diabetic patients. The second affected mechanism is the reduced activity of the cellular immunity functions of chemotaxis, phagocytosis, and killing of polymorphonuclear cells as well as monocytes/macrophages that have been shown to occur in the acute hyperglycemic state.

7. Postsurgical adverse outcomes related to diabetes mellitus are believed to be related to the preexisting complications of chronic hyperglycemia, which include vascular atherosclerotic disease and peripheral as well as autonomic neuropathies (Geerlings et al., 1999).

8. Suppression of the immune system by disease, medication, or age can delay wound healing (Cheadle, 2006).

9. Chronic alcohol exposure causes impaired wound healing and enhanced host susceptibility to infections. Wounds from trauma in the presence of acute alcohol exposure have a higher rate of postinjury infection due to decreased neutrophil recruitment and phagocytic function (Guo & DiPietro, 2010).

BRADEN SCALE FOR PREDICTING PRESSURE SORE RISK

Patient's Name _____ Evaluator's Name _____ Date of Assessment _____

SENSORY PERCEPTION ability to respond meaningfully to pressure-related discomfort

1. Completely Limited
Unresponsive (does not moan, flinch, or grasp) to painful stimuli, due to diminished level of consciousness or sedation OR limited ability to feel pain over most of body.

2. Very Limited
Responds only to painful stimuli. Cannot communicate discomfort except by moaning or restlessness OR has a sensory impairment which limits the ability to feel pain or discomfort over ½ of body.

3. Slightly Limited
Responds to verbal commands, but cannot always communicate discomfort or the need to be turned OR has some sensory impairment which limits ability to feel pain or discomfort in 1 or 2 extremities.

4. No Impairment
Responds to verbal commands. Has no sensory deficit which would limit ability to feel or voice pain or discomfort.

MOISTURE degree to which skin is exposed to moisture

1. Constantly Moist
Skin is kept moist almost constantly by perspiration, urine, etc. Dampness is detected every time patient is moved or turned.

2. Very Moist
Skin is often, but not always moist. Linen must be changed at least once a shift.

3. Occasionally Moist
Skin is occasionally moist, requiring an extra linen change approximately once a day.

4. Rarely Moist
Skin is usually dry, linen only requires changing at routine intervals.

ACTIVITY degree of physical activity

1. Bedfast
Confined to bed.

2. Chairfast
Ability to walk severely limited or non-existent. Cannot bear own weight and/or must be assisted into chair or wheelchair.

3. Walks Occasionally
Walks occasionally during day, but for very short distances, with or without assistance. Spends majority of each shift in bed or chair.

4. Walks Frequently
Walks outside room at least twice a day and inside room at least once every two hours during waking hours.

MOBILITY ability to change and control body position

1. Completely Immobile
Does not make even slight changes in body or extremity position without assistance.

2. Very Limited
Makes occasional slight changes in body or extremity position but unable to make frequent or significant changes independently.

3. Slightly Limited
Makes frequent though slight changes in body or extremity position independently.

4. No Limitation
Makes major and frequent changes in position without assistance.

NUTRITION usual food intake pattern

1. Very Poor
Never eats a complete meal. Rarely eats more than $\frac{1}{3}$ of any food offered. Eats 2 servings or less of protein (meat or dairy products) per day. Takes fluids poorly. Does not take a liquid dietary supplement OR is NPO and/or maintained on clear liquids or IVs for more than 5 days.

2. Probably Inadequate
Rarely eats a complete meal and generally eats only about $\frac{1}{2}$ of any food offered. Protein intake includes only 3 servings of meat or dairy products per day. Occasionally will take a dietary supplement OR receives less than optimum amount of liquid diet or tube feeding.

3. Adequate
Eats over half of most meals. Eats a total of 4 servings of protein (meat, dairy products) per day. Occasionally will refuse a meal, but will usually take a supplement when offered OR is on a tube feeding or TPN regimen which probably meets most of nutritional needs.

4. Excellent
Eats most of every meal. Never refuses a meal. Usually eats a total of 4 or more servings of meat and dairy products. Occasionally eats between meals. Does not require supplementation.

FRICTION & SHEAR

1. Problem
Requires moderate to maximum assistance in moving. Complete lifting without sliding against sheets is impossible. Frequently slides down in bed or chair, requiring frequent repositioning with maximum assistance. Spasticity, contractures or agitation leads to almost constant friction.

2. Potential Problem
Moves feebly or requires minimum assistance. During a move skin probably slides to some extent against sheets, chair, restraints or other devices. Maintains relatively good position in chair or bed most of the time but occasionally slides down.

3. No Apparent Problem
Moves in bed and in chair independently and has sufficient muscle strength to lift up completely during move. Maintains good position in bed or chair.

Total Score _____

Scoring: The Braden Scale is a summated rating scale made up of six subscales scored from 1–3 or 4, for total scores that range from 6–23. A lower Braden Scale Score indicates a lower level of functioning and, therefore, a higher level of risk for pressure ulcer development. A score of 19 or higher, for instance, would indicate that the patient is at low risk, with no need for treatment at this time. The assessment can also be used to evaluate the course of a particular treatment.

Bibliography

Author's Notes
Classic publications are designated with an asterisk (*)
Citations listed under the general category are used throughout the book

GENERAL REFERENCES

American Nurses Association. (2012). *ANA social policy statement.* Washington, DC: Author.

American Psychiatric Association. (2014). *DSMV: Diagnostic and statistical manual of mental disorders* (4th ed., text revision). Washington, DC: Author.

Alfaro-Lefevre, R. (2014). *Applying nursing process: The foundation for clinical reasoning* (8th ed.). Philadelphia: Wolters Kluwer.

Andrews, M., & Boyle, J. (2012). *Transcultural concepts in nursing* (8th ed.). Philadelphia: Lippincott Williams & Wilkins.

Arcangelo, V. P., & Peterson, A. (2016). *Pharmacotherapeutics for advanced practice* (4th ed.). Philadelphia: Wolters Kluwer.

Barnsteiner, J., Disch, J., & Walton, M. K. (2014). *Person and family-centered care.* Indianapolis, IN: Sigma Theta Tau International.

Boyd, M. A. (2012). *Psychiatric nursing: Contemporary practice* (5th ed.). Philadelphia: Lippincott Williams & Wilkins.

Carpenito, L. J. (1986). *Nursing diagnosis: Application to clinical practice.* Philadelphia: Lippincott Williams & Wilkins.

Carpenito, L. J. (1989). *Nursing diagnosis: Application to clinical practice* (3rd ed.). Philadelphia: Lippincott Williams & Wilkins.

Carpenito, L. J. (1995). *Nurse practitioner and physician discipline specific expertise in primary care.* Unpublished manuscript.

Carpenito, L. J. (1999). *Nursing diagnosis: Application to clinical practice* (5th ed.). Philadelphia: Lippincott Williams & Wilkins.

Carpenito-Moyet, L. J. (2007). *Understanding the nursing process: Concept mapping and care planning for students.* Philadelphia: Lippincott Williams & Wilkins.

Carpenito-Moyet, L. J. (2010). Teaching nursing diagnosis to increase utilization after graduation. *International Journal of Nursing Terminologies and Classifications, 21*(10), 124–133.

Carpenito-Moyet, L. J. (2014). *Nursing care plans/Transitional patient & family centered care* (6th ed.). Philadelphia: Wolters Kluwer.

Carpenito-Moyet, L. J. (2016). *Handbook of nursing diagnoses* (15th ed.). Philadelphia: Wolters Kluwer.

Centers for Disease Control and Prevention (CDC). (2015a). *Vaccines & immunizations*. Retrieved from www.cdc.gov/vaccines/

CDC. (2015b). *Sexually transmitted diseases* (STDS). Retrived from www.cdc.gov/std/

*Clemen-Stone, E., Eigasti, D. G., & McGuire, S. L. (2001). *Comprehensive family and community health nursing* (6th ed.). St. Louis, MO: Mosby-Year Book.

Coulter, A. (2012). Patient engagement—What works? *Ambulatory Care Manage, 35*(2), 80–89.

*Cunningham, R. S., & Huhmann, M. B. (2011). Nutritional disturbances. In C. H. Yarbro, D. Wujcik, & B. H. Gobel (Eds.), *Cancer nursing: Principles and practice* (7th ed.). Boston: Jones and Bartlett.

DeWalt, D. A., Callahan, L., Hawk, V. H,. Broucksou, K. A., & Hink, A. (2010). *Health literacy universal precautions tool kit* (Prepared by North Carolina Network Consortium, The Cecil G. Sheps Center for Health Services Research, The University of North Carolina at Chapel Hill, under Contract No. HHSA290200710014.) AHRQ Publication No. 10-0046-EF). Rockville, MD: Agency for Healthcare Research and Quality. Retrieved from www.ahrq.gov/professionals/quality-patient-safety/quality-resources/tools/literacy-toolkit/healthliteracy-toolkit.pdf

Dudek, S. (2014). *Nutrition essentials for nursing practice* (7th ed.). Philadelphia: Wolters Kluwer.

Edelman, C. L., & Mandle, C. L. (2014). *Health promotion throughout the life span* (8th ed.). St. Louis, MO: Mosby-Year Book.

Giger, J. (2013). *Transcultural nursing: Assessment and intervention* (6th ed.). St. Louis, MO: Mosby-Year Book.

*Gordon, M. (1982). Historical perspective: The National Group for Classification of Nursing Diagnoses. In M. J. Kim & D. A. Moritz (Eds.), *Classification of nursing diagnoses: Proceedings of the fourth national conference*. New York: McGraw-Hill.

Grossman, S., & Porth, C. A. (2014). *Porth's pathophysiology: Concepts of altered health states* (9th ed.). Philadelphia: Wolters Kluwer.

Halter, M. J. (2014). *Varcarolis' foundations of psychiatric mental health nursing* (7th ed.). Philadelphia: W. B. Saunders.

Herdman, H., & Kamitsuru, S. (Eds.). (2014). *Nursing diagnoses/definitions and classification 2015–2017*. Ames, IA: Wiley Blackwell.

Hickey, J. (2014). *The clinical practice of neurological and neurosurgical nursing* (5th ed.). Philadelphia: Wolters Kluwer.

Hockenberry, M. J., & Wilson, D. (2015). *Wong's essentials of pediatric nursing* (10th ed.). New York: Elsevier.

Jenny, J. (1987). Knowledge deficit: Not a nursing diagnosis image. *The Journal of Nursing Scholarship, 19*(4), 184–185.

Joint Commission. (2010). *Achieving effective communication, cultural competence, and patient-family-centered care: A roadmap for hospitals*. Oakbrook Terrace, IL: Author.

Labs on Line. (2014). Retrieved from https://labtestsonline.org

Lutz, C., Mazur, R., & Litch, N. (2015). *Nutrition and diet therapy*. Philadelphia: F.A. Davis.

Lutz, C., & Przytulski, K. (2011). *Nutrition and diet therapy* (5th ed.). Philadelphia: F.A. Davis.

McCaffery, M., & Beebe, A. (1989). *Pain: Clinical manual for nursing practice*. St. Louis: CV Mosby.

Miller, C. (2015). *Nursing for wellness in older adults* (7th ed.). Philadelphia: Wolters Kluwer.

Morse, J. M. (1997). *Preventing patient falls*. Thousand Oaks: Sage Broda.

*Murray, R. B., Zentner, J. P., & Yakimo, R. (2009). *Health promotion strategies through the life span* (8th ed.). Upper Saddle River, NJ: Pearson Prentice Hall.

*Norris, J., & Kunes-Connell, M. (1987). Self-esteem disturbance: A clinical validation study. In A. McLane (Ed.), *Classification of nursing diagnoses: Proceedings of the seventh NANDA national conference*. St. Louis, MO: C.V. Mosby.

North American Nursing Diagnosis Association. (2002). *Nursing diagnosis: Definitions and classification 2001–2002*. Philadelphia: Author.

Pasero, C., & McCaffery, M. (2011). *Pain assessment and pharmacologic management*. St. Louis: Mosby.

Pasero, C., Paice, J., & McCaffery, M. (2014). Basic mechanisms underlying the causes and effects of pain. In M. McCaffery & C. Pasero (Eds.), *Clinical pain manual* (pp. 15–34). New York: Mosby.

Pillitteri, A. (2014). *Maternal and child health nursing* (7th ed.). Philadelphia: Wolters Kluwer.

Procter, N., Hamer, H., McGarry, D., Wilson, R., & Froggatt, T. (2014). *Mental health: A person-centered approach*. Sydney: Cambridge Press.

*Ratzan, S. C. (2001). Health literacy: Communication for the public good. *Health Promotion International, 16*(2), 207–214.

Soussignan, R., Jiang, T., Rigaud, D., Royet, J., & Schaal, B. (2010). Subliminal fear priming potentiates negative facial reactions to food pictures in women with anorexia nervosa. *Psychological Medicine, 40*(3), 503–514. Retrieved from ProQuest Health and Medical Complete (Document ID: 1961359321).

Underwood, P. W. (2012). Social support. In V. H. Rice (Ed.), *Handbooks of stress, coping and health* (2nd ed.). Thousand Oaks, CA: SAGE Publications.

Varcarolis, E. M. (2011). *Manual of psychiatric nursing care planning* (4th ed.). St. Louis, MO: Saunders.

Varcarolis, E. M., & Halter, M. J. (2010). *Foundations of psychiatric mental health nursing* (6th ed.). Philadelphia: W. B. Saunders.

Weiss, B. D. (2007). *Health literacy and patient safety: Help patients understand*. Retrieved from http://med.fsu.edu/userFiles/file/ahec_health_clinicians_manual.pdf. American Medical Association.

*White, S., & Dillow, S. (2005). Key concepts and features of the 2003 National Assessment of adult literacy. National Center for Education Statistics. Retrieved from http://nces.ed.gov/NAAL/PDF/2006471.PDF.

Yarbro, C., Wujcik, D., & Gobel, B. (2013). *Cancer nursing: Principles and practice* (17th ed.). Boston: Jones & Bartlett.

SECTION 1: NURSING DIAGNOSES

Activity Intolerance

Bauldoff, G. S. (2015). When breathing is a burden: How to help patients with COPD. *American Nurse Today, 10*(2).

*Bauldoff, G., Hoffman, L., Sciurba, F., & Zullo, T. (1996). Home based upper arm exercises training for patients with chronic obstructive pulmonary disease. *Heart and Lung, 25*(4), 288–294.

*Breslin, E. H. (1992). Dyspnea-limited response in chronic obstructive pulmonary disease: Reduced unsupported arm activities. *Rehabilitation Nursing, 17*, 12–20.

Risk for Adverse Reaction to Iodinated Contrast Media

American College of Radiology Committee on Drugs and Contrast Media. (2013). *ACR manual on contrast media: Version 9*. Reston, VA: American College of Radiology. Retrieved from www.acr.org/quality-%20safety/resources/~/media/37D84428BF1D4E1B9A3A2918DA9E27A3.pdf/

Pasternak, J., & Williamson, E. (2012). Clinical pharmacology, uses, and adverse reactions of iodinated contrast agents: A primer for the non-radiologist. *Mayo Clinical Proceedings, 87*(4), 390–402. Retrieved from www.ncbi.nlm.nih.gov/pmc/articles/PMC3538464/

Robbins, J. B., & Pozniak, M. A. (2010). *Contrast media tutorial.* Retrieved from www.radiology.wisc.edu/fileShelf/contrastCorner/files/ContrastAgentsTutorial.pdf

Siddiqi, N. (2011). Contrast medium reactions. In *Medscape.* Retrieved from http://emedicine.medscape.com/article/422855-overview

Siddiqi, N. (2015). Contrast medium reactions. In *Medscape.* Retrieved from http://emedicine.medscape.com/article/422855-overview

Singh, J., & Daftary, A. (2008). Iodinated contrast media and their adverse reactions. *Journal of Nuclear Medicine Technology, 36*(2), 69–74.

Risk for Allergy Response

Asthma and Allergy Foundation of America. (2011). *Reducing allergens in the home: A room-by-room guide.* Retrieved from msdh.ms.gov/msdhsite/_static/resources/2111.pdf

Mayo Clinic Staff. (2011). *Allergy-proof your house.* Retrieved from www.mayoclinic.com/health/allergy/HQ01514

Anxiety

*Grainger, R. (1990). Anxiety interrupters. *American Journal of Nursing, 90*(2), 14–15.

*Grealish, L., Lomasney, A., & Whiteman, B. (2000). Foot massage. A nursing intervention to modify the distressing symptoms of pain and nausea in patients hospitalized with cancer. *Cancer Nursing, 23,* 237–243.

Guardino, C. M., & Dunkel Schetter, C. (2014). Coping during pregnancy: A systematic review and recommendations. *Health Psychology Review, 8*(1), 70–94.

Gurung, R. A., Dunkel-Schetter, C., Collins, N., Rini, C., & Hobel, C. J. (2005). Psychosocial predictors of prenatal anxiety. *Journal of Social and Clinical Psychology, 24*(4), 497.

*Jones, P. E., & Jakob, D. F. (1984). Anxiety revisited from a practice perspective. In M. J. Kim, G. K. McFarland, & A. M. McLane (Eds.), *Classification of nursing diagnoses: Proceedings of the fifth national conference.* St. Louis, MO: C.V. Mosby.

*Lobel, M., DeVincent, C. J., Kaminer, A., & Meyer, B. A. (2000). The impact of prenatal maternal stress and optimistic disposition on birth outcomes in medically high-risk women. *Health Psychology, 19*(6), 544.

*Lugina, H. I., Christensson, K., Massawe, S., Nystrom, L., & Lindmark, G. (2001). Change in maternal concerns during the 6 weeks postpartum period: A study of primiparous mothers in Dar es Salaam, Tanzania. *Journal of Midwifery and Women's Health*, *46*(4), 248–257.

*May, R. (1977). *The meaning of anxiety.* New York: W.W. Norton.

*Stephenson, N. L., Weinrich, S. P., & Tavakoli, A. S. (2000). The effects of foot reflexology on anxiety and pain in patients with breast and lung cancer. *Oncology Nursing Forum*, *27*, 67–72.

*Taylor-Loughran, A., O'Brien, M., LaChapelle, R., & Rangel, S. (1989). Defining characteristics of the nursing diagnoses fear and anxiety: A validation study. *Applied Nursing Research*, *2*, 178–186.

*Whitley, G. (1994). Concept analysis in nursing diagnosis research. In R. Carroll-Johnson & M. Paquette (Eds.), *Classification of nursing diagnosis: Proceedings of the tenth conference*. Philadelphia: J.B. Lippincott.

*Yokom, C. J. (1984). The differentiation of fear and anxiety. In M. J. Kim, G. K. McFarland, & A. M. McLane (Eds.), *Classification of nursing diagnoses: Proceedings of the fifth national conference*. St. Louis, MO: C.V. Mosby.

Death Anxiety

Braun, M., Gordon, D., & Uziely, B. (2010). Associations between oncology nurses' attitudes toward death and caring for dying patients. *Oncology Nursing Forum*, *37*(1), E43–E49.

Yakimo, R. (2008). Mental health promotion of the young and middle-aged adult. InM.A. Boyd (Ed.), *Psychiatric nursing: Contemporary perspectives* (4th ed.). Philadelphia: Lippincott Wilkins & Williams.

Ineffective Breastfeeding

Amir, L. H., & The Academy of Breastfeeding Medicine Protocol Committee. (2014). ABM clinical protocol #4: Mastitis. *Breastfeeding Medicine*, *9*(5), 293–243.

Arizona Department of Health Services (AZDHS). (2010). Model Hospital Policy Resource Guide. www.azdhs.gov/phs/bnp/gobreastmilk/documents/AzBSBS-Model-Hospital-Policy-Guide.pdf/

AZDHS. (2012). *Arizona baby steps to breastfeeding success*. Retrieved from www.azdhs.gov/phs/gobreastmilk/BFAzBabySteps.htm

Evans, A., Marinelli, K. A., Taylor, J. S., & The Academy of Breastfeeding Medicine. (2014). ABM clinical protocol #2: Guidelines for hospital discharge of the breastfeeding term newborn an mother " The going home protocol" (revised 2014). *Breastfeeding Medicine*, *9*(1), 3–8.

Hale, T. (2010). *Breastfeeding and medications*. Retrieved from www
.breastfeedingonline.com/meds.shtml#sthash.bx7EQILt
.dpbs

Lawrence, R. A., & Lawrence, R. M. (2010). *Breastfeeding—A
guide for the medical professional* (7th ed.). Philadelphia: Elsevier
Health Services.

*Walker, M. (2006). *Breastfeeding management for the clinician: Using
the evidence*. Boston: Jones and Bartlett.

Caregiver Role Strain

American Association of Retired Persons. (2009). *AARP statement
to the 53rd session of the United Nations Commission on the Status
of Women*. Retrieved from www.un.org/womenwatch/daw/
csw/53sess.htm

Gambert, S. R. (2013). Why do i always feel tired? Evaluating older
patients reporting fatigue. *Consultant, 53*(11), 785–789.

Hagen, B. (2001). Nursing home placement: Factors affecting
caregivers' decisions to place family members with dementia.
Journal of Gerontological Nursing, 27(2), 44–53.

Miller, B., Townsend, A., Carpenter, E., Montgomery, R. V., Stull,
D., & Young, R. F. (2001). Social support and caregiver distress
a replication analysis. *The Journals of Gerontology Series B:* Psychological *Sciences and Social Sciences, 56*(4), S249–256.

*Pearlin, L., Mullan, J., Semple, S., & Skaff, M. (1990). Caregiv-
ing and the stress process: An overview of concepts and their
measures. *The Gerontologist, 30*, 583–594.

*Shields, C. (1992). Family interaction and caregivers of Alzheim-
er's disease patients: Correlates of depression. *Family Process,
31*(3), 19–32.

*Winslow, B., & Carter, P. (1999). Patterns of burden in wives
who care for husbands with dementia. *Nursing Clinics of North
America, 34*(2), 275–287.

Impaired Comfort

*D'Arcy, Y. (2008). Pain in older adults. *Nurse Practitioner, 38*(3),
19–25.

*Dewar, A. (2006). Assessment and management of chronic pain in
the older person living in the community. *The Australian Journal
of Advanced Nursing, 24*(1), 33.

Institute of Medicine. (2011). *Relieving pain in America: A blueprint
for transforming prevention, care, education, and research*. Washington, DC: National Academies Press.

*Simkin, P., & Bolding, A. (2004). Update on nonpharmacologic approaches to relieve labor pain and prevent suffering. *Journal of midwifery & women's health*, *49*(6), 489–504.

Singh, M. (2014). Chronic pain syndrome treatment & management. In *Medscape*. Retrieved from http://emedicine.medscape.com/article/310834-treatment

*Von Korff, M., & Simon, G. (1996). The relationship between pain and depression comorbidity of mood. *The British Journal of Psychiatry*, *168*(30), 101–108.

Williams, H., Svensson, A., & Diepgen, T. (2006). Epidemiology of skin diseases in Europe. *European Journal of Dermatology*, *16*(2), 209–14.

Labor Pain

*Association of Women's Health, Obstetric and Neonatal Nurses (AWHONN). (2008a). *Nursing care and management of the second stage of labor: Evidence-Based Clinical Practice Guideline* (2nd ed.). Washington, DC: Author.

*Association of Women's Health, Obstetric and Neonatal Nurses (AWHONN). (2008b). *Nursing care of the woman receiving regional analgesia/anesthesia in labor: Evidence-based clinical practice guideline* (2nd ed.). Washington, DC: Author.

Association of Women's Health, Obstetric and Neonatal Nurses (AWHONN). (2011). *Nursing support of laboring women*. Position Statement. Washington, DC: Author.

Burke, C. (2014). Pain in labor: Nonpharmacologic and pharmacologic management. In K. R. Simpson & P. Creehan (Eds.), *AWHONN's perinatal nursing* (4th ed., pp. 493–529). Philadelphia: Wolters Kluwer.

Simkin, P., & Ancheta, R. (2011). *The labor progress book: Early interventions to prevent and treat dystocia* (3rd ed.). New York: Wiley-Blackwell.

Impaired Communication

*Bauman, R. A., & Gell, G. (2000). The reality of picture archiving and communication systems (PACS): A survey. *Journal Digit Imaging*, *13*(4), 157–169.

DeWalt, D. A., Callahan, L., Hawk, V. H,. Broucksou, K. A., & Hink, A. (2010). *Health literacy universal precautions tool kit*. Rockville, MD: Agency for Healthcare Research and Quality. Retrieved from www.ahrq.gov/professionals/quality-patient-safety/quality-resources/tools/literacy-toolkit/healthliteracytoolkit.pdf

Grossbach, I., Stranberg, S., & Chlan, L. (2011). Promoting effective communication for patients receiving mechanical ventilation. *Critical Care Nurse*, *31*(3), 46–60.

Office of Student Disabilities Services, University of Chicago. (2014). *Teaching students with disabilities resources for instructors 2014–2015*. Chicago, IL: Author. Retrieved from https://disabilities.uchicago.edu/sites/disabilities.uchicago.edu/files/uploads/docs/Teaching%20Students%20with%20Disabilities%20201415.pdf

Confusion (Acute & Chronic)

Francis, J., & Young, G. B. (2014). *Diagnosis of delirium and confusional*. Retrieved from www.uptodate.com/contents/diagnosis-of-delirium-and-confusional-states

*Hall, G. R., & Buckwalter, K. C. (1987). Progressively lowered stress threshold: A conceptual model for care of adults with Alzheimer's disease. *Archives of Psychiatric Nursing*, *1*, 399–406.

Khachiyants, N., Trinkle, D., Son, S. J., & Kim, K. Y. (2011). Sundown syndrome in persons with dementia: An update. *Psychiatry investigation*, *8*(4), 275–287.

*Rasin, J. (1990). Confusion. *Nursing Clinics of North America*, *25*, 909–918.

*Roberts, B. L. (2001). Managing delirium in adult intensive care patients. *Critical Care Nurse*, *21*(1), 48–55.

Smith, G. (2010). *What is sundowning? Answer to question "Sundowning: Late day confusion"*. Retrieved from www.mayoclinic.com/health/sundowning/HQ01463

Chronic Functional Constipation

Erichsén, E., Milberg, A., Jaarsma, T., & Friedrichsen, M. (2015). Constipation in specialized palliative care: Prevalence, definition, and patient-perceived symptom distress. *Journal of Palliative Medicine*, *18*(7), 585–592.

McCay, S. L., Fravel, M., & Scanlon, C. (2012). Evidence-based practice guideline: Management of constipation. *Journal of Gerontological Nursing*, *38*(7), 9–15.

*Shua-Haim, J., Sabo, M., & Ross, J. (1999). Constipation in the elderly: A practical approach. *Clinical Geriatrics*, *7*(12), 91–99.

Wald, A. (2015). Patient information: Constipation in adults (Beyond the Basics). In *UpToDate*. Retrieved from www.uptodate.com/contents/constipation-in-adults-beyond-the-basics#H1

*Wisten, A., & Messner, T. (2005). Fruit and fibre (Pajala porridge) in the prevention of constipation. *Scandinavian Journal of Caring Sciences*, *19*(1), 71–76.

Coping

Acquired Brain Injury Outreach Service. (2011). *Understanding emotional lability*. Buranda: State of Queensland (Queensland Health). Retrieved from www.health.qld.gov.au/abios/behaviour/professional/lability_pro.pdf

Ahmed, A., & Simmons, Z. (2013). Pseudobulbar affect: Prevalence and management. *Therapeutics and Clinical Risk Management, 9,* 483.

Allender, J., Rector, C., &Warner, K. (2010). *Community & public health nursing: Promoting the public's health* (8th ed.). Philadelphia: Lippincott Williams & Wilkins,

American Academy of Pediatrics. (2015). *Attention-deficit/hyperactivity disorder (ADHD)*. Retrieved from www.cdc.gov/ncbddd/adhd/guidelines.html

*Carson V. M., & Smith-DiJulio, K. (2006). Sexual assault. In E. Varcarolis, V. M. Carson, & N. C. Shoemaker (Eds.), *Foundations of psychiatric-mental health nursing* (5th ed.). Philadelphia: W. B. Saunders.

Centers for Disease Control and Prevetion. (2015). *Vaccines & immunizations*. Accessed at www.cdc.gov/vaccines/

*Cowen, P. S. (1999). Child neglect: Injuries of omission. *Pediatric Nursing, 25*(4), 401–418.

*Finkelman, A. W. (2000). Self-management for psychiatric patient at home. *Home Care Provider, 5*(6), 95–101.

*Fulmer, T., & Paveza, G. (1998). Neglect in the elderly. *Nursing Clinics of North America, 33*(3), 457–466.

Grant, J. E. (2011). *Gambling and the brain: Why neuroscience research is vital to gambling research*. Beverly, MA: National Center for Responsible Gaming. Retrieved from www.ncrg.org/sites/default/files/uploads/docs/monographs/ncrgmonograph6final.pdf

Kaakinen, J. R., Gedaly-Duff, V., Coehlo, D., & Hanson, S. (2010). *Family health care nursing, theory, practice, and research* (4th ed.). Philadelphia: F.A. Davis.

*Shah, K. R., Potenza, M. N., & Eisen, S. A. (2004). Biological basis for pathological gambling. In J. E. Grant & M. N. Potenza (Eds.), *Pathological gambling: A clinical guide to treatment* (pp. 127–142). Washington, DC: American Psychiatric Publishing.

Videbeck, S. (2013). *Psychiatric-mental health nursing* (6th ed.). Philadelphia: Lippincott Williams & Wilkins.

World Health Organization. (2014). *Mental health: A state of well-being*. Retrieved from www.who.int/features/factfiles/mental_health/en/

Wortzel, H. S., Filley, C. M., Anderson, C. A., Oster, T., & Arciniegas, D. B. (2008). Forensic applications of cerebral single photon emission computed tomography in mild traumatic brain injury. *Journal of the American Academy of Psychiatry and the Law Online, 36*(3), 310–322.

Labile Emotional Response

Beauchaine, T., Gatze-Kopp, L., & Mead, H. (2007). Polyvagal theory and developmental psychopathology: Emotion dysregulation and conduct problems from preschool to adolescence. *Biological Psychology, 74*, 174–184.

Olney, N. T., Goodkind, M. S., & Lomen-Hoerth, C. (2011). Behavior, physiology and experience of pathological laughing and crying in amyotrophic lateral sclerosis. *Brain, 134*(12), 3455–3466. Retrieved from www.ncbi.nlm.nih.gov/pmc/articles/PMC3235565

Decisional Conflict

Danis, M., Southerland, L. I., Garrett, J. M., Smith, J. L., Hielema, F., Pickard, C. G., . . . Patrick, D. L. (1991). A prospective study of advance directives for life-sustaining care. *New England Journal of Medicine, 324*(13), 882–888.

Lilley, M., Christian, S., Hume, S., Scott, P., Montgomery, M., Semple, L., . . . Somerville, M. J. (2010). Newborn screening for cystic fibrosis in Alberta: Two years of experience. *Paediatrics & Child Health, 15*(9), 590.

*Soholt, D. (1990). *A life experience: Making a health care treatment decision* (Unpublished master's thesis). South Dakota State University, Brookings, SD.

Diarrhea

Clay, P. G., & Crutchley, R. D. (2014). Noninfectious diarrhea in HIV seropositive individuals: A review of prevalence rates, etiology, and management in the era of combination antiretroviral therapy. *Infectious Diseases and Therapy, 3*(2), 103–122.

Elseviers, M. M., Van Camp, Y., Nayaert, S., Duré, K., Annemans, L., Tanghe, A., & Vermeersch, S. (2015). Prevalence and management of antibiotic associated diarrhea in general hospitals. *BMC Infectious Diseases, 15*(1), 129. Retrieved from www.biomedcentral.com/1471-2334/15/129

Food and Drug Administration. (2014). While you're pregnant—What is foodborne illness? Retrieved from www.fda.gov/Food/ResourcesForYou/HealthEducators/ucm083316.htm

*Goodgame, R. (2006). A Bayesian approach to acute infectious diarrhea in adults. *Gastroenterology Clinics, 35*(2), 249–273.

MacArthur, R. (2014). Understanding noninfectious diarrhea in HIV-infected individuals. *GI Digest*. Retrieved from www.salix.com/healthcare-professionals-resources/gi-digest-newsletter/gi-digest-archive/id/432/understanding-noninfectious-diarrhea-in-hiv-infected-individuals

*Ravry, M. J. (1980). Dietic food diarrhea. *JAMA, 244*(3), 270.

Siegal, K., Schrimshaw, E. W., Brown-Bradley, C. J., & Lekas, H. M. (2010). Sources of emotional distress associated with diarrhea among late middle-age and older HIV-infected adults. *Journal of Pain and Symptom Management, 40*(3), 353–369.

Spies, L. (2009). Diarrhea A to Z: America to Zimbabwe. *Journal of the American Academy of Nurse Practitioners, 21*(6), 307–313.

*Tramarin, A., Parise, N., Campostrini, S., Yin, D. D., Postma, M. J., Lyu, R., . . . Palladio Study Group. (2004). Association between diarrhea and quality of life in HIV-infected patients receiving highly active antiretroviral therapy. *Quality of Life Research, 13*(1), 243–250.

Wanke, C. A. (2016a). Epidemiology and causes of acute diarrhea in resource-rich countries. In *UpToDate*. Retrieved from www.uptodate.com/contents/epidemiology-and-causes-of-acute-diarrhea-in-resource-rich-countries

Wanke, C. A. (2016b). Acute diarrhea in adults (beyond the basics). In *UpToDate*. Retrieved from www.uptodate.com/contents/acute-diarrhea-in-adults-beyond-the-basics

Weller, P. (2015). Patient information: General travel advice (beyond the basics). In *UpToDate*. Retrieved from www.uptodate.com/contents/general-travel-advice-beyond-the-basics?source=see_link

Disuse Syndrome

*Maher, A., Salmond, S., & Pellino, T. (2006). *Orthopedic nursing* (3rd ed.). Philadelphia: W. B. Saunders.

Zomorodi, M., Topley, D., & McAnaw, M. (2012). Developing a mobility protocol for early mobilization of patients in a surgical/trauma ICU. *Critical Research and Practice, 2012*, 10. Retrieved from www.hindawi.com/journals/ccrp/2012/964547/

Deficient Diversional Activity

*Rantz, M. (1991). Diversional activity deficit. In M. Maas, K. Buckwalter, & M. Hardy (Eds.), *Nursing diagnoses and interventions for the elderly*. Redwood City, CA: Addison-Wesley Nursing.

Dysreflexia

*McClain, W., Shields, C., & Sixsmith, D. (1999). Autonomic dysreflexia presenting as a severe headache. *American Journal of Emergency Medicine*, *17*(3), 238–240.

Interrupted Family Process

Kaakinen, J. R., Gedaly-Duff, V., Hanson, S. M. H., & Padgett, D. (2010). *Family health care nursing: Theory, practice, and research* (4th ed.). Philadelphia: F.A. Davis.

*Lindeman, M., Hokanson, J., & Batek, J. (1994). The alcoholic family. *Nursing Diagnosis*, *5*(2), 65–73.

US Census Bureau. (2013). *America's families and living arrangements: 2012*. Retrieved from www.census.gov/prod/2013pubs/p20-570.pdf

Varcarolis, E. M., Carson, V. B., & Shoemaker, N. C. (2010). *Foundations of psychiatric mental health nursing* (6th ed.). Philadelphia: W. B. Saunders.

Deficient and Excess Fluid Volume

American Academy of Pediatrics. (2011). Policy statement— Climatic Heat Stress and Exercising Children and Adolescents. Council on Sports Medicine and Fitness and Council on School Health. *Pediatrics*, *128*(3), e741–e747.

Grieving

Ball, J., Bindler, R., & Cowen, K. (2015). *Principles of pediatric nursing: Caring for children* (6th ed.). Upper Saddle River, NJ: Pearson.

Block, S. (2013). Grief and bereavement. In *UpToDate*. Retrieved from www.uptodate.com

*Hooyman, N. R., & Kramer, B. J. (2006). *Living through loss: Interventions across the life span*. New York: Columbia University Press.

*Mina, C. (1985). A program for helping grieving parents. *Maternal-Child Nursing Journal*, *10*, 118–121.

*Vanezis, M., & McGee, A. (1999). Mediating factors in the grieving process of the suddenly bereaved. *British Journal of Nursing*, *8*(14), 932–937.

Worden, J. W. (2009). *Grief counseling and grief therapy :A handbook for the mental health practitioner* (4th ed.). New York : Springer Publishing.

Risk Prone Health Behavior

Kann, L., Kinchen, S., Shanklin, S. L., Flint, K. H., Kawkins, J., Harris, W. A., ... Whittle, L. (2014). Youth risk behavior surveillance—United States, 2013. *MMWR Surveill Summ*, *63*(Suppl 4), 1–168.

Tyler, D. O., & Horner, S. D. (2008). Family-centered collaborative negotiation: A model for facilitating behavior change in primary care. *Journal of the American Academy of Nurse Practitioners, 20*(4), 194–203.

Ineffective Health Maintenance

Ineffective Health Management

DeWalt, D. A., Callahan, L. F., Hawk, V. H., Broucksou, K. A., Hink, A, Rudd, R., & Brach, C. (2010). *Health literacy universal precautions tool kit*. Retrieved from www.ahrq.gov/professionals/quality-patient-safety/quality-resources/tools/literacy-toolkit/index.html

Iuga, A. O., & McGuire, M. J. (2014). Adherence and health care costs. *Risk Management and Healthcare Policy, 7*, 35.

Impaired Home Maintenance

Edelman, C. L., Kudzma, E. C., & Mandle, C. L. (2014). Health promotion throughout the life span (8th ed.). CV Mosby: St. Louis.

Hopelessness

Brothers, B. M., & Anderson, B. L. (2009). Hopelessness as a predictor of depressive symptoms for breast cancer patients coping with recurrence. *Psycho-Oncology, 18*, 267–275. doi:10.1002/pon.1394

*Herth, K. (1993). Hope in the family caregiver of terminally ill people. *Journal of Advanced Nursing, 18*, 538–547.

*Hinds, P., Martin, J., & Vogel, R. (1987). Nursing strategies to influence adolescent hopefulness during oncologic illness. *Journal of the Association of Pediatric Oncology Nurses, 4*(1/2), 14–23.

Risk for Compromised Human Dignity

*Walsh, K., & Kowanko, I. (2002). Nurses' and patients' perceptions of dignity. *International Journal of Nursing Practice, 8*(3), 143–151.

Disorganized Infant Behavior

*American Academy of Pediatrics (AAP) Committee on Fetus and Newborn, American Academy of Pediatrics Section on Surgery, Canadian Paediatric Society Fetus and Newborn Committee. (2006). Prevention and management of pain in the neonate: An update. *Pediatrics, 118*(5), 2231–2241.

Askin, D., & Wilson, D. (2007). The high risk newborn and family. In M. J. Hockenberry & D. Wilson (Eds.), *Wong's nursing care of infants and children* (8th ed.). St. Louis: Mosby Elsevier.

*Bozzette, M. (1993). Observations of pain behavior in the NICU: An exploratory study. *Journal of Perinatal and Neonatal Nursing, 7*(1), 76–87.

Holditch-Davis, D., & Blackburn, S. (2007). Neurobehavioral development. In C. Kenner & J. W. Lott (Eds.), *Comprehensive neonatal care: An interdisciplinary approach* (4th ed., pp. 448–479). St. Louis: Saunders Elsevier.

Kenner, C. & McGrath, J. M. (Eds.) (2010). Developmental care of newborns and infants, *The Neonatal Intensive Care Unit Environment* (pp.63–74). Glenview, IL: NANN.

*Merenstein, G. B. & Gardner, S. L. (Eds.). (2002). The neonate and the environment: Impact on development. In *Handbook of neonatal intensive care* (pp. 219–282). St. Louis, MO: Mosby.

*Thomas, K. A. (1989). How the NICU environment sounds to a preterm infant. *MCN: American Journal of Maternal-Child Nursing, 14*, 249–251.

*Vandenberg, K. (1990). The management of oral nippling in the sick neonate, the disorganized feeder. *Neonatal Network, 9*(1), 9–16.

VandenBerg, K. (2007). State systems development in high-risk newborns in the neonatal intensive care unit: Identification and management of sleep, alertness, and crying. *Journal Perinatal & Neonatal Nursing, 21*(2), 130–139.

Risk for Infection & Infection Transmission

Armstrong, D. G., & Mayr, A. (2014). Wound healing and risk factors for non-healing. In *UpToDate*. Retrieved from www.uptodate.com/contents/wound-healing-and-risk-factors-for-non-healing.

Centers for Disease Control and Prevention. (2013). *Guidance for the Selection and Use of Personal Protective Equipment (PPE) in Healthcare Settings*. CDC. Retrieved from www.google.com/webhp?sourceid=chrome-instant&ion=1&espv=2&1e=UTF-8#q=www.cdc.gov%20gloves.

Centers for Disease Control and Prevention. (2015). *Hand Hygiene in Healthcare Settings*. CDC. Retrieved from www.cdc.gov/handhygiene/.

Diaz, V., & Newman, J. (2015). Surgical site infection and prevention guidelines: A primer for certified registered nurse anesthetists. *AANA Journal, 83*(1), 63.

O'Grady, N. P., Alexander, M., Burns, L. A., Dellinger, P. E., Garland, J., Heard, S. O., . . . The Healthcare Infection Control Practices Advisory Committee (HICPAC). (2011). *Guidelines for the prevention of intravascular catheter-related infections*. Atlanta, GA: Centers for Disease Control and Prevention. Retrieved from www.cdc.gov/hicpac/pdf/guidelines/bsi-guidelines-2011.pdf

Internet Resources

Association for Professionals in Infection Control, www.apic.org

Centers for Disease Control and Prevention, www.cdc.gov

National Center for Infectious Disease, www.cdc.gov/ncidod/nicid.htm

Risk for Injury

American Association of Critical Care Nurses. (2011). *Prevention of aspiration.* Aliso Viejo, CA: Author. Retrieved from www.aacn.org/wd/practice/docs/practicealerts/prevention-aspiration-practice-alert.pdf?menu=aboutus

Kaufman, H., & Kaplan, N. M. (2015). Mechanisms, causes, and evaluation of orthostatic hypotension. In *UpToDate*. Retrieved from www.uptodate.com/contents/mechanisms-causes-and-evaluation-of-orthostatic- hypotension.

Perlmuter, L. C., Sarda, G., Casavant, V., & Mosnaim, A. D. (2013). A review of the etiology associated comorbidities and treatment of orthostatic hypotension. *American Journal of Therapeutics, 20,* 279.

*Riefkohl, E. Z., Bieber, H. L., Burlingame, M. B., & Lowenthal, D. T. (2003). Medications and falls in the elderly: A review of the evidence and practical considerations. *Pharmacy & Therapeutics, 28*(11), 724–733.

*Rothrock, J. C. (2003). *Alexander's care of the patient in surgery* (12th ed.). St. Louis: Mosby.

*Schoenfelder, D. P. (2000). A fall prevention program for elderly individuals. *Journal of Gerontological Nursing, 26*(3), 43–45.

Webster, K. (2012). *Peripheral nerve injuries and positioning for general anesthesia.* London: World Federation of Societies of Anesthesiologists. Retrieved from www.frca.co.uk/Documents/258 Peripheral Nerve Injuries and Positioning for Anaesthesia.pdf

Internet Sources

Centers for Disease Control and Prevention. (2011). Retrieved August 8, 2011 from www.cdc.gov/tobacco/data_statistics/

Professional Assisted Cessation Therapy (PACT), www.endsmoking.org

Tobacco.org, www.tobacco.org

Latex Allergy Response

American Association of Nurse Anesthetists. (2014). Latex allergy management (Guidelines). Retrieved from www.aana.com/resources2/professionalpractice/Pages/Latex-Allergy-Protocol.aspx

DeJong, N. W., Patiwael, J. A., de Groot, H., Burdorf, A., & Gerth van Wijk, R. (2011). Natural rubber latex allergy among health-care workers: Significant reduction of sensitization and clinical relevant latex allergy after introduction of powder-free latex gloves. *Journal of Allergy and Clinical Immunology, 127*(2), AB70.

Jenny, J. (1987). Knowledge deficit: Not a nursing diagnosis image. *The Journal of Nursing Scholarship, 19*(4), 184–185.

Impaired Memory

*Maier-Lorentz, M. (2000). Effective nursing interventions for the management of Alzheimer's disease. *Journal of Neuroscience Nursing, 32*(3), 153–157.

Impaired Physical Mobility

*Addams, S., & Clough, J. A. (1998). Modalities for mobilization. In A. B. Mahler, S. Salmond, & T. Pellino (Eds.), *Orthopedic nursing*. Philadelphia: W. B. Saunders.

Adler, J., & Malone, D. (2012). Early mobilization in the intensive care unit: A systematic review. *Cardiopulmonary Physical Therapy Journal, 23*(1), 5. Accessed at www.ncbi.nlm.nih.gov/pmc/articles/PMC3286494/table/T3/

American Association of Critical Care Nurses . (2012). *Early progressive mobility protocol*. ACCNPearl. Retrieved from www.aacn.org/wd/practice/docs/tool%20kits/early-progressive-mobility-protocol.pdf

American Hospital Association, & USDHHS. (2014). *Health Research & Educational Trust, American Hospital Association, partnership for patients ventilator associated events (VAE) change package: Preventing harm from VAE 2014 update*. Retrieved from www.hret-hen.org/index.php?option=com_content&view=article&id=10&Itemid=134

Gillis, A., MacDonald, B., & MacIssac, A. (2008). Nurses' knowledge, attitudes, and confidence regarding preventing and treating deconditioning in older adults. *The Journal of Continuing Education in Nursing, 39*(12), 547–554.

Halsstead, J., & Stoten, S. (2010). Orthopedic nursing: Caring for patients with musculoskeletal disorders. Brockton, MA: Western Schools.

King, L. (2012). Developing a progressive mobility activity protocol. *Orthopaedic Nursing, 31*(5), 253–262.

Levin, R. F., Krainovitch, B. C., Bahrenburg, E., & Mitchell, C. A. (1989). Diagnostic content validity of nursing diagnoses. Image: *Journal of Nursing Scholarship, 21*(1), 40–44.

Timmerman, R. A. (2007). A mobility protocol for critically ill adults. *Dimensions of Critical Care Nursing, 26*(5), 175–179. Retrieved from www0.sun.ac.za/Physiotherapy_ICU_algorithm/Documentation/Rehabilitation/References/Timmerman_2007.pdf

Vollman, K. M. (2012). Hemodynamic instability: Is it really a barrier to turning critically ill patients? *Critical care nurse, 32*(1), 70–75.

Zomorodi, M., Topley, D., & McAnaw, M. (2012). Developing a mobility protocol for early mobilization of patients in a surgical/trauma ICU. *Critical Care Research and Practice*. Article ID 964547. doi:10.1155/2012/964547

Moral Distress

*American Association of Critical Care Nurses. (2004). *The 4 A's to rise above moral distress.* AACN Ethics Work Group. Aliso Viejo, CA: AACN.

American Nurse's Association. (2010a). *Just culture.* Retrieved from www.justculture.org/Downloads/ANA_Just_Culture.pdf

American Nurses Association. (2010b). *Nursing: Scope and standards of practice* (2nd ed.). Silver Springs, MD: Author.

*Beckstrand, R. L., Callsiter, L. C., & Kirchhoff, K. T. (2006). Providing a "Good Death": Critical care nurse's suggestions for improving end-of-life care. *American Journal of Critical Care, 15*(1), 38–45.

Gallup Poll. (2009). *Honesty and ethics poll finds congress' image tarnished.* Retrieved from www.gallup/poll124625/honesty-ethics-pol

LaSala, C. A., & Bjarnason, D. (2010). Creating workplace environments that support moral courage. *The Online Journal of Issues in Nursing, 15*(3), 1–11. Retrieved from www.nursingworld.org/OJIN

Lusardi P., Jodka, P., Stambovsky, M., Stadnicki, B., Babb, B., Plouffe, D., . . . Montonye, M. (2011). The going home initiative: Getting critical care patients home with hospice. *Critical Care Nurse, 31*(5), 46–57.

Zuzelo, P. R. (2007). Exploring the moral distress of registered nurses. *Nursing Ethics, 14*(3), 344–359.

Noncompliance

Gruman, J. (2011). Engagement does not mean compliance. *Center for Advancing Health.* Retrieved from www.cfah.org/blog/2011/engagement-does-not-mean-compliance

Imbalanced Nutrition

*Chima, C. (2004). *The nutrition care process: Driving effective intervention and outcomes*. Retrieved from www3.uakron.edu/.../ Screening%20Nutrition%20Ca

Fass, R. (2014). Overview of dysphagia in adults. In *Up to Date*. Retrieved from www.uptodate.com/contents/overview-of-dysphagia-in-adults

Gröber, U., & Kisters, K., (2007). Influence of drugs on vitamin D and calcium metabolism. *Dermatoendocrinology, 4*(2), 158–166.

*Hammond, K. A. (2011). Assessment: Dietary and clinical data. In L. Kathleen Mahan, J. L Raymond, & S. Escott-Stump (Eds.), Krause's food & the nutrition care process (13th ed.). St. Louis: Elsevier.

*Hunter, J. H. & Cason, K. L. (2006). Nutrient density clemson university cooperative extension service. Retrieved from www .clemson.edu/extension/hgic/food/nutrition/nutrition/dietary_ guide/hgic40 62.html

Sura, L., Madhavan, A., Carnaby, G., & Crary M. A. (2012). Dysphagia in the elderly: Management and nutritional considerations. *Clinical Interventions in Aging, 7,* 287–298.

Impaired Swallowing

*Emick-Herring, B., & Wood, P. (1990). A team approach to neurologically based swallowing disorders. *Rehabilitation Nursing, 15,* 126–132.

Obesity & Overweight

*Hunter, J. H., & Cason, K. L. (2006). *Nutrient density*. Clemson University Cooperative Extension Service. Retrieved at www. clemson.edu/extension/hgic/food/nutrition/nutrition/dietary_ guide/hgic40 62.html

Institute of Medicine. (2009). *Weight gain during pregnancy: Reexamining the guidelines*. Retrieved from www.nap.edu

*Martin, L. R., Williams, S. L., Haskard, K. B., & DiMatteo, M. R. (2005). The challenge of patient adherence. *Therapeutic Clinincal Risk Management, 1*(3), 189–199.

Pelzang, R. (2010). Time to learn: Understanding patient-centered care. *British Journal of Nursing, 19*(14), 912–917.

Impaired Parenting

Ball, J., Bindler, R., & Cowen, K. (2015). *Principles of pediatric nursing: Caring for children* (6th ed.). Upper Saddle River, NJ: Pearson.

*Gage, J., Everett, K., & Bullock, L. (2006). Integrative review of parenting in nursing research. *Journal of Nursing Scholarship, 38*(1), 56–62. Retrieved from CINAHL Plus with Full Text database.

Post-Trauma/Rape-Trauma Syndrome

Acierno, R., Hernandez, M. A., Amstadter, A. B., Resnick, H. S., Steve, K., Muzzy, W., & Kilpatrick, D. G. (2010). Prevalence and correlates of emotional, physical, sexual, and financial abuse and potential neglect in the United States: The National Elder Mistreatment Study. *American Journal of Public, 100*(2), 292–297.

*Burgess, A. W. (1995). Rape-trauma syndrome: A nursing diagnosis. *Occupational Health Nursing, 33*(8), 405–410.

Centers for Disease Control and Prevention. (2008). *HIV transmission rates in US*. Retrieved February 25, 2009, from www.cdc.gov/hiv/topics/surveillance/resources/fact-sheets/

Dudek, S. G. (2014). *Nutrition essentials for nursing practice* (7th ed.). Philadelphia: Wolters Kluwer.

Friedman, M. J. (2016). PTSD history and overview. Retrieved from www.ptsd.va.gov/professional/PTSD-overview/ptsd-overview.asp

*Ledray, L. E. (2001). Evidence collection and care of the sexually assault survivor: SANE-SART response. Retrieved from www.vaw.umn.edu/documents/commissioned/2forensicvidence.htlm

U.S. Department of Justice. (2014). *Rape and sexual assault*. Retrieved from www.bjs.gov/index.cfm?ty=tp&tid=317

Powerlessness

Orzeck, T., Rokach, A., & Chin, J. (2010). The effects of traumatic and abusive relationships. *Journal of Loss & Trauma, 15*(3), 167–192. doi:10.1080/15325020903375792

Ineffective Protection

Risk for Corneal Injury/Risk for Red Eye

Mayo Clinic. (2010). *Red eye*. Retrieved from www.mayoclinic.org/symptoms/red-eye/basics/definition/sym-20050748

Impaired Oral Mucous Membrane

Eilers, J., Harris, D., Henry, K., & Johnson, L. A. (2014). Evidence-based interventions for cancer treatment-related mucositis: Putting evidence into practice. *Clinical Journal of Oncology Nursing, 18*, 80–96.

Feider, L. I., Mitchell, P., Bridges, E. (2010). Oral care practices for orally intubated critically ill adults. *American Journal of Critical Care, 19*(2), 175–183.

National Comprehensive Cancer Network. (2008). *Oral mucositis is often underrecognized and undertreated*. Retrieved from www.nccn.org/professionals/meetings/13thannual/highlights

Perry, S. E., Hockenberry, M. J., Lowdermilk, D. L., & Wilson, D. (2014). *Maternal child nursing care* (5th ed.). St. Louis, MO: Elsevier.

Quinn, B., Baker, D. L., Cohen, S., Stewart, J. L., Lima, C. A., & Parise, C. (2014). Basic nursing care to prevent nonventilator hospital-acquired pneumonia. *Journal of Nursing Scholarship*, 46 (1), 11–17.

Risk for Impaired Tissue Integrity/Pressure Ulcer

Agency for Healthcare Research and Quality. (2011). *Are we ready for this change? Preventing pressure ulcers in hospitals: A toolkit for improving quality of care*. Rockville, MD: Author. Retrieved from www.ahrq.gov/professionals/systems/long-term-care/resources/pressure-ulcers/pressureulcertoolkit/putool1.html

Armstrong, A., & Meyr, D. (2014). Clinical assessment of wounds. In *Up to Date*. Retrieved from www.uptodate.com/contents/clinical-assessment-of-wounds

*Bennett, M. A. (1995). Report of the task force on the implications for darkly pigmented intact skin in the prediction and prevention of pressure ulcers. *Advances in Skin & Wound Care*, 8(6), 34–35.

*Bergstrom, N., Allman, R., Alvarez, O., Bennett, M., Carlson, C., Frantz, R., . . . Yarkony, G. (1994). *Treatment of pressure ulcers*. Clinical practice guideline (No. 15). Rockville, MD: Agency for Health Care Policy and Research, AHCPR Publication No. 95-0652.

Berlowitz, D. (2014). Epidemiology, pathogenesis and risk assessment of pressure ulcers. In *UpToDate*. Retrieved from www.uptodate.com/contents/epidemiology-pathogenesis-and-risk-assessment-of-pressure-ulcers?source=search_result&search=pressure+ulcers&selectedTitle=4~120

Berlowitz, D. (2015). Clinical staging and management of pressure ulcers. In *UpToDate*. Retrieved from www.uptodate.com/contents/clinical-staging-and-management-of-pressure-ulcers?

Brem, H., Maggi, J., Nierman, D., Rolnitzky, L., Bell, D., Rennert, R., . . . Vladeck, B. (2010). High cost of stage IV pressure ulcers. *American Journal of Surgery*, 200(4), 473–477. Retrieved from www.ncbi.nlm.nih.gov/pmc/articles/PMC2950802/

Clark, M. (2010). Skin assessment in dark pigmented skin: A challenge in pressure ulcer prevention. *Nursing Times*, 106(30), 16–17.

Dorner, B., Posthauer, M. E., & Thomas, D. (2009). The role of nutrition in pressure ulcer prevention and treatment: National Pressure Ulcer Advisory Panel white paper. *Advances in Skin & Wound Care*, 22(5), 212–221.

*Fore, J. (2006). A review of skin and the effects of aging on skin structure and function. *Ostomy Wound Manage*, 52(9), 24–35.

Guo, S., & DiPietro, L. A. (2010). Factors affecting wound healing. *Journal of dental research*, *89*(3), 219–229.

Ling, S. M., & Mandl, S. (2013). *Pressure ulcers: CMS update and perspectives*. National Pressure Ulcer Advisory Panel Biennial Conference, Houston, TX. Retrieved from www.npuap.org/wp-content/uploads/2012/01/NPUAP2013-LingMandl-FINAL2-25-131.pdf

*Maklebust, J., & Sieggreen, M. (2006). *Pressure ulcers: Guidelines for prevention and nursing management* (3rd ed.). Springhouse, PA: Springhouse.

National Pressure Ulcer Advisory Panel, European Pressure Ulcer Advisory Panel. (2014). *Clinical practice guideline*. Retrieved from www.npuap.org/resources/educational-and-clinical-resources/prevention-and-treatment-of-pressure-ulcers-clinical-practice-guideline/

*Wound Ostomy Continence Nursing (WOCN). (2003). *Guideline for prevention and management of pressure ulcers*. Glenview, IL: Author.

Relocation Stress

Chrisitie, L. (2014). *Foreclosures hit six-year low in 2013*. Retrieved from http://money.cnn.com/2014/01/16/real_estate/foreclosure-crisis/

Whittenhall, J. (2008). *Helping an adolescent student cope with moving*. The College of Information Sciences and Technology. Retrieved from http://citeseerx.ist.psu.edu/viewdoc/download?doi=10.1.1.509.86&rep=rep1&type=pdf

Risk for Ineffective Respiratory Function

*Chan, L. (1998). Effectiveness of a music therapy intervention on relaxation and anxiety for patients receiving ventilation assistance. *Heart and Lung, 27*(3), 169–176.

Epstien, S. (2015). Weaning from mechanical ventilation: Readiness testing. In *UpToDate*. Retrieved from www.uptodate.com/contents/weaning-from-mechanical-ventilation-readiness-testing

Institute for Healthcare Improvement. (2008). Implement the ventilator bundle: Elevation of the head of the bed. Retrieved from www.ihi.org/IHI/Topics/CriticalCare/IntensiveCare/Changes/IndividualChanges/Elevationoftheheadofthebed.htm

*Jenny, J., & Logan, J. (1991). Analyzing expert nursing practice to develop a new nursing diagnosis: Dysfunctional ventilatory weaning response. In R. M. Carroll-Johnson (Ed.), *Classification of nursing diagnoses: Proceedings of the ninth conference*. Philadelphia: J. B. Lippincott.

*Logan, J., & Jenny, J. (1990). Deriving a new nursing diagnosis through qualitative research: Dysfunctional ventilatory weaning response. *Nursing Diagnosis, 1*(1), 37–43.

*Morton, P., Fontaine, D., Hudak, C., & Gallo, B. (2005). *Critical care nursing* (8th ed.). Philadelphia: Lippincott Williams & Wilkins.

Nance-Floyd, B. (2011). Tracheostomy care: An evidence-based guide to suctioning and dressing changes. *American Nurses Today, 6*(7), 14–16.

Schwartzstein, R. M., & Richards, J. (2014). *Hyperventilation syndrome*. Retrieved from www.uptodate.com/contents/hyper-ventilation-syndrome

Sharma, S., Sarin, J., & Bala, G. K. (2014). Effectiveness of endotracheal suctioning protocol, In terms of knowledge and practices of nursing personnel. *Nursing and Midwifery Research Journal, 10*(2), 47–60.

Swadener-Culpepper, L. (2010). Continuous lateral rotation therapy. *Critical Care Nurse, 30*(2), S5–S7. Retrieved from Medline Database.

WebMD. (2012). *Hyperventilation*. Retrieved from www.webmd.com/a-to-z-guides/hyperventilation-credits

Internet Resources

Agency for Healthcare Research and Quality, www.ahrq.gov/

Asthma and Allergy Foundation of America, www.aafa.org/

Asthma Management Model, www.nhlbi.nih.gov/health/public/lung/index.htm

Global Initiative for Chronic Obstructive Lung Disease, www.goldcopd.org

Joint Council of Asthma, Allergy, and Immunology, www.jcaai.org/

Quitting Smoking Guidelines, www.surgeongeneral.gov/tobacco/default.htm

QuitNet, www.quitnet.com

Disturbed Self-Concept

*Atherton, R., & Robertson, N. (2006). Psychological adjustment to lower limb amputation amongst prosthesis users. *Disability and Rehabilitation, 28*(9), 1201–1209.

*Camp-Sorrell, D. (2007). Chemotherapy: Toxicity management. In C. Yarbro, M. H. Frogge, M. Goodman, & S. Groenwald, *Career nursing* (6th ed.). Boston: Jones and Bartlett.

Holzer, L. A., Sevelda, F., Fraberger, G., Bluder, O., Kickinger, W., & Holzer, G. (2014). Body image and self-esteem in lower-limb amputees. *PLoS One, 9*(3), e92943. Retrieved from www.ncbi.nlm.nih.gov/pmc/articles/PMC3963966/

*Johnson, B. S. (1995). *Child, adolescent and family psychiatric nursing*. Philadelphia: J.B. Lippincott.

*Leuner, J., Coler, M., & Norris, J. (1994). Self-esteem. In M. Rantz & P. LeMone (Eds.), *Classification of nursing diagnosis: Proceedings of the eleventh conference*. Glendale, CA: CINAHL.

Martin, B. (2013). Challenging negative self-talk. In *Psych Central*. Retrieved on August 26, 2015, from psychcentral.com/lib/challenging-negative-self-talk/

*Murray, M. F. (2000). Coping with change: Self-talk. *Hospital Practice, 31*(5), 118–120.

Risk for Self-Harm

American Foundation for Suicide Prevention. (2015). *Facts and figures*. Retrieved from www.afsp.org/understanding-suicide/facts-and-figures

*Carscadden, J. S. (1993). *On the cutting edge: A guide for working with people who self injure*. London, Ontario: London Psychiatric Hospital.

Tofthagen, R., Talsethand, A. G., & Fagerström, L. (2014). Mental health nurses' experiences of caring for patients suffering from self-harm. *Nursing Research and Practice*. doi:10.1155/2014/905741

Ineffective Sexuality Patterns

*Annon, J. S. (1976). The PLISST model: A proposed conceptual scheme for the behavioral treatment of sexual problems. *Journal of Sex Education and Therapy, 2*, 211–215.

Ginsburg, K. R. (2015). *Talking to your child about sex*. Retrieved from www.healthychildren.org/English/ages-stages/gradeschool/puberty/Pages/Talking-to-Your-Child-About-Sex.aspx.

Kazer, M. W. (2012a). Issues regarding sexuality. In: M. Boltz, E. Capezuti, T. Fulmer, & D. Zwicker (Eds.), *Evidence-based geriatric nursing protocols for best practice* (4th ed., pp. 500–515). New York: Springer.

Kazer, M. W. (2012b). *Sexuality assessment for older adults best practices in nursing care to older adults*. Retrieved from http://consultgerirn.org/uploads/File/trythis/try_this_10.pdf

Disturbed Sleep Pattern

Arthritis Foundation. (2012). *Sleep problems with arthritis*. Retrieved from www.arthritis.org/living-with-arthritis/comorbidities/sleep-insomnia/

Bartick, M. C., Thai, X., Schmidt, T., Altaye, A., & Solet, J. M. (2010). Decrease in as-needed sedative use by limiting nighttime sleep disruptions from hospital staff. *Journal of Hospital Medicine, 5*(3), E20–E24.

Cole, C., & Richards, K. (2007). Sleep disruption in older adults: Harmful and by no means inevitable, it should be assessed for and treated. *AJN The American Journal of Nursing, 107*(5), 40–49.

Faraklas, I., Holt, B., Tran, S., Lin, H., Saffle, J., & Cochran, A. (2013). Impact of a nursing-driven sleep hygiene protocol on sleep quality. *Journal of Burn Care & Research, 34*(2), 249–254.

Chronic Sorrow

*Burke, M. L., Hainsworth, M. A., Eakes, G. G., & Lindgren, C. L. (1992). Current knowledge and research on chronic sorrow: A foundation for inquiry. *Death Studies, 16*(3), 231–245.

Gordon, J. (2009). An evidence-based approach for supporting parents experiencing chronic sorrow. *Pediatric Nursing, 35*(2), 115–119.

*Melnyk, B., Feinstein, N., Moldenhouer, Z., & Small, L. (2001). Coping of parents of children who are chronically ill. *Pediatric Nursing, 27*(6), 548–558.

*Monsen, R. B. (1999). Mothers' experiences of living worried when parenting children with spina bifida. *Journal of Pediatric Nursing, 14*(3), 157–163.

Rhode Island Department of Health. (2011). *Resource guide for families of children with autism spectrum*. Retrieved from www.health.ri.gov/publications/guidebooks/2011ForFamiliesOfChildrenWithAutismSpectrumDisorders.pdf

*Teel, C. (1991). Chronic sorrow: Analysis of the concept. *Journal of Advanced Nursing, 16*(11), 1311–1319.

Spiritual Distress

*Burkhart, L., & Solari-Twadell, A. (2001). Spirituality and religiousness: Differentiating the diagnoses through a review of the nursing diagnosis. *12*(2), 44–54.

*Kendrick, K. D., & Robinson, S. (2000). Spirituality: Its relevance and purpose for clinical nursing in the new millennium. *Journal of Clinical Nursing, 9*(5), 701–705.

*O'Brien, M. E. (2010). *Spirituality in nursing: Standing on holy ground* (4th ed.). Boston: Jones and Bartlett.

Puchalski, C. M., & Ferrell, B. (2010). *Making Health Care Whole: Integrating Spirituality into Patient Care*. West Conshohocken, PA: Templeton Press.

Swift, C., Calcutawalla, S., & Elliot, R. (2007). Nursing attitudes towards recording of religious and spiritual data. *British Journal of Nursing, 16*(20), 1279–1282.

*Wright, L. M. (2004). Spirituality, suffering, and illness: Ideas for healing. Philadelphia: F.A. Davis Co.

Stress Overload

*Bodenheimer, T., MacGregor, K., & Sharifi, C. (2005). *Helping patients manage their chronic conditions*. Retrieved from www.chef.org/publications

Peaceful Parenting Institute. (2015). *Avoiding stress overload*. Retrieved from www.peacefulparent.com/avoiding-stress-overload/

U.S. Department of Health and Human Service. (2015). *Healthy people 2020*. Retrieved from www.healthypeople.gov/2020/topics-objectives

Risk for Sudden Infant Death Syndrome

Anderson, J. E. (2000). Co-sleeping: Can we ever put the issue to rest? *Contemporary Pediatrics*, *17*(6), 98–102, 109–110, 113–114.

Corwin, M. J. (2015). Sudden infant death syndrome. In *UpToDate*. Retrieved from www.uptodate.com/contents/sudden-infant-death-syndrome-risk-factors- and-risk-reduction-strategies

Edelman, C. L., Kudzma, E. C., & Mandle, C. L. (2014). *Health promotion throughout the life span* (8th ed.). St. Louis: C.V. Mosby.

Risk for Delayed Surgical Recovery

Price, C. S., Williams, A., Philips, G., Dayton, M., Smith, W., & Morgan, S. (2008). *Staphylococcus aureus* nasal colonization in preoperative orthopaedic outpatients. *Clinical Orthopaedics and Related Research*, *466*(11), 2842–2847.

Impaired Urinary Elimination

Davis, N. J., Vaughan, C. P., Johnson, T. M., Goode, P. S., Burgio, K. L., Redden, D. T., & Markland, A. D. (2013). Caffeine intake and its association with urinary incontinence in United States men: Results from National Health and Nutrition Examination Surveys 2005–2006 and 2007–2008. *The Journal of Urology*, *189*(6), 2170–2174.

Derrer, D. (2014). Diet, drugs and urinary incontinence. WebMD. Retrieved from www.webmd.com/urinary-incontinence-oab/urinary-incontinence-diet-medications-chart?page=2

DuBeau, C. E. (2014). Treatment and prevention of urinary incontinence in women. In *UpToDate*. Retrieved from www.uptodate.com/home

DuBeau, C. (2015). Epidemiology, risk factors, and pathogenesis of urinary incontinence in women. In *UpToDate*. Retrieved from www.uptodate.com/contents/epidemiology-risk-factors-and-pathogenesis-of-urinary-incontinence-in-women

Gleason, J. L., Richter, H. E., Redden, D. T., Goode, P. S., Burgio, K. L., & Markland, A. D. (2013). Caffeine and urinary incontinence in US women. *International Urogynecology Journal*, *24*(2), 295–302.

Holroyd-Leduc, J., Tannenbaum, C., Thorpe, K., & Straus, S. (2008). What type of urinary incontinence does this woman have? *Journal of the American Medical Association, 299*, 1446–1456.

Lukacz, E. (2015). Treatment of urinary incontinence in women. In *UpToDate*. Retrieved from www.uptodate.com/contents/treatment-of-urinary-incontinence-in-women

Mayo Clinic. (2012). Kegel exercises: A how-to guide for women. In *Healthy lifestyle/women's health*. Retrieved from www.mayo-clinic.org/healthy-lifestyle/womens-health/in-depth/kegel-exercises/art-20045283?pg=1

*Morant, C. A. (2005). ACOG guidelines on urinary incontinence in women. *American Family Physician, 72*(1), 175–178.

National Clinical Guideline Centre. (2010). *Nocturnal enuresis: The management of bedwetting in children and young people*. London, UK: National Institute for Health and Clinical Excellence (NICE) (Clinical Guideline No. 111). Retrieved from www.guideline.gov/content.aspx?id=25680

*Nygaard, I. E., Thompson, F. L., Svengalis, S. L., & Albright, J. P. (1994). Urinary incontinence in elite nulliparous athletes. *Obstetrics & Gynecology, 84*(2), 183–187.

Smeltzer, S., Bare, B., Hinkle, J., & Cheever, K. (2010). *Brunner & Suddarth's textbook of medical-surgical nursing* (12th ed.). Philadelphia: Lippincott Williams & Wilkins.

*Smith, D. B. (2004). Female pelvic floor health: A developmental review. *Journal of Wound Ostomy & Continence Nursing, 31*(3), 130–137.

Testa, A. (2015). Understanding urinary incontinence in adults. *Society of Urologic Nurses and Associates, 35*, 82–86.

Tu, N. D., Baskin, L. S., & Amhym, A. M. (2014). Nocturnal enuresis in children: Etiology and evaluation. In *UpToDate*. Retrieved from www.uptodate.com/contents/nocturnal-enuresis-in-children-etiology-and-evaluation

Wilkinson, J., & Van Leuven, K. (2007). *Fundamentals of nursing: Theory, concepts & applications*. Philadelphia: F.A. Davis.

Wilson, P., Berghmans, B., Hagen, S., Hay-Smith, J., Moore, K., Nygaard, I., . . . Wyman, J. (2005) Adult conservative management in incontinence. In: *Incontinence Volume 2: Management*. Paris: International Continence Society Health Publication.

SECTION 2: HEALTH PROMOTION/WELLNESS NURSING DIAGNOSES

Allender, J. A., Rector, C., & Warner, K. (2014). *Community health nursing* (8th ed.). Philadelphia, PA: Wolters Kluwer.

*Bodenheimer, T., MacGregor, K., & Sharifi, C. (2005). *Helping patients manage their chronic conditions.* Retrieved January 10, 2007, from www.chef.org/publications

*Blackburn, S. (1993). Assessment and management of neuralgic dysfunction. In C. Kenner, A. Brueggemeyer, & L. Gunderson (Eds.), *Comprehensive neonatal nursing.* Philadelphia: W. B. Saunders.

*Breslow, D., & Hron, B. G. (2004). Time-extended family interviewing. *Family Process, 16(1),* 97–103 (reprint, March 1977).

Edelman, C. L., Kudzma, E. C. & Mandle, C. L. (2014). *Health promotion throughout the Life span* (8th ed.). St. Louis: C.V. Mosby.

*Gordon, M. (2002). *Manual of nursing diagnosis.* St. Louis: Mosby-Year Book.

*Vandenberg, K. (1990). The management of oral nippling in the sick neonate, the disorganized feeder. *Neonatal Network, 9*(1), 9–16.

SECTION 3: MANUAL OF COLLABORATIVE PROBLEMS

Barbar, S., Noventa, F., Rossetto, V., Ferrari, A., Brandolin, B., Perlati, M., . . . Prandoni, P. (2010). A risk assessment model for the identification of hospitalized medical patients at risk for venous thromboembolism: The Padua Prediction Score. *Journal of Thrombosis and Haemostasis, 8*(11), 2450–2457.

Barrisford, G., & Steele, G. S. (2014). Acute urinary retention. In *UpToDate.* Retrieved from www.uptodate.com/contents/acute-urinary-retention

Bordeianou, L., & Yeh, D. D. (2015). Epidemiology, clinical features, and diagnosis of mechanical small bowel obstruction in adults. In *UpToDate.* Retrieved from www.uptodate.com/contents/epidemiology-clinical-features-and-diagnosis-of-mechanical-small-bowel-obstruction-in-adults

Chow, E., Bernjak, A., Williams, S., Fawdry, R. A., Hibbert, S., Freeman, J., . . . Heller, S. R. (2014). Risk of cardiac arrhythmias during hypoglycemia in patients with type 2 diabetes and cardiovascular risk. *Diabetes, 63*(5), 1738–1747.

Chu, Y. F., Jiang, Y., Meng, M., Jiang, J. J., Zhang, J. C., Ren, H. S., & Wang, C. T. (2010). Incidence and risk factors of gastrointestinal bleeding in mechanically ventilated patients. *World J Emergency Medicine, 1*(1), 32–36.

Deegens, J. K., & Wetzels, J. F. (2011). Nephrotic range proteinuria. In John T. Daugirdas (Ed.), *Handbook of chronic kidney disease management* (pp. 313–332). Philadelphia: Lippincott Williams & Wilkins.

Eriksson, E. A., Schultz, S. E., Cohle, S. D., & Post, K. W. (2011). Cerebral fat embolism without intracardiac shunt: A novel presentation. *Journal of Emergencies, Trauma, and Shock, 4*(2), 309–312.

Fazia, A., Lin, J., & Staros, E. (2012). *Urine sodium.* Retrieved December 28, 2012, from http://emedicine.medscape.com/article/2088449-overview#showall

Halloran, R. S. (2009). Caring for the patient with inflammatory response, shock, and severe sepsis caring for the patient with inflammatory response, shock, and severe sepsis (Chap. 61). In Osborn, K. (Ed.), *Medical surgical nursing: Preparation for practice* (Vol. 1). Upper Saddle River, NJ: Prentice Hall.

Heist, E. K., & Ruskin, J. N. (2010). Drug-induced arrhythmia. *Circulation, 122*(14), 1426–1435.

Institute for Clinical System Improvement [ICSI]. (2008). *Health care guideline: Venous thromboembolism prophylaxis* (5th ed.). Bloomington, MN: Author. Retrieved from www.icsi.org

Kovesdy, C. P., Kopple, J. D., & Kalantar-Zadeh, K. (2015). Inflammation in renal insufficiency. In *UpToDate.* Retrieved from www.uptodate.com/contents/inflammation-inrenal-insufficiency

Labs on Line. (2014). Retrieved from https://labtestsonline.org/

Mabvuure, N. T., Malahias, M., Hindocha, S., Khan, W., & Juma, A. (2012). Acute compartment syndrome of the limbs: Current concepts and management. *The Open Orthopaedics Journal, 6*(1), 535–543.

McCutcheon, T. (2013). The Ileus and Oddities After Colorectal Surgery. *Gastroenterology Nursing, 36*(5), 368–375.

National Qualitty Forum. (2011). *Serious reportable events in healthcare—2011 update: A consensus report.* Retrieved from www.qualityforum.org/projects/hacs_and_sres.aspx

Neviere, R. (2015). Sepsis and the systemic inflammatory response syndrome: Definitions, epidemiology, and prognosis. In *UpToDate.* Retrieved from www.uptodate.com/contents/sepsis-and-the-systemic-inflammatory-response-syndrome-definitions-epidemiology-and-prognosis

O'Dowd, L. C., & Kelle, M. A. (2015). Air embolism. In *UpToDate.* Retrieved from www.uptodate.com/contents/air-embolism

*Lynn-McHale Wiegand, D. J., & Carlson, K. K. (2005). *AACN procedure manual for critical care.* St. Louis, MO: Elsevier.

Payne, A. B., Miller, C. H., Hooper, W. C., Lally, C., & Austin, H. D. (2014). High factor VIII, von Willebrand factor, and fibrinogen levels and risk of venous thromboembolism in blacks and whites. *Ethnicity & Disease, 24*(2), 169–174.

Pereira de Melo, R., Venícios de Oliveira Lopes, M., Leite de Araujo, T., de Fatima da Silva, L., Aline Arrais Sampaio Santos, F., & Moorhead, S. (2011). Risk for decreased cardiac output: Validation of a proposal for nursing diagnosis. *Nursing in Critical Care, 16*(6), 287–294.

The Renal Association. (2013). *Clinical practice guidelines.* Retrieved at www.renal.org/information-resources/the-uk-eckd-guide/ckd-stages#sthash.B1UX7gPz.3q8WiJDw.dpbs

Schmidt, A., & Mandel, J. (2012). Management of severe sepsis and septic shock in adults. In *UpToDate.* Retrieved January 19, 2013, from www.uptodate.com/contents/management-of-severe-sepsis-and-septic-shock-in-adults

Shadgan, B., Menon, M., Sanders, D., Berry, G., Martin, C., Duffy, P., Stephen, D., O'Brien, P. J. (2010). Current thinking about acute compartment syndrome of the lower extremity. *Canadian Journal of Surgery, 53*(5), 329–334.

Shaughnessy, K. (2007). Massive pulmonary embolism. *Critical Care Nurse, 27*(1), 39–51.

Stracciolini, A., & Hammerberg, E. M. (2014). Acute compartment syndrome of the extremities. In *UpToDate.* Retrieved from www.uptodate.com/contents/acutecompartment-syndrome-of-the-extremities

Urinary Retention. (2012,). Retrieved from http://kidney.niddk.nih.gov/kudiseases/pubs/UrinaryRetention/

Weinhouse, G. L. (2016). Fat embolism syndrome. In *UpToDate.* Retrieved from www.uptodate.com/contents/fat-embolism-syndrome

APPENDICES

*Cornish, P. L., Knowles, S. R., Marchesano, R., Tam, V., Shadowitz, S., Juurlink, D. N., & Etchells, E. E. (2005). Unintended medication discrepancies at the time of hospital admission. *Archives of Internal Medicine, 165*(4), 424–429.

DeWalt, D. A., Callahan, L., Hawk, V. H,. Broucksou, K. A., & Hink, A. (2010). *Health literacy universal precautions tool kit.* Rockville, MD: Agency for Healthcare Research and Quality. Retrieved from www.ahrq.gov/professionals/quality-patient-safety/quality-resources/tools/literacy-toolkit/healthliteracytoolkit.pdf

Entwistle, V. A., McCaughan, D., Watt, I. S., Birks, Y., Hall, J., Peat, M., . . . Wright, J. (2010). Speaking up about safety concerns: Multi-setting qualitative study of patients' views and experiences. *Quality and Safety in Health Care, 19*(6), e33–e33.

Franz, M. G., Robson, M. C., Steed, D. L., Barbul, A., Brem, H., Cooper, D. M., . . . Wiersema-Bryant, L. (2008). Guidelines to aid healing of acute wounds by decreasing impediments of healing. *Wound Repair and Regeneration*, *16*(6), 723–748.

Frosch, D. L., & Elwyn, G. (2014). Don't blame patients, engage them: Transforming health systems to address health literacy. *Journal of Health Communication*, *19*(Suppl 2), 10–14.

Frosch, D. L., May, S. G., Rendle, K. A., Tietbohl, C., & Elwyn, G. (2012). Authoritarian physicians and patients' fear of being labeled 'difficult' among key obstacles to shared decision making. *Health Affairs*, *31*(5), 1030–1038.

*Hibbard, J. H., & Cunningham, P. J. (2008). How engaged are consumers in their health and health care, and why does it matter? Findings from HSC No. 8: Providing insights that contribute to better health policy. Washington, DC: HSC

*Kutner, M., Greenberg, E., Jin, Y., & Paulsen, C. (2006). *The health literacy of America's adults: Results from the 2003 National Assessment of Adult Literacy.* U.S. Dept. of Education. Washington, DC: National Center for Education Statistics. Retrieved from http://nces.ed.gov/pubs2006/2006483.pdf

Morse, J. M. (1997). *Preventing patient falls.* Thousand Oaks: Sage Broda

*National Association of Adult Literacy. (2003). Health literacy of America's adults: Results of the National Assessment of Adult Literacy (NAAL). Retrieved from https://nces.ed.gov/naal/

Pear, S. M. (2007). *Managing infection control: Patients risk factors and best practices for surgical site infection prevention* (pp. 56–63). Tucson, AZ: University of Arizona.

*Podsiadlo, D., & Richardson, S. (1991). The timed 'Up and Go' test: A test of basic functional mobility for frail elderly persons. *Journal of American Geriatric Society.* 1991, 39:142–148 Retrieved August 2, 2012, www.fallrventiontaskforce.orgpdf. Timed UpandGoTest.pdf

Price, C. S., Williams, A., Philips, G., Dayton, M., Smith, W., & Morgan, S. (2008). *Staphylococcus aureus* nasal colonization in preoperative orthopaedic outpatients. *Clinical Orthopaedics and Related Research*, *466*(11), 2842–2847.

*Ratzan, S. C. (2001). Health literacy: Communication for the public good. *Health Promotion International*, *16*(2), 207–214.

*Roter, D. L., Rune, R. E., & Comings, J. (1998). Patient literacy: A barrier to quality of care. *Journal General Internal Medicine*, *13*(12), 850–851.

Sofaer, S., & Schumann, M. J. (2013). *Fostering successful patient and family engagement.* This White Paper was prepared for the Nursing Alliance for Quality Care with grant support from the Agency for Healthcare Research and Quality (AHRQ); Approved. Retrieved from www.naqc.org/WhitePaper-PatientEngagement

Sørensen, L. T. (2012). Wound healing and infection in surgery: The pathophysiological impact of smoking, smoking cessation, and nicotine replacement therapy: A systematic review. *Annals of Surgery, 255*(6), 1069–1079. Retrieved from http://archsurg jamanetwork.com/article.aspx?articleid=1151013

Weiss, B. D. (2007). *Health literacy and patient safety: Help patients understand.* American Medical Association. Retrieved from http://med.fsu.edu/userFiles/file/ahec_health_clinicians_ manual.pdf

*White, S., & Dillow, S. (2005). Key concepts and features of the 2003 National Assessment of Adult Literacy. National Center for Education Statistics. Retrieved from http://nces.ed.gov/ NAAL/PDF/2006471.PDF

*Williams, M. V., Parker, R. M., Baker, D. W., Parikh, N. S., Pitkin, K., Coates, W. C., & Nurss, J. R. (1995). Inadequate functional health literacy among patients at two public hospitals. *JAMA, 274*(21), 1677–1682.

INDEX

Note: Page numbers followed by *t* or *b* indicate tables and boxes, respectively. Nursing diagnoses are in **bold**.